FIFTY YEARS OF NEUROSURGERY

Golden Anniversary
of the Congress
of Neurological Surgeons

FIFTY YEARS OF NEUROSURGERY

Golden Anniversary of the Congress of Neurological Surgeons

Editors

Daniel L. Barrow, M.D
MBNA/Bowman Professor and Chairman
Department of Neurosurgery
Emory University School of Medicine
Atlanta, Georgia

Douglas Kondziolka, M.D., M.Sc., F.R.C.S. (C)
Professor of Neurological Surgery and Radiation Oncology
Co-Director
Center for Image-Guided Neurosurgery
University of Pittsburgh Medical Center
Pittsburgh, Pennsylvania

Edward R. Laws, M.D., F.A.C.S.
W. Gayle Crutchfield Professor of Neurosurgery
Professor of Medicine
University of Virginia
Charlottesville, Virginia

Vincent C. Traynelis, M.D.
Professor of Surgery
Division of Neurosurgery
The University of Iowa
Iowa City, Iowa

Sponsored by the Congress of Neurological Surgeons

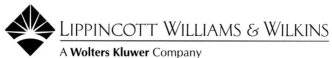

LIPPINCOTT WILLIAMS & WILKINS
A **Wolters Kluwer** Company
Philadelphia • Baltimore • New York • London
Buenos Aires • Hong Kong • Sydney • Tokyo

LW&W

Printed in the United States of America
(ISBN 0-781-72757-X)

PREFACE

In the years immediately following World War II, unprecedented numbers of neurosurgeons were swelling our professional ranks. Many were young and partially trained, and were not members of the restricted membership neurosurgical societiesof the day. These young, energetic surgeons, just home from the war, desired participation in a member service organization which would allow them collegial interaction, educational exchange and professional development. They desired an organization, which might serve the needs of all neurosurgeons, from trainee to practitioner, to professor young or old, board certified or not. The stage was set for the formation of a new professional organization in neurosurgery, one which would be called the Congress of Neurological Surgeons (CNS). Nine men established the Congress of Neurological Surgeons and held the First Annual Meeting at the Peabody Hotel in Memphis, Tennessee, November 15–17, 1951. Thus the CNS became the first non-exclusive international neurosurgical organization with ostensibly no limitations to membership.

During the fifty-year history of the CNS, we have witnessed some of the most astounding advances in science as compared to any previous period of similar length. The specialty of Neurosurgery has benefited immensely from this scientific renaissance and has been transformed from a fledgling branch of general surgery into a comprehensive and rewarding subspeciality that the neurosurgeons of 1951 would have difficulty recognizing.

In celebration of the Golden Anniversary of the CNS, the principal participants of the 50th Annual Meeting chose to edit this monograph that reviews the state of the science, art and practice of neurosurgery in 1951 and traces the progress in each of the neurosurgical subspecialty areas over the past five decades.

The editors followed the advice of one of the Century's greatest men, Winston Churchill, who said, ''The farther back you look, the farther forward you can see.'' Understanding our history and the lessons of our predecessors is vital if we are to continue the outstanding advances in our specialty.

The Editors

CONTRIBUTORS

Issam A. Awad, MD, MsC, FACS
The Nixdorff-German Professor of
Neurosurgery
Head, Neurovascular Surgery Program
Yale University School of Medicine
New Haven, Connecticut

T. Forcht Dagi, MD, FACS, FCC
Clinical Professor of Neurosurgery
Medical College of Georgia;
Professor
Georgia Institute of Technology
Atlanta, Georgia

Igor de Castro, MD
Department of Neurosurgery
University of Arkansas for Medical Sciences
Little Rock, Arkansas

Robert E. Florin, MD, FACS
Clinical Professor of Neurosurgery
Department of Neurosurgery
University of Southern California School of
Medicine
Los Angeles, California

Philip L. Gildenberg, MD, PhD
Director
Houston Stereotactic Center
Houston, Texas

David G. Kline, MD
Boyd Professor and Chairman
Department of Neurosurgery
Louisiana State University Health Science
Center
New Orleans

Thomas Kretschmer, MD
Department of Neurosurgery
University of Ulm
Gunzburg, Germany

Edward R. Laws, MD, FACS
W. Gayle Crutchfield Professor of
Neurosurgery
Department of Neurosurgery
University of Virginia Health System
Charlottesville, Virginia

Sunghoon Lee, MD
Resident in Neurosurgery
Department of Neurosurgery
Yale University School of Medicine
New Haven, Connecticut

Louis Marroti, BS
Medical Student
Yale University School of Medicine
New Haven, Connecticut

Robert G. Ojemann, MD
Professor of Surgery
Massachusetts General Hospital;
Visiting Neurosurgeon
Massachusetts General Hospital
Boston, Massachusetts

T. Glenn Pait, MD, FACS
Associate Professor
Department of Neurosurgery
University of Arkansas for Medical Sciences
Little Rock, Arkansas

Mark Preul, MD
Director, Neurosurgery Research
Division of Neurological Surgery
Barrow Neurological Institute
St. Joseph's Hospital and Medical Center
Phoenix, Arizona

Theodore S. Roberts, M.D.
Professor
Department of Neurological Surgery
University of Washington School of Medicine
Seattle, Washington

Harold Rosegay, PhD, MD
Professor
Department of Neurological Surgery
University of California San Francisco
San Francisco, California

Volker K. H. Sonntag, MD
Vice Chairman
Division of Neurological Surgery;
Director, Residency Program
Chairman, BNI Spine Section
Barrow Neurological Institute
St. Joseph's Hospital and Medical Center
Phoenix, Arizona

Christina Spetzler
Neurosurgery Research Laboratory
Division of Neurological Surgery
Barrow Neurological Institute
St. Joseph's Hospital and Medical Center
Phoenix, Arizona

Ronald R. Tasker, MD, MA, FRCS(C)
Professor
Department of Surgery
Division of Neurosurgery
University of Toronto
Toronto, Ontario, Canada

Nicholas Theodore, MD
Chief Resident
Division of Neurological Surgery
Barrow Neurological Institute
St. Joseph's Hospital and Medical Center
Phoenix, Arizona

John Morgan Thompson, MD
Clinical Professor of Neurological Surgery
University of South Florida School of
Medicine
Tampa, Florida

Marion L. Walker, MD
Professor & Chairman
Division of Pediatric Neurosurgery
University of Utah and
Primary Children's Medical Center
Salt Lake City, Utah

Charles B. Wilson, MD, DSc, MSHA
Professor
Department of Neurological Surgery
University of California San Francisco
San Francisco, California

M. Gazi Yasargil, MD
Professor
Department of Neurosurgery
University of Arkansas College of Medicine
Little Rock, Arkansas

CONTENTS

1

History of the Congress of Neurological Surgeons

John Morgan Thompson, MD

1992 Honored Guest Robert G. Ojemann
1993 Honored Guest Albert L. Rhoton, Jr.
1994 Honored Guest Robert F. Spetzler
1995 Honored Guest John Anthony Jane
1996 Honored Guest Peter Joseph Jannetta
1997 Honored Guest Nicholas T. Zervas
1998 Honored Guest John M. Tew, Jr.
1999 Honored Guest Duke S. Samson
2000 Honored Guest Edward R. Laws, Jr.

1992 CNS President William F. Chandler
1993 CNS President Arthur L. Day
1994 CNS President Richard Arthur Roski
1995 CNS President Ralph G. Dacey, Jr.
1996 CNS President Stephen Haines
1997 CNS President Marc R. Mayberg
1998 CNS President William Allan Friedman
1999 CNS President H. Hunt Batjer
2000 CNS President Daniel Louis Barrow

The birth certificate of neurological surgery in the United Stated was issued on November 18, 1904, when Dr. Harvey Cushing presented a paper at the Academy of Medicine in Cleveland entitled "The Special Field of Neurological Surgery" (2). A small number of general surgeons in large academic centers gradually started doing more cranial and brain surgery. The large number of head injuries, spine injuries, and peripheral nerve injuries seen in World War I further stimulated interest in neurological surgery. There developed a need to share experiences. In March 1920, the Society of Neurological Surgeons was founded by 11 neurosurgeons attending a meeting in Boston. These 11 neurosurgeons, plus other neurosurgeons who were not members of the Society, trained young associates who were not invited to join the Society. The Society of Neurological Surgeons limited its membership. Drs. Temple Fay, Eustice Semmes, Glen Spurling, and W. E. Van Wagenen met in Washington, DC, on October 10, 1931, to plan a new neurosurgical society. Dr. Fay suggested the name "Harvey Cushing Society" after Dr. Cushing expressed his approval of the new

group. Thirty charter members were chosen, and the Harvey Cushing Society held its first meeting in Boston on May 6, 1932. Membership was initially limited to 35, which meant that only 5 additional members could be inducted into the new Society. It was felt that a small group was desirable to allow exchange of ideas and to facilitate visits to members' operating rooms. Cushing welcomed the new Society to his clinic and remarked that in another 10 years another neurosurgical group would be formed that would look on the members of the Harvey Cushing Society as senile and antiquated. Cushing's prediction proved to be somewhat conservative, because in 1938, seven young neurosurgeons who had not been elected into the Harvey Cushing Society met in Memphis, Tennessee, and organized the American Academy of Neurological Surgery. The Academy vowed to keep its doors open to newcomers, but the need for close fellowship and education eventually caused this group, too, to restrict membership. Dr. Walter Dandy, Sr., refused to join any of these neurosurgical societies but he did enjoy membership in the American Neurological Association, which was founded in 1874, 46 years before the first American neurosurgical society was founded.

The Great Depression during the 1930s had a profound effect on the practice of neurological surgery. The annual net income for physicians in the United States had fallen to $2,900 by 1939. Dr. James G. Lyerly had joined his mentor, Dr. Claude C. Coleman, in practice in Richmond, Virginia, and they had a very successful practice for some years. However, by 1934 the income of the practice had declined so severely that Lyerly felt it was his duty to leave the partnership so that Coleman would have enough income to support his family. Lyerly moved from Richmond to Jacksonville, Florida, in 1934, and became the first and only neurological surgeon in Florida in the 1930s.

It was actually World War II that sowed the seeds for the founding of the Congress of Neurological Surgeons (CNS). The United States sustained numerous casualties, including 405,399 dead and 670,846 wounded. Medical school was reduced to 3 calendar years, and internship was reduced to 9 months. Most young physicians joined the Armed Forces before completing their residency training, and many young surgeons developed their skills by caring for the enormous number of war casualties. Many of these young surgeons were assigned to neurosurgical units, where they developed an interest in the specialty under the tutelage of experienced neurosurgeons. Most of these young men matured far more rapidly than they might have with an equal number of years of experience in civilian life. After their release from active duty, these mature but young and partially trained surgeons applied for civilian residencies. Grateful and patriotic program directors accepted many more people into their programs than they had been accustomed to training. The American Board of Neurological Surgery, which was founded in 1940, required only 2 years of neurosurgical residency training. However, few men completed their training in less than 6 or 7 years after graduating from medical school.

Before World War II, most neurological surgeons were associated with academic centers, where there were opportunities to discuss problem cases with colleagues. After World War II, many young neurological surgeons completing their training went into solo private practice in areas that previously had no neurosurgeons. These young men felt the need for continuing education, and felt the need to belong to a national group of neurological surgeons. The Neurosurgical Society of America (NSA) was founded in June 1948, but this group also chose to limit its membership. The Harvey Cushing Society opened its membership in 1949 and expanded into an organization of national scope with 148 members. However, the Harvey Cushing Society would not consider applicants until they were board certified, and the board required a waiting period of at least 2 years of practice before the certifying examination could be taken. Therefore, the time lag between completing training and being accepted into membership in the Harvey Cushing Society was at least 3 years, and frequently longer. The young, war-matured neurosurgeons were not willing to wait this long; thus, the stage was set for the establishment of another national neurosurgical society.

Several neurosurgeons met at Sea Island, Georgia, in September 1950 and discussed the possibility of forming a new national society. This discussion continued in February 1951 at the meeting of the Southern Neurosurgical Society in New Orleans. Nine neurological surgeons met in a room at the Palmer House in Chicago on February 24, 1951, just after the conclusion of the Interurban Neurosurgical Society. The meeting was attended by Drs. Floyd S. Barringer, Bland W. Cannon, James R. Gay, Louis J. Gogela, Nathaniel R. Hollister, Wilber A. Muehlig, David Roth, Elmer C. Schultz, and Emil P. Pelan. They discussed in more detail the formation of a new society. Dr. Cannon was appointed chairman pro tem, and Dr. Gay was appointed secretary pro tem. This group decided to hold an organizational meeting on May 10, 1951, just after the examination of the American Board of Neurological Surgery. The meeting initially was planned for Chicago and then was changed to St. Louis. Letters were sent out to approximately 50 neurosurgeons, inviting their suggestions about the formation of a new neuro-surgical society. This letter explained that the proposed new group had no intentions of competing with the existing neurosurgical societies. Cannon, the first secretary of the CNS and the sixth president of the CNS, sent to me all of his historical material. I also received much historical material from Dr. James R. Gay and from Dr. Richard DeSaussure, the first historian, of the CNS. The archives indicated that the CNS was founded on May 11, 1951, but information received recently from Dr. A. Roy Tyrer indicates that the meeting actually took place on May 10, 1951. Tyrer sent to me his bill from the Hotel Jefferson, indicating that he checked into the hotel on May 9 and that he paid his hotel bill of $8 with a tax of 0.16¢ at 5:41 PM on May 10th. However, his expense account indicated lodging at $16.32, which is exactly twice the 1-day rate, so I strongly suspect that the meeting extended over into May 11th. Further review of the archives sent by Cannon indicated that five neurosurgeons met in Cannon's room at the Jefferson Hotel at 3:30 PM on May 9th. The name, Congress of Neurological Surgeons, was selected with great care. The word ''American'' was deliberately omitted because the founders wanted the new organization to be international in scope with unlimited membership. Many of these young neurosurgeons had served overseas in World War II and already had an international outlook. It was recognized that the initials of the CNS were the commonly used abbreviation for the central nervous system—the target of many neurosurgical operations. The CNS was designed to be an association of neurosurgeons organized to study and discuss the principles of neurological surgery, to study developments in scientific fields allied to neurosurgery, and to honor living leaders in the field of neurosurgery. These principles have been adhered to diligently ever since, with the single exception that a deceased neurological surgeon, Dr. Walter E. Dandy, Sr., was an honored guest at the 1984 meeting in New York. Dandy shared the honored guest position with his pupil, Dr. Hugo Victor Rizolli. It is of interest that our honored guest at the 50th anniversary meeting, Dr. Edward Laws, was the president of the CNS at that time.

At the time of the founding meeting in St. Louis, Dr. Elmer C. Schultz was elected president, Dr. Carrol A. Brown was elected vice president, and Dr. Bland W. Cannon was elected secretary. Memphis, Tennessee, was chosen as the first scientific meeting site. Committees were appointed and the enthusiastic members of the CNS worked long and hard to ensure the success of the 1st annual meeting. The 11 members of the Steering Committee were asked to donate $50 each to provide funds to meet expenses until the time of the 1st annual meeting. The members of the CNS will forever owe a debt of gratitude to these men for subsidizing the organization at such a critical period in its history. Remember that $50 was more than six times the cost of one night at the Hotel Jefferson and would be equivalent to the donation of $1000 today. It was decided that there would be no initiation fee. The dues were set at $25 a year and were not increased for more than 20 years. The founding members of the CNS had many unique talents. Dr. Hendrik Svien became the national strategist, putting out fires started by older neurosurgeons. Cannon was the internal strategist, selling ideas to members and proposing candidates for membership. Gay was the logistics person—planner and organizer. Figure 1.1 lists the founding members on a certificate presented to them at the Silver Anniversary Meeting in Atlanta in 1975.

The Congress had 69 members by August 1951 and already was an international organization with active members in United States, Canada, Mexico, Chile, and Cuba. The 1st annual meeting of the CNS was held at the Peabody Hotel in Memphis, Tennessee, from Thursday, November 15 to Saturday, November 17, 1951, and was attend by 63 of its 121 members. The meeting was also attended by 17 guests and 9 guest speakers. The archives include the program of the first meeting, and a review of the papers presented at the scientific sessions reveals how much the art and science of diagnosis in the neurosciences has changed. The first paper presented was ''Diagnosis of Brain Tumor with Plain Roentgenogram of Skull'' by a radiologist. The next paper presented was ''Homonymous

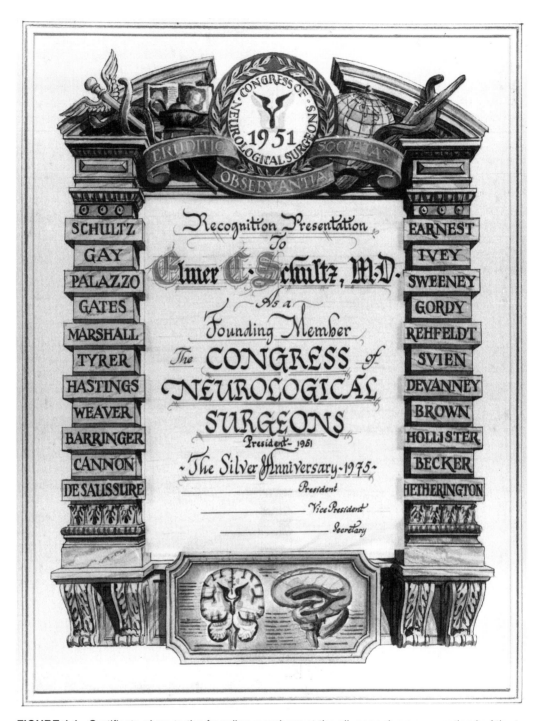

FIGURE 1.1. Certificate given to the founding members at the silver anniversary meeting in Atlanta in 1975. All the founding members are listed.

Visual Field Defects'' by an ophthalmologist, and then ''Electro-encephalographic Localization in Brain Tumor.'' There was another paper on ''Interpretation of Cerebral Angiogram,'' because angiograms were then performed by neurological surgeons. A review of the schedule of fees at this meeting reveals the extent of inflation that has taken place since 1951. Luncheon tickets were $2.50 per person and banquet tickets were $5. The banquet ticket included dancing and was labeled ''formal banquet (dress optional).'' Figure 1.2 is a photograph of the men who attended this 1st annual meeting. It should be noted that there are no women in the photograph because there were no female neurosurgeons at that time.

The legal advisor, Mr. Dunlap Cannon, Jr., was a brother of Dr. Bland Cannon. Mr. Cannon prepared the charter for the CNS, which was incorporated in the state of Tennessee on November 15, 1951. A Ladies Auxiliary was organized at the meeting in Memphis. Before that meeting in Memphis, neurosurgical meetings were ''bachelor'' affairs; wives were not invited. CNS leaders were sensitive to the loneliness spouses faced as a result of the long hours and erratic schedules of their husbands, and felt that bachelor meetings out of town only aggravated marital problems. Therefore, spouses were encouraged to attend and engage in interesting programs of their own during the day, and to attend social functions with their spouses in the evening. This policy resulted in making the annual meetings much more fun for everyone. The annual meetings became important social events as well as much-needed professional experiences. The members of the Auxiliary contributed an enormous amount of free labor during the past 50 years and worked side by side with their neurosurgical spouses on CNS activities. The only reason the annual dues of the CNS could remain at $25 for more than 20 years was because of this free labor. The wives manned the registration desk and did much of the secretarial work. It wasn't until 1968 that the CNS secretary had a paid secretary to handle just the CNS work. Up until then, most of the work was completed with donated time.

The Executive Committee authorized publication of *The Congress Newsletter* in February 1952, and Dr. Tyrer was appointed the first editor. The 2nd annual meeting of the CNS was held at the Palmer House in Chicago, November 5 through 8, 1952. For the first time, the CNS had an honored guest—Dr. Hurbert Olivecrona. Dr. Olivecrona was a world-class neurosurgeon who had a brilliant career at the Karolinska Institute in Sweden. A famous Chicago neurosurgeon wanted to host Olivecrona during the CNS meeting, but the Executive Committee of the CNS refused the invitation, claiming that Olivecrona belonged only to them during the meeting. Figure 1.3 shows the men who attended that meeting. Figure 1.4 presents the members of the Auxiliary. Note the fashion styles.

The Executive Committee authorized publication of *Clinical Neurosurgery* in November 1953, with Dr. Raymond A. Thompson as the first editor-in-chief. A leather-bound volume of *Clinical Neurosurgery Vol. I,* was presented to the honored guest, Prof. Sir Geoffrey Jefferson, at the 3rd annual meeting in New Orleans in 1953. This volume was presented to K. James Hardman, FRCS, by Michael and Antony Jefferson, the sons of Sir Geoffrey. Later, the book was auctioned, and Dr. A. Norman Guthkelch bought the book and presented it to the CNS archives. Guthkelch knew Sir Geoffrey and his family personally. We are very grateful to Dr. Guthkelch for his generosity.

The first postconvention tour followed the 1953 New Orleans meeting. Dr. Jorge Picaza, a Cuban neurosurgeon and member of the CNS, led the postconvention tour to Cuba. This was the last time that the CNS has had a meeting in Cuba.

The CNS seal was officially adopted in November 1954. In June 1956, the Executive Committee authorized the chairman of the Survey Committee, Dr. John R. Russell, to publish a *Directory of Neurological Surgeons in the United States.* Dr. Russell published the first directory in 1958, and in 1960 he published the directory in two parts: *Part I, Directory of Neurological Surgeons in the United States,* and *Part II, The Neurological Surgeons of the World*

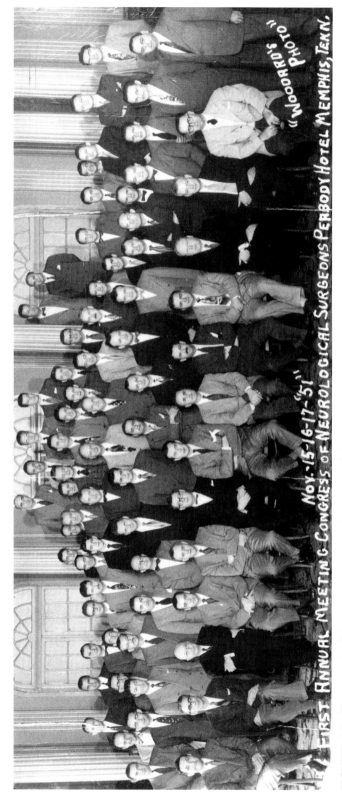

FIGURE 1.2. Photograph of the neurosurgeons who attended the 1st annual meeting in Memphis in 1951.

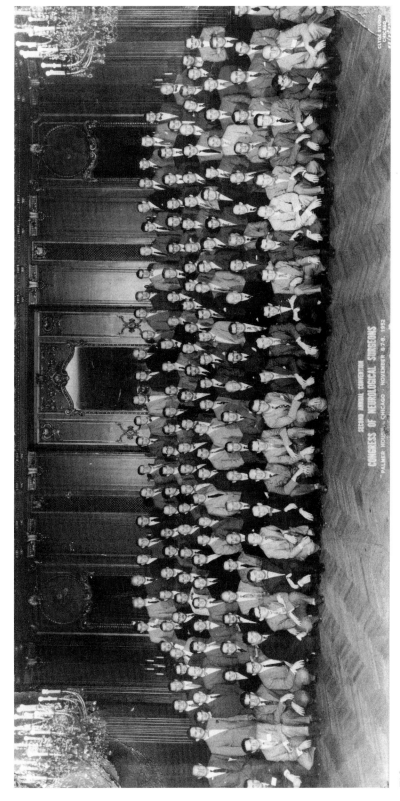

FIGURE 1.3. Photograph of the neurosurgeons who attended the 2nd annual meeting in Chicago in 1952.

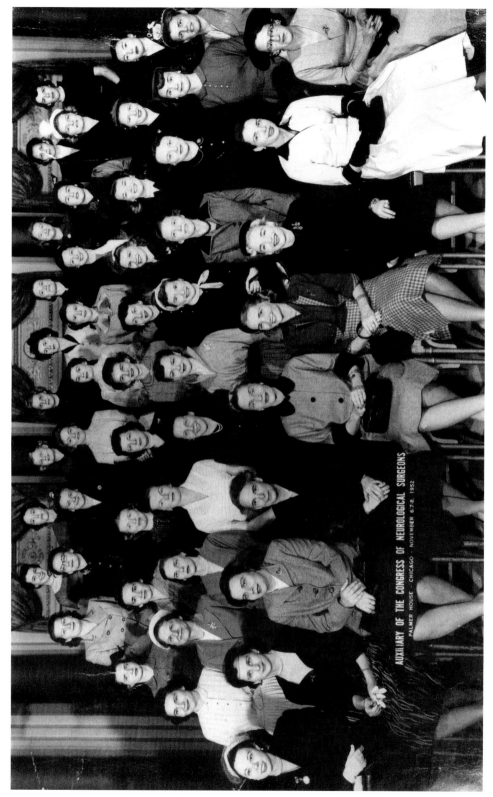

FIGURE 1.4. Photograph of the Auxiliary members attending the 2nd annual meeting in Chicago in 1952.

(Exclusive of the United States). Russell prepared part II, and part I was prepared by Karl L. Manders. Part I of the directory was expanded in 1961 to include the United States and Canada. Dr. George Ablin in Bakersfield, California, became editor in 1965, and he appointed Dr. Theodore S. Roberts as the editor of part I (United States and Canada). Ablin continued to be the editor of the World Directory for the next 30 years. He traveled extensively in many parts of the world and became friends with neurosurgeons in practically every country that had neurosurgeons. He produced superb directories that were used by neurological surgeons throughout the world. Ablin spread the name of the CNS worldwide and recruited many of the international members of the CNS. Ablin continued to be editor of the World Directory through the 7th edition. Ablin wrote to Dr. H. Hunt Batjer, president of the CNS, on May 20, 1999, and sent him a history of the *World Directory of Neurological Surgeons.* Ablin also sent a copy to me for the archives. Ablin knew that he had metastatic carcinoma of the pancreas at the time and that this would probably be his last contribution to the CNS. Dr. Ablin died on June 8, 1999, 3 days after his 50th wedding anniversary, which he attended. Dr. Richard Perrin of Toronto, Canada, became editor of the 8th edition, which was published in 1998. Dr. LaVerne S. Erickson became editor of the directory of the United States and Canada after the 15th edition, and continued to be editor of part I until 1993, when the American Association of Neurological Surgeons (AANS) and the CNS then started publishing jointly a directory for the United States, Canada, and Mexico. Advertising pages were added for the first time. The first directory, printed in 1958, contained the names of 1040 neurosurgeons. The 7th edition, published in 1993, contained the names of approximately 23,900 neurosurgeons, and it is now estimated (in 1999) that there are approximately 26,000 neurological surgeons in the world. Many of the directory editions provided demographic manpower statistics via tables and charts, and listed the ratios of neurosurgeons to population and land areas. The directory also highlighted those countries with

a population of more than one million with no known practicing neurological surgeons. The World Directory is certainly a memorial to Dr. George Ablin and to the other editors who worked so diligently for the benefit of neurological surgeons throughout the world.

The CNS was founded as an international neurosurgical society, and its history in international neurosurgical involvement is impressive, in addition to the World Directory. Dr. Tyrer made a trip to India in June 1963 and laid the groundwork for the participation of CNS volunteers in the neurosurgical programs in India. Dr. William Mosberg, the CNS representative on the Advisory Board of Care–Medico, traveled the world and visited every Care–Medico installation except the one in Honduras. Under the leadership of Mosberg, president of the CNS in 1965, the International Committee was established, which was chaired by Tyrer. Mosberg and Tyrer left for India immediately after the CNS meeting in 1966. The CNS actively supported the formation of the Foundation for International Education in Neurological Surgery (FIENS). The CNS is a member society of the World Federation of Neurosurgical Societies (WFNS) and has participated actively in its international congresses. The CNS has continued very active involvement in the international scene. Exchange visits have been carried out between the officers of the CNS and the officers of the Japanese Congress of Neurological Surgeons. During the presidency of Dr. Arthur Day (1992–1993), the CNS International Committee was rejuvenated. Dr. Stephen Giannotta was appointed chairman, and he worked closely with FIENS and WFNS to ensure that efforts among these three organizations would not be duplicated. Dr. Batjer replaced Dr. Giannotta as chairman in 1995, followed by Dr. Richard Perrin. The International Committee is currently developing educational and support programs in Zimbabwe, Ghana, Peru, and Nepal. The CNS, working with WFNS and FIENS, established the Federation for International Neurosurgical Development (or FIND). This organization has secured millions of dollars worth of equipment and has distributed it to needy target sites. The CNS approved international fellowships in 1994. Fellows from the following countries have served fellowships in the United States: Uruguay, Albania, the Slovak Republic, India, the People's Republic of China, Armenia, Ethiopia, Egypt, and Nepal.

An international luncheon is held each year during the CNS annual meeting. Excellent international speakers are featured at these luncheons. Each year, an increasing number of international CNS members attend our annual meeting.

The CNS was the first neurosurgical society to recognize that socioeconomics were important to practicing neurosurgeons. The Socioeconomic Committee was appointed, and in 1966 this committee—under the chairmanship of Dr. Edward Bishop—published *Tabulation of the Results of a National Neurosurgical Fee Survey* (1). This publication became one of the most widely used neurosurgical books ever published. The Utilization Guidelines Committee, under the chairmanship of Dr. Walter S. Lockhart, Jr., published the *Neurosurgical Hospital Utilization Guidelines Manual* (3) in 1969. The AANS recognized that, in its role as spokesman for United States neurosurgeons, it also should be involved in socioeconomics. Thus, the Socioeconomic Committee became a joint committee in the early 1970s. This joint committee invited representatives from the various state neurosurgical societies to join the committee. Eventually, the Joint Socioeconomic Committee evolved into the Joint Council of State Neurosurgical Societies. This provided even more grass roots representation to the CNS and to the AANS.

The Washington Committee, supported by both the CNS and the AANS, has become increasingly important. Under the chairmanship of Dr. Arthur L. Day, a past president of the CNS, the Washington Committee provided valuable insight into the Health Care Financing Administration (HCFA) initiative to establish practice expense relative value units (RVUs) and to decrease markedly the neurosurgical reimbursement for practice expenses. Organized neurosurgery was a major source in the establishment of the Practice Expense Coalition, which lobbied

successfully against the HCFA proposal. This struggle is certainly not over, but thus far organized neurosurgery has put up a good fight.

The CNS was founded to provide high-quality continuing education for neurological surgeons. This continues to be the main mission of the CNS. The scientific programs at all of our meetings have been superb. The Scientific Committee program chairmen have done excellent work. The meetings have expanded to scientific sessions both before and after the regular scientific programs. In 1959, we had a "postgraduate day," which was the day before the regular meeting. Dr. Louise Eisenhardt, a neuropathologist and an associate of Dr. Harvey Cushing, presented a course on neuropathology. I was fortunate to be able to take this course, and I still have the Kodachrome pathology slides that Eisenhardt prepared for those taking the course. Eisenhardt examined me in neuropathology when I took my oral neurosurgical boards. There were no written boards at that time. The CNS now sponsors practical courses each Saturday and Sunday before the annual scientific meetings start on Monday. Postconvention tours were offered for many years and were resumed at the 1998 meeting in Seattle during the presidency of Dr. William Friedman. The joint sessions have scientific programs in the afternoons during the annual meeting. Luncheon seminars provide opportunities to participate in small groups to discuss a large variety of topics. Scientific posters enhance the educational opportunities. The scientific, historical, and commercial exhibits provide valuable knowledge of the past, present, and future of neurological surgery.

Continuing education is also enhanced by the many publications of the CNS. *Clinical Neurosurgery* continues to be published each year, incorporating the papers presented at the annual meeting. All members of the CNS receive this publication. The CNS started publishing its own neurosurgical journal, *Neurosurgery,* in 1977 with Dr. Robert H. Wilkins as the first editor. Dr. Bruce Sorensen kindly donated to the CNS archives an autographed, bound copy of the first edition of *Neurosurgery. Concepts in Neurosurgery* is a series of topical monographs that has provided in-depth information on many topics in our field. The *CNS Newsletter* was published for many years and was incorporated into *Neurosurgery News* this past year to expand the ability of the CNS to communicate socioeconomic news and related stories. The CNS has also published a *Young Neurosurgeons Directory,* with Dr. Joel D. MacDonald as editor. Neurosurgery://On-Call (http://www.neurosurgery.org/directory/), organized neurosurgery's Web site, is sponsored jointly by the CNS and the AANS, and is currently edited by Dr. Joel MacDonald.

The CNS has always been very interested in neurosurgical residents, and on May 19, 1958, the Executive Committee authorized the expenditure of CNS funds to provide free lodging for residents attending the annual meeting. This continued for many years and fortunately was reinstated in 1998 at the meeting in Seattle during the presidency of Dr. William Friedman, and continues to this day. At the same time, a structural program of CNS fellowships was developed for residents and young neurosurgeons. The CNS has matured and now has members varying in age from 20 to 80 years old. The CNS has chosen its presidents and officers from all types of neurosurgical practice, including private practice, clinic practice, and academic practice. Many of our presidents have been full professors and chairmen of their own departments. Many of our members and past presidents have become presidents of the AANS, and we now have honored guests who have been former presidents of the CNS.

The CNS has become one of the largest neurosurgical societies in the world. At the time of our 20th anniversary meeting in St. Louis, the CNS had 1260 members in all 50 states, 7 Canadian provinces, and 28 other nations on every continent except Antarctica. At the time of our 1991 annual meeting, the CNS had 3636 members, including 615 resident members and 243 international members. At the time of our 1998 annual meeting in Seattle, the total membership was 4505, including 745 resident members and 432 international members. The international members now come from at least 63 countries.

There has been some discussion in the past of merging the AANS and the CNS. Some have complained that there are too many neuro-surgical meetings, but actually the number of neurosurgical meetings has increased with the separate meetings of the joint sections. The joint officers of the CNS and the AANS work very well together, and I and many others feel that there is strength in two separate major neurosurgical societies. The CNS has provided the model for neurosurgical societies, and many new concepts have originated in the CNS. There is a great need for two major neurosurgical society meetings in the United States each year because only approximately 40% of neurosurgeons can attend meetings at any one time. Each practicing neurosurgeon in the United States needs to be able to attend at least one major neurosurgical meeting per year, and obviously somebody needs to stay home to take care of the patients. I am a loyal, active member of the AANS and plan to remain so. I am also a loyal, active member of the CNS and plan to remain so. The massive volunteer effort in the CNS has allowed the annual dues to remain extremely low.

The Future Meeting Sites Committee has done superb work in choosing excellent sites for our annual meetings. Sites must be chosen many years in advance. Sites are chosen in practically every region of the United States and Canada to make the meetings convenient to a different segment of our members each year. Sites are also chosen on the basis of facilities and general interest. Figure 1.5 shows the sites of the founding meeting and the 50 annual meetings since. The numbers of meetings at each city are indicated.

The Long-Range Planning Committee (strategic planning) has the responsibility for looking to the future, including the distant future. Figure 1.6 shows the projections made by the Long-Range Planning Committee 30 years ago in 1969. These projections extend to the year 2000 and have proved to be very accurate.

The CNS was the first neurosurgical society to be family friendly. Spouses were invited to the 1st annual meeting. In 1999, during the presidency of Dr. H. Hunt Batjer, the CNS became even more family friendly by providing child care during the meeting. This was another first for the CNS.

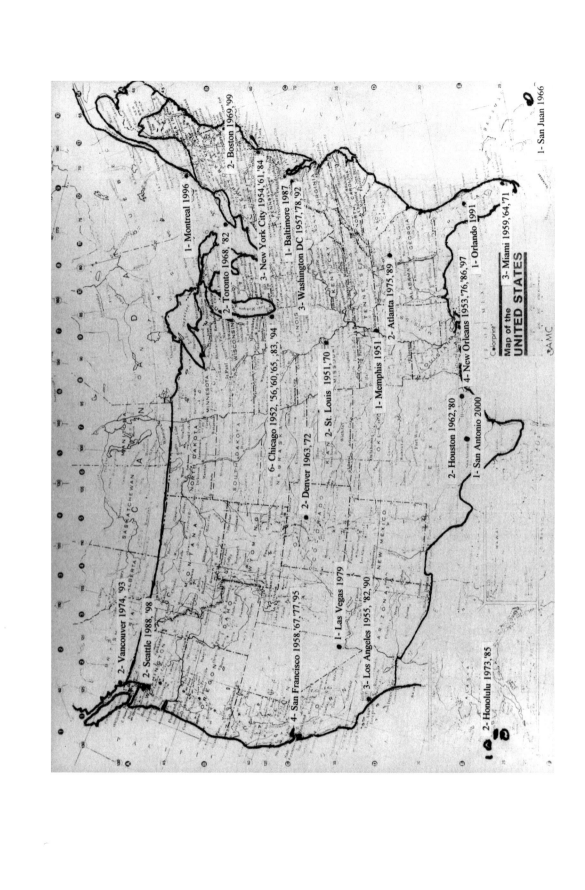

Map of the
UNITED STATES

2- Vancouver 1974, '93

2- Seattle 1988, '98

4- San Francisco 1958, '67, '77, '95

3- Los Angeles 1955, '82, '90

1- Las Vegas 1979

2- Denver 1963, '72

6- Chicago 1952, '56, '60, '65, '83, '94

2- St. Louis 1951, 70

1- Memphis 1951

2- Houston 1962, 80

1- San Antonio 2000

4- New Orleans 1953, '76, '86, '97

2- Atlanta 1975, '89

2- Honolulu 1973, '85

1- Montreal 1996

2- Toronto 1968, '82

2- Boston 1969, '99

3- New York City 1954, '61, '84

1- Baltimore 1987

3- Washington DC 1957, 78, '92

1- Orlando 1991

3- Miami 1959, '64, '71

1- San Juan 1966

Congress of Neurological Surgeons
Projected membership growth with annual meeting attendamce

Jan.	Number mbrs.	Attend Annual Meeting 30%	Number equal 40%	# of residents	Total at Scientific sessions	Hotel Rms Members & guests	Hotel Rms Residents 3 per Rm	Total Rooms
1969	1123	337	449	150	749	599	50	649
1970	1213	344	485	155	795	640	52	692
1971	1303	391	521	160	841	681	54	735
1972	1393	418	557	165	887	722	55	777
1973	1483	445	593	170	933	763	57	820
1974	1573	472	629	175	979	804	59	863
1975	1663	499	665	180	1025	845	60	905
1976	1753	526	701	185	1071	886	62	948
1977	1843	553	737	190	1117	927	64	991
1978	1933	580	773	195	1163	968	65	1033
1979	2023	607	809	200	1209	1009	67	1076
1980	2113	633	845	205	1255	1050	69	1119
1985	2563	769	1025	230	1485	1255	77	1332
1990	3013	904	1205	255	1715	1450	85	1545
2000	3913	1174	1565	305	2175	1870	102	1972

FIGURE 1.6. Projected membership growth and annual meeting attendance prepared by the Long-Range Planning Committee in 1969. These projections extended to the year 2000 and proved to be very accurate.

It is not possible to list all the people who have made important contributions to the CNS, but it does seem appropriate to list the Resident Award Winners, the Clinical Fellowship Award Winners, and the Distinguished Service Award Winners, which are shown in Figure 1.7. The first 41 presidents of the CNS and the first 41 honored guests were featured in a previous publication, *History of the Congress of Neurological Surgeons 1951–1991* (4). The biographies of these people will not be presented again. The names of these past honored guests and past presidents are listed in Figure 1.8.

It seems appropriate to present biographies of the nine honored guests and nine presidents of the CNS who have served since 1991, to bring the biographies up to date. These are now presented in the following pages.

FIGURE 1.5. Map of the United States and Canada showing the sites of the founding meeting and the 50 annual meetings held since, and the number of meetings held in each city.

PAST AWARD WINNERS

Distinguished Service Award Winners

Lycurgus M. Davey	1966	Ronald I. Apfelbaum	1987
Walter S. Lockhart, Jr.	1969	E. Fletcher Eyster	1988
Edward J. Bishop	1970	Fremont P. Wirth	1989
George Ablin	1971	Merwyn Bagan	1990
William S. Coxe	1973	Roy Black	1992
J. F. Ross Fleming	1975	Russell L. Travis	1993
Perry Black	1977	Steven Giannotta	1995
William A. Buchheit	1979	John Morgan Thompson	1996
Edwin Amyes	1980	Charles L. Plante	1997
Edward F. Downing	1984	Robert H. Wilkins	1998
J. Charles Rich	1986		

CNS Resident Award Winners

Arthur I. Kobrine	1974	Lew Disney	1987
Stephen Brem	1975	Martin E. Weinand	1988
Philip H. Gutin	1976	Nayef R. F. Al-Rodhan	1989
Robert F. Spetzler	1977	Ivar Mendez	1990
Martin G. Luken, III	1978	Captain Charles Miller	1991
George R. Prioleau	1979	Dante J. Morassutti	1992
Larry V. Carson	1980	Stephen E. Doran	1993
Ted S. Keller	1981	E. Antonio Chiocca	1994
Mervin P. Kril	1982	Grant P. Sinson	1995
J. F. Graham	1983	David Pincus	1996
Fredric Meyer	1984	Andrew K. Metzger	1997
Emily D. Friedman	1985	Robert M. Friedlander	1998
Victoria C. Neave	1986	Kelly Foote	1999

CNS Clinical Fellowship Award Winners

Brian Andrews	1987	Gregory Przybylski	1994
Charles Branch	1987	Jason A. Brodkey	1995
Randall Poweli	1987	Folios D. Vrionis	1995
Eric Zager	1988	Bruce Pollock	1996
Jonathan Hodes	1989	John Wong	1996
James Rutka	1989	Ali R. Rezai	1997
Claudio Feler	1990	Fernando L. Vale	1997
Mazen Khayata	1990	Giancarlo Vishtch	1997
Prem Pillay	1991	Nozipo Marnire	1998
Isabelle Germano	1992	Ghassan Bejjani	1998
Howard Chandler	1993	Daniel Yoshor	1999
Nayef Al-Rodhan	1993	Odette Harris	1999
John Day	1994		

FIGURE 1.7. Resident Award Winners, the Clinical Fellowship Award Winners, and the Distinguished Service Award Winners.

Past Honored Guests

Past Presidents

Past Honored Guests	Year	Past Presidents
	1951	Elmer S. Schultz
Herbert Olivecrona	1952	Hendrik J. Svien
Sir Geoffrey Jefferson	1953	Nathaniel R. Hollister
Kenneth G. McKenzie	1954	James R. Gay
Carl W. Rand	1955	Donald B. Sweeney
Wilder G. Penfield	1956	Bland W. Cannon
Francis Grant	1957	Frederick C. Rehfeldt
A. Earl Walker	1958	Raymond K. Thompson
William J. German	1959	Philip D. Gordy
Paul C. Bucy	1960	Thomas M. Marshall
Eduard A. V. Busch	1961	Martin P. Sayers
Bronson S. Ray	1962	Richard L. DeSaussure
James L. Poppen	1963	A. Roy Tyrer, Jr.
Edgar A. Kahn	1964	Edward C. Weiford
James C. White	1965	Gordon van den Noort
Hugo Krayenbuhl	1966	William H. Mosberg, Jr.
W. James Gardner	1967	John R. Russell
Norman M. Dott	1968	John Shillito, Jr.
Wallace B. Hamby	1969	Paul C. Sharkey
Barnes Woodhall	1970	John Morgan Thompson
Elisha S. Gurdjian	1971	Donald F. Dohn
Francis Murphey	1972	John N. Meagher
Henry G. Schwartz	1973	Bernard S. Patrick
Guy L. Odom	1974	George T. Tindall
William H. Sweet	1975	James T. Robertson
Lyle A. French	1976	Robert G. Ojemann
Richard C. Schneider	1977	Bruce F. Sorensen
Charles G. Drake	1978	Albert L. Rhoton, Jr.
Frank H. Mayfield	1979	David L. Kelly, Jr.
Eben Alexander, Jr.	1980	Robert H. Wilkins
J. Garber Galbraith	1981	J. Fletcher Lee
Keiji Sano	1982	Donald H. Stewart, Jr.
C. Miller Fisher	1983	John M. Tew, Jr
Hugo V. Rizzoli and Walter F. Dandy	1984	Edward R. Laws, Jr.
Sidney Goldring	1985	Robert A. Ratcheson
M. Gazi Yasargil	1986	Joseph C. Maroon
Thomas W. Langfitt	1987	Donald O. Quest
Lindsay Symon	1988	Christopher B. Shields
Thoralf M. Sundt, Jr.	1989	J. Michael McWhorter
Charles B. Wilson	1990	Hal L. Hankinson
Bennett M. Stein	1991	Michael Salcman

FIGURE 1.8. Past honored guests and past presidents, 1951 through 1991.

1992 HONORED GUEST ROBERT G. OJEMANN

Robert G. Ojemann (Fig. 1.9) was born in Iowa City, Iowa. He attended the University of Iowa, where he received his BS degree and was elected to Phi Beta Kappa. He also attended medical school at the same university, where he was awarded the MD degree and was elected to Alpha Omega Alpha (AOA). He completed his internship at Cincinnati General Hospital, followed by a year of assistant residency in general surgery at Baylor University Hospital. He also performed his neurological surgery residency at Baylor University Hospital. Bob then became a fellow at Massachusetts General Hospital, and

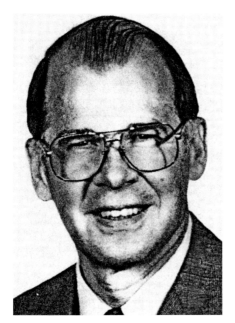

FIGURE 1.9. 1992 Honored Guest Dr. Robert G. Ojemann.

he has now been associated with that hospital for almost 40 years. He is a full professor of neurological surgery at Harvard Medical School. By 1992 he had published more than 170 articles and book chapters, and had authored several books. He has made important contributions in normal pressure hydrocephalus, cerebellar infarction and hemorrhage, acoustic neuroma surgery, cerebrovascular surgery, and in many other areas.

Dr. Ojemann is the first past president of the CNS to be selected as an honored guest. He has demonstrated superb leadership ability and has served as president of the Society of Neurological Surgeons (SNS), the AANS, the American Academy of Neurological Surgeons, and the Society of University Neurosurgeons. He has been chairman of the American Board of Neurological Surgery and chairman of the Washington Committee.

Bob has been devoted to his wife, Jean, for more than 44 years. They have raised four fine sons. Bob has been so efficient that he has been able to strike a happy balance between patient care, research, teaching, leadership, and family.

The CNS is proud that one of its own has been able to contribute so much to the human race.

1993 HONORED GUEST
ALBERT L. RHOTON, JR.

Albert L. Rhoton, Jr. (Fig. 1.10), was born in Parvis, Kentucky. He graduated from Washington University School of Medicine *cum laude,* with the highest academic standing in the class of 1959. He then served 2 years at Columbia Presbyterian Medical Center, one in general surgery and one in neurosurgery. He returned to Washington University at Barnes Hospital, where he completed his neurosurgery residency under Dr. Henry Schwartz. He remained at Washington University for 1 year as a Research Fellow in neuroanatomy and began using the surgical microscope. He joined the staff of the Mayo Clinic in January 1966, and began his microanatomic studies. He accepted the offer to become Professor of Surgery, Chief of the Division of Neurological Surgery, University of Florida College of Medicine in 1972. Al was named the RD Keene Family Professor and

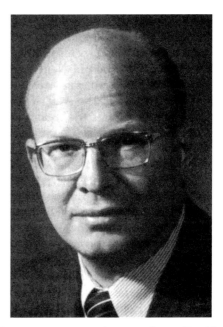

FIGURE 1.10. 1993 Honored Guest Dr. Albert L. Rhoton, Jr.

Chairman of the Department of Neurological Surgery in 1981, when the division was awarded departmental status. Al has been very successful in raising funds for his department, and obtained funds for 10 endowed chairs in neurosurgery. He also helped raise funds for the creation of a Brain Institute, which was completed in 1996. Al was president of CNS in 1978. During his presidency he strengthened the relationship of the national and state neurosurgical societies. He played a key role in the founding of the Joint Section on Disorders of the Spine and Peripheral Nerves of the AANS and the CNS. He served as chairman of the Joint Section on Cerebrovascular Surgery. He has served as president of the AANS, the SNS, and the North American Skull Base Society. He served as vice-chairman of the American Board of Neurological Surgery. He has been the honored guest or honorary member of 16 neurosurgical societies throughout the United States, Latin American, Europe, Asia, and Africa. He has served on the editorial board of six journals and has been the author of more than 200 articles and book chapters.

Al not only has been an inspiration to hundreds of medical students and neurosurgical residents, but he has also been an inspiration to his own four children, all of whom chose medicine as a career. One son is a neurosurgeon, one son specializes in internal medicine, one daughter specializes in obstetrics and gynecology, and one daughter is a pediatric nurse. Al will be the first to admit that his wife, Joyce, deserves much of the credit for his success and for the successful rearing of their four children.

1994 HONORED GUEST
ROBERT F. SPETZLER

Robert F. Spetzler (Fig 1.11) was born in Germany and came to the United States, where he attended Knox College in Galesburg, Illinois, and graduated *cum laude*. Before graduation he spent a year at the Free University of Berlin on a scholarship. He received his MD degree from Northwestern University and served his internship at Wesley Memorial Hospital on the Northwestern service. He completed his neurosurgical residency at the University of California at San

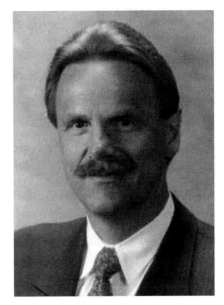

FIGURE 1.11. 1994 Honored Guest Dr. Robert F. Spetzler.

Francisco under Dr. Charles B. Wilson. He developed a keen interest in neurovascular surgery under the expert tutelage of Dr. Wilson. He received the Annual Resident Award at the 27th annual meeting of the CNS. He also was awarded a Trauma Fellowship from the National Institutes of Health (NIH).

Dr. Spetzler joined the Department of Neurosurgery, Case Western Reserve University, Cleveland, Ohio, where he conducted excellent research on cerebrovascular disease. He was recruited in 1983 to assume the J. N. Harber Chair of Neurological Surgery at the Barrow Neurological Institute in Phoenix, Arizona, and 2 years later he was promoted to the position of director of the Institute. Under Dr. Spetzler's leadership, the Institute grew from a regional center to an internationally recognized center of excellence. The neurosurgical residency program at Barrow became one of the most highly sought programs. Dr. Spetzler has published more than 100 articles in peer-reviewed journals and more than 83 book chapters. His work on stroke, arteriovenous malformations, and skull base surgery is well known. At the time of the 1994 annual meeting, Dr. Spetzler was the youngest person ever to receive the position of honored guest of the CNS.

1995 HONORED GUEST
JOHN ANTHONY JANE

John Anthony Jane (Fig 1.12) was born and raised in the Chicago area. He received his BA degree *cum laude* from the University of Chicago, as well as his MD degree. He then moved to Canada, where he did his internship at the Royal Victoria Hospital in Montreal. He began his neurosurgical residency at the University of Chicago under Dr. Sean Mullan. His residency included important research and clinical fellowships. He was a Fellow in neurophysiology at the Montreal Neurological Institute, and a Senior Fellow and Demonstrator in neuropathology at McGill University in Montreal. He went to London in 1961 to serve as a research assistant to Mr. Wylie McKissock at St. George's Hospi-

tal and the National Hospital at Queen's Square. He conducted his seminal work on the natural history of intracranial aneurysms while in London. He was awarded a PhD degree from the University of Chicago in 1967. His Chicago training also included a neurosurgical residency at the University of Illinois Neuropsychiatric Institute with Drs. Oscar Sugar and Eric Olberg.

Dr. Jane joined Dr. Frank Nulsen at Case Western Reserve University and served on the neurosurgery faculty for 4 years. He then, at the age of 37, was named Alumni Professor and Chairman, Department of Neurological Surgery, University of Virginia, Charlottesville, Virginia. He became the David D. Weaver Professor in 1987. He was selected as editor of the *Journal of Neurosurgery*. He has served as president of the SNS and as director of the American Board of Neurological Surgery. Many of the neurosurgeons he has trained have become full professors of neurosurgery, and many of them are now chairmen of their own departments. Dr. Jane is an expert on comparative neuroanatomy and comparative neurophysiology. He has done a great deal of pediatric neurosurgery, and originated the modern techniques for treatment of craniofacial disorders. He has done much clinical and basic research on the treatment of severe head injuries and disorders of the spine. Dr. Jane has published more than 250 peer-reviewed articles.

Dr. Jane married the former Miss Noella Fortier of Montreal. The Janes have four grown children (three daughters and one son). Dr. Jane had the unique privilege of training his own son in his neurosurgical residency. Dr. Jane obviously had a profound influence on his son, who knew that the residents who trained with Dr. Jane respected his immense capacity for work, his surgical skill and judgment, and his unselfish commitment to his patients, his residents, and his nurses. His residents also appreciated his sense of humor.

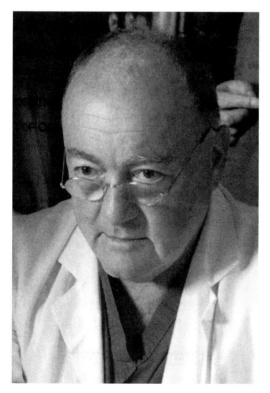

FIGURE 1.12. 1995 Honored Guest Dr. John Anthony Jane.

1996 HONORED GUEST
PETER JOSEPH JANNETTA

Peter Joseph Jannetta (Fig. 1.13) was born in Philadelphia and grew up in Haddonfield, New

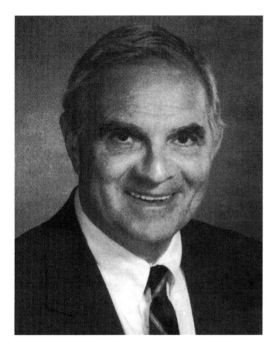

FIGURE 1.13. 1996 Honored Guest Dr. Peter Joseph Jannetta.

Jersey, and York, Pennsylvania. He was a high school All-American swimmer. He received both his AB and MD degrees from the University of Pennsylvania, and was president of his class at the University of Pennsylvania. Dr. Jannetta trained in general surgery at the University of Pennsylvania and became an NIH Fellow in neurophysiology. He completed his residency in neurosurgery at the University of California at Los Angeles Center for Health Sciences. He was recruited to Louisiana State University Medical Center, where he was named chairman of the section of neurological surgery and was promoted to full professor. He next was recruited to the University of Pittsburgh School of Medicine and was named professor and director of neurological surgery in 1971. The section became a department in 1973, and Dr. Jannetta was made professor and chairman of the new department. He was honored in 1992 when he became the first Walter Dandy Professor of neurological surgery at the University of Pittsburgh. The Peter J. Jannetta Chair in neurological surgery has also been established. At the time of the 1996

annual CNS meeting in Montreal, Dr. Jannetta had published 172 refereed articles, 2 books, 68 book chapters, and 77 abstracts. He is a recognized pioneer in the treatment of cranial nerve compression syndromes, especially those related to facial pain. He is also a pioneer in the etiology of hypertension. He was elected to the position of second vice-president-at-large of the WFNS. He has received an honorary DSc degree from Washington and Jefferson College, and in 1990 was selected as the Vectors–Pittsburgh Man of the Year in Sciences. He was one of the recipients of the 1990 Horatio Alger Award, and he became a member of the Horatio Alger Association. He received the Herbert Olivecrona Award. Dr. Jannetta created one of the outstanding schools of neurological surgery in the world at the University of Pittsburgh. Five of the 17 Van Wagenen Fellows named since 1980 were trained by Dr. Jannetta.

Dr. Jannetta has demonstrated considerable musical talent. He was schooled on the piano and has mastered the tenor banjo. He also has a keen interest in art and has sculpted in plaster. He is a proud father of six children: two physicians, two international business executives, a historian, and an actor. His wife, Diana, is an art collector and art critic.

Dr. Jannetta was named Secretary of Health of the Commonwealth of Pennsylvania by Governor Tom Ridge in March 1995, with senate confirmation of the nomination on May 2, 1995.

1997 HONORED GUEST
NICHOLAS T. ZERVAS

Nicholas T. Zervas (Fig. 1.14) was born in Lynn, Massachusetts. He demonstrated a talent for music while a child and won the Young Artist's Award of the American Piano Teacher's Federation in 1946. He attended Harvard University, and received his MD degree from the University of Chicago. His surgical internship was performed at the Cornell Service of New York Hospital, where he had the privilege of serving on the neurosurgical service under the direction of Dr. Bronson Ray. He next spent a year at the Montreal Neurological Institute working as a resident in both neurology and neu-

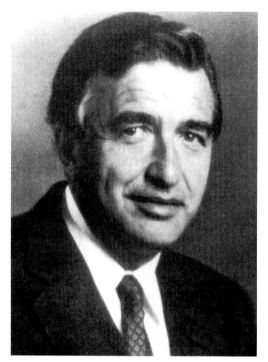

FIGURE 1.14. 1997 Honored Guest Dr. Nicholas T. Zervas.

ropathology. He spent 1 year in 1960 at the Hospital St Anne in Paris working under Dr. Jean Talairach and Dr. Gabor Szikla, learning stereotactic surgery. He completed his neurosurgical training at Massachusetts General Hospital in 1962 under the direction of Dr. William Sweet. He was appointed assistant professor of neurological surgery at Jefferson Medical College in 1962, and remained there until 1967, when he became chief of neurosurgery at Beth Israel Hospital in Boston, and was appointed assistant professor of surgery at Harvard Medical School. He was appointed chief of the neurosurgical service at Massachusetts General Hospital in 1977, where he succeeded Dr. Sweet.

Dr. Zervas has published more than 250 articles on a variety of research and clinical topics including cerebral vasospasm, stroke, stereotactic neurosurgery, pituitary disorders, radiosurgery, and spinal disorders. He has been an innovator in the application of technology to neurosurgery including stereotaxis, telemetric intracranial pressure monitoring, pulsed-dye

laser vasodilatation, and intraoperative radiosurgery. Under Dr. Zervas' guidance, the neurosurgical service at Massachusetts General Hospital has flourished and continues to be one of the premier training and research programs in the world.

Dr. Zervas has served as chairman of the editorial board of *The Journal of Neurosurgery,* president of the AANS, chairman of the American Board of Neurological Surgery, and vice-chairman of the AANS Research Foundation Executive Council. He also is a member of the Institute of Medicine of the National Academy of Sciences, and is a Fellow of the American Academy of Arts and Sciences.

Dr. Zervas and his wife, Thalia, hold a great affection for the arts. He has served as chairman of the Massachusetts Council of the Arts and Humanities of the Commonwealth of Massachusetts, and he has also served as president of the Boston Symphony Orchestra.

1998 HONORED GUEST
JOHN M. TEW, JR.

John McLellan Tew, Jr. (Fig. 1.15), was born and raised on a farm in eastern North Carolina.

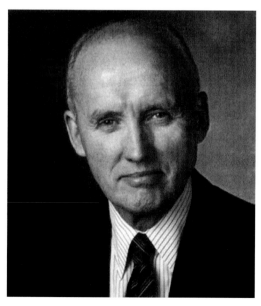

FIGURE 1.15. 1998 Honored Guest Dr. John M. Tew, Jr.

He graduated from Campbell and Wake Forest University *cum laude* in 1957. He attended the Bowman Gray School of Medicine of Wake Forest University. He was elected to AOA and received his MD degree in 1961. His internship in general surgery was at the Cornell–New York Hospital Center, and he then went to the Peter Bent Brigham Hospital, where he worked with Dr. Francis Moore in transplantation research. He became a Fellow in neurophysiology at NIH, where he worked with Dr. Cho Lu Li. They developed techniques to acquire intracellular recordings in the human cerebral cortex and thalamus. Dr. Tew returned to Boston in 1965 for a research fellowship and a neurosurgical residency at Massachusetts General Hospital under the direction of Dr. William Sweet. He also worked with Drs. Kjellberg and Ballantine. Dr. Tew spent a year at the Boston Children's Hospital with Dr. Donald Matson in 1967, where he learned pediatric neurological surgery. He worked with Dr. Robert Ojemann during his final years of residency, when microneurosurgery was being born. Dr. Tew was awarded the second Van Waganen Fellowship, which allowed him to study with Prof. Gazi Yaşargil in Zurich, Switzerland.

Dr. Tew joined Drs. Frank Mayfield and Stewart Dunsker at the Mayfield Clinic, where he came under the wise mentorship of Mayfield. An outstanding community-based neurosurgical program developed, and this was merged with the University of Cincinnati in 1983. Dr. Tew became the first Frank Mayfield Chairman of Neurological Surgery, University of Cincinnati, Ohio, in 1992. The neurological services were integrated into The Neuroscience Institute in 1998, with Dr. Tew as medical director. Dr. Tew is especially proud of the residents and fellows he has trained who now have outstanding careers at many of the leading academic institutions in the United States and other countries. Dr. Tew has served as president of the CNS and the AANS. He received the Papal Pro Ecclesia et Pontifica Medal from Pope John Paul II, which was delivered by Archbishop Daniel Pilarczyk in 1990, and he received the Distinguished Service Citation from the National Conference of Christians and Jews in 1995.

Dr. Tew has published more than 250 articles, including not only his research on facial pain, cerebrovascular disease, brain tumors, and disorders of the spine, but also papers on history and biography, which were written as a member of the Literary Club of Cincinnati. Dr. Tew and his wife have been very active in community affairs, and he has served as president of the Cincinnati Symphony.

1999 HONORED GUEST DUKE S. SAMSON

Dr. Duke S. Samson (Fig. 1.16) was born in Odessa, Texas. He moved with his family frequently during his early childhood because his father was an officer in the Army Corps of Engineers. The family returned to Odessa in 1949, where Duke received his primary and secondary education in the Odessa public school system. He was active in athletics and entered Stanford University in 1961 on a football scholarship. He played both football and rugby until he sustained a knee injury in 1963. He excelled in the honors psychology program with a minor in philosophy.

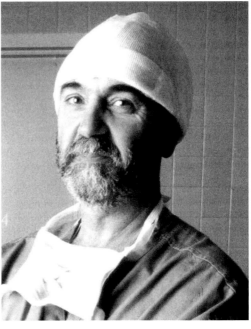

FIGURE 1.16. 1999 Honored Guest Dr. Duke S. Samson.

He spent 6 months at Stanford-in-France, and there he substituted parachute jumping for collegiate football. He graduated from Stanford in 1965. He attended Washington University School of Medicine and was named Outstanding Student in Surgery. He graduated in 1969 and served as a surgical intern at Duke University from 1969 to 1970. He returned to Texas and served his neurosurgical residency at the University of Texas Southwestern Medical Center at Dallas. He spent 6 months with Gerard Guiot in Paris and 7 months with Dr. Gazi Yaşargil in Zurich, Switzerland, while he was a senior resident. He focused his physical prowess on the martial arts of Tae Kwon Do and Judo. He achieved the rank of brown belt in Judo.

Dr. Samson enlisted in the United States Army Medical Corps after he completed his neurosurgical residency, and was stationed at the Western Pacific Neurosurgical Service at Clark Air Base in the Republic of Philippines. He later was transferred to the Walter Reed Medical Center, where he served on the neurosurgical service. He then returned to Dallas and has been on the faculty of the University of Texas Southwestern Medical School ever since. He was promoted to professor in 1985 and was named chairman of the division of neurosurgery in 1985. He engineered the complex transition to departmental status in 1989, and was appointed director of the University of Texas Center for Clinical Research in Stroke and Spinal Cord Injury in 1998.

Dr. Samson has had a keen interest in microvascular neurosurgery. He has directed a large department consisting of 9 faculty members, 10 residents, and 26 employees. He is committed to patient welfare without compromise.

Dr. Samson is married to Patricia Bergen, MD, who served as chief of surgical services at the Dallas Veterans Administration Hospital. They have two sons—Lome Daniel (age 10) and Gabriel Stanford (age 8). Duke has continued his interest in western horsemanship and is a burgeoning novelist.

2000 HONORED GUEST EDWARD R. LAWS, JR.

Edward R. Laws, Jr. (Fig 1.17), was born in New York City, the son of a physician. He en-

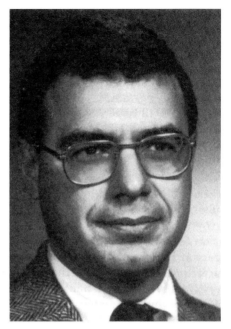

FIGURE 1.17. 2000 Honored Guest Dr. Edward R. Laws, Jr.

tered Princeton University at the age of 17 and received an AB degree with honors in the special program in American Civilization. He received his MD degree from Johns Hopkins School of Medicine. He did elective work in the department of neurosurgery with studies on the histochemistry and cytochemistry of brain tumors. He was a surgical intern at Johns Hopkins under Dr. Alfred Blalock and then spent 2 years in the United States Public Health Service. He was assigned to the National Communicable Disease Center in Atlanta, where he was responsible for a research program in pesticide toxicology. He then returned to Johns Hopkins for residency training in neurological surgery under Dr. A. Earl Walker. After completing his residency he remained on the faculty of Johns Hopkins with major responsibility for pediatric neurosurgery. He left Baltimore in September 1972 to join the staff of the Mayo Clinic, where he became deeply involved in pituitary surgery and epilepsy surgery. He continued his research interest in experimental biology of malignant brain tumors at the Mayo Clinic. He became a recipient of an endowed chair at the Mayo Clinic. Dr. Laws was selected in 1987 to succeed Dr. Hugo Rizzoli as

Professor and Chairman, Department of Neurosurgery, George Washington University Medical Center, Washington, DC. He built a superb residency training program there. He then moved to Charlottesville, Virginia, where he is professor of neurological surgery and continues to be very active in research, teaching, and clinical practice.

Dr. Laws became president of the CNS in 1984, when the annual meeting was held in New York City, his place of birth. Dr. Walter Dandy was a posthumous honored guest and Dr. Hugo Rizzoli was a living honored guest. Dr. Laws became president of the AANS for the year 1997 to 1998. We were proud to have Dr. Laws as the honored guest for our 50th anniversary meeting in San Antonio, Texas.

Dr. Laws married Peggy in 1962 between his third and fourth years of medical school. She was an instructor in the school of nursing. Ed and Peggy are justly proud of their four daughters. They have worked closely together in the broad profession of medicine. Dr. Laws was editor of *Neurosurgery,* and Peggy served as managing editor of the same journal using her maiden name, Margaret Anderson. We are happy to honor Peggy as well as Ed.

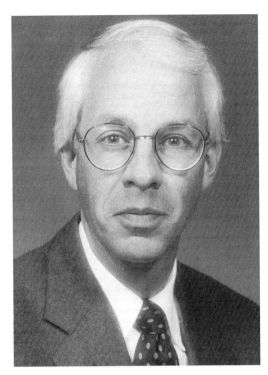

FIGURE 1.18. 1992 CNS President Dr. William F. Chandler.

1992 CNS PRESIDENT
WILLIAM F. CHANDLER

William F. Chandler (Fig. 1.18) was born in Chicago just as World War II was coming to a close in July 1945. His family moved 1 year later, and he spent his entire childhood in the same house in suburban Detroit. He attended Ferndale High School and graduated at the top of his class. He attended Northwestern University in Evanston, Illinois, majoring in psychology in a pre-med program and graduated in 1967. He returned to Michigan as a medical student at the University of Michigan. It was there that his interest in the neurosciences developed. During his first 3 years he worked on research projects involving spinal cord regeneration with a senior neurologist. His interest in neurosurgery was sparked by working with Drs. Richard Schneider, Eddie Kahn, Glenn Kindt, Jim Taren, and Elizabeth Crosby. He was drawn into the ''Michigan Way,'' and signed up for internship

and residency. During medical school he became reacquainted with an old high school friend, Susan Plesscher, and within a year they were happily married. Their first son, Scott, was born near the end of his residency training.

During his residency he had the privilege of doing research with the legendary neuroanatomist Dr. Elizabeth Crosby. He had an early interest in intracranial pressure monitoring and, along with Dr. Glenn Kindt, documented the first cases of elevated intracranial pressure in Reyes syndrome. At the end of his residency in 1977, he received the Van Wagenen Fellowship and spent 6 months in Stockholm, Sweden, working with Dr. Nicolas Zwetnow. He also developed a strong interest in cerebrovascular neurosurgery and arranged for a visit with Prof. Yaşargil in 1977. An interest in pituitary surgery led to a visit with Prof. Guiot in Paris, also in 1977.

Dr. Chandler and his wife, Susan, returned from the Van Wagenen experience with a second son, Jesse, born at the Karolinska Institute. Dr.

Chandler joined Drs. David Kline and Michael Carey at Louisiana State University in 1978 and had a wonderful experience in New Orleans. In 1979, he and his young family returned to the University of Michigan, where he rose through the ranks to professor. He was instrumental in developing the use of intraoperative ultrasound in 1980 for both the brain and spinal cord. He pursued his interest in pituitary lesions and has become a leader in pituitary surgery. He and his family took a 4-month sabbatical to Zurich, Switzerland, in 1986, where he worked with Dr. Alex Landolt in basic pituitary research. Once again he had the opportunity to observe Prof. Yaşargil. He has had a sustained interest in brain tumors and was the chairman of the Joint Section on Tumors for 2 years.

He joined the Executive Committee of the CNS in 1986. He was the scientific program chairman in 1990, and annual meeting chairman in 1991. He was vice-president in 1991, and president in 1992. During his presidency, joint officers' meetings with the AANS were encouraged and established on a regular schedule. Joint task forces were established, and a positive working relationship with the AANS continued to be cultivated.

Dr. Chandler plays tennis once or twice a week and loves to ski with his family each winter.

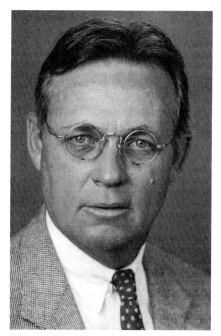

FIGURE 1.19. 1993 CNS President Dr. Arthur L. Day.

1993 CNS PRESIDENT
ARTHUR L. DAY

Arthur L. Day (Fig 1.19) was born in Red Chute, Louisiana, and graduated from medical school at Louisiana State University in 1972. He interned in Birmingham, Alabama. He completed his neurological surgery residency training at the University of Florida in 1977 under the direction of Dr. Albert Rhoton. After a fellowship in brain tumor immunology at the University of Florida, he joined the neurosurgery faculty in 1978 and is currently professor, co-chairman, resident program director, and the James and Newton Eblen Eminent Scholar Chair in cerebrovascular surgery of the department of neurological surgery at the University of Florida.

Dr. Day's clinical interests are in cerebrovascular disease and sports medicine. His research activities focus on cerebral ischemia and protection. Dr. Day currently serves on the editorial boards of the *Journal of Stroke and Cerebrovascular Disease, Neurosurgery,* and *Operative Techniques in Neurosurgery.*

He has served as president of the Florida Neurosurgical Society, the CNS, the Joint Section of Cerebrovascular Surgery of the AANS/CNS, the Sports Medicine Section of the AANS/CNS, and the Alachua County Medical Society. He has recently completed a term as a member of the board of directors of the AANS and chairman of the AANS/CNS Washington Committee. He has also recently been appointed as a director on the American Board of Neurological Surgery.

Dr. Day married Dana while he was in medical school, and they have three children—Lauren (age 23), Steven (age 20), and Lindsey (age 13). When they are able to get away together as a family, they enjoy walking or working out at the track, skiing, or spending time at Amelia Island, Florida.

1994 CNS PRESIDENT
RICHARD ARTHUR ROSKI

Richard A. Roski (Fig. 1.20) was born December 6, 1949, in Cleveland, Ohio. One of five children, he was raised in Cleveland Heights, Ohio. While at Cleveland Heights High School, Richard set the state record in the 2-mile run and received an athletic scholarship to attend Purdue University in West Lafayette, Indiana. He received his BS degree in engineering sciences from the School of Aeronautical Engineering in 1971. It was during this time that he developed an interest in pursuing a career in medicine. He was accepted into Case Western Reserve School of Medicine in Cleveland, Ohio, graduating in 1976. He continued his training at the University Hospitals of Cleveland, completing both his internship and residency program in neurosurgery. His neurosurgical training was under the direction of Dr. Frank Nulsen. Another attending physician, Dr. Robert Spetzler, had a profound influence on Richard's subsequent interest in cerebrovascular surgery. He received the Dudley P. Allen Surgical Research Scholarship in 1980, and carried out research with Drs. Robert Spetzler and Warren Selman in studying the protective effects of barbiturates in focal cerebral ischemia.

After completing his residency, Dr. Roski accepted a position on the faculty at the University of Louisville School of Medicine as an assistant professor of surgery. While working with Drs. Henry Garretson and Christopher Shields, he recognized the importance of being actively involved in the volunteer efforts with the national neurosurgical societies. Their influence fostered a longstanding commitment to both the CNS and the AANS, which continues today.

In 1983 Richard left academics to pursue a career in private practice. He practiced for more than 1 year in Lumberton, North Carolina, and then moved to Davenport, Iowa, in 1985 to start Quad City Neurosurgical Associates, PC.

The challenges of running a private practice, and the increasing national efforts of cost containment in medicine, influenced him to return to Purdue University to obtain an MBA degree in business management. With this background, Richard recognized that there was a growing need for neurosurgeons to understand the changing health care environment and the factors that affect physician reimbursement. Dr. Roski's efforts in this area of medicine have included positions as president of his local Independent Practice Association, a current procedure terminology (CPT) advisor to the American Medical Association (AMA), and a lecturer on CPT coding and reimbursement.

Married in 1981 to Debbie, Richard has four children. In recent years, he has renewed his longtime interest in motorcycles and enjoys riding on a regular basis. He also enjoys playing golf and has been fortunate enough to play on many courses around the world. Other interest include recreational skiing and running.

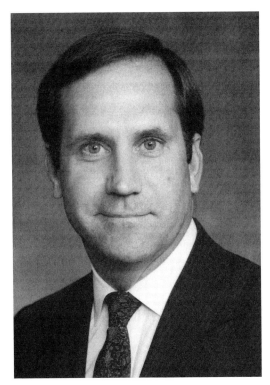

FIGURE 1.20. 1994 CNS President Dr. Richard Arthur Roski.

1995 CNS PRESIDENT
RALPH G. DACEY, JR.

Ralph G. Dacey, Jr. (Fig. 1.21), was born in Massachusetts on August 7, 1948. He received

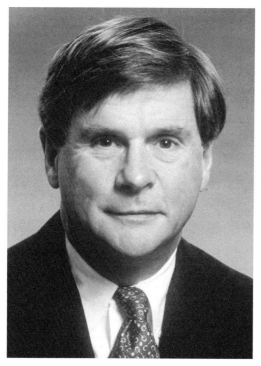

FIGURE 1.21. 1995 CNS President Dr. Ralph G. Dacey, Jr.

his BA degree from Harvard University in 1970 and his MD degree from the University of Virginia School of Medicine in Charlottesville in 1974. He served as a resident in internal medicine from 1974 to 1976 and subsequently became board certified in internal medicine. He served as a general surgery resident at the University of Virginia in 1975. He did his neurosurgical training with Dr. John Jane at the University of Virginia. During his residency at the University of Virginia he did a postdoctoral fellowship in microvascular physiology in the laboratory of Dr. Brian Duling, and was an American College of Surgeons (ACS) Schering Scholar. Also during his residency he worked as a neurosurgical registrar in Plymouth, England.

After his postgraduate training, he became an assistant professor of neurological surgery at the University of Washington in Seattle. He subsequently became Professor and Chief, Division of Neurosurgery, University of North Carolina, Chapel Hill, North Carolina. He then came to

Washington University at St. Louis. He is now the Henry G. and Edith R. Schwartz professor and chairman of neurological surgery and co-chairman of the Department of Neurology and neurological surgery.

Dr. Dacey was president of the CNS in 1995. He is a member of the AANS, American Academy of Neurological Surgery, American Board of Neurological Surgery, ACS, American Heart Association, AMA, American Surgical Association, CNS, Neurology Study Section NIH, NSA, Research Society of Neurological Surgeons, SNS, Society of University Neurosurgeons, and the Southern Neurosurgical Society. He is the consultant neurosurgeon for the St. Louis Rams, St. Louis Blues, and the St. Louis Cardinals.

Dr. Dacey has a special interest in cerebrovascular neurosurgery and has an active general practice in neurosurgery as well. His research activities have concentrated primarily in the area of physiology of the intracerebral microcirculation. He was awarded a Clinician Investigator Development Award by NIH.

While at Washington University, Dr. Dacey has served on many committees, including the Executive Faculty (1989–present), Board of Directors, Washington University Physician Network, Neurosurgeon-in-Chief Barnes Hospital, Executive Committee, Barnes/Jewish Christian Inc. Medical Executive Committee (1989–present), Medical Executive Committee Chairman (1995–1998), Practice Plan Board of Directors–Chairman (1997, 1998), and the Practice Plan Finance Committee Chairman (1997, 1998).

Dr. Dacey married Corinne Holland Mears in 1975. They have one daughter, Elizabeth Campbell, born in 1979, and one son, Ralph G. Dacey, III, born in 1983. His nonmedical interests include golf and sailing.

1996 CNS PRESIDENT
STEPHEN HAINES

A native of Burlington, Vermont, Steve Haines (Fig. 1.22) studied at Dartmouth College with highest distinction in mathematics and social sciences, earning his BS degree *magna cum laude* in 1971. He received his medical degree

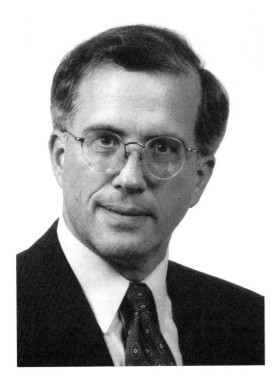

FIGURE 1.22. 1996 CNS President Dr. Stephen Haines.

from the University of Vermont College of Medicine in 1975, and after a year's internship in surgery at the University of Minnesota, he completed his neurological surgery residency at the University of Pittsburgh in 1981. In that year, the AANS awarded him the Van Wagenen Fellowship, a prize that allowed him to study at Oxford University under the tutelage of Dr. Charles Warlow.

Dr. Haines joined the faculty at the University of Minnesota in 1982 as assistant professor of neurosurgery, then moved up to the rank of full professor in 1993. He was also appointed to professorships in the otolaryngology and pediatric departments. In 1997 he was appointed professor of neurological surgery, otolaryngology, and pediatrics, and chairman of the department of neurological surgery at the Medical University of South Carolina.

Dr. Haines' primary clinical interests lie in pediatric neurosurgery, and surgery of the skull base and posterior fossa. He has participated in several multidisciplinary programs involving pediatric brain tumors, myelodysplasia (both adult and pediatric), craniofacial disorders, spasticity treatment, and skull base surgery. He headed the University of Minnesota division of pediatric neurosurgery for more than 12 years, and he managed his department's participation in the University's highly respected Craniofacial and Skull Base Surgery Center.

Dr. Haines' major research interest focuses on the development of resources for the evidence-based practice of neurosurgery, including application of epidemiological and statistical methods to neurosurgical outcomes studies. He has published and lectured extensively on the subject. He has participated in several industry-sponsored clinical trials, was the University of Minnesota Clinical Center principal investigator for the NASCET trial, and was principal investigator of an NIH- and AHCPR-funded multicenter trial comparing percutaneous discectomy with conventional discectomy techniques.

Dr. Haines' bibliography includes more than 260 peer-reviewed articles, books, chapters, reviews, abstracts, and invited presentations on topics ranging from pediatric and skull base surgical techniques to infections and antibiotic prophylaxis in neurosurgery. He has served as a course instructor on a wide range of continuing medical education topics relating to neurosurgical techniques and the application of outcome analysis.

In addition to his academic and clinical pursuits, Dr. Haines is very active in national organized neurosurgery. He served on the Executive Committee of the CNS from 1991 to 1997. He also served as the neurosurgical representative to the ACS Young Surgeons' Committee and was the committee chairman for 2 years.

Dr. Haines is listed in *Who's Who in America* (1997) and *Best Doctors in America* (1997). He is married to Jennifer Plombon and has two grown children, Christopher and Jeremy.

1997 CNS PRESIDENT
MARC R. MAYBERG

Marc R. Mayberg (Fig. 1.23) spent his childhood in Edina, Minnesota. He attended Harvard

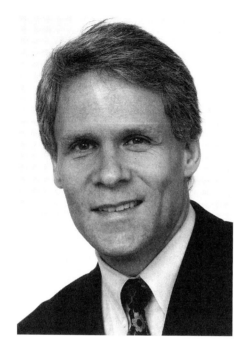

FIGURE 1.23. 1997 CNS President Dr. Marc R. Mayberg.

University and played varsity football. He received his degree from Harvard University in 1974 and received his MD degree from the Mayo Medical School. He worked in the laboratory of Dr. Thoralf Sundt while he was in medical school. He completed his residency training in neurological surgery at Massachusetts General Hospital under the direction of Dr. Nicholas T. Zervas. He did a research fellowship with Dr. Michael Moskowitz. He was a Van Wagenen Fellow at the National Hospital for Nervous Diseases in London, England, in 1985, and he worked in the laboratory of Prof. Lindsay Symon. He joined the faculty of the University of Washington in 1986 and became professor of neurosurgery and chief of the clinical services at the University of Washington Medical Center. He now is chief of neurological surgery at the Cleveland Clinic.

Dr. Mayberg has done considerable research on cerebral vessel wall biology including research on cerebral vasospasm, mechanisms of smooth muscle proliferation, and the response of arteries to radiation. He has had a special interest in acoustic neuromas, pituitary tumors, and carotid endarterectomy. He has authored approximately 100 scientific journal articles and more than 50 book chapters.

Before his election as president of the CNS, Dr. Mayberg served the CNS as vice-president, Executive Committee member, Scientific Program Committee chairman, Annual Meeting Committee chairman, and chairman of the Education Committee. He has served on the Joint Officers Committee, Washington Committee, and was chairman of the Devices and Drugs Committee. He has been active in NIH, the Veterans Administration (VA) Research Council, the National Stroke Association, the American Heart Association, and the Brain Attack Coalition. He is a member of the AANS, the NSA, the American Academy of Neurosurgeons, and the ACS. He has served on the editorial boards of several journals.

Dr. Mayberg is married to Theresa (Terry), who is a neuroanesthesiologist. She was associate professor in the department of anesthesia and neurological surgery at the University of Washington. Her research interest includes the effect of anesthetic agents on cerebral blood flow. Marc and Terry have a son, Matthew, who is now 5 years old, and a daughter, Katherine, who is 1 year old.

1998 CNS PRESIDENT
WILLIAM ALLAN FRIEDMAN

William Allan Friedman (Fig. 1.24) was born in Dayton, Ohio, and attended high school in Cincinnati, Ohio. He graduated in 1970 as a National Merit Scholar and attended Oberlin College, where he was elected to Phi Beta Kappa. He graduated *summa cum laude* from Ohio State University College of Medicine, where he was elected to the Alpha Omega Alpha Honor Society and received the Maurice B. Rusoff Award for excellence in medicine.

Dr. Friedman served a surgical internship at the University of Florida in Gainesville and completed his residency there under the direction of Dr. Albert Rhoton. During his residency training he did basic neurophysiology research as an NIH Postdoctoral Fellow. He was invited

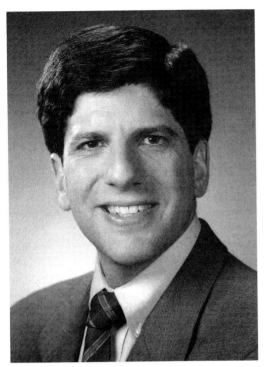

FIGURE 1.24. 1998 CNS President Dr. William Allan Friedman.

to join the faculty of the department of neurosurgery as assistant professor and has continued on the faculty ever since. He received the NIH Teacher Investigator Award, and held that award from July 1982 to July 1987. He studied basic neurophysiology of spinal cord injuries. He also developed one of the first intraoperative neurophysiology monitoring laboratories, which was used to monitor thousands of neurosurgical and orthopedic surgical cases.

Dr. Friedman is the author of more than 150 articles and book chapters, and has authored a book on radiosurgery. He has conducted excellent courses on stereotactic radiosurgery. He developed the University of Florida radiosurgery system working with Dr. Frank Bova. Drs. Friedman and Bova received the 1990 University of Florida College of Medicine Clinical Research Prize in recognition of this accomplishment. Dr. Friedman is currently professor and chairman of the department of neurological surgery at the University of Florida. Dr. Friedman

is a past president of the Florida Neurosurgical Society. Before his election as president of the CNS, Dr. Friedman served as a member of the Executive Committee, Scientific Program Committee chairman, Annual Meeting Committee chairman, and treasurer. He served as editor of both Neurosurgery://On-Call and SANS V.

Dr. Friedman is married to Ransom LaRoche, and they are very proud of their three children—Daniel, Abigail, and David.

1999 CNS PRESIDENT
H. HUNT BATJER

H. Hunt Batjer (Fig. 1.25) was born in Burlington, Vermont, in 1951. His father was called to active duty by the United States Navy during the Korean conflict and served as Lt. Commander. The family moved to California during the war. The family later settled in San Angelo, Texas, where Hunt excelled in varsity basketball as well as varsity baseball. He was an excellent left-handed pitcher and was drafted by the Balti-

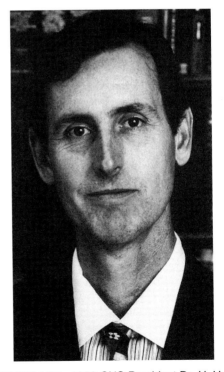

FIGURE 1.25. 1999 CNS President Dr. H. Hunt Batjer.

more Orioles as a free agent in 1970, but he declined in order to attend the University of Texas on a baseball scholarship. He received his MD degree in 1977 from the University of Texas Southwestern Medical School in Dallas. He was elected to Alpha Omega Alpha. He served an internship in general surgery at University of Texas Southwestern and continued as a neurosurgical resident at the same institution. Dr. Kemp Clark was chief of neurological surgery at that time. Dr. Batjer was closely associated with Dr. Duke Samson, who was already an excellent cerebrovascular neurosurgeon. Dr. Batjer served a fellowship at the National Hospital, Institute of Neurology, University of London at Queen's Square, and a second fellowship at the University of Western Ontario under the supervision of Dr. Charles Drake. These fellowships were served during his period of neurosurgical residency. Dr. Batjer was invited to join the faculty at University of Texas Southwestern, and he coordinated basic laboratory studies with clinical work. He had a particular interest in cerebral ischemia, ischemic brain protection, cerebral vasospasm, and autoregulatory disturbance associated with vascular malformations.

Dr. Batjer was recruited to Northwestern Medical School in Chicago, where he became chief of neurological surgery and director of the neurosurgical training program in 1995. He was appointed as director of the Feinberg Clinical Neuroscience Research Institute in 1997, and in 1998 he became the Michael J. Marchese professor and chairman of the department of neurological surgery. He has received numerous academic awards including Outstanding Teacher Awards, and has been a visiting professor at more than 25 institutions worldwide. He serves on the editorial boards of *Neurosurgery* and *Perspectives in Neurological Surgery,* and as an ad hoc reviewer for a dozen other scientific publications. He also serves as co-editor of *Techniques in Neurosurgery* with Dr. Chris Loftus. He has published more than 175 scientific papers and chapters, and 4 books.

Dr. Batjer was elected to the Executive Committee of the CNS in 1990 and has served on many committees. He was Scientific Program Committee chairman in 1993 and Annual Meet-

ing Committee chairman in 1994. He was elected secretary of the CNS in 1995, and president-elect in 1997.

Dr. Batjer married Janet Eileen Wright in 1989. The Batjers have four wonderful daughters, including a set of twins born in August 1998. It is obvious that Janet and Hunt lead very busy lives.

2000 CNS PRESIDENT
DANIEL LOUIS BARROW

Daniel Louis Barrow (Fig. 1.26) was raised in west central Illinois, the first of four children of Dr. and Mrs. Warren C. Barrow. During high school, Dan was active in varsity sports, including football, golf, and track. He was named an Illinois State Scholar and appeared in *Who's Who in High School Dramatics.* Dan graduated *magna cum laude* from Westminster College in 1976 and began his medical education at Southern Illinois University School of Medicine in the summer of 1976. He received his MD degree from Southern Illinois University in 1979 and

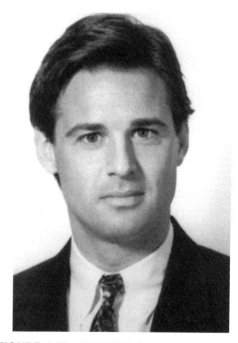

FIGURE 1.26. 2000 CNS President Dr. Daniel Louis Barrow.

moved to Atlanta, Georgia, to obtain his postgraduate training in neurosurgery at Emory University School of Medicine.

Dr. Barrow completed his general surgery internship and neurosurgical residency at Emory University affiliated hospitals and obtained his neurology training at Massachusetts General Hospital. On completing his neurosurgical residency, Dr. Barrow completed a fellowship in cerebrovascular surgery at the Mayo Clinic in Rochester, Minnesota. He returned to Emory University in 1985 as an assistant professor in the department of neurosurgery. In 1990, Dr. Barrow was promoted to associate professor, and in 1991 was named vice-chairman of the department of neurosurgery at Emory University School of Medicine. In 1995, Dr. Barrow was named MBNA/Bowman professor and chairman of the department of neurosurgery. In 1998 he was appointed to the board of directors of Emory Clinic, Inc.

Dr. Barrow has authored more than 200 scientific articles and chapters in medical textbooks. He has authored or edited 12 monographs, including a major text book of neurosurgery, *The Practice of Neurosurgery*. He has been a visiting professor at major universities throughout the United States, Europe, and Asia. His research interests have focused on cerebrovascular disease and stroke. During his career in medicine, he has won many awards, including induction into the honorary medical society, Alpha Omega Alpha. He has been named in *Who's Who in America* and has been chosen by his peers to appear in the publication *The Best Doctors in America*. In 1997 Dr. Barrow received the Distinguished Alumnus Award from Southern Illinois University School of Medicine, one of only four recipients of this prestigious honor. In 1998

he received the Alumni Achievement Award from Westminster College.

Dr. Barrow has been active in organized neurosurgery, holding a variety of leadership and editorial positions. He has been on the Executive Committee of the CNS since 1990 and served as Scientific Program Committee chairman (1991), Annual Meeting Committee chairman (1992), secretary (1992–1995), and president (1999–2000). He was president of the Georgia Neurosurgical Society and member of the AANS/CNS Washington Committee (1997–present). Dr. Barrow has been on the editorial boards of *Clinical Neurosurgery* (1988–1992), *Neurosurgery* (1993–present), *Neurosurgical Consultations* (1989–1995), *Neurologia Medico Chirurgica* (1996–present); has coedited *Contemporary Neurosurgery* (1985–1995); edited *Perspectives in Neurological Surgery* (1989–1992); and chaired the AANS Publications Committee.

Dr. Barrow is an avid outdoorsman who enjoys hunting, fishing, and other outdoor sporting activities. He is married to Mollie Winston Barrow, a practicing oral and maxillofacial surgeon. They live in Atlanta with their three children—Emily (age 12), Jack (age 10), and Tom (age 8).

REFERENCES

1. Bishop EJ. *Tabulation of the Results of a National Neurosurgical Fee Survey 1963–1966.* Congress of Neurological Surgeons, Socio-Economic Committee, 1966.
2. Fulton JF. *Harvey Cushing A Biography.* Springfield, IL, Charles C. Thomas, 1946.
3. Lockhart WS Jr. *Neurosurgical Hospital Utilization Guidelines Manual.* Congress of Neurological Surgeons, Utilization Guidelines Committee, 1969.
4. Thompson JM. *History of the Congress of Neurological Surgeons 1951–1991.* Baltimore, Williams & Wilkins, 1992.

2

Status of Neurosurgery in 1951: Science

Robert G. Ojemann, MD

INTRODUCTION

The remarkable improvement in neurosurgical treatment in the last 50 years has depended to a great extent on basic and clinical investigations. After World War II, neuroscience research began to expand and increasingly involved neurosurgeons. Wilder Penfield (36,40) had published his outstanding clinical research, and others were pursuing exciting investigations. Support for research came from many sources including the NIH, Department of the Army, National Cancer Institute, Atomic Energy Commission, Public Health Service, American Cancer Society, National Foundation for Infantile Paralysis, and many named private funds.

In 1951, when the CNS was founded, I entered medical school at the University of Iowa. We had no rotation on the neurosurgical service, but I have a vivid recollection during a surgical rotation of seeing Dr. Russell Meyers, who had been investigating methods to treat patients with movement disorders, making a stereotactic lesion using ultrasound (32,33). Neurosurgeons were reporting an increasing number of basic investigations in areas such as cerebrospinal fluid physiology, cerebrovascular physiology, and the use of radioactive isotopes in the central nervous system. By reviewing the *Journal of Neurosurgery* and the *Index Medicus* for 1950, 1951, and 1952, as well as several book chapters related to the history of neurological surgery, we can gain some insight into what neurosurgeons in North America were doing in the early 1950s.

We are fortunate that some of the leaders in neurosurgery at that time were concerned about research in neurosurgical training programs. In his presidential address in 1952 to the then Harvey Cushing Society, Paul Bucy (12), in speaking on "Our Training Programs and the Future of Neurological Surgery," said,

We must never forget that training in research has a two-fold advantage. There are a few men who will make important discoveries and will go on to become leaders in the field of neurological investigation. Unfortunately, the number of such men is not great. However, training in basic research is of value not only to these select few. It can be of the greatest value to those who will carry on clinical research and clinical observation. All too many of those who publish on clinical subjects have little appreciation of the scientific method, or its inherent importance in the evaluation of clinical observations. They fail to appreciate the importance of adequate controls, and of multiple observations. They often do not recognize the difference between those statistical variations that are insignificant and those that are valid. The most profitable way in which to correct these deficiencies and to improve the level of clinical research in the field of neurological surgery is to extend the opportunity for basic research under leaders with a thorough understanding of scientific principles. Furthermore, it is of importance to the advancement of neurological surgery that its devotees be thoroughly conversant with developments in the basic neurological sciences and be sufficiently well trained in scientific methods to evaluate and understand the works of others in these fields.

It is also of importance that interest in research into the structure and function of the nervous system be kept alive among neurological surgeons. Only in that way will our specialty remain alive as a vital growing field of medicine. Furthermore, there are many problems in the field of fundamental neurology that can be investigated only by or through the active cooperation of a neurological surgeon. (p. 541)

CENTRAL NERVOUS SYSTEM FUNCTION

In 1934, Wilder Penfield established the Montreal Neurological Institute and developed a well-planned program of clinical research. Rasmussen (40), in writing about Penfield's life, said the Montreal Neurological Institute

> was planned by Dr. Penfield as a clinically oriented institute with basic research laboratories and scientists grouped around the patient and the neurological and neurosurgical team. Both the organization and the physical plant were planned to provide maximum opportunities for constant cross-fertilization between research oriented clinic and clinically oriented basic research scientists, and for continuing stimulation of both by the patients' clinical diagnostic and therapeutic problems. (p. 139–140)

In 1950, Penfield and Rasmussen (36) published their book *The Cerebral Cortex of Man. A Clinical Study of Localization of Function.* The findings in this publication were based on studies of approximately 400 craniotomies performed under local anesthesia using electrocorticography and careful evaluation of the effects of brain stimulation. Investigations continued at that institution in the early 1950s. Penfield and

Welch (37) reported clinical and experimental studies of the supplementary motor area of the cerebral cortex. Jasper and Penfield (27) studied the effect of voluntary movement on the electrical activity of the precentral gyrus. Penfield (35) presented his theories on memory mechanisms. Rasmussen (40) summarized the major contributions of Penfield and those who worked with him. These included

> (t)he role of the medial temporal structures in memory, the refined localization and interrelationships of the cerebral speech areas and of somatosensory and motor function in the human pre- and postcentral gyri, the identification of the second somatosensory area in the lower central region, and the identification of the supplementary motor area on the medial aspect of the intermediate frontal region. (p. 140)

Other neurosurgeons reported clinical investigations in the early 1950s to increase understanding of how the central nervous system functioned. Ward (54), from the University of Washington, discussed somatic function of the nervous system. Pool and Ransohoff (39), from Columbia, reported the autonomic effects of stimulating the rostral portion of the cingulate gyri in man. Glumann et al. (23), from Columbia, studied electrical excitability of the human motor cortex to determine the most effective parameters for eliciting motor response with a square wave pulse.

LOCALIZATION OF INTRACRANIAL PATHOLOGY

In 1951 there was great interest in improving the diagnosis and localization of intracranial pathology. At the first meeting of the CNS, the first five papers all related to this topic:

1. "Diagnosis of Brain Tumors with Plain Roentgenogram of the Skull"
2. "Homonymous Visual Field Defects in Localization of Brain Tumors"
3. "Electroencephalographic Localization in Brain Tumors"
4. "Neurologic Diagnosis—False Localizing Signs in Brain Tumors"
5. "Interpretation of Cerebral Angiogram"

Angiography

In 1951, angiography was performed by direct puncture of the carotid and vertebral arteries in the neck. An editorial in the January 1951 issue of the *Journal of Neurosurgery* written by Paul Bucy (11) noted that

> the most recent advance in cerebral angiography has been the development of several different methods for the taking of serial pictures, demonstrating the various degrees of filling and visualization of the arterial, capillary and venous systems of the brain. None of these methods have as yet been thoroughly perfected, although several show great promise. There is undoubtedly much advantage in being able to study the various parts of the cerebral circulation as compared with single cerebral angiography. (p. 1–2)

He went on to say that many problems related to angiography remained to be solved, the most important being the development of a contrast medium that "will be readily available, reasonable in cost, provide excellent visualization, be non-irritating to the vascular wall and generally innocuous." (11, p. 2)

Many investigations during that time period related to angiography. Sugar (47), from the University of Illinois Neuropsychiatric Institute, reported the "Pathological Anatomy and Angiography of Intracranial Vascular Anomalies." He noted that a "more careful consideration of the embryologic features of the vessels of the brain may give a better understanding of intracranial vascular anomalies" (p. 22). Bloor et al. (9), from Duke, reported "An Experimental Method for the Evaluation of Contrast Media Used in Cerebral Angiography," which discussed using indicator dye injection and electroencephalography. They concluded that this was a useful technique to evaluate contrast media. Subsequently, they reported studies of three contrast media (8). Smith et al. (44), from the University of Minnesota, presented an experimental study in rabbits on the toxicity of Diodrast as a contrast agent for angiography. Foltz, Thomas, and Ward (20), from the University of Washington, studied the effects of intracarotid Diodrast in monkeys. Their study showed this contrast medium to be far from ideal because of its toxicity.

Radioactive Isotope Scanning

In 1951, the localization of many brain tumors remained a challenge. Use of plain skull films, pneumoencephalography, ventriculography, and angiography combined with careful clinical examinations were the principle methods available. Many tumors were missed, and a frequent operation was an exploratory craniotomy.

In 1947, Moore et al. (14), from the University of Minnesota, found that intravenous fluorescein concentrated in brain tumors and other lesions of the central nervous system. Studies on tagging this and other compounds with a radioactive label were conducted at that institution and were reported by Chou et al. (14,15) and by Peyton et al. (38), who reported the localization of intracranial lesions by radioactive isotopes using radioactive diodofluorescein and single-shield window-type Geiger–Mueller counters.

Other institutions also studied intracranial localization with radioactive compounds. Ashkenazy, Davis, and Martin (3), from the University of Chicago, reported an evaluation of the technique and results of the radioactive diodofluorescein test for the localization of intracranial lesions. They found they had the ability to localize accurately 95% of intracranial tumors. Bakay (6), from Massachusetts General Hospital, evaluated the blood–brain barrier with radioactive phosphorus.

Ultrasound

French, Wild, and Neal (22), from the University of Minnesota, reported the experimental application of ultrasound to the localization of brain tumors at the time of operation. The use of pulsed ultrasound was studied in rabbits, and no damage to normal tissue was found. They also were able to locate subcortical neoplasms in postmortem brains.

ANEURYSMS AND ARTERIOVENOUS MALFORMATIONS

In his 1951 editorial in the *Journal of Neurosurgery*, Paul Bucy (11) stated the following:

> Cerebral angiography has made it possible to plan and execute suitable treatment for various

intracranial vascular lesions. However, only a beginning has been made in this therapeutic field. These lesions still remain serious and carry with them a high mortality and morbidity. Certainly, it is reasonable to believe that with further study of cerebral circulation, increased utilization of cerebral angiography and continued clinical experience with lesions of this type, our ability to deal with them successfully will steadily improve. (p. 2)

Because many intracranial aneurysms were treated by carotid ligation in 1951, there were clinical investigations on the hemodynamic effects of this ligation by Sweet et al. (50,51) from Massachusetts General Hospital and Shenkin et al. (43), from the University of Pennsylvania.

Margolis et al. (31), from Duke, discussed the role of small angiomatous malformations in the production of intracerebral hematomas. They pointed out that these small angiomatous malformations may play a more important role as the cause of intracerebral hemorrhage than had been previously suspected.

BRAIN TUMORS

Horrax and Wu (26), from the Lahey Clinic, evaluated postoperative survival of patients with intracranial oligodendroglioma with special reference to radical tumor removal and found that there was a longer survival after radical removal.

Investigations of new treatments for malignant brain tumors were being pursued in the early 1950s. Sweet and Javid (48,49) proposed the possible use of neutron-capturing isotopes such as boron-10 in the treatment of neoplasms. They presented background information on this technique and its proposed use in humans. French et al. (21), from the University of California at Los Angeles, investigated the effect of intracarotid administration of nitrogen mustard on the normal brain in cats and monkeys. It was concluded that this drug was too toxic to normal endothelium when administered in this manner.

HEAD TRAUMA

Serial electroencephalographic studies were performed on patients with acute head injuries by Dawson, Webster, and Gurdjian (18), from Wayne State University. They attempted to cor-

relate their findings with the prognosis. Aird et al. (2), from the University of California at San Francisco, reported neurophysiological studies on cerebral concussion in cats. These studies showed cerebral concussion increased the permeability of the blood–brain barrier, as measured by the increase in cocaine in the cerebral cortex, and caused dysrhythmia on electroencephalography. The dysrhythmia was markedly lessened by the preliminary use of Trypan red. Ward (53), from the University of Washington, reported a clinical study on the use of atropine in the treatment of closed head injuries. Initial results were encouraging.

Gurdjian, Webster, and Lissner (25), from Wayne State University, reported the mechanism of skull fracture from studies of cadaveric skulls. They described the deformation patterns that occurred with impact. A comparison of polyethylene and tantalum for cranioplasty in 24 patients from the Korean War was reported by Lockhart et al. (30), from Valley Forge Army Hospital. This was not a controlled study, and no real difference was found except that several patients with the tantalum plates complained about the effect of the hot sun.

Evans (19), from the University of Cincinnati, presented experimental and clinical studies on increasing intracranial pressure. He worked on the development of a method to record continuous intracranial pressure in the monkey. During this study he found that the rate of cerebral blood flow was the most important variable in determining intracranial pressure.

HYDROCEPHALUS AND CEREBROSPINAL FLUID PHYSIOLOGY

In the early 1950s, experimental studies were being performed to learn about normal cerebrospinal physiology and the changes that occurred in hydrocephalus. Adams (1), from the University of California at San Francisco, reported tracer studies with radioactive phosphorous (P32) on the absorption of cerebrospinal fluid under normal conditions and then in hydrocephalus, initially in dogs and later in patients. Bering (7), from the Children's Medical Center in Boston, studied water exchange of central nervous system and cerebrospinal fluid in both animals and humans in normal and hydrocephalic brains using deuterium oxide (heavy water) as a tracer. He found that water was exchanged freely at all surfaces by free diffusion, and several conclusions were drawn from his study.

EPILEPSY

Penfield's (36) careful clinical investigations had established cortical excision as a method of treating medically refractory focal epilepsy. Studies related to epilepsy were also being conducted at other institutions. Pacella et al. (34), from New York University, presented the results of precentral motor cortical ablation in experimental epilepsy in the monkey. Electroencephalographic results in psychomotor epilepsy were investigated by Green, Duisberg, and McGrath (24), from The Barrow Neurological Institute.

FUNCTIONAL NEUROSURGERY

In 1949, Egas Moniz received the Nobel Prize for his initiation of psychosurgery. According to Wilkins (56), Moniz's development of prefrontal leukotomy as an operation to modify abnormal behaviors began in 1935, when he heard a presentation by John Fulton and others about frontal lobe function at a meeting where he was presenting his experience on angiography.

Others reported experimental investigations in the early 1950s. Bailey, Small, and Ingraham (5), of the Children's Medical Center in Boston, studied the use of a procaine block of frontal lobe white fibers as a means of predicting the effect of prefrontal lobotomy in cats and monkeys. They found that on histological examination there were only slight tissue changes that were no different from those seen after saline injection. Van Waganan and Liu (52), from the Strong Memorial Hospital in Rochester, New York, reported the results of this technique in 26 patients. They concluded that this procedure predicted the effect of prefrontal lobotomy on the behaviors of psychotic patients in two-thirds of the patients, and was most reliable when the patient was in a period of overactivity. This test was also very useful in predicting relief from unusual complaints of pain.

STEREOTACTIC SURGERY

In 1947, Spiegel et al. (29,45), from Temple University, were the first to use ventriculography for localization to make a stereotactic lesion. They were attempting to find an alternative to frontal lobotomy. In 1951 they reported improvements in their equipment (46). Stereotactic procedures were continuing to be developed throughout the world in the early 1950s (29).

MOVEMENT DISORDERS

Several neurosurgeons were investigating ways to treat various movement disorders. Surgical procedures had been tried, but none were very effective. Meyers et al. (32,33), at the University of Iowa, were describing experiments to make lesions to treat patients with hemiballismus and other movement disorders.

In 1952, Irving Cooper performed a craniotomy to divide the left cerebral peduncle in a patient incapacitated by tremor and rigidity. He accidentally tore the left anterior choroidal artery and it was occluded. The pedunculotomy was not performed and the patient had an excellent result (56). Subsequent results of anterior choroidal artery occlusion were variable, but this led Cooper to investigate what a lesion would do in an area supplied by the anterior choroidal artery—the globus pallidus.

SPINE

The number of investigations related to the spinal cord and peripheral nerves were few. Johnson, Roth, and Craig (28), from the Mayo Clinic, studied autonomic pathways in the spinal cord after anterolateral cordotomy. They evaluated vasomotor and sweating functions. White (55), from Massachusetts General Hospital, studied the conduction of visceral pain.

Davis, Martin, and Goldstein (17), from Northwestern, described the sensory changes with herniated nucleus pulposus in 500 patients. They concluded that there was no correlation between the sensory patterns and the level of the disc protrusion.

OTHER INVESTIGATIONS

The results of animal investigations into the characteristic changes produced in the brain by coagulator current as demonstrated by the fluorescein technique were reported by Caudill et al. (13), from the University of Minnesota. Boldrey, Giansiracusa, and Beltran (10), from the University of California at San Francisco, studied the effects of cortisone and adrenocorticotropic hormone on scarring in the brain and peripheral nerves. Cooper et al. (16) reported the "Catabolic Effect of Craniotomy and Its Investigative Treatment with Testosterone Propronite." They studied patients undergoing craniotomy for brain tumor and found that the catabolic reaction was less marked in those patients who received testosterone.

Scheuerman, Pacheco, and Groff (42), from the University of Pennsylvania, reported an experimental study on the use of Gelfoam as a dural substitute in dogs and patients, and concluded that this was a satisfactory substitute. Bailey et al. (4), from the Children's Medical Center in Boston, studied tissue reactions to powdered tantalum in the central nervous system in cats and monkeys. Their findings showed that "the reactions to tantalum powder within the cerebral tissues were considerable in microsurgery preparations, but they would not be of great clinical significance" (4, p. 92).

CONCLUSION

As we look back to the early 1950s, we see the foundation being laid for the great advances in neuroscience that were to come during the next half century. Neurosurgeons were becoming increasingly involved in research, and more training programs were offering opportunities to gain research experience. It must also be emphasized that a large number of individuals in many disciplines were turning their attention to the neurosciences, and they would have a great impact on advancing our specialty.

REFERENCES

1. Adams JE. Tracer studies with radioactive phosphorus (P32) on the absorption of cerebrospinal fluid and the problem of hydrocephalus. *J Neurosurg* 8:279–288, 1951.
2. Aird RB, Strait LS, Zealear D, et al. Neurophysiological studies on cerebral concussion. *J Neurosurg* 9:331–347, 1952.
3. Ashkenazy M, Davis L, Martin J. An evaluation of the technique and results of the radioactive di-iodo-fluoroscein test for the localization of intracranial lesions. *J Neurosurg* 8:300–314, 1951.
4. Bailey OT, Ingraham FD, Weadon PS, et al. Tissue reactions to powdered tantalum in the central nervous system. *J Neurosurg* 9:83–92, 1952.
5. Bailey OT, Small WT, Ingraham FD. Procarie block of frontal lobe white fibers as a means of predicting the effect of prefrontal lobectomy. 1. Experimental studies. *J Neurosurg* 9:21–29, 1952.
6. Bakay L. Studies on blood–brain barrier with radioactive phosphorus. *AMA Arch Neurol Psychiatry* 66:419–426, 1951.
7. Bering EA Jr. Water exchange of central nervous system and cerebrospinal fluid. *J Neurosurg* 9:275–287, 1952.
8. Bloor BM, Wrenn FR Jr, Hayes GJ. An experimental method for evaluation of contrast media used in cerebral angiography. *J Neurosurg* 8:425–440, 1952.
9. Bloor BM, Wrenn FR Jr, Margolis G. An experimental evaluation of certain contrast media used for cerebral angiography. Electroencephalographic and histopathological correlations. *J Neurosurg* 8:585–594, 1951.
10. Boldrey EB, Giansiracusa JE, Beltran P. Effect of cortisone and ACTH on scanning in brain and in peripheral nerves: Preliminary report. *Surg Forum*:386–388, 1952.
11. Bucy PC. Editorial: To Egas Moniz. *J Neurosurg* 8:1–2, 1951.
12. Bucy PC. Our training programs and the future of neurological surgery. *J Neurosurg* 9:538–543, 1952.
13. Caudill CM, Smith GA, French LA, et al. Experimental studies of the effect of coagulating currents upon the brain when applied to the intact dura and directly on the cortex. *J Neurosurg* 8:423–434, 1951.
14. Chou SN, Aust JB, Peyton WT, et al. Radioactive isotopes in localization of intracranial lesions; survey of various types of isotopes and "tagged compounds" useful in diagnosis and localization of intracranial lesions with special reference to use of radioactive iodine-tagged human serum albumin. *AMA Arch Surg* 63:554–560, 1951.
15. Chou SN, Moore GE, Marvin JF. Localization of brain tumors with radioiodine 131. *Science* 115:119–120, 1952.
16. Cooper IS, Rynearson EH, MacCarty CS, et al. The catabolic effect of craniotomy and its investigative treatment with testosterone propionate. *J Neurosurg* 8:295–299, 1951.
17. Davis L, Martin J, Goldstein SL. Sensory changes with herniated nucleus pulposus. *J Neurosurg* 9:133–138, 1952.
18. Dawson RE, Webster JE, Gurdjian ES. Serial electroencephalography in acute head injuries. *J Neurosurg* 8:613–630, 1951.
19. Evans JP. Experimental and clinical observations on rising intracranial pressure. *AMA Arch Surg* 63:107–114, 1951.
20. Foltz EL, Thomas LB, Ward AA Jr. The effect of intracarotid Diodrast. *J Neurosurg* 9:68–82, 1952.
21. French JD, West PM, Von Amerongen FK, et al. Effects

of intracarotid administration of nitrogen mustard on normal brain and brain tumors. *J Neurosurg* 9:378–389, 1952.

22. French LA, Wild JJ, Neal D. The experimental application of ultrasonics to the localization of brain tumors. *J Neurosurg* 8:198–203, 1951.

23. Glumann M, Ransohoff J, Pool JL, et al. Electrical excitability of the human motor cortex. *J Neurosurg* 9:461–471, 1952.

24. Green JR, Duisberg REH, McGrath WB. Electrocorticography in psychomotor epilepsy. *Electroencephalogr Clin Neurophysiol* 3:292–299, 1951.

25. Gurdjian ES, Webster JE, Lissner HR. The mechanism of skull fracture. *J Neurosurg* 7:106–114, 1950.

26. Horrax G, Wu WQ. Postoperative survival of patients with intracranial oligodendroglioma with special reference to radical tumor removal. A study of 26 patients. *J Neurosurg* 8:473–479, 1951.

27. Jasper H, Penfield W. Electrocorticograms in man: Effect of voluntary movement upon electrical activity of precentral gyrus. *Arch Psychiatry* 183:163–174, 1949.

28. Johnson DA, Roth GM, Craig WM. Autonomic pathways in the spinal cord. *J Neurosurg* 9:599–605, 1952.

29. Kelly PJ. Stereotactic surgery: What is past is prologue. *Neurosurgery* 46:16–27, 2000.

30. Lockhart WS Jr, Van Den Noort G, Kimsey WH, Groff RA. A comparison of polyethylene and tantalum for cranioplasty. *J Neurosurg* 9:254–257, 1952.

31. Margolis G, Odom GL, Woodhall B, et al. The role of small angiomatous malformations in the production of intracerebral hematoma. *J Neurosurg* 8:564–575, 1951.

32. Meyers R. Surgical experiments in therapy of certain "extrapyramidal" disease: Current evaluation. *Acta Psychiatiet Neurol* (Suppl 67):5–42, 1951.

33. Meyers R, Sweeney DB, Schwiddle JT. Hemiballismus: Etiology and surgical treatment. *J Neurol Neurosurg Psychiatry* 13:115–126, 1950.

34. Pacella BL, Kennard MA, Lopeloff LM, et al. Precentral motor cortical ablation in experimental epilepsy in the monkey. *J Neurosurg* 7:390–397, 1950.

35. Penfield W. Symposium on brain and mind; memory mechanisms. *AMA Arch Neurol Psychiatry* 67:178–191, 1952.

36. Penfield W, Rasmusson T. The cerebral cortex of man. A clinical study of localization of function. New York, The Macmillan Co, 1950.

37. Penfield W, Welch K. Supplementary area of cerebral cortex: Clinical and experimental study. *AMA Arch Neurol Psychiatry* 66:289–317, 1951.

38. Peyton WT, Moore GE, French LA, et al. Localization of intracranial lesions by radioactive isotopes. *J Neurosurg* 9:443–442, 1952.

39. Pool JL, Ransohoff J. Autonomic effects on stimulating rostral portion of cingulate gyri in man. *J Neurophysiol* 12:385–392, 1949.

40. Rasmussen T. Wilder Penfield 1891–1976, in Bucy PC (ed): *Neurosurgical Giants: Feet of Clay and Iron.* New York, Elsevier, 1985, pp 139–141.

41. Ryder HW, Espey FF, Kristoff FV, et al. Observations on the interrelationships of intracranial pressure and cerebral blood flow. *J Neurosurg* 8:46–58, 1951.

42. Scheuerman WG, Pacheco F, Groff RA. The use of Gelfoam films as a dural substitute. Preliminary report. *J Neurosurg* 8:608–612, 1951.

43. Shenkin HA, Cabieses F, VanDen Nort G, et al. The hemodynamic effect of unilateral carotid ligation on the cerebral circulation of man. *J Neurosurg* 8:38–45, 1951.

44. Smith GS, Caudill CM, Moore GE, et al. Experimental evaluation of cerebral angiography. *J Neurosurg* 8:556–563, 1951.

45. Spiegel EA, Wyeis HT, Marks M, et al. Stereotaxic apparatus for operations on the human brain. *Science* 106:349–359, 1947.

46. Spiegel EA, Wycis HT, Thur C. The stereoencephalotome: Model III of our stereotaxic apparatus for operations on the human brain. *J Neurosurg* 8:452–453, 1951.

47. Sugar O. Pathological anatomy and angiography of intracranial vascular anomalies. *J Neurosurg* 8:3–22, 1951.

48. Sweet WH. Uses of nuclear disintegration in diagnosis and treatment of brain tumor. *N Engl J Med* 245:875–878, 1951.

49. Sweet WA, Javid M. The possible use of neutron-capturing isotopes such as boron 10 in the treatment of neoplasms. *J Neurosurg* 9:200–209, 1952.

50. Sweet WH, Bennett HS. Changes in internal carotid pressure during carotid and jugular occlusion and their clinical significance. *J Neurosurg* 5:178–195, 1948.

51. Sweet WH, Sarnoff SJ, Bakay L. Clinical method for recording internal carotid pressure; significance of changes during carotid occlusion. *Surg Gynecol Obstet* 90:327–334, 1950.

52. Van Wagenen WP, Liu CT. Procaine block of frontal lobe white fibers as a means of predicting the effect of prefrontal lobotomy II. Clinical evaluation. *J Neurosurg* 9:30–51, 1952.

53. Ward AA Jr. Atropine in the treatment of closed head injury. *J Neurosurg* 7:398–402, 1950.

54. Ward AA Jr. Somatic functions of nervous system. *Ann Rev Physiol* 12:421–444, 1950.

55. White JC. Conduction of visceral pain (Osler Society lecture). *N Engl J Med* 246:686–691, 1952.

56. Wilkins RH. History of neurosurgery, in Wilkins RH, Rengachary SS (eds): *Neurosurgery.* New York, McGraw–Hill, 1996, pp 25–36.

3

The Status of Neurosurgery in 1951: Clinical Practice

Charles B. Wilson, MD, DSc, MSHA, and Harold Rosegay, PhD, MD

GENERAL CONSIDERATIONS

In 1951, a patient suspected of having an intracranial mass lesion would undergo assessment for localization of the mass and for increased intracranial pressure. The assessment would have included evaluation of the medical history and vital signs; physical, neurological, and funduscopic examinations; radiographic films of the skull or spine and chest; perimetry; and consultation with other services if necessary. No house officer would dare to call his chief about an admission until he had accomplished this workup expeditiously, had given it some thought, and was prepared to discuss the next step—radiographic studies performed with a contrast agent.

In 1951, all contrast studies were performed by neurosurgeons, and they accounted for ap-proximately 50% of the neurosurgeon's work and income. In 1953, the radiologist Sven Seldinger (58) introduced the transfemoral catheter technique for cerebral angiography. This technique gradually replaced percutaneous carotid puncture, and angiography became a neuroradiological procedure. The replacement of pneumoencephalography, ventriculography, and pantopaque myelography with computed tomography (CT) began in 1972. The transition to modern radiographic diagnostic methods was complete in 1980, when magnetic resonance imaging (MRI) was introduced.

Pneumoencephalography and Ventriculography

Pneumoencephalography and ventriculography were the principal procedures used to confirm or rule out mass lesions in 1951, although angiography was being introduced in large medical centers. Relying mainly on the displacement of vessels to disclose a mass, angiography was less informative than ventriculography initially, but the situation changed dramatically during the next decade as automatic seriography and subtraction techniques, introduced by Ziedes des Plantes (68), and catheter angiography, introduced by Seldinger (58) in 1953, came into general use.

Pneumoencephalography was used mainly to study the epilepsies and post-traumatic syndromes, in which there was little clinical suspicion of a mass lesion. It was almost never used if increased intracranial pressure was documented. The patient, sedated and monitored for vital signs, was seated in an open-back chair. A lumbar puncture was performed, and as the spinal fluid dripped into a basin it was replaced, volume for volume, by room air that had been drawn into a 10-cc syringe through a gauze filter. The process was repeated until the return of spinal fluid ceased. The needle was withdrawn and the chair was wheeled into position in front of the Bucky diaphragm. The patient often experienced headaches, vomiting, and sweating, which could only be lessened by taking care to inject the air slowly. Several years were to elapse before fractional pneumoencephalography, introduced by Graeme Robertson (49) in 1946, provided a technique that caused less morbidity.

The roentgenographic criteria for a normal pneumoencephalographic study were ventricles of normal and equal size, not displaced from the midline, and without focal deformity, and equal distribution of air over both hemispheres in sulcal markings of normal size.

Ventriculography was the procedure used most often to locate a mass lesion. It was the best technique for elucidating the clinical problem of choked discs with no localizing signs. The procedure was performed in the operating room with the patient sitting or semirecumbent and under local anesthesia. Occipital burr holes were made 7 cm above the inion and 3 cm to each side, and the dura was opened. From this position a ventricular cannula was used, puncturing the ependyma at approximately the junction of the tri-

gone and occipital horn. The cannulas were stabilized by packing cotton pledgets or bone wax around them in the burr holes. Indigo carmine (1 ml) was injected on one side, and as both ventricles drained, the fluid from each side was collected separately and measured. Knowing that a normal ventricle holds approximately 20 ml, the surgeon could, at this point, draw certain conclusions: First, if the volumes were clearly unequal in a patient who had papilledema, the mass was on the side of the smaller ventricle. Second, if the volumes were equal but more than 30 ml each, hydrocephalus was present. Third, if indigo carmine crossed to the opposite ventricle, the obstruction was not at the interventricular foramina, but rather was in the third ventricle, aqueduct, or fourth ventricle. Walter Dandy (10) called the steps taken thus far ventricular estimation. He used this observation confidently to shorten the time needed for ventriculography, especially if herniation was impending. For example, the finding of hydrocephalus by ventricular estimation alone in a patient who had papilledema and cerebellar signs not resulting from acoustic neuroma was sufficient reason for him to perform a suboccipital craniectomy directly without additional study involving injection of air into the ventricles. This practice was generally accepted in 1951, but because it was a refinement of limited application, most patients underwent the full procedure, including air injection. After the burr holes were closed in the operating room, the patient was taken to the radiology department, where close monitoring was continued and a ventricular tap tray was available to release injected air if the patient's neurological status declined because of a rise in intracranial pressure as a reaction to the presence of air. In the meantime, the operating room was prepared for the patient's return.

Cerebral Angiography

By 1951, angiography was an established procedure in the diagnosis of cerebrovascular lesions and was beginning to play a role in identifying supratentorial tumors. For example, the displacement of the anterior and middle cerebral arteries around olfactory groove and sphenoid wing meningiomas respectively were recognizable features, as was the increased and irregular vascularity of glioblastomas. These characteristics had been elusive in the days of single-exposure angiography, but by 1951 better definition of the tumor blush could be achieved with the use of hand-pull cassette changers, which permitted a series of three exposures to be made after a single injection of contrast agent. The first exposure, which showed the arterial phase, was made at the precise end of the percutaneous injection of 8 ml of 35% Diodrast. The exposure showing the capillary phase was made 1 second later, and the venous phase was recorded at 3 seconds. Automatic motor-driven cassette changers, which had been available for more than 10 years but generally had not been adopted, were being replaced in 1950 by cinefluorography—a procedure that provided continuous arteriographic records. Angiography also had the advantage of not altering intracranial dynamics. In summary, the introduction of rapid seriography, the Seldinger catheter technique for selective angiography, and subtraction techniques fundamentally changed the way tumors were localized, and led to the assimilation of angiography into the practice of neuroradiology.

RADIOACTIVE ISOTOPE SCREENING

It had been known for some time that fluorescein was taken up preferentially by neoplastic, infarcted, and inflammatory tissue, and was detectable under ultraviolet light during craniotomy. By 1951, fluorescein was being used in the radioactive form (131I-diodofluorescein) for the diagnosis and localization of brain tumors. The less costly isotope tracer, iodinated human serum albumin, was introduced at approximately the same time. Its activity was recorded from 24 positions on the cranium by a scintillation counter. Isotope scanning of the brain was a useful addition in the screening of suspected brain tumors, but it never attained more than ancillary status. When isotope screening showed positive results, confirmation was required by other tests before surgery was recommended.

Anesthesia

The year 1951 was the middle of a broad period of transition in neurosurgical anesthesia.

Local anesthesia had been popular until the mid 1940s, when endotracheal intubation (with tubocurarine used for smooth induction) became an accepted procedure, permitting the safer use of general anesthesia. Senior surgeons were uneasy with the new science of anesthesiology, with its complex pharmacology and its use of respiratory control. For decades they had been accustomed to using local anesthesia with the knowledge that their favorite nurse anesthetist was monitoring the patient, keeping the airway clear for spontaneous respiration, and administering 5 mg of morphine and open drop ether as necessary. However, 1951 was the year that hypercapnia was proved experimentally to increase intracranial pressure. From that point, intubation, controlled respiration, and the use of gas ether or intravenous sodium Pentothal became standard practice, with local anesthesia as an adjuvant rather than the primary anesthetic technique.

Positioning the Patient

Devices for head fixation were not in general use in 1951, and improvised combinations of straps and adhesive tape were used to stabilize the head. Three positions were in use for operations on the posterior fossa: the prone, the upright, and the recumbent lateral (now called the park bench) positions. Cerebellar tumors in children were always operated with the patient placed prone in a padded horseshoe frame. For operations on adults, the upright position was popular, with the patient's face cushioned in a holder attached to the table in front of the patient. The upright position was always used for a subtemporal trigeminal root section. Section of cranial nerve (CN) IX, cervical rhizotomy, and acoustic neuroma surgery were usually performed with the patient upright, but some neurosurgeons preferred to use the lateral position because of the added exposure provided by gravity.

The Operating Room

Neurosurgeons scrubbed their hands with bar soap, timed by a 10-minute hourglass. The forearms were then immersed in cylinders of alcohol, followed by immersion in 0.5% bichloride of mercury, which turned the fingernails brown. After being dried, the hands were dusted with a packet of talc and were gloved. The patient's newly shaved scalp was then prepared with many gauze wipes of ether followed by alcohol, and the area for incision was marked and injected with procaine.

The materials and instruments on the table reflected the era. Cottonoid pledgets had been prepared the previous day by sewing suture tails on 1-inch squares cut from a sheet. Black silk sutures and cotton sutures were still cut from spools and were pulled through bone wax to make knot-tying easier. Likewise, the silver clips used for hemostasis were still cut and crimped with a special instrument from 23-gauge flattened silver wire wound on a spool.

Other aids to hemostasis were cotton pledgets, bits of crushed temporal muscle held in readiness for use as stamps, Gelfoam (which had been introduced in 1944) (24), and bone wax. Bleeding from the incised surface of the scalp was stopped by finger pressure, flat Michel clips, Adson–Fincher spring clips, and Kolodny clamps. The tips of the Kolodny clamps were bent downward to grasp and tent the galea over the skin without perforating the galea, as did straight hemostats. Coagulation with the electrosurgical unit was effective when used correctly: The coagulating forceps had to pinpoint the bleeding source, because applying the current indiscriminately to clumps of tissue led to charring without hemostasis. The Bovie loop used with the cutting current was quite effective in resecting solid tumors, such as meningiomas. Bipolar coagulation was not available in 1951. Although Greenwood had been experimenting with bipolar coagulation since 1940, it was not until 1954 that he reported its essential role in the total removal of intramedullary spinal cord tumors (20).

Osteoplastic craniotomy was performed with hand-operated instruments—burrs, the Gigli saw and guide, and the Stille double-action rongeur. The use of motor-driven tools was a departure from standard practice, although a combined perforator and burr that worked equally well as a manual or a power tool was exhibited before the Society of Neurological Surgeons in 1949 (59)—a harbinger of things to come. An electrically driven spiral osteotome used to connect burr holes by cutting down onto a Gigli guide was unsafe but was still in use.

A set of Hudson burrs consisted of a perforator, a drill, and an enlarging burr. The principle underlying the operation of the burr, as stated by Hudson (15), is that as long as there is resistance in the bottom of the opening, the burr will cut. When resistance ceases, it will move no farther. Hudson (15) also introduced the cerebellar extension and a biting connecting forceps that cut a 2.4-mm channel between burr holes.

Getting adequate light to a deep exposure within or beneath the brain was the same problem in 1951 that it had been in 1907, when Herman Schloffer (54) described how he had moved an operating table to a window so that his head mirror could direct reflected daylight into the cavity leading to the patient's sella. Overhead lights, spotlights, and headlights all had limitations. The Frazier lighted retractor was of great help in illuminating the interior of cavities and cysts that contained a mural nodule; but if bleeding occurred, the small bulb became coated and was rendered useless.

Intracranial Pressure and Postoperative Care

Nothing illustrates the differences between the years before 1951 and the years afterward as clearly as a review of the management of increased intracranial pressure. In 1951, continuous monitoring of intracranial pressure was first described by Guillaume and Janny (21), and the strain gauge was used by Eli Goldensohn (19) to establish experimentally that hypercarbia raises intracranial pressure. These advances were the key to an explosion of laboratory and clinical work during the next decade on measuring and controlling intracranial pressure so that impending herniation could be diagnosed and treated early. Only brief reflection on the surgery of uncal herniation introduced in the 1930s—resection of the uncus and division of the tentorium—is needed to appreciate its replacement by medical management with hyperventilation, urea, and mannitol in the decade after 1951. Hyperventilation by controlled respiration became an important intraoperative aid in reducing brain swelling. Reported in 1960, the finding that cortisone was beneficial in experimental cerebral edema (31) led to clinical trials of steroids and their subsequent use in 1961.

In 1951, however, those advancements were still in the future, and the reality was stark. A patient was nursed in a ward bed close to the nurses' station. The hyperosmolar agent in use was a 50-ml ampule of 50% dextrose administered intravenously. Ventricular tapping was the principal measure for reducing intracranial pressure, but it was not as effective for supratentorial tumors as it was for infratentorial tumors. Diagnosing a postoperative clot was difficult, and such a case could be settled only by exploration. Decisions also had to be made about the need for transfusion and for intubation or tracheotomy. The patient's head dressing had to be changed after a few hours because it was typically wet with bloody fluid from the extradural drain. Nurses' duties included continuous observation and reporting of vital signs, keeping the airway clear, controlling fever with alcohol-soaked sheets or ice-water enemas, and administering oxygen by nasal catheter, nourishment by stomach tube, and penicillin. Caring for the patient was arduous, but it was the best care that could be provided at the time.

NEOPLASMS

Intrinsic Tumors

The principal problem presented by intrinsic tumors was diagnostic—identifying small tumors that did not deform the ventricles and subarachnoid spaces or the cerebral vessels, and defining precisely the anatomic location and relationships of large gliomas. In rare cases, intratumoral calcification indicated tumor location, but too often the approach to an intrinsic tumor was based on localization derived from "soft" information provided by the displacement and deformity of normal structures and, less often, by neovascularity. Angiography was a superb technique for delineating and predicting the pathology of glioblastomas and hemangio-

blastomas; but for other intrinsic tumors, the information it provided on vessel displacement and a faint, nonspecific tumor blush were too often less useful. Radionuclide brain scans were beginning to evolve into a valuable tool for the diagnosis and localization of many intrinsic cerebral and cerebellar tumors, but the technology was crude by modern standards and was restricted to major academic medical institutions. The localization of intrinsic tumors was grounded in the neurological examination and details of the patient's history (for example, an observer's description of the onset of a seizure) in localizing intrinsic tumors continued until CT and later MRI provided images that permitted greater precision.

The surgical removal of intrinsic tumors involved finding the tumor during surgery and achieving hemostasis—a very real problem before the introduction of bipolar coagulation and synthetic hemostatic material. Much of the time required to remove a glioblastoma involved sealing opened vessels with silver clips and electrocautery delivered through a forceps or sucker-tip. When all else failed, the surgeon sometimes resorted to the use of muscle stamps or fluffed cotton, which were left in the tumor bed. Removal of intrinsic tumors in the posterior fossa ranged from relatively simple, in the case of cystic cerebellar astrocytomas, to exceedingly difficult, in the case of vermian medulloblastomas, fourth ventricular ependymomas, or large cerebellar hemangioblastomas.

Although technology for precise localization of the tumor and hemostasis were crude by present standards, the greatest concern of neurosurgeons 50 years ago was the management of brain swelling. In less than a decade, urea and Decadron would be introduced, but for the surgeon dealing with cerebral gliomas in 1951, the principal means of handling postoperative edema were mechanical rather than chemical. There were several surgical tricks of the trade, depending on the circumstances: 1) polar lobectomies, principally of the frontal or temporal poles contiguous with the tumor; 2) leaving the dura open and hinging the bone flap so that it could "ride out" as the brain swelled beneath it; 3) removing most of the squamous portion of the temporal bone with open dura so that the brain could swell beneath the temporalis muscle (i.e., the temporal decompression advocated by Cushing (6)); and 4) leaving the dura open and removing the bone flap altogether for possible replacement later.

Few neurosurgeons practicing today have had to treat a cerebral fungus, the consequence of sustained intracranial hypertension, a large defect in the dura and adjacent skull, and no muscle buffer between the brain and the scalp, which, because of its inelasticity, will stretch to the point of becoming ischemic, necrotic, and ultimately eroded to expose angry, fungating brain. The inherent elasticity of the closed muscle layers in subtemporal and suboccipital craniectomies prevents the scalp from breaking down. Imagine the near miracle made possible by urea and corticosteroids in managing intrinsic tumors during the course of an operation and afterward.

Meningiomas

In the 1950s, as now, meningiomas were surrounded by the aura given to them by Harvey Cushing and Louise Eisenhardt, and later by Sir Geoffrey Jefferson, Leo Davidoff, and other neurosurgical legends. In 1951, much attention was given to classic syndromes related to meningiomas at favorite sites, such as the outer sphenoid wing with orbital involvement, the olfactory groove, the tuberculum sellae, the cerebellopontine angle, and the middle-third parasagittal skull. Skull radiographs were scrutinized carefully for enlarged vascular grooves, erosion, hyperostosis, pneumosinus dilatans, erosion of the dorsum sellae, and intratumoral calcification, although calcification was more likely to be seen in the classic thoracic meningioma in women. In 1951, a higher proportion of meningiomas seemed to have visible and palpable calvarial hyperostosis, possibly reflecting late diagnosis in many patients. Angiography was extremely helpful in identifying a tumor as a meningioma. Embolization of external carotid arteries came much later. At the time, enlarged arteries supplying a meningioma were occluded extracranially by ligating the external carotid artery or securing the middle meningeal artery intracranially early in the operation.

The surgical principles were simple and inviolable: Get to the dural base and interrupt the blood supply as early as possible in the operation, then remove the tumor by gently separating it from the adjacent brain, preserving the pia arachnoid and all cerebral veins if possible. Postoperative brain edema was a major problem in patients with large meningiomas or meningiomas at the skull base requiring deep and prolonged retraction. The potential for the adjacent brain to swell and to remain swollen, often for weeks afterward, is still a problem today. It is not difficult to imagine the problems it presented in the years before surgeons could use urea and corticosteroids. In some patients, large meningiomas were removed in stages, leaving out the bone flap after the first procedure until swelling resolved completely. The benign histology and innocent gross appearance of meningiomas seemed inconsistent with the morbidity and mortality resulting from surgery to remove them—an inconsistency still observed, but resolving rapidly, a decade later.

Acoustic Neuromas and Meningiomas of the Cerebellopontine Angle

Preoperatively, these two common tumors of the cerebellopontine angle were identified correctly in most patients on the basis of four observations: erosion of the internal auditory meatus, deafness, statistical probability favoring the diagnosis of an acoustic tumor, and, in contrast, the prediction of a meningioma associated with hyperostosis of the petrous bone with preserved hearing.

The surgical approach to the angle in 1951 was through a ''hockey stick'' or straight lateral incision and a suboccipital craniectomy. It was only later that electrical drills were applied to the distal exposure of CN VII. Overall, except for frequent injury to the facial nerve, the morbidity of the operation was low. Preservation of the facial nerve was possible in the hands of skilled and experienced surgeons, but the salvage rate was low and most patients had permanent facial palsy and often were told before the operation that a hypoglossal–facial anastomosis would be done electively after their recovery from the primary operation. When offered the option, many patients chose subtotal intracapsular removal of acoustic tumors because of the much greater likelihood of saving CN VII.

Meningiomas in the angle presented the same problems that they present today: a vascular tumor with a broad base, situated in a confined space that is traversed by major blood vessels and cranial nerves, and almost certainly intimately related to the brainstem, principally the pons. Petroclival meningiomas shared these anatomic and pathological features with an even greater risk of brainstem injury. Meningiomas in the angle were rarely if ever cured by the operation, and regrowth was a matter of time.

A neurosurgeon ''exploring'' the angle—a fairly common operation—was delighted to find an epidermoid, for which an incomplete and bloodless removal would be much easier and more satisfying. Managing the chemical meningeal reaction was not simple, and some patients developed chronic hydrocephalus as a consequence of inflammatory arachnoiditis, a serious problem until the introduction of satisfactory shunts and the use of corticosteroids several years later.

Pituitary Adenomas

One of us (H. R.) has described why and when Harvey Cushing abandoned the transsphenoidal removal of pituitary adenomas to return to earlier intracranial approaches (50). The reason had little to do with outcomes but was a matter of his growing interest in intracranial approaches to the sella and parasellar region. Dott, in Europe, and Hirsch, an otorhinolaryngological surgeon in Vienna and later in Boston, were masters of transnasal removal of these adenomas, but their influence in setting the standard for pituitary surgery paled in relation to Cushing's. Consequently, in 1951, the accepted operation for pituitary adenomas was intracranial, either subfrontal or pterional. The pterional approach had the disadvantage of exposing the tumor from its lateral aspect, and the subfrontal approach required deeper retraction with a greater risk for postoperative brain edema. The transcranial operation achieved excellent results with accept-

able morbidity and mortality rates when performed by an experienced surgeon.

In 1951 we saw the first use of therapeutic hypophysectomy for breast and prostate cancer, two endocrine-responsive cancers. For more than two decades, hypophysectomy was used as second- or third-line palliation of patients with advanced breast or prostate cancer. Ray (48) was the unquestioned leader of this approach, and at the time, an untold number of patients who had exhausted other endocrine-based and drug-directed therapies obtained excellent and prolonged palliation after hypophysectomy. The procedure became obsolete with the later introduction of more effective medical therapies.

CEREBROVASCULAR DISEASE

Aneurysms

The recognition of aneurysms, at least those of the carotid circulation, was not difficult after the widespread adoption of carotid angiography with direct needle puncture. Vertebral angiography was more difficult technically and was used less often, in part because of the difficulties of dealing with aneurysms in the posterior circulation. In 1951, most aneurysms located on the intracranial internal carotid and anterior cerebral arteries were treated by carotid ligation. Proponents of abrupt occlusion of the cervical internal carotid artery argued with proponents of incremental occlusion, and both camps argued with those surgeons who favored occlusion of the common carotid artery because of its usually lower frequency of neurological deficits. Aneurysms of the anterior communicating artery often were treated by proximal intracranial clipping of the dominant anterior cerebral artery. Reinforcement of aneurysms with muscle and muslin was favored by some surgeons.

Few aneurysms were treated by direct clipping. Exposure of an aneurysm of the anterior circulation was less difficult than applying the clips available at the time. Spring clips were unknown in 1951. The clip most commonly applied was the flat, V-shaped silver clip, which was held in a straight clip applier or a hemostat. Both this clip and the clips beginning to appear in surgical catalogs tended to jam in the longitudinal groove of the applying forceps. An instrument for applying clips introduced in 1953 (13) corrected this problem by replacing the longitudinal groove with coarse, transverse striations. Olivecrona designed an excellent straight clip applier, but the clips, once applied, could not be readjusted. He then designed a removable clip (37)—a V-shaped flat clip with "wings" at the base. An applied clip that was not well positioned could be removed by grasping the two wings in a hemostat and gently squeezing the tips of the wings. The base of the clip at the V acted as a fulcrum. Reapplying a misapplied clip was not a maneuver for the faint of heart, but the winged clip was a major advance. The giant step in improving clip technology occurred in 1952, however, with the introduction of the Mayfield spring clip, designed by Frank Mayfield (35). The closing force of this clip resided in its cross-leg design. It was the first of a long succession of spring clips.

The British neurosurgeons were fond of ligating rather than clipping intracranial aneurysms and had introduced ligature carriers that failed to gain popularity in this country. Dandy (9) and Poppen (44) were leaders in this field, but the results were poor by current standards. Improved outcomes had to await the availability of urea and corticosteroids, and an understanding of cerebral vasospasm.

Mistaking an aneurysm for a pituitary adenoma or a parasellar tumor led to well-publicized warnings, and it was customary to puncture suspected parasellar and intrasellar masses to exclude the possibility. Few events in the course of an operation compare with the drama of confidently entering an aneurysm mistaken for a tumor.

Arteriovenous Malformations

Dandy (12) and Olivecrona (40) were among the first to take an interest in excising arteriovenous malformations. Carotid angiography was crude. Subtraction techniques and serial cassette changers had yet to be developed, but with patience and multiple injections of contrast medium, early filling and late drainage could be studied with a few intervening phases to indicate the general speed of flow within the fistulas. At this point, the futility of distal ligation (cervical carotid artery) and proximal clipping of one or several major arteries entering the malformation was recognized, but removing an arteriovenous malformation of any size was a daunting prospect for a surgeon armed with silver clips, Bovie coagulation, and muscle stamps or cotton balls to arrest bleeding. All except the boldest and most experienced surgeons recognized that the natural history of a ruptured or an unruptured arteriovenous malformation carried a better prognosis than an attempt to remove it. To state that surgery for the removal of arteriovenous malformation was in its infancy would be accurate.

CRANIAL NERVE DISORDERS

Trigeminal neuralgia, almost 100 years ago, was one of the first disorders treated successfully with neurosurgery. The approach then, and through most of the next 100 years, was the extradural subtemporal operation that became known as the *Frazier procedure* (16), named after Charles Frazier of Philadelphia. The procedure could be performed under general or local anesthesia through a vertical incision in front of the ear, extending from the zygomatic arch to the temporal line, which came to be known as the tic incision. The circular opening in the temporal squama permits an extradural exposure of the foramen spinosum, which was plugged with the tip of a wooden matchstick. An incision was then made through the dura to enter Meckel's cave and to identify the postganglionic roots in their characteristic pattern. We have both seen the operation performed skin to skin in less than 30 minutes. Peet performed the operation under local anesthesia with the patient sitting upright, which puts him in a special class of master surgeons. Dandy (7), the master of posterior fossa surgery, approached the trigeminal root through a laterally placed suboccipital craniectomy.

Glossopharyngeal neuralgia was recognized as distinct from trigeminal neuralgia and was treated by sectioning the CN IX rootlets. Later, division of the upper two vagal rootlets was added. In certain cases of head and neck cancer associated with pain, section of CNs V and IX, and the C1–C3 posterior roots was advocated. That procedure did not gain favor because of failure to relieve pain in many cases and because of the complicating anesthesia dolorosa caused by total interruption of the sensory rootlets of CN V.

SPINAL DISORDERS

Spinal Cord Tumors

Spinal cord tumors could be localized with contrast medium, and in 1951 the removal of spinal meningiomas and schwannomas was quite successful and one of the brighter aspects of neurosurgical practice. The treatment of intrinsic tumors was less successful. Intramedullary tumors were exposed by dorsal myelotomy with removal of ependymomas and, for astrocytomas, partial removal or simply drainage of a cyst if present. Elsberg (14) proposed a two-stage operation comprising a midline dorsal myelotomy at the first stage and a second exposure later, at which time the tumor would "deliver itself" to the surface, but the procedure was not practiced widely. In general, patients with intramedullary tumors had only temporary relief of symptoms.

Anterolateral cordotomy for pain was performed by exposing the spinal cord and cutting a dentate ligament at the level of the planned cordotomy. After the spinal cord was rotated by grasping the ligament, an incision was made through the anterolateral quadrant to interrupt the spinothalamic fibers. The majority of cordotomies were performed in the upper thoracic cord. Later, Schwartz (56) introduced direct anterolateral cordotomy in the upper cervical cord at C1–C2. The success of this approach was the impetus for the later introduction of radiofrequency high cervical cordotomy.

Cervical Disc Disease

The spectrum of cervical disc disease was clearly defined in the early 1950s by Scoville (57) as follows: central soft disc, often presenting with paraplegia; central spondylosis–multiple transverse ridges of osteophytes related to discal degeneration causing a chronic presentation with anterior root or long tract signs; the lateral intraforaminal osteophyte causing neck and arm pain; and the soft, lateral ruptured disc, with radiculopathy, removable through a keyhole facetectomy.

Because of poor outcomes, the spondylotic forms of cervical disc disease were approached surgically only after prolonged conservative management. With regard to the central soft disc, Kahn (26) had proposed in 1947 that posterior displacement of the anterior columns stretches the pial attachments of the dentate ligaments and produces a zone of stress involving the pyramidal tracts. Accordingly, bilateral section of the dentate ligaments became part of a surgical procedure that included wide laminectomy and transdural removal of soft disc (55).

In 1952, Brain (4) reported the neurological manifestations of spondylotic radiculopathy and myelopathy, and described the successful procedure practiced by his surgical colleagues that included complete laminectomy and unroofing of the foramina by removing the overlying inner border of the articular facets. Wide laminectomy for multiple levels of spondylosis and the keyhole facetectomy for focal radiculopathy were standard procedures for these conditions. Although anterior approaches to cervical disc disease were introduced during the 1950s by Smith and Robinson (60), and by Cloward (5), in 1951 they were unknown to American neurosurgeons.

Thoracic Disc Disease

Around 1951, the results of surgery for thoracic disc disease were dismal. Locked into performing laminectomy for decompression, surgeons were reporting not only lack of improvement for most patients but also new postoperative deficits that were often profound (32).

Hulme (23), in 1960, operated through a costotransversectomy, removing the adjacent pedicle. The introduction of the transthoracic approach by Perot (43) and Ransohoff in (47) 1969 improved the line of vision across the anterior surface of the dura from side to side and was the final step in the evolution of this operation. Both Perot and Ransohoff recommended that selective spinal angiography be performed to identify the great radicular artery if the operation was to be conducted below T8 on the left side. The operations of Hulme, Perot, and Ransohoff changed the surgical prognosis from grim to excellent.

Lumbar Spondylosis

The operation for herniated lumbar disc was an established procedure in 1951, but the literature of the period also indicated that another cause of sciatica, namely spondylosis or hard disc, had to be considered. In 1950, Hadley (22) wrote that any operation to relieve the compression of nerve roots must include inspection of the intervertebral foramen for encroachment caused by hypertrophic changes that, if found, would be an indication for facetectomy. Verbiest (65) later expanded this to include the other features of spondylotic encroachment on the cauda equina, which when superimposed on a developmentally small canal caused a characteristic syndrome. He went on to describe all the features of intermittent claudication of the cauda equina, so named by Blau and Logue (3) in 1961. Because the neurological examination was usually normal, Verbiest (64) thought the syndrome was subject to misinterpretation as vascular claudication, and he recommended myelography by cisternal or lateral puncture if lumbar puncture was not successful. If myelography showed narrowing with blockage, decompressive laminectomy was indicated. The many aspects of this syndrome were reviewed later (67).

INFANTILE HYDROCEPHALUS

In 1951, the steps taken after the clinical diagnosis was made included puncturing the anterior fontanel to rule out chronic subdural hematoma, advancing the needle until clear fluid was obtained so that an estimation of the thickness of the cortex could be made, injecting a few cubic centimeters of air for a brow-up lateral film (bubble ventriculogram), and instilling 1 ml of indigo carmine for a Blackfan test. The Blackfan test, although not used universally, differentiated between communicating hydrocephalus (dye appearing within minutes after a lumbar puncture and soon afterward in the urine) and obstructive hydrocephalus (no dye in the spinal fluid and delayed appearance in the urine). The common causes of obstructive hydrocephalus were atresia of the aqueduct or of the basal foramina and tumor. Treatment of the hydrocephalus, if an obstructing tumor could not be removed, was third ventriculostomy as performed by Dandy (8) and Scarff (51) or ventriculocisternostomy as performed by Torkildsen (63).

The only procedure still in use for communicating hydrocephalus before 1951 was coagulation of the choroid plexus performed by Dandy (11) and Putnam (45). About that time, however, several new procedures became available. Matson introduced spinal subarachnoid ureterostomy in 1949 (33) and ventriculoureterostomy in 1951 (34). Nosik (38) described ventriculomastoidostomy in 1950, and Nulsen and Spitz (39) described valve-regulated ventriculovenous shunting (internal jugular vein/superior vena cava) in 1951, stating that their first shunt had been placed in May 1949. Since then, shunting has remained the mainstay of treatment for hydrocephalus. A point that deserves mention is that the glass ventriculoscope used by Putnam (45) to coagulate the choroid plexus was wired for bipolar coagulation.

BRAIN ABSCESS

From the early 1930s to the early 1950s, the management of brain abscess reflected the unsettled question of drainage or excision. The only initial step on which surgeons agreed was tapping done through a burr hole after the lesion was localized. Paths then diverged. For subacute abscess, Vincent (66), in 1936, turned an osteoplastic flap for decompression, and several weeks later resected the thickened abscess capsule. Adson (1) incised the cortex overlying the abscess through a craniectomy, aspirated it, unroofed it, and placed drainage tubes and gauze packing into it. In 1938, Kahn (27) put 5 ml of Thorotrast in the abscess after tapping, enlarged the burr hole to a small craniectomy, coagulated the overlying cortex, and covered the wound with medicated gauze. Radiographs taken during the next 14 days showed migration of the capsule toward the surface, where it could be either excised or packed with Metaphen gauze for drainage. Grant (18) placed a rubber tube into the abscess through the largest of a series of nested silver tubes used as cannulas. The rubber tube was cut flush with the skin and was held with a suture, which was cut after several days. The tube then slowly extruded and was trimmed back as the capsule contracted, ideally leaving behind a collagenous and glial scar. In 1946, LeBeau (29), Vincent's junior colleague, described one-stage radical surgery, which he said was made possible only by penicillin coverage. Regardless of the degree of encapsulation, he removed the abscess complex much in the fashion of removal of an infiltrating tumor.

Around 1951, Kahn (28) settled on repeated aspiration and excision as the most desirable management. The patient was given antibiotics (penicillin and sulfadiazine), and the lesion was localized by ventriculography, angiography, or radionuclide scan. A burr hole was made directly over the abscess, which was tapped, drained, and cultured. Thorotrast (2–5 ml) was instilled, and the wound was closed with a single layer of sutures. Radiographs were then acquired to check the position of the burr hole with regard to the abscess and to follow changes in the size of the capsule. If it increased despite additional tapping, and if the patient's status deteriorated, then open drainage was instituted as described. To control edema, Kahn (28) used 100 ml of 50% dextrose administered twice over 2 to 4 hours. If the capsule became smaller, aided as necessary by repeated tapping under radiographic control, nothing more was done for 2 to 4 weeks. The residual lesion was then excised through a small craniectomy. A series of cases managed similarly was reported by Pennybacker (25) in 1951.

ABLATIVE SURGERY FOR MOVEMENT DISORDERS

The surgical treatment of movement disorders that started in the late 1930s was the subject of the 1942 meeting of the Association for Re-

search in Nervous and Mental Disease. A review of the operations in use in 1951 follows.

Athetosis

Because rhizotomy and peripheral neurectomy were not effective in treating athetosis, area 6 was targeted for excision because of its strong connections with the basal ganglia. Area 6 was identified by stimulation begun anteriorly and carried backward until the arm area was found in the extreme anterior edge of the excitable cortex.

Cordotomy was an alternative operation for athetosis, but it involved greater risk and difficulty. It was used for patients with severe, generalized involvement of the extremities. The incision was made in the anterior surface of the spinal cord between the exiting anterior roots and the median sulcus. Postoperative flaccid paralysis usually improved within a few weeks.

Torticollis

The treatment of torticollis started with section of the spinal accessory nerve in the neck. If this failed, bilateral section of the C1–C3 anterior roots and intradural section of the spinal accessory nerve were performed. In addition, if the arm was athetotic, the anterior column was sectioned. If the torticollis persisted, the C2–C3 posterior primary rami were sectioned extraspinally as they curved backward over the transverse processes.

Paralysis Agitans

Surgery for paralysis agitans was new and not yet standardized. For one extremity with alternating tremor, the following were performed: a subpial cortical excision of areas 6 and 4 in the depth of the central sulcus; section of the pyramidal tract at C2 (46) between the posterior roots and the pial attachment of the dentate ligaments, to a depth of 4 mm; or partial removal of the contralateral head of the caudate nucleus, as reported in 1942 by Meyers (36).

Ojemann (41) pointed out that the risk of the open operations for movement disorders performed in the 1940s and the desire to retain their benefits, however small, led to the development of stereotaxy around 1951. Spiegel and Wycis (62), in 1947, reported a stereotactic apparatus for operating on the human brain. The procedures that followed from this report in the 1950s targeted the globus pallidus and its outflow systems, and the thalamus with ablative lesions (30). The next advance—stereotactic stimulation—was to come in the 1970s.

Prefrontal Lobotomy

This operation, practiced in the mid 1930s to treat agitated depression, was used to relieve pain and suffering in cancer patients in the mid 1940s (17,53). A 3.8-mm trephine opening was made 3.5 cm in front of the coronal suture and 3.5 cm to either side of the midline. A ventricular needle was used to locate the edge of the sphenoid wing. The lobotomy was performed in this coronal plane, which is just anterior to the frontal horn, by coagulating and dividing the cortex, pushing a flat spatula to a depth of 5 to 6 cm, and sweeping it from side to side, more medially than laterally. An alternate method was the use of a thin suction tube to divide the white matter, a brain retractor to expose the plane of the section, and electrocoagulation to follow closely for hemostasis.

The operation either relieved pain or made it more controllable for approximately 60% of patients (52). For those who had poor results, the same operation on the second side provided relief, but the respite was accompanied by apathy and deterioration of personality.

Sympathectomy

In 1951, sympathectomy was a standard procedure in the practice of neurosurgery. The indications for sympathectomy were few but definite, having been culled from dozens of conditions for which it did no good. Essential hypertension responded to thoracolumbar sympathectomy and to supradiaphragmatic splanchnicectomy (61), usually with effective control. Upper thoracic sympathectomy, stellate ganglionectomy, and lumbar sympathectomy were indicated in painful syndromes of the upper and lower extremities such as causalgia, selected cases of reflex sympathetic dystrophy, and Raynaud's disease. Cure of the wracking pain of major causalgia was a triumph of sympathectomy.

In managing pain syndromes in the extremities, it was usual to perform sympathetic blocks to predict the outcome of operation. In some patients, repeated blocks became therapeutic in themselves. In others, especially in those with sympathetic dystrophy, a diminishing response raised a note of caution about operating.

In his presidential address to the Harvey Cushing Society in 1954, Kahn reflected on Peet's (42) experiences with supradiaphragmatic sympathectomy for hypertension, an indication of the place occupied by sympathectomy in neurosurgical practice at the time, and a stark reminder of the practice of medicine before the evolution of powerful pharmaceuticals.

CONCLUSION

"How did you manage?" is a question residents of the current generation sometimes ask neurosurgeons who worked in the days before imaging was introduced. The question reflects mild disbelief about a clinical era that has since been transformed by technological change. In a biographical sketch, written in 1963, of the German master Fedor Krause—who worked at the turn of the century—Behrend remarked, "If we think of the diagnostic and therapeutic results he achieved without the indispensable aids available to us today, we must be filled with admiration" (2, p. 206). This wonderment notwithstanding, we may say that neither Krause nor the neurosurgeons of the 1950s ever felt deprived. All things being relative, they worked with the tools of neurosurgery available to them, and in doing so they contributed to the foundation of our discipline that we enjoy today.

REFERENCES

1. Adson AW, Craig W McK. The surgical management of brain abscess. *Ann Surg* 101:7–26,1935.
2. Behrend CM. Fedor Krause (1857–1937). In Kolle K (ed): Grasse Nervenarzte. Stuttgart: Thieme, 1963, vol 3, p 206.

3. Blau JN, Logue V. Intermittent claudication of the cauda equina. An unusual syndrome resulting from central protrusion of a lumbar intervertebral disc. *Lancet* I: 1081–1086, 1961.

4. Brain R, Northfield D, Wilkinson M. The neurological manifestations of cervical spondylosis. *Brain* 75: 187–225, 1952.

5. Cloward RB. The anterior approach for removal of ruptured cervical discs. *J Neurosurg* 15:602–617, 1958.

6. Cushing H. A method of combining exploration and decompression for cerebral tumors which prove to be inoperable. *Surg Gynecol Obstet* 9:1–5, 1909.

7. Dandy W. An operation for the cure of tic douloureaux. Partial section of the sensory root at the pons. *Arch Surg* 18:687–734, 1929.

8. Dandy W. Diagnosis and treatment of strictures of the aqueduct of Sylvius (causing hydrocephalus). *Arch Surg* 51:1–14, 1945.

9. Dandy W. Intracranial arterial aneurysms. Ithaca NY: Comstock, 1944

10. Dandy W. Surgery of the brain. In: Lewis D (ed). Lewis' Practice of Surgery. Hagerstown: WF Prior, 1944, vol XII, p 117.

11. Dandy W. The operative treatment of communicating hydrocephalus. *Ann Surg* 108:194–202, 1938.

12. Dandy WE, Arteriovenous aneurysm of the brain. *Arch Surg* 17:190–243, 1928.

13. Drew J. An applicating forceps in which clips cannot stick or jam. *J Neurosurg* 10:439–440, 1953.

14. Elsberg CA. The surgical treatment of intramedullary affections of the spinal cord. *Surg Gynecol Obstet* 18: 170–179, 1914.

15. Fincher EF. William Henry Hudson, M.D. Itinerant neurosurgeon. 1862–1917. *J Neurosurg* 16:123–134, 1959.

16. Frazier CH. Subtotal resection of sensory root for relief of major trigeminal neuralgia. *Arch Neurol Psychiatr* 13:378–384, 1925.

17. Freeman W, Watts JW. Pain of organic disease relieved by prefrontal lobotomy. *Lancet* I:953–955, 1946.

18. Grant FC. End results in 100 consecutive cases of brain abscess. *Surg Gynecol Obstet* 75:465–467, 1942.

19. Goldensehn E, Whitehead R, Parry T, Spencer J, Grover R, Dreper W. Effect of diffusion respiration and high concentrations of CO_2 on cerebrospinal fluid pressure of anesthetized dogs. *Am J Physiol* 165:334–340, 1951.

20. Greenwood J. Total removal of intramedullary tumors. *J Neurosurg* 11:616–621, 1954.

21. Guillaume J, Janny P. [Continuous intracranial manometry]. *Rev Neurol* 84:131–142, 1951. [Article in French.]

22. Hadley LA. Intervertebral foramen studies. I. Foramen encroachment associated with disc herniation. *J Neurosurg* 7:347–356, 1950.

23. Hulme A. The surgical approach to thoracic intervertebral disc protrusions. *J Neurol Neurosurg Psychiatr* 23: 133–137, 1960.

24. Ingraham FD, Bailey OT, Nielsen FE. Studies in fibrin foam as a hemostatic agent in neurosurgery, with special reference to its comparison with muscle. *J Neurosurg* 1:171–181, 1944.

25. Jooma OV, Pennybacker JB, Tutton GK. Brain abscess: aspiration, drainage or excision? *J Neurol Neurosurg Psychiatr* 14:308–313, 1951.

26. Kahn EA. The role of the dentate ligaments in spinal cord compresson and the syndrome of lateral sclerosis. *J Neurosurg* 4:191–199, 1947.

27. Kahn EA. The treatment of encapsulated brain abscess with visualization by colloidal thorium dioxide. *Univ Hosp Bull Ann Arbor* 4:17–19, 1938.

28. Kahn EA, Bassett RC, Schneider RC, Crosby EC. Correlative Neurosurgery. Springfield IL: Charles C Thomas, 1955, pp 118–120.

29. LeBeau J. Radical surgery and penicillin in brain abscess. A method of treatment in one stage with special reference to the cure of three thoracogenic cases. *J Neurosurg* 3:359–374, 1946.

30. Leksell L. The stereotaxic method and radioscopy of the brain. *Acta Chir Scand* 10:316–319, 1951.

31. Lippert RG, Svien HJ, Grindlay JH, Goldstein NP, Gastineau CF. Effect of cortisone on experimental cerebral edema. *J Neurosurg* 17:583–589, 1960.

32. Logue V. Thoracic intervertebral disc prolapse with spinal cord compression. *J Neurol Neurosurg Psychiatr* 15:127–241, 1952.

33. Matson DD. A new operation for the treatment of communicating hydrypocephalus. *J Neurosurg* 6:238–247, 1949.

34. Matson DD. Ventriculoureterostomy *J Neurosurg* 8: 398–404, 1951.

35. Mayfield FH, Kees G. A brief history of the development of the Mayfield clip. *J Neurosurg* 35:97–100, 1971

36. Meyers R. The modification of alternating tremors, rigidity and festination by surgery of the basal ganglia. *Assoc Res Nerve Mental Dis Proc* 21:602–665, 1942.

37. Norlen G, Olivecrona H. The treatment of aneurysms of the circle of Willis. *J Neurosurg* 10:404–415 [*illustration* Fig. 6.7, p 414], 1953.

38. Nosik WA. Ventriculomastoidostomy. *J Neurosurg* 7: 236–239, 1950.

39. Nulsen F, Spitz E. Treatment of hydrocephalus by direct shunt from ventricle to jugular vein. *Surg Forum* 2: 399–403, 1951.

40. Olivecrona H, Landenheim J. Congenital arteriovenous aneurysms of the carotid and vertebral arterial systems. Berlin: Springer Verlag, 1957.

41. Ojemann G, Ward AA. Abnormal movement disorders. In Youmans JR (ed): Neurological Surgery. Philadelphia: Saunders, 1982, vol 6, p 3823.

42. Peet M. Splanchnic section for hypertension. Univ Hosp Bull Ann Arbor 1:17–18, 1935.

43. Perot PL, Munro DD. Transthoracic removal of midline thoracic disc protrusions causing spinal cord compression. *J Neurosurg* 31:452–458,1969.

44. Poppen J. Diagnosis of intracranial aneurysms. *Am J Surg* 75:178–186, 1948.

45. Putnam TJ. Treatment of hydrocephalus by endoscopic coagulation of the choroid plexus. Description of a new instrument and preliminary report of results. *N Engl J Med* 210:1373–1376, 1934.

46. Putnam TJ. Treatment of unilateral paralysis agitans by section of the lateral pyramidal tract. *Arch Neurol Psychiatr* 44: 950–976, 1940.

47. Ransohoff J, Spencer F, Siew F, Gage L. Transthoracic removal of thoracic disc. *J Neurosurg* 31:459–461, 1969.

48. Ray BS. Intracranial hypophysectomy. *J Neurosurg* 28: 180–186, 1968.

49. Robertson EG. A method of encephalography. *Surgery* 19:810–824, 1946.

50. Rosegay H. Cushing's legacy to transsphenoidal surgery. *J Neurosurg* 54:448–454, 1981.

51. Scarff JE. Treatment of obstructive hydrocephalus by puncture of the lamina terminalis and floor of the third venricle. *J Neurosurg* 8:204–213, 1951.

52. Scarff JE. Unilateral prefrontal lobotomy for the relief of intractable pain. *J Neurosurg* 7:330–336, 1950.

53. Scarff JE. Unilateral prefronatal lobotomy with relief of ipsilateral, contralateral, and bilateral pain. *J Neurosurg* 5:288–293, 1948.

54. Schloffer H. Erfolgreiche operation eines hypophysentumors auf nasalen wege. *Wien Klin Wochenschr* 20: 621–624, 1907.

55. Schneider RC. A syndrome in acute cervical spine injuries for which early operation is indicated. *J Neurosurg* 8:360–367, 1951.

56. Schwartz HG. High cervical cordotomy. *J Neurosurg* 26:452–455, 1967.

57. Scoville WB. Discussion [of Cloward RB. The anterior approach for removal of ruptured cervical discs. J Neurosurg 15:602–617, 1958]. *J Neurosurg* 15:615, 1958.

58. Seldinger S, Catheter replacement of the needle in percutaneous angiography. A new technique. *Acta Radiol* 39:368–376, 1953.

59. Smith GW. An automatic drill for craniotomy. *J Neurosurg* 7:285–286, 1950.

60. Smith GW, Robinson RA. The treatment of certain cervical-spine disorders by anterior removal of the intervertebral disc and interbody fusion. *J Bone Joint Surg* 40A: 607–617, 1958.

61. Smithwick R. A technique for splanchnic resection for hypertension. *Surgery* 7:1–8, 1940.

62. Spiegel EA, Wycis HT. Stereotaxic apparatus for operating on the human brain. *Science* 106:349–350, 1947.

63. Torkildsen A. Should extirpation be attempted in cases of neoplasm in or near the third ventricle of the brain? Experiences with a palliative method. *J Neurosurg* 5: 249–275, 1948.

64. Verbiest H. A radicular syndrome from developmental narrowing of the lumbar vertebral canal. *J Bone Joint Surg* 36B:230–237, 1954.

65. Verbiest H. Further experiences on the pathological influence of a developmental narrowness of the bony lumbar vertebral canal. *J Bone Joint Surg* 37B:576–583, 1955.

66. Vincent C. Sur une méthode de traitement des abcès subaigus des hémisphères cérébraux. Large décompression, puis ablation en masse sans drainage. *Gaz Méd Fr* 43:93–96, 1936.

67. Wilson CB. Significance of the small lumbar spinal canal: cauda equina compression syndrome due to spondylosis. *J Neurosurg* 31:499–506, 1969.

68. Ziedes des Plantes BG. Subtraktion. Stuttgart: Thieme, 1961.

4

Status of Neurosurgery in 1951: A Socioeconomic Perspective

Robert E. Florin, MD, FACS

The status of neurosurgery in 1951, the year in which the Congress of Neurological Surgeons (CNS) was formed, can be defined by the social, political, and economic circumstances of that time. The place of neurosurgery in medicine was already well established, with official recognition of neurosurgery as a specialty during a meeting of the American College of Surgeons in 1920. The growth of the specialty as well as the various neurosurgical societies that formed during the next 30 years are examined in this chapter. The state-of-the-art and practice in the 1950s are also reviewed after setting the background in terms of the various social, political, and economic issues that influenced the larger practice of medicine in the United States.

Because this chapter deals with the socioeconomic issues surrounding neurosurgery in 1951, it is helpful to examine just what may be encompassed in these issues. First, the term *socioeconomic* refers to the interaction of a combination of social and economic factors. The social aspect deals with the tendency to form cooperative and interdependent relationships with one's fellows. The economic aspect relates to the production, distribution, and consumption of commodities or services, including consideration of costs and returns. Applied to the practice of neurosurgery, socioeconomics represents a rather broad group of factors that influence the place and role of neurosurgery in our society and economy.

It is difficult to separate neurosurgery from the broader view of the practice of medicine before 1940 because it was represented by a very small part of the physician population and was not organized to influence and shape policy and attitudes at critical junctures.

HISTORICAL PERSPECTIVES

Review of the patterns of social and economic relations by examining the historical as well as the structural changes in American medicine provides insight into the socioeconomic issues of major concern during the 20th century. The interaction of physicians with the forces of social and economic reform reveals a number of key factors that allowed physicians to develop their professional authority, and use it to exercise control over the market and potential competition. This frequently focused on efforts by the government to develop some form of a national health insurance program, and the battles on just this one issue serve to illuminate the major players and factors in the development of our medical care delivery system. Accommodations made by both sides during the 1940s initiated a series of major changes that had a substantial impact on medical practice in the 1950s, including some unforeseen consequences that are still evolving.

BY DECADE

1890 to 1900

At the end of the 19th century there was considerable effort to control market forces by a number of groups. Among these were labor unions, corporations developing monopoly power and the medical profession. As hospitals emerged from their history as charitable institutions that cared for ill patients to their new role as medical institutions that cured ill patients, the increasing authority of physicians had the effect of increasing their market by moving the care of the sick from the family and lay practitioners to the domain of professional service. At the same time, it supported imposing limits on the uncontrolled supply of medical services by giving political support for licensing laws. The combination of increased demand and control of supply (read competition) served to ensure better compensation for physicians (1).

Some attention to professionalism is also relevant to this review because it serves as a base of solidarity in resisting forces that threaten the social and economic position of an occupational group such as physicians. A profession is an occupation that regulates itself through systematic and required training and collegial discipline, is based on technical and specialized knowledge, and has a service orientation supported by a code of ethics. The development and growth of professionalism from 1900 to 1935 helped to resist competition from other practitioners, and subsequently to resist corporate and governmental competition and control.

The market power of physicians was augmented further by the increasing dependence of patients on physicians. This accelerated as the differences between lay practice and professional knowledge widened. Adding to market power was the fact that medical services were sold to individual patients rather than to an organization. This was supported by a policy of strong resistance by physicians and the American Medical Association (AMA) to any third-party participation in the doctor–patient relationship, which had its roots in some basic precepts widely held by the medical profession during the early decades of the 20th century. These precepts included a deep distrust of any corporate involvement in medical care as a direct threat to their autonomy. It also included a fear that a third party might retain the profits of medical transactions, thereby cutting the physician out of the revenue stream. The AMA supported this position in their 1934 code of ethics, stating it was ''unprofessional'' to permit others to profit from physicians' work. In other words, the AMA opposed anyone other than a physician from making a return from physician labor (14).

1900 to 1920

During the first two decades of the 20th century, a variety of plans were developed that attempted to spread the cost of medical care over a broad base of subscribers, employees, or beneficiaries. Doctors were able to resist these moves because of their strategic position in health care. The power of the profession originated in the dependence of patients on the knowledge of and trust in their physicians, as well as their psychological dependence on the superior competence of the profession. This developed as a direct consequence of the advances in science and technology, which led to improved therapeutic competence of physicians. Public trust in this arrangement was bolstered by the development of standardized training and licensing requirements for medical practitioners, which had the effect of assuring the public regarding the quality and reliability of their ''product'' (15).

The professional authority that developed from these interrelationships served the physicians well and was a key factor in the ability to resist threats from the evolving bureaucratic organizations that either employed physicians or provided facilities or financing of medical care. Doctors claimed that such arrangements for payment of services by other than the patient to the providing physician were unethical—a position supported by the collective political organization of the profession.

In dealing with hospitals and insurance companies, the doctors shaped their own interests by setting the terms for controlling their work while setting their own prices. The gatekeeping authority of physicians gave them a strategic advantage in relation to organizations because it put the purchasing power of patients at the disposal of the doctor. The physician's authority to decide when and where to hospitalize patients or to prescribe drugs and supplies provided great leverage over hospital policy and insurance companies. As doctors developed this type of control, the hospitals and insurers developed financial arrangements that allowed them to pass through the higher costs of a physician's autonomy. This accommodation became a key factor in the ongoing maintenance of the profession's economic position (i.e., for physicians to keep their patients and maintain their fees).

1930s

In the context of the Depression and the hard times experienced by both the general population as well as patients, the physicians also experienced dramatic reductions in payment for services. Despite these pressures, the fear of socialization of the health care system drove medical and then public opinion to resist inclusion of such provisions in the Social Security program. However, by the mid 1930s, the AMA began to ease its resistance to any type of insurance because of the growing perception among physicians that private physicians, charities, and even hospitals could no longer afford to meet the demand for free services.

1940s

During the 1940s, the issue of a national health care plan received a boost that put it at the center of national attention when the United States Supreme Court indicated acceptance of a national health insurance program, putting to rest concerns about a states rights violations by such a policy. This led proponents to recommend that health insurance be operated as part of Social Security without limitations on coverage. The Wagner–Murray–Dingel bill incorporated these notions plus a system of life-long coverage, emulating the National Health plan being discussed in Britain. Roosevelt's death precluded his plan to ask Congress to approve such a bill, and Truman was unable to overcome continued opposition from the AMA. However, Truman did follow through with some important changes. He proposed to expand the program by shifting its focus to improve access to medical care by increasing the national medical resources and lowering the financial barriers to their use. He also called for the expansion of hospitals and increased support of public health plus federal aid to medical research and education (16).

The budding Cold War also provided new ammunition in the fight against ''socialized medicine.'' Fear of socialism was used as a symbolic issue in the crusade against communistic influence in American politics that arose in the postwar years with the Alger Hiss trial for espionage and the Joseph McCarthy hearings in the Senate regarding communists in government positions. Branding any proposal for national health insurance as ''socialistic'' carried the implicit taint of communistic influence and made the fight easier for organized medicine (17).

The AMA continued its resistance, adding a public relations campaign in 1949 that was the most expensive lobbying effort in American history. It effectively blocked the efforts at expanding medical school enrollment by federal assistance despite the growing shortage of physicians through the 1950s. While this was happening, Social Security was quietly expanding during the postwar period to include additional citizens as well as shared state funding for medical services to welfare recipients.

1950s

The Growth of Private Health Insurance

By 1950, the nation had a system of private insurance for those who could afford it and public welfare services for the poor. Further efforts to pass national health insurance were eclipsed by the onset of the Korean war in 1951. The repeated defeats of national health insurance proposals left the insurance of health to private interests, which began to grow slowly in the 1930s. A few of them continued to grow through the 1940s and settled into a recognizable pattern by the 1950s (18).

Blue Cross began during the Depression, when it was clear that hospitals would not be able to rely on patients to pay all their bills for hospital services. In 1932, the community hospitals of Sacramento offered contracts for hospital services to employed persons, and this plan soon spread across the country. It was rapidly recognized as a solution to the problem of distributing the costs of hospital care, and was approved by the American Hospital Association, with some caveats. The plans were to be nonprofit, to emphasize the public welfare, and were to limit themselves to hospital charges, thereby avoiding the turf of the private practitioners. They also provided free choice of physicians and hospital that effectively ruled out the single-hospital model.

Capitalization was provided by *hospital underwriting,* which backed the promise of hospital services by agreement among the member hospitals to provide service regardless of the payments they would receive. This made a key difference and underwrote the success of the Blue Cross, because this underwriting plan provided a basis of legal support for the long-term control of Blue Cross by the voluntary hospitals.

The Blues grew rapidly, reaching 6 million subscribers in 39 plans by 1940, surpassing the enrollment of commercial indemnity plans of 3.7 million (6). Blue Shield was formed in 1942 after the AMA approved physician service benefits in a plan that remained under medical society control as a preferred alternative to compulsory insurance that was again threatening. The California Blue Shield plan, called *California Physi-*

cians Service, initiated a unit value system that represented the forerunner of our present relative value systems. Once stabilized, the payments reached a value of $2.25 per unit of service. These service benefit insurance plans that were set up by hospitals and doctors achieved an effective monopoly because no other group could commit to pay for services without an agreement with providers about their prices.

The key differences between the Blue plans was that Blue Cross offered service benefits on a prepayment approach, with the same premium for all income levels, whereas Blue Shield operated more like indemnity insurance. The Blue Shield plans that offered service benefits restricted them to low-income subscribers, which allowed physicians to use their time-honored sliding scale of fees pegged to the income of their patients. They were willing to provide service benefits for their low-income patients because they were ensured of at least some payment and because it served to reduce the prospects of government insurance (19).

By 1945, Blue Cross had more than 19 million subscribers nationally, whereas Blue Shield had approximately 2 million (18). The only serious competition came from commercial insurance on an indemnity basis, which imposed no controls on hospitals or physicians. The competition was restrained by the accommodations to the provider interests inherent in the Blue plans, which effectively limited the growth of other types of coverage. However, this began to change after the war, with the inclusion of health insurance as a fringe benefit in various employee health plans. After labor unions gained the right to include health benefits in their collective bargaining, the great expansion of these plans began.

During the postwar years, the success of the labor movement in acquiring health benefits began to alarm the union officials as they faced the rapidly rising costs of excess hospitalization that third-party insurance encouraged. They also began to realize the shortcomings of a fee-for-service payment system when they shifted their focus to full coverage for their members. The prepaid group practice plans that had emerged during those same years began to look attractive to the unions, and they gradually began using

Kaiser, Group Health Cooperative of Puget Sound, and the Health Insurance Plan of New York.

Commercial indemnity insurance was not far behind. By 1950, commercial insurers had more subscribers than Blue Cross and Blue Shield, but they were forcing the Blues to change their business to more commercial terms. Coverage of individuals by commercial insurers in 1949 was estimated at 28 million, compared with more than 31 million by Blue Cross (18). By 1953, commercial insurers provided hospital insurance to 29% of the population; Blue Cross, 27%; and other independent plans, 7% (18).

Two other factors helped shape the insurance plans during the 1950s. One was experience rating, which was begun by the commercial plans to match risk to premiums in their population of insured patients. This was gradually adopted by even the Blues, who had traditionally "community rated" their premiums, and found they could not compete with actual experience rating. The second was a tax ruling in 1954 that employers' contributions to health benefit plans were tax exempt, thereby providing a subsidy to people with private insurance policies.

By 1958, two-thirds of the population had some coverage for hospital costs, which was the most common type of insurance. The private insurance system had provided enough protection that there was no great demand for national health insurance during the 1950s. The new system of financing health care had increased the share of national income allotted to health care and stabilized the financing of the whole industry.

Advancement of Scientific/Medical Research

Before World War II, the principal sources of funding of medical research were private foundations and universities. The pharmaceutical companies also sponsored an increasing amount of research, but this was directed toward applied research.

The war gave scientific research priority. In 1941, Roosevelt set the new Office of Scientific Research and Development on two tracks: one for national defense and one for medical re-

search of problems related to the war. Results of applied medical research produced not only a new drug for malaria—atabrine—but vastly improved the production of penicillin. This proved the value of such research and led to additional support for government-sponsored research performed in independent institutions rather than government laboratories. Political support and funding for these ideas took until 1950 to be realized, with the formation of the National Science Foundation.

Medicine, in particular, was a beneficiary of this popular view that recognized science as a national asset, with the demonstrated successes of drugs that could overcome infection, vaccines that could eradicate disease, and advances in surgery that could even reduce the death rate during war. This occurred concomitantly with a shift in focus from concern about infectious illnesses to chronic diseases such as cancer and heart disease. The combination of success stories and examples from applied scientific research such as the atomic bomb and nuclear energy added to the public's expectations that a combination of money and scientific effort could overcome most obstacles. This was one of the reasons that the success of the Salk vaccine for polio was such an important national event in the early 1950s, and led to even greater support of medical research (21).

The rate at which federal support for medical research grew between 1941 and 1951 was from $3 million to $76 million (19). The degree of control over research was largely managed by the scientific community. Basic policy issues as well as approval of grant applications were determined by scientists not in governmental positions. The autonomy and freedom enjoyed by the individual investigator was largely a result of the public trust in science coupled with the acceptance by the government that scientists be left to follow their own rules and research. One example from the 1950s confirmed the public's faith in the value of focused research against specific diseases. Poliomyelitis was widely feared in those years, with research funded by the March of Dimes, which raised more money than any other health campaign. When the Salk vaccine proved effective in a nationwide double-blind clinical trial that involved millions of citizens, it gave hope that chronic diseases could also be stopped. Congress was supportive of this feeling and the NIH budget rose from $81 million in 1955 to $400 million by 1960 (19). Federal aid to medical education would have been an expected beneficiary of the attitude toward expanding medical science and research. However, the AMA blocked a bill that would have provided a 5-year program of grants and scholarships for medical schools to increase the number of physicians. This was based on a perception and fear that such federal support for medical schools would set a dangerous precedent regarding the controls that usually accompany federal money. It also served to limit the competition among practitioners already in practice. The consequence of this action was to restrain the growth in the number of physicians needed to meet the rapidly increasing demand for medical care. The consequences of this restraint on the supply of physicians would have a major impact on health care policy in the ensuing two decades.

Support for Growth of Hospitals: VA and Hill–Burton

The support of science and technology in postwar health policy was paralleled by an effort to improve access to medical services. This effort took the form of aid for hospital construction, to create employment and an alternative to national health insurance. The first part of this initiative was directed to the revitalization of the Veterans Administration, building new hospitals in metropolitan areas and affiliating them with medical schools. Clinical research and training programs were developed that enhanced the role of the medical schools in running hospitals.

The second part of this effort was the passage of a bill (Hill–Burton) in 1946 that provided public funds for the construction of community hospital beds with remarkably few strings. In fact, in both the programs for medical research and community hospital construction, there was a respect for the sovereignty of the medical institutions as well as the profession, which further supported the case that public aid to medicine should not bring public control (22).

The Growth of Medical Education and Its Consequences

The federal support programs to expand medical research and build hospitals had a large influence on the development of medical care in the 1950s. The research funds created new opportunities for medical schools, which increased their annual income from $1.5 million in 1950 to $3.7 million by 1959 (21). The schools identified their missions as research, education, and patient care. The full-time faculty increased 51% during the 1940s and doubled from 4,200 in 1950 to more than 11,000 in 1960 (23).

The expanding staff, coupled with the rapid growth of specialties and subspecialties, broke down the old hierarchical pyramid system that had operated since the 1920s to restrain the promotion of physicians in training programs. With the infusion of funds from NIH research and training grants, the demand for academic physicians grew along with their income. The medical schools became interested in expanding their research space and clinical facilities to attract new talent, and the hierarchy began to change.

With growth of faculty in the clinical departments paralleling that in research, local physicians who had enjoyed admitting their patients to the teaching hospital and who served as instructors were displaced. Control of staff appointments fell to the medical school rather than the hospital, in the interest of maintaining the quality of graduate medical education. This displacement of the local "town" practitioners by the "gown" members of the faculty led to much resentment as well as loss of prestige and even income. Some of this was moderated by the prosperity during those years along with the migration of patients and their private physicians to the suburbs, leaving behind the urban-based medical school with its faculty.

Increasing Specialization and Certification

The growth of specialization was widespread during the 1940s and 1950s, with 24% of doctors reporting a full-time practice in a specialty in 1940. This grew to 37% by 1949, 44% by 1955, and 55% by 1960. The biggest growth was in the surgical specialties, starting at 10% of physicians in 1931 and increasing to 26% by 1960 (21).

The reasons for this trend generally include the growth of knowledge and the desire to become expert in at least a portion of medical practice as a key factor leading medical students to become specialists. However, another factor is probably a better explanation for the choice: The economic rewards of specialization are greater than those acquired from general practice.

The certification of medical specialists that developed in the 1930s contributed to the rising rate of specialization. This ostensibly set limits on entry into a specialty, which had the potential to create a monopoly position. However, this was limited by the absence of regulation of the size or distribution of the specialties involved. The specialty boards backed off from imposing limits on hospital privileges when the risk of anticompetitive actions was raised. The general practitioners also opposed any limits on specialty practice or specialty training, so the definitions of a specialist remained deliberately vague.

The growing value of certification was becoming obvious to most physicians and was supported by such actions as the higher rank assigned to military physicians with specialty certification. After the war, the VA would not recognize a doctor as a specialist without board certification (23).

The advantage hospitals derived from graduate training programs also played a role in the move toward greater specialization. Hospitals with interns and residents could provide inexpensive professional labor that aided the hospital-oriented specialties, such as surgery, by adding to the productivity of these specialists. The bottom line was that specialty incomes varied directly with the percentage of work reimbursed by third parties. With better insurance coverage for hospital services plus inexpensive support services by house staff, hospital-based services were promoted over those in the office. As a consequence, the surgical specialties benefited directly from this policy.

The Results of the Changes in Medicine During the 1950s

Despite the many changes that occurred during the postwar period in medical practice, education, and research, the ratio of physicians to the population remained relatively stable. Doctors in private practice declined from 108 to 91 per 100,000 people between 1940 and 1957, whereas those employed in hospitals and other institutions increased from 12.8% to 26.5% of all physicians (22). The volume of practice for each physician increased substantially as a result of the growth in demand for health services, the concentration of work in hospitals and offices, and the declining availability of private practitioners. The average workload in a private office per week in 1930 was 50 patients, which grew to 100 patients by 1950 (22).

In 1950, most doctors served at least 3 years after internship in a specialty resident program compared with before the war, when a 1-year internship was the only postgraduate training before entering general practice. The role of the house staff was an important one in the relationship between the hospitals and their attending staff, because the profit to the hospitals and doctors from the labor of the house staff was a major force in the economics of the postwar medical system. The shortfall in ability to staff house officer positions by the hospitals with new beds created a demand for additional candidates that by 1957 reached 5000 unfilled positions annually (22). The medical schools were graduating 7,000 students each year whereas the hospitals sought to fill more than 12,000 intern positions in the same year (22). This ultimately led Congress to help by allowing foreign trained physicians to enter the United States and work in these positions. The result was an increase in the number of foreign medical graduates from 10% to 26% of all house staff during the 1950s (25). The result of this policy of expanding hospital capacity while restraining medical school enrollment was to create a new lower tier of medical practice with physicians recruited from third-world countries.

Another consequence of this shortfall was that the community hospitals with house staff training positions that were not affiliated with a medical school or university were at a serious disadvantage in attracting American interns and residents. As a result, the community hospitals sought ties with medical schools, and during the late 1950s and the 1960s, the major metropolitan medical schools and universities developed affiliations with many community hospitals that helped to secure the house staff positions while building major medical conglomerates that functioned as regional medical centers.

1960s

By the 1960s, American medicine had developed three identifiable sectors. The first included the physicians who worked in the medical schools and their associated hospitals, including house staff and faculty. Their primary focus was on research and training, and the basic feature of their patient relations was the absence of a long-term commitment to them. Physicians involved in research and training depend on the opinions of their colleagues rather than patient goodwill or referrals from colleagues, which contributes to the aura of autonomy of physicians and the sense of a loss of power by the patients when in such settings.

The second group included the private practitioners, mostly office based and located in the suburbs. They still had a dominant role in community hospitals and were prospering. Because consumer demand remained high, hospital resources had expanded rapidly and there was little competition. They did depend on the goodwill of patients and colleagues for referrals as well as their staff privileges. These interrelationships promoted professional solidarity, which was reflected in the positions of the AMA, whereas part of this group was growing closer to their specialty societies, at the expense of the AMA.

The last group included the doctors working in inner-city or rural areas, or state hospitals. These doctors tended to be older general practitioners or foreign medical graduates. This was the smallest group and most professionally isolated, frequently working in the same service area as the major medical centers. These contrasts among physicians were representative of the variations in the overall medical care system, which ranged from the most advanced centers of excellence to medically abandoned areas with no doctors and scant public health services. This disparity was one of the forces that ultimately led to the reformation of the system and to the introduction of parts of the national health insurance program under Social Security in 1965 (24).

SOCIAL SETTING IN 1951

Demographics

The national population in 1951 was 155 million, an increase of more than 3 million from 1950, which was the peak year in population growth after World War II, which gave rise to the phrase *baby boom*. Only 63.1% of the population were native to the United States, whereas 0.6% were born abroad. Compare this with 1990, when 92% of the population were born in the United States and 2.6% were born abroad (30). There were only five cities with more than 1 million people: New York, Chicago, Philadelphia, Los Angeles, and Detroit (31).

The western migration, especially to California, was marked by an influx of more than 8.8 million residents in the two decades beginning in 1940, with the population rising from 6.9 million in 1940 to 15.7 million in 1960. Once the migration began, it accelerated, with more than 5 million people moving west in the 1950s alone (10).

There was another migration in progress at that time. The exodus from central cities to the suburbs began in earnest during the war years, and as it accelerated, it required a change in social policy to support the infrastructure required by this shift in population. This extended to dealing with the inadequate supply of housing, transportation, and other areas in which supply failed to match demand. Federal mortgage guarantees, highway trust funds, and aid for hospital construction were all programs designed to meet such demands. The federal government support of medicine for both medical research and mental health were specific targets of these policies.

Politics

Party in Power:
Democrat/Truman 1945 to 1952

After the death of President Roosevelt during the closing days of World War II in the spring of 1945, Harry Truman became president and presided over the end of the conflict with Germany and Japan after the use of the atomic bomb at Hiroshima and Nagasaki. The next decade marked the era of the Cold War with the Soviet Union. Early political problems were located in the eastern European countries that were dominated by the USSR, and included the blockade of Berlin, which was overcome by a United States airlift to supply Berlin during the ensuing year.

The Truman administration extended until 1952, and the focus of foreign policy during that time was the containment of communism. This included the Truman Doctrine, the Marshall Plan (1947), the creation of the North Atlantic Treaty Organization (NATO), and support of nationalist China. There was much public concern over charges of communist infiltration of the federal government, which was supported by the conviction and execution of Julius and Ethel Rosenberg on charges of giving atomic secrets to the USSR, and the conviction of Alger Hiss, a former employee of the state department, of charges of perjury regarding his relations with the communist party. Senator Joseph McCarthy made extravagant claims about communist agent infiltration into the government that were not substantiated.

During this same period there was widespread communist aggression in eastern Europe, the eastern Mediterranean, and China. The Soviet blockade of Berlin in 1948 to 1949 represented the degree of aggression the communists were willing to deploy. With a victory by the communists in China, followed in 1949 by a Soviet atomic test explosion, the fear of communist expansion and plans to contain it became the dominant theme in United States foreign policy.

This was further aggravated by the invasion of South Korea by North Korea in 1950, with support from the Soviet Union. The United States government promptly obtained support from the United Nations Security Council to mount a United Nations response under the command of General Douglas MacArthur that repelled the invasion. However, when Chinese communist troops joined North Korea, the United Nations' force was driven back and the situation became critical. Truman initiated a large program for defense, declared a national emergency, and placed the nation back on a war basis. He also authorized development of the hydrogen bomb. Several months later, MacArthur was recalled by Truman over differences in conduct of the war and Far East policy, and was replaced by General Matthew Ridgeway. An armistice began several months later but dragged on for more than a year.

The social and economic programs during this period included Truman's *Fair Deal*. The only part that survived Congress was the Employment Act of 1946, which stated that the government was responsible for maintaining full employment, and it established the Council of Economic Advisers. The postwar conversion to a peacetime economy included the GI Bill of Rights, which provided benefits of educational support and mortgage finance assistance to veterans. The pressure of consumer buying power was not matched by the output of consumer goods, which sparked steep rises in prices. This was aggravated by union activity that was now allowed to organize and strike under the Taft Hartley Act of 1947. This resulted in spikes in certain basic commodity prices.

Truman used the United States Army to seize all the railroads in 1950 to prevent a general strike, and returned control to the railroad companies in 1952 when the labor dispute had been resolved. By the end of 1951, the Truman administration was beset by charges of corruption directed toward a number of cronies who Truman appointed to government office. In addition, the Korean War and the public dispute with General MacArthur did not serve to garner support for Truman (3,29).

Party in Power:
Republican/Eisenhower 1953 to 1960

After 2 years as commander-in-chief of NATO, Eisenhower was elected in the 1952 presidential campaign, defeating Adlai Stevenson with a platform of modern republicanism, promising to "clean out the mess in Washington" and end the Korean war. He accomplished both of these feats and went on slowly to strengthen a number of federal social programs including an expansion of Social Security coverage. He also supported an increased minimum wage and inaugurated a massive highway-building program. The program of farm product supports begun to reduce farm bankruptcies in the 1930s was also revised to a system of flexible rather than rigid/mandated supports. The Civil Rights unrest began during Eisenhower's second term, followed by turmoil in Suez and Lebanon (3,29).

Economy

The United States' receipts in 1951 were $48 billion compared with expenditures of $44 billion (26).

Stock Market

In January 1951, the New York Stock Exchange covered 1472 stock issues representing 2.3 billion shares with a total market value of $93 billion (26).

Cost of Living for Reference Items

Examples of a few costs were $2000 for a new Ford sedan, $0.20 for a pair of socks, and $15,000 to 30,000 for a three-bedroom, two-bath home in the suburbs. Loans averaged approxi-

TABLE 4.1. *Consumer price index from Bureau of Labor Statistics, United States Department of Labor (1967 = 100)*

Year	Consumer price index
1915	30.4
1940	42.0
1950	72.1
1960	88.7
1970	116.3
1980	248.8
1990	391.4
1999	495.5

mately 4.5% for a 20-year mortgage. Average retail food prices were as follows: 1 lb. round steak, $1.05; 1 lb. butter, $0.80; 1 lb. sliced bacon, $0.68; one dozen eggs, $0.69; 1 quart of milk, $0.23; 1 lb. sugar or flour, $0.10; and 1 lb. potatoes, $0.05 (26).

The Consumer Price Index comparisons in table 4.1 allows for comparison of relative costs across the decades (26). A 1999 dollar would be worth only approximately 15 cents in 1950.

Income

The average per capita income in the United States in 1950 was $1436. Median income in the United States in 1998 was $26,732.

The average net profit from a medical practice in 1945 was $8,000, whereas in 1969 it had increased to $32,000. The consumer price index rose at an annual rate of 2.8% during the postwar period, whereas physician fees rose 3.8% and income rose 5.9% per year.

Miscellaneous

The Xerox copying machine was introduced, and Charles Schulz's Peanuts comic strip first appeared in late 1950.

Television

The first transcontinental TV broadcast occurred in September 1951, when President Truman addressed the Japanese Peace Conference in San Francisco. The existing network linked 52 cities by means of 107 relay stations, each 30 miles away from its neighbors.

In television, Sid Caesar and Imogene Coca in *Your Show of Shows,* and Groucho Marx in *You Bet Your Life* were the prime shows.

Movies

The major films of 1951 were *An American in Paris* with Gene Kelly, *A Streetcar Named Desire* with Marlon Brando and Vivien Leigh, *Show Boat* with Kathryn Grayson and Howard Kiel, *Alice in Wonderland* from Walt Disney, and the *Lavender Hill Mob* with Alec Guinness.

Books

The books of 1951 included *The Caine Mutiny* by Herman Wouk, *From Here to Eternity* by James Jones, and *The Sea Around Us* by Rachael Carson.

Theater

The theatrical hits of the year were *Mister Roberts, Born Yesterday, Call Me Madam* with Ethel Merman, *Guys and Dolls* with Robert Alda and Vivian Blaine, *The King and I* with Yul Brynner and Gertrude Lawrence, and *A Tree Grows in Brooklyn* with Shirley Booth and Johnny Johnston.

Sports

In 1951, Joe DiMaggio announced his retirement from baseball and Ben Hogan won the Masters golf tournament.

Transportation

A key to the extraordinary mobility of the American people was the automobile. During the two decades after 1950, the number of bus and subway rides dropped annually from 17 billion to 7 billion, whereas the rate of auto registration more than doubled. This occurred in the face of a large increase in urban population, which attests to the close bond between the people and their cars (8).

This mobility made possible the large metropolitan centers with their rings of suburbs, the expansion of commuter travel, as well as a number of untoward effects. The latter include air pollution, urban decay, traffic congestion, and a decline in the public transportation system in certain areas.

Air travel was growing, including overseas routes, and Pan American reported one of their Stratocruisers made the trip from New York to London, 3500 miles, in only 8 hours 35 minutes.

Science

Noteworthy events included the first hydrogen bomb explosion and the first time power was generated by nuclear fission reactor.

Insurance

Blue Cross enrollees totaled 32,921,212.

Hospitals

There were 6,430 hospitals with 1,456,912 beds and an annual census of 17,023,000 patients. The average hospital cost per patient per day was $16.77, with a length of stay of 8.3 days (8). The total average cost per patient stay was $138.73 (5).

Medicine

General versus Specialty

The total number of physicians in the United States in the early 1950s is shown in Table 4.2 (26) compared with the total in 1998, which increased by almost threefold. Neurosurgeon numbers increased tenfold over the same period, from 400 in 1950 to 4739 in 1998. Much of this was the result of the rapid accelertion in

TABLE 4.2. *Number of physicians*

Parameter	1952	1954	1998
Total no. of physicians	214,667	218,522	600,829
No. in private practice	151,363	156,333	
No. in research/teaching	6,677		
No. hospital-based services	28,366		
No. of retired or inactive	8,166	9311	
No. in government service	20,095	17,040	
No. of women	0	177,030	
No. in training programs	0	29,161	

specialization that occurred following the end of the War in 1946. However, the growth of specialization had its roots much earlier.

The practice of surgery during the first two decades of the 20th century was a period of transition in which surgeons gradually implemented techniques of gentle and careful control of bleeding and tissue handling that followed patterns developed by a small group of prominent surgeons. As surgical applications expanded beyond the abdomen, the eye, the musculoskeletal system, and gynecology, the widening scope of surgery led to more specialization.

Neurosurgery was one of the first of these subspecialties to emerge, probably because the techniques and principles of general surgery were inadequate for work within the nervous system. Harvey Cushing was the pioneer in the United States who consolidated neurosurgery as a specialty. His methods of meticulous dissection, gentle handling of the tissues, careful hemostasis, antisepsis, and continuous review of his techniques advanced the specialty rapidly. His success provided visible proof of the value of surgery on the nervous system and helped to counter the common notion that all neurosurgery was linked to a high rate of surgical mortality. From 1905 onward, his contributions to the surgical management of tumors, pituitary disorders, epilepsy, and trigeminal neuralgia led an increasing number of his students to spread his ideas and methods among a small but growing group of surgeons specializing in surgery of the nervous system.

From a socioeconomic viewpoint, the value of certification in a specialty became increasingly evident during the Depression in the 1930s. The potential of limiting entry into a specialty by establishing a specialty credentialing process represented a response to increased competition by noncertified practitioners. The roots of this movement can be traced to the first examining board for ophthalmology in 1916, followed by the otolaryngologists in 1924, and the obstetricians and gynecologists in 1930. There were no limits set on the number or distribution of certified specialists, and hospitals had strong incentives to set up specialty training programs after the war because of the public funding and sup-

TABLE 4.3. *Medical schools*

Parameter	1950	1951
No. of medical schools	71	72
Total enrollment	23,670	27,076
Veterans, %	66	42.2
No. of women enrolled	89	
Median student cost/yr	$1473	$1800
No. of graduates/ no. of female graduates		6080/351

port available to expand hospital services. When the effect of government subsidies and the better returns to specialists from health insurance plans became evident, the value of certification to young physicians was confirmed, and further strengthened the move to certification (23).

When the move to divide medicine into ever smaller specialty groups accelerated, the AMA in 1933 formed what has become the American Board of Medical Specialties to set general standards for the examining boards and various jurisdictional disputes among specialties. The American Board of Neurological Surgery was formed in 1940, joining a growing list of specialties so recognized.

Medical Schools

The number of medical schools and their enrollment and annual cost per student are shown in Table 4.3 (26). It was not sufficient just to graduate with an MD degree to meet the public and state mandated requirements for opening a practice. Certain requirements had to be met to satisfy the licensing authorities, which represented a degree of regulation of the practice of medicine by the state.

Control and Regulation of Medical Practice

State licensing and medical boards provided the structure and authority for reviewing the credentials of applicant physicians to assure the public (the consumers) that the minimum standards set by the boards had been met for physicians holding a valid license. At the local level, hospital credential committees, peer review committees, surgical privilege committees, use review committees, and mortality reviews provided oversight among peers of the proper exercise of a physician's capabilities. Medical society grievance and fee complaint committees were designed to provide a forum for patient and professional problems to be reviewed by a group of impartial physicians who represented the local medical establishment.

Neurosurgery

In 1951, there were approximately 400 neurosurgeons practicing in the United States (9). This means that there was one neurosurgeon for every 387,000 people in the nation. Most were in major metropolitan areas, with very few practicing without proximate access to a medical school.

In 1960, there were 1142 United States neurosurgeons plus 39 in the military reported by the Survey Committee of the CNS (26). The national ratio for 1960 was one neurosurgeon per 153,000 people. The move to the suburbs had begun in the mid 1950s, and new graduates were following the tide into the suburbs.

By 1998, the number of neurosurgeons had grown to 4739, 225 of whom were women. The national ratio for 1998 was one neurosurgeon per 55,000 general population (12). The distribution had been driven by increasing competition and declining lifestyle problems in the large cities, so there were neurosurgeons practicing in many small communities, even in the mountain states and central plains states. The popularity of certain areas such as Portland, Oregon, and California had attracted a disproportionate share of neurosurgeons, which led to major problems when the health maintenance organizations began competitive bidding for their contracts.

Resident Training Programs

There were 80 neurosurgical training programs in 1952, with a total of 241 residents in all years of training. By 1998, the number of programs had grown to 94, with a total of 818 residents. The length of the programs early in the 1950s varied, ranging from 4 years for ''general

neurosurgery'' to 6 years when a research program was included (10).

Neurosurgical Certification

In 1951, there were 337 board-certified neurosurgeons in the United States. By June 1952, this had increased to 393 (1), and in May 1954, there were 454. In 1989, the number reached 3500, where it has remained for the past decade (8,10).

NEUROSURGICAL PRACTICE

We don't have a good source of data regarding the specific mix of cases and the frequency within an average neurosurgical practice for 1951. However, we can infer some differences from current practices when we examine the procedures used for the CNS fee surveys during the early 1960s (13). These practices included a group of cranioplasty-related procedures that would be uncommon today and may have some relationship to the number of veterans who may have had long-term complications with their cranial repairs dating back to the 1940s. There was a collection of procedures that dealt with drainage or removal of abscesses, which may correlate with the development of antibiotic therapies during the 1950s. Diagnostic tests of the preaxial imaging era prevailed, including open carotid angiography, pneumoencephalography, and ventriculography when intracranial pressure was elevated or suspected.

The state of cerebrospinal fluid shunting was still in its early development phase, with subarachnoid–ureteral and–peritoneal shunting listed along with the early version of the Holter valve ventriculo-auriculostomy. The spectrum of spine surgery was rather limited in its scope compared with modern listings, although disc surgery was quite common. The number of sympathectomy codes suggest that this was a big part of the business of neurosurgery, soon to be eclipsed by the development of effective antihypertensive medications.

The most common procedure performed in practices and programs with a busy trauma service was emergency tracheostomy. The advent of common endotracheal intubation for airway access occurred approximately 5 years later. The second most common procedure was exploratory burr holes. In an era before easy access to other imaging modalities that could provide information about the intracranial contents and possible hematomas, skull films were usually performed with the hope of visualizing a calcified pineal to assess the possibility of a lateralized mass effect.

PHARMACEUTICALS

A list of 11 different sulfonamides appears in the Merck Manual, 8th edition (7), whereas the antibiotics were limited to penicillin, streptomycin, aureomycin, and chloromycetin. Drugs used for epilepsy included diphenylhydantoin, phenobarbital, mesantoin, tridione, and bromides.

FEES

The Executive Committee of the CNS authorized in 1963 the Socioeconomic Committee of the CNS to prepare and distribute a questionnaire regarding customary fees for a selection of neurosurgical procedures. The actual survey was performed in 1964, supplemented by additional surveys performed in 1965. The results were sent to all the members of the CNS. Some samples of the then extant fees for selected procedures are listed in Table 4.4 (13).

Use of Relative Value Scales as a Basis for Reimbursement

The California Medical Association (CMA) initiated a project to develop a Relative Value Study (RVS) based on physician fees in 1953. A report was produced during 1956 that was delivered to the CMA Committee on Fees (1). They forwarded the work to the council of the CMA, which approved the project and emphasized that the RVS was not a fee schedule but simply a tool to determine the relative value of one procedure to another. This occurred in the absence of standardized procedural terminology and required adoption of some new standards for describing specific services.

The RVS was divided into four section—medicine, surgery, radiology, and pathology—each with its own conversion factor to translate the RVUs into dollars. The 1st edition of this project appeared in 1956, followed in 1957 by a 2nd edition, which included pediatrics, plastic surgery, anesthesiology, and assistant surgeons (1). There were only 12 visit codes included in the medicine section. Of more interest were the RVUs assigned to the most complex surgical procedures. There appeared to be an upper limit of 100 RVUs for procedures that included

- Spinal fusion with partial excision of intervertebral disc

TABLE 4.4. *CNS Fee schedule survey 1965[a]*

Procedure, current CPT code	Average fee, $					Range of fees (high/Low)
	New York	Ohio	Illinois	Texas	California	
Lumbar puncture, 62270	28	17	22	18	21	75/5
Open reduction skull fracture with reparative brain surgery, 62010	705	464	497	579	694	1500/300
Carotid endarterectomy, 35301	474	465	376	397	552	1000/150
Exploration for or excision of herniated disc, lumbar, 63030	525	380	427	385	557	1500/250
Excision of brain cyst or neoplasm, 61510	2500	592	610	678	905	2500/350
Intracranial clipping or trapping of aneurysm, 61700	1017	732	693	788	1031	2500/275
Sympathectomy, thoracolumbar, unilateral, 64809	508	404	450	433	559	1500/225
Neurolysis: freeing of nerve and/or transposition of nerve, 64721	380	331	278	295	335	1000/150

[a] CPT, current procedural terminology.

- Total pneumonectomy
- Pericardiectomy
- Repair of abdominal aorta
- Esophagoplasty
- Pancreatectomy, subtotal (Whipple type)
- Nephrectomy with ureterectomy
- Excision of brain cyst, neoplasm, or abscess
- Scleral resection, lamellar

This relativity no longer applies, but at that time, these procedures represented equivalence at the maximum conceived by the originators of the RVS.

Subsequently, the California RVS went through a series of revisions in which both the coding nomenclature improved and the work in the usual global follow-up periods was included in the RVUs. Eventually, the AMA began the current procedural terminology process, and Dr. Byron Pevehouse was on the leading edge of that activity on behalf of neurosurgery. He established a collection of codes and descriptors for neurosurgical procedures in 1974 to 1975 with a five-digit numerical code (2), some of which are still in use. The logic and system imposed by these changes improved the RVS enormously, and set the foundation for both tracking and coding medical and surgical services for reimbursement into our current decade.

Revenue

Average physician income in private practice in 1949 was $11,058, led by neurosurgeons with an average of $28,628. Income was highest in the West and lowest in New England. Samples of income from a poll of senior neurosurgeons who had active practices during the 1950s revealed that the annual income during the mid 1950s for a solo neurosurgeon was $28,000, which rose to $92,000 by 1978 (26).

Early in the decade, the fee-for-service mode of billing was dominant, and the schedule for payments was very elastic. In many cases, the care was uncompensated, and in some practices, the first 30 to 40 hours of practice each week would be written off as charity service. Nevertheless, neurosurgeons were busy, with caseloads of surgery ranging from 100 to several hundred per year. The case mix included many

sympathectomies for hypertension, disc excisions, and a scattering of craniotomies. Many air studies were conducted in pursuit of the cause of headaches. The typical hospital census for a neurosurgeon in California during the early 1950s was 20 to 30 patients per week. In many suburban areas, neurosurgeons also provided a full spectrum of neurology services as well.

Fees for these services generally ranged below $1000, and $750 was considered a generous fee for a service. This is generally consistent with the fee survey conducted by the CNS approximately 10 years later. Only approximately 20% of charges were covered by health insurance during that period, whereas the remainder of charges were at the discretion of the providing physician (7).

Many of the senior neurosurgeons interviewed for this chapter were frank in describing the remarkable flexibility in their billing and collections during the early 1950s. A common thread was a personal "means testing" when it came to stating a fee for a surgical service. Equally common was the comment that when no means were available, the service was provided at no charge. Payment in noncash media was also relatively common, especially when provided in settings outside of major cities. Receipt of produce of various sorts, sometimes over extended periods of time, was not rare. On occasion, a barter system of trading services occurred, such as trading a room addition for a discectomy.

Cash payments, frequently in installments, were a common mode of reimbursement. Insurance payments to physicians for office and surgical services were still infrequent, although as the Blue Shield plan expanded and other commercial insurers joined in covering the employees of corporations, insurance payments became more frequent. Industrial insurance was another source of income, although the relative amount could not be determined.

Malpractice

The problem of malpractice was relatively small in the 1950s, as reflected by the premiums paid for coverage. In California in the mid

1950s, the annual premium for $10,000 of coverage was less then $50. In Florida, it was only $36 for the same coverage (A. Raney and J.M. Thompson, personal communication).

Medical Organizations and Associations

National

American Medical Association

Much has already been presented regarding the role of the AMA and its influence on socioeconomic issues during the first 50 years of the 20th century. Its educational and informational objectives have not been stressed in this chapter. It seems clear at the beginning of the 21st century that the AMA had a sustained and pivotal role in shaping the model of medical practice.

The roots of the AMA go back to its formation in 1847, with progressively more involvement in issues of ethics, licensing, and efforts at establishing standards for medical education and training. In 1905, the AMA Council on Medical Education published minimum standards for medical schools. These were updated following the *Flexner Report on Medical Education* in the United States and Canada in 1910, and cited examples of diploma mills turning out poorly qualified practitioners. This was followed in 1914 by standards for hospital internships and a list of approved hospitals in 1927. In 1934, the AMA Judicial Council amended the Principles of Medical Ethics, stating that it would be unethical for a third party to profit from a doctor's services. By 1936, AMA membership had reached 100,000. It participated in the formation of the Joint Commission on Accreditation of Hospitals in collaboration with the American Hospital Association, the ACS, and the Canadian Medical Association. In 1952, the House of Delegates condemned fee splitting.

American College of Surgeons

The ACS was established in 1913 with the aim of improving the standard of practice by surgeons and of providing a means by which the public could better select a qualified surgeon from those with lesser qualifications. Dr. Cush-

ing strongly supported this development, even over the objections of the AMA, which for a time tried to suppress the formation of the college. Speculation suggests that the AMA may have viewed another national group, representing only surgeons, as a threat to their solidarity and power, but details of their differences are not available. The ACS did go on to become an umbrella organization for many of the then developing surgical specialities, and provided useful representation until the growth of individual specialty organizations began to take over political and socioeconomic issue management themselves. Currently, general surgeons appear to be the major constituency in the ACS, while providing representation for a number of surgical subspecialties.

State and County

The state and county medical organizations began to organize later than the AMA. They played lesser roles in the politics at their respective levels, while supporting the AMA with the collective power of their aggregate memberships.

Neurosurgical Organizations: Social, Fraternal, Educational, and Political

The recurring emergence of new professional associations designed to serve neurosurgeons is well documented and analyzed in a paper written by Carl Hauber and Chris Philips published in 1995 (5). They examined the reasons that led successive generations of neurosurgeons to develop these organizations by studying the early phases of these associations, including the historical records, their minutes, and personal correspondence among the founders when available. They observed that each association was designed to pursue the same general goals, primary among which was that of providing universal access to significant organizational activities and relationships among colleagues in neurosurgery. However, they reported a pattern in each of the associations in which limits on membership were established that prevented young neurosurgeons from participating in the organized activities of the existing societies. It seems that the members of these societies valued the professional and social intimacy provided by the virtue of their small memberships more than their original desires to help younger neurosurgeons in their professional growth. This was the pattern manifest in the first four neurosurgical organizations.

The Society of Neurological Surgeons (SNS), established in 1920 when neurosurgery was recognized as a specialty, gradually grew from the initial 11 founders to a total of 45 members. During the next decade, when younger neurosurgeons found they had no access to the forum inherent to the SNS in which to discuss their professional work as well as have a voice in the development of the specialty and the training of neurosurgeons, they formed the Harvey Cushing Society in 1931. The SNS, during the following three decades, concomitant with major increases in research, medical education, and medical science, gradually included all the North American neurosurgical academics as members, thereby becoming the society that represented academic interests for the specialty.

Despite its goal of promoting the advancement of the various fields of organic neurology, the Harvey Cushing Society also held to a strict limit of 40 members, and within just 7 years of its inception, it was followed by still another neurosurgical organization.

The American Academy of Neurological Surgeons began in 1938 with the same self-imposed limitation on total membership as its predecessors, and with the same results. At the 10th annual meeting, Frank Mayfield launched a discussion within the Academy about the problem of multiple associations designed to represent the interests of neurosurgeons. Unfortunately, his initiative met the same fate as in the previous associations, and the Academy remained a club exclusive of younger neurosurgeons.

The final member of the group of limited-access neurosurgical societies was the Neurosurgical Society of America, founded in 1948 with the express commitment to a young membership. It limited active membership to neurosurgeons younger than 45 years age and required transfer to senior (and nonactive) status when

older than 45. This lasted until the oldest members reached 45, whereupon the by-laws were changed to allow continued active membership.

Because the number of young neurosurgeons was increasing faster than available memberships in the then active societies, and the number of neurosurgeons grew at a rapid pace after World War II, the pressure to have a principal forum for discussion and publication of important developments in neurosurgery became quite strong. During this postwar period, the Harvey Cushing Society gradually accepted these obligations, expanded its membership, and became the de facto forum for neurosurgery, despite the membership requirement of board certification adopted in 1942. In 1948, it had 148 members; by 1954, the Harvey Cushing Society had 305 members.

The issue of board certification became a key part of membership policy in the association begun by the founders of the CNS in May 1951. It imposed no evident limitations on membership for neurosurgeons, such as board certification. It did emulate the NSA with a policy that limited the age of its leadership to 45 years, which still remains in effect. A measure of the success of this strategy was the rapid growth of the CNS, which grew to nearly 70 members in its first year, second only to the Harvey Cushing Society. The subsequent growth of the CNS proved the need for a neurosurgical organization without the restrictions imposed by the other societies. This policy continues to date, to encourage membership by any neurosurgeon while strongly supporting the value of board certification as a measure of the quality of neurosurgical training. The primary focus of the CNS has remained the education of neurosurgeons, with a tilt toward the younger members (27).

The Joint SocioEconomic Committee was formed in 1972, with members from both the CNS and the American Association of Neurological Surgeons, to deal with the increasing problems of socioeconomics and their impact on neurosurgery. This committee was subsequently renamed as the Joint Council of State Neurosurgical Societies, because state organizations formed to deal with both local and regional problems. Currently, this operates as the Council of

State Neurosurgical Societies, which meets twice annually as a representative assembly in conjunction with the annual meetings of the AANS and the CNS.

Another committee to deal with economic and governmental issues was formed in 1976 under the heading of the Washington Committee for Neurosurgery. This was based in Washington, DC, and was staffed by Charles Plante (28). Both the AANS and the CNS provided representatives to this committee, which had considerable influence on policy matters that impacted neurosurgery during the 1970s and later. During the 1950s, there were few issues that affected neurosurgeons of a regulatory or governmental nature. The turf battles of later decades had not yet developed and there was little need for intervention on behalf of the specialty interests by neurosurgical organizations. The escalation in malpractice premiums that began during the growth in the plaintiffs bar in the 1960s came to crisis levels in the 1970s, and was a focal point for a major increase in political involvement of neurosurgical organizations. A number of state neurosurgical organizations mobilized and formed effective groups that had varying degrees of success in combating the malpractice threat. As a consequence, the state organizations continued to function after the crisis, dealing with the myriad problems that followed during the next several decades. These organizations now comprise the basis for the Council of State Neurosurgical Societies, which addresses both regional and national issues.

FINAL OBSERVATIONS

Social Aspects

The role of neurosurgery in the socioeconomic arena during the years leading up to 1951 was small, more like a passenger than a driver. The principal driver of the policies and politics that influenced the social and economic issues for medicine was the AMA, which dated back to the end of the 19th century. The AMA was clearly effective in realizing the goals of securing the authority and autonomy of physicians while maneuvering into a position to exercise control over their health care market, and thereby controlling competition. This was a truly remarkable achievement of informed self-interest mixed with altruistic goals that included ethical as well as quality issues. It is even more remarkable in the context of the fact that these developments ran counter to a major effort in the United States to break up monopolies during those decades. When viewed from a corporate perspective, what the AMA achieved represents the enthronement of medicine in a special place, insulated from the antitrust sentiments of federal prosecutors, all with public and congressional support.

Economic Aspects

A basic trend during the first half of the 20th century in the economics of medicine was that economic dynamics provided the "compelling force" that influenced the number and distribution of physicians above all other factors. Other trends such as demographics, technological and scientific advances, productivity, professionalism, and ethics were important, but all were eclipsed by the underlying economic factors (11).

Time and again, the pivotal consideration on which some issue or policy stood or fell was economic (14). This may disappoint some analysts who hoped for higher motives in the decisions made. The reality does seem clear from this point in time, and can be helpful when viewing and dealing with current socioeconomic issues. The human animal will usually act in terms of economic self-interest when challenged. Choices among different plans or policies eventually come down to a consideration of the economic risks and benefits for the group or individual concerned in the transaction. An old saying attributed to Willie Sutton, a notorious bank robber in the 1940s, when apprehended, was in response to the question, "Why do you rob banks?" to which Willie replied, "That's where the money is."

Ethical Aspects

This conclusion should serve to alert our professional organizations that the tendency for economic matters to drive policy and actions must be considered in the context of the mission of the organizations. The conflict between protecting the economic interests of members in negotiations with payers, plans, and even government should be balanced against the ethical obligations of a profession that requires the trust of its patients and its desire to maintain a privileged place in our society. Because our ability to influence change in the current health care system depends primarily on these ethical considerations, it is important that a balance be achieved between our economic advocacy and the public interest.

REFERENCES

1. Committee on Fees of the Commission on Medical Services: Relative Value Study. 2nd ed. Committee on Fees of the Commission on Medical Services, California Medical Association, 1957.
2. Committee on Task and Terminology and the Joint Socioeconomic Committee of the AANS and CNS: Procedural terminology for neurological surgeons. Baltimore, Williams & Wilkins, 1975.
3. Encyclopedia Britannica. 15th ed. Chicago, IL, Encyclopedia Britannica Inc., 1978.
4. Flexner A. Medical education in the United States and Canada, Bulletin No. 4. New York, Carnegie Foundation for the Advancement of Teaching, 1910.
5. Hauber C, Philips C. The evolution of organized neurological surgery in the United States. *Neurosurgery* 36: 814–826, 1995.
6. Herman N, Somer A. Doctors, patients and health insurance. Washington, DC, The Brookings Institution, 1961, p 548.
7. Merck manual. 8th ed. Rahway, NJ, Merck & Co., 1950.
8. Minutes of the meeting of the Harvey Cushing Society, Hollywood, FL, April. Park Ridge, IL, AANS Archives, 1951.
9. Author: Minutes of the meeting of the Harvey Cushing Society. Victoria, BC, AANS archives, June 5–7, 1952.
10. New York Times encyclopedic almanac 1970. New York, New York Times, 1970.
11. Pellegrino E, Relman A. Professional medical associations: Ethical and practical guidelines. *JAMA* 282: 984–986, 1999.
12. Popp J. Neurosurgical workforce: Examining the physician supply controversy. *AANS Bull* 9:7–9, 2000.
13. Socioeconomic Committee of the Congress of Neurological Surgeons: Neurosurgical fee survey, 1963–66. Socioeconomic Committee of the Congress of Neurological Surgeons, 1965.
14. Starr P. The social transformation of American medicine. New York, Basic Books, 1982, pp 3–29.
15. Starr P. The social transformation of American medicine. New York, Basic Books, 1982, pp 215–220.
16. Starr P. The social transformation of American medicine. New York, Basic Books, 1982, pp 229–232.
17. Starr P. The social transformation of American medicine. New York, Basic Books, 1982, pp 270–279.
18. Starr P. The social transformation of American medicine. New York, Basic Books, 1982, pp 280–289.
19. Starr P. The social transformation of American medicine. New York, Basic Books, 1982, pp 290–300.
20. Starr P. The social transformation of American medicine. New York, Basic Books, 1982, pp 306–331.
21. Starr P. The social transformation of American medicine. New York, Basic Books, 1982, pp 339–347.
22. Starr P. The social transformation of American medicine. New York, Basic Books, 1982, pp 348–351.
23. Starr P. The social transformation of American medicine. New York, Basic Books, 1982, pp 352–358.
24. Starr P. The social transformation of American medicine. New York, Basic Books, 1982, pp 359–363.
25. Stevens R, Vermeulin J. Foreign trained physicians and American medicine. Washington, DC, Department of Health, Education and Welfare, 1972, p 112.
26. Survey Committee of the Congress of Neurological Surgeons: Directory of Neurological Surgeons in the United States. Survey Committee of the Congress of Neurological Surgeons, October 1960.
27. Thompson J. History of the Congress of Neurological Surgeons 1951–1991. Baltimore, Williams & Wilkins, 1992.
28. Travis R, Orrico K. Neurosurgery and politics: Neurosurgery in transition, the socioeconomic transformation of neurological surgery. Baltimore, Williams & Wilkins, 1998, pp 211–219.
29. United States Census Bureau: State level census data, 1940, 1950, 1960. Washington, DC, Census Bureau, United States.
30. United States Census Bureau: Historical national population estimates: July 1900 to July 1998. Washington, DC, United States Census Bureau.
31. United States Census Bureau. Table 18 population of the 100 largest urban places: 1950. Washington, DC, United States Census Bureau, 1950.
32. World almanac & book of facts for 1950, 1952, 2000. New York, New York World Telegram, 1950, 1952, 2000.

5

Historical Perspectives of Imaging the Nervous System

T. Glenn Pait, MD, FACS, and Igor de Castro, MD

FOUNDATIONS

The foundations from which radiology would arise were the discoveries in 1643 of the barometric vacuum by Evangelista Torricelli (1608–1647) and the air pump of Otto von Guericke in 1654 (Fig. 5.1) (34). The air pump was used to evacuate air slowly from enclosed containers. In 1855 at the University of Bonn, Heinrich Geissler (1814–1879), a glassblower, developed a mercury vacuum pump with which he evacuated his glass tubes. Julius Plucker (1801–1868), a professor of physics also at Bonn, refined the Geissler tubes. These tubes, when filled with various gases, showed beautiful colors when high-tension discharges from an induction coil were passed through them. Plucker's observation of an emanation from the cathode end of the tubes when a discharge was passed through them was one of the earliest to be made of the so-called cathode rays (34).

In 1876, William Crookes (1832–1919), an English chemist, called these cathodic rays a new "fourth state of matter" (34,50). During the 1890s, Philipp Lenard (1862–1947) equipped glass cathode tubes with very thin aluminum windows through which the cathodic rays could penetrate to the outside. He noted that the rays made the air electrically conductive;

however, the rays traveled only a few centimeters. Lenard also discovered that these rays produced luminescent effects on fluorescent salts and darkened a photographic plate (34). It was these cathode rays that interested Wilhem–Conrad Röntgen (1845–1923), a physicist at the University of Würzburg. On November 8, 1895, using a cathode tube enclosed in a tightly fitting black cardboard coat and a Ruhmkorff induction coil, Röntgen (Fig. 5.2) discovered an entirely new type of ray (34,50). He was investigating cathode ray fluorescence by passing electricity through vacuum tubes filled with rarified gas. He soon observed a strange glow emanating from a small photographic plate lying on a nearby table. He realized that he was observing a previously undiscovered kind of ray. He devoted himself exclusively to identifying more properties of the emanation from the tubes. He ate and slept in his laboratory. He named the rays "X," because "X" is used in mathematics to indicate an unknown quantity. He soon learned that metals and lead stopped the rays from penetrating. To test further the ability of lead to stop the penetration of the rays, he held with his hand a small lead disc between the rays and a photographic plate. He suddenly saw the outline of his thumb and finger, within which were other shadows—the bones of his hand. This was the

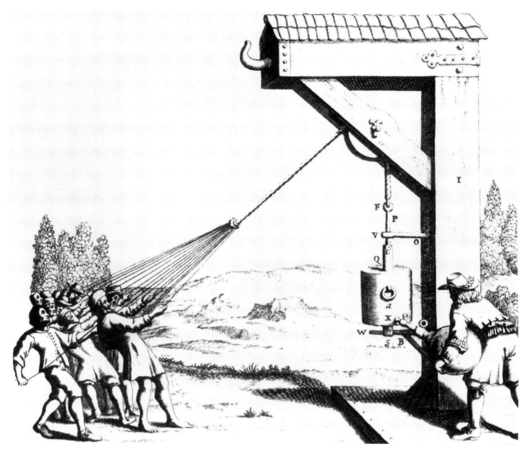

FIGURE 5.1. 1654, the von Guericke vacuum pump, Magdeburg, Germany. In 1654, Otto von Guericke lifted 50 men from the earth with his invention, an air pump that created an invisible vacuum. The people thought that Guericke had magical powers.

first picture of the human skeleton within living tissue (34,35,50). One can easily appreciate Röntgen's amazement and excitement—the first to see what no other has ever witnessed.

On December 22, 1895, Röntgen persuaded Frau Röntgen to place her left hand with her wedding ring onto a cassette loaded with a photographic plate, on which he directed rays from his cathode tube for 15 minutes. This became the hand and ring seen around the world. Röntgen realized that early publication of his work was essential. On December 28, 1895, he sent his manuscript—"On a New Kind of Rays, a Preliminary Communication"—to the *Würzburg Physical Medical Society Journal* (34,35,38, 40,50,74). It was printed in the very next issue

of the *Sitzungsberichte der Physikalisch-Medizinischen Gesellschaft zu Würzburg* (74). In January 1896, Professor Röntgen presented his work before his colleagues. Soon his discovery was applauded and praised worldwide by both scientists and others. Within only a few months of their discovery, X rays proved their usefulness as a diagnostic and therapeutic tool in medicine. These new rays allowed physicians their first noninvasive look inside the human body. So enthusiastic was the scientific community over Röntgen's discovery that more than 1000 papers and more than 50 books about the newly named "Röntgen Ray" appeared in the literature in the first year, 1896 (50). Wilhem Röntgen was given numerous awards, one of which included the

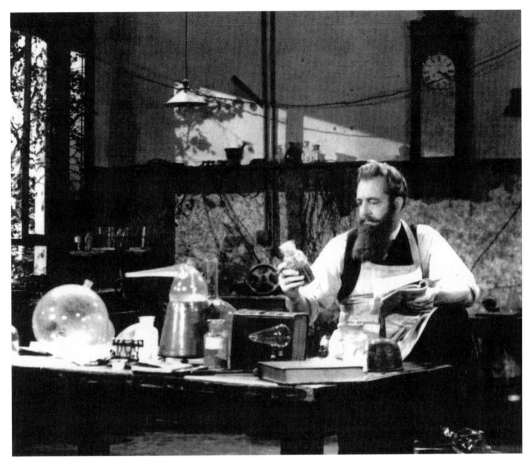

FIGURE 5.2. Wilhem Conrad Röntgen (1845–1923) in his laboratory. (Courtesy of the National Library of Medicine)

first Alfred Nobel Prize in Physics, in 1901 (35). The discovery of X rays revolutionized medicine and science.

EARLY APPLICATIONS: 19TH CENTURY

Thomas Alva Edison (1847–1931), the great American inventor, learned of Röntgen's discovery only weeks after the official scientific announcement. Edison, having a severe attack of Röntgenmania, immediately built himself a machine to emit the unknown rays (35,40). The task was no great challenge for the experienced experimenter. The cathode tube was not very different from his electric light bulb. He began

to undertake studies to make the rays practical and profitable. Edison's West Orange, New Jersey, laboratory was soon hard at work on improving Röntgen's procedure and instrumentation. They made the glass tube thinner, which allowed more X rays through faster. The platinum wires inside the tube were replaced with aluminum disks. Such improvements allowed Edison and his team to develop the first fluoroscope (Fig. 5.3) (50).

Not unlike today, the press became excited about a new scientific discovery. William Randolph Hearst (1863–1951), the newspaper giant, became very interested in the X ray. An X ray image of the human brain would be a sensational story, not to mention that it would sell newspa-

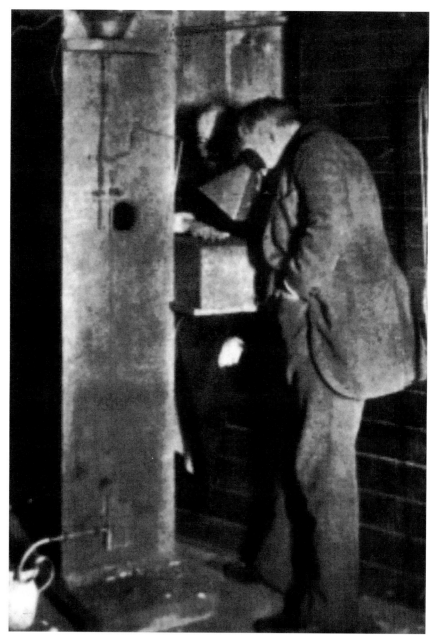

FIGURE 5.3. Edison with his fluoroscope, examining the hand of his glassblower, Clarence Dalby, in 1896. Dalby later became one of the first to die as a result of repeated x-ray exposure. (Courtesy of the Burdy Library, Dibner Institute, Cambridge, MA)

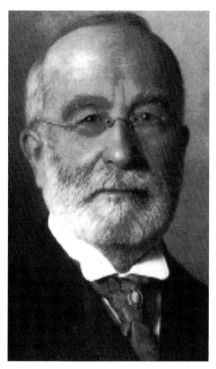

FIGURE 5.4. William Williams Keen (1837–1932) in 1905. (Courtesy of the National Library of Medicine)

pers, a lot of papers. In 1896, after learning about Edison's radiological work, Hearst challenged Edison to produce an X ray image of the human brain. Edison readily accepted. However, after only a few weeks of trying to photograph the brain, he and his team acknowledged defeat (32,50). For many scientists, Edison's failure meant that the brain was beyond the reach of X rays. In the same year, William Williams Keen (1837–1932), a pioneering Philadelphia neurological surgeon (Fig. 5.4), expressed doubt about the use of the new X ray technology: ''In tumors of the brain, the bones of the head (especially as the rays would have to penetrate two thickness of bone) will absolutely preclude any use of this method in diagnosis'' (44,47). It was true that X rays would not allow viewing of the brain itself; however, they did provide pictures of the ''brainpan'' and could reveal certain objects that had passed through the skull.

On January 8, 1896, Professor Arthur Schus-ter, a physicist and one of only two men in Great Britain who received a reprint from Dr. Röntgen of his original paper, wrote a letter in the *Manchester Guardian* newspaper. He gave a very concise report of the X ray and offered to discuss the exciting new discovery. Dr. Little of Nelson, a small town north of Manchester, read the communication. He attended a patient, Mrs. Hartley, whom he believed might benefit from the new system of photography. On April 25, 1896, her insane husband, who committed suicide afterward by jumping into a canal and drowning, shot his wife in the head. Dr. Little contacted Professor Schuster requesting him to use X rays to help locate the four bullets lodged in the poor woman's head. Schuster was not available; however, he sent his assistant, Dr. Staunton. The studies were performed at the home of the patient. This was the first occasion that X rays were obtained outside an institution or hospital. The first photograph took 1 hour to complete; the second required even longer. The studies were very helpful; the experiment was a success. Three of the bullets were appreciated; the whereabouts of the fourth was undetermined. Shortly thereafter, Professor Schuster traveled to Nelson and again photographed Mrs. Hartley. All four bullets were visualized. She apparently progressed satisfactorily for a time, but died on May 9, 1896 (56,77).

The first case in which an intracranial lesion was localized exactly with X rays and then attacked successfully with surgery occurred on February 2, 1897. A patient with headaches who presented after a gunshot wound to the head consulted Dr. Stenbeck, a Swedish physician. On September 10, 1897, Stenbeck acquired lateral and frontal views of the patient's skull. A bullet was appreciated in the occipital region. Dr. Lannander confirmed at surgery that the bullet was in the position suggested by the radiological photograph. The headache-producing bullet was extracted without complication (56). Most assuredly, the patient was very grateful. In 1897, this remarkable case was presented by Dr. S. E. Henschen at the XII International Congress of Medicine in Moscow (42). In 1899, Church (11) reported a case of a ''cerebellar tumor which was recognized clinically, demonstrated by the X ray, and proved by autopsy.'' In the same

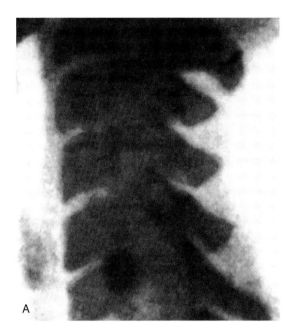

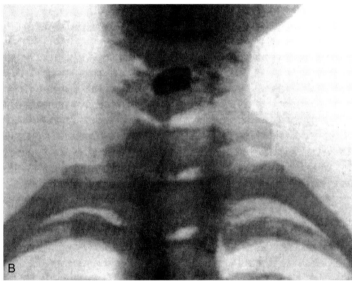

FIGURE 5.5. (A) Lateral cervical spine radiograph made by Cushing of Baltimore from a woman who had been shot in the neck in 1896 (from Cushing (13)). (B) Cushing's radiograph of a bullet wound of the cervical spine, 1898 (from Cushing (14)).

year, Oppenheim presented an X ray image of a pituitary tumor at a gathering of the Society of Psychiatric and Nervous Diseases in Berlin (30). Other reports of radiographs of gunshot wounds of the head and neck (Fig. 5.5) appeared between 1896 and 1900 (13,14).

EARLY APPLICATIONS: 20TH CENTURY

During the early part of the 20th century, special photographic attention was directed to the normal and abnormal anatomy of the skull. Exposure times were long, often 30 minutes of direct exposure (56). In 1902, G. E. Pfahler developed detailed photographic plates of the skull showing the scalp, the inner and outer tables, the diploe, the sinuses, the coronal suture, the meningeal artery grooves, and the skull base. In one patient, Pfahler noted findings suggestive of a tumor. At surgery, a lesion was found that supported the preoperative X ray image. This prompted him to begin cadaveric experiments. He removed sections of the brain and filled the defects with known, embalmed tumors (56,71). Even though Pfahler's work produced some degree of enthusiasm, his X ray results failed to provide a consistent avenue of preoperative intracranial pathological diagnosis. In the same year, Beclère, in Paris, compared the roentgenograms of a normal, healthy young woman with a 24-year-old woman affected with acromegaly. This was the first diagnosis of acromegaly using X ray images. He demonstrated characteristic bony changes produced by acromegaly: an irregular thickening of the cranium, an exaggerated development in the height and depth of the frontal and maxillary sinuses, and an increase in the dimensions of the pituitary fossa (5,56).

Arthur Schüller (1874–1957) of Vienna continued radiological investigations to elucidate the anatomy of the skull. He developed extraordinary skill in the interpretation of skull X ray images. He closely correlated the clinical findings, anatomic structures, and previous autopsies to formulate a diagnosis. His radiological labors resulted in two monumental works in radiology whose principles form the basis of X ray examinations of the skull. His first book, published in 1905, was entitled *Die Schädelbasis im Röntgen-bilde* (75), and in 1912 he published *Röntgen-Diagnostik der Erkrankungen des Kopfes* (76). He was the first to demonstrate calcification of the pineal gland and to recognize its value as an intracranial landmark. He summarized, ''One may, for instance, conclude that displacement of the pineal shadow to the right or left of the midline in symmetric skulls is due to pressure by a tumor or to traction from cerebral scarring'' (56,76). Schüller and Erdheim studied patients with suspected pituitary tumors. Schüller encouraged Oscar Hirsch to operate for the relief of pituitary adenoma using the trans-

sphenoidal approach (56). Prof. Schüller continued his work at the Viennese School of Röntgenology until Hitler's regime forced him and his wife to leave their home in 1938. They spent a few months in England until securing a position in Melbourne, Australia. Walter E. Dandy became quite upset after learning of Schüller's departure from Vienna. He wondered about the distinguished radiologist moving to the United States. On February 14, 1939, Dandy wrote to Schüller offering his assistance, including money (31). Schüller's colleagues from all over the world learned of his new home and sent him films to interpret. In Australia, Schüller carried on his work. He described cephalohematoma deformans, osteoporosis circumscripta, and Schüller–Christian disease (30,56,74,75). Schüller's dedication to understanding cranial pathology made him an early neuroradiological pioneer (Fig. 5.6).

In 1910, Fedor Krause, a German pioneering neurosurgeon, included a chapter on radiology in his classic three-volume surgical textbook *Surgery of the Brain and Spinal Cord Based on Personal Experiences* (51). Krause stated that X rays offered assistance with certain neurological problems:

> Above all other means of diagnosis it furnished the most useful in tumours with calcareous or bony deposits, as for instance in exostosis . . . any injury to the skull may bring on epileptic seizures . . . whenever possible X ray examination should be made. It is frequently a great aid in clearing up the diagnosis. Even in other forms of epilepsy Röntgenography is of urgent need. (51, vol. 1, p. 278)

Folke Henschen, a Swedish pathologist, observed that acoustic tumors had a tendency to widen the internal auditory meatus. He had the insight that this feature could be appreciated on X ray images of patients suspected of such lesions. On February, 1910, Henschen consulted Forssell, a radiological colleague, about a patient with a possible tumor. Unfortunately only one side of the patient's head was subjected to the photographic plates. For the next patient with a possible tumor, a full set of X ray images was acquired in March 1911. These studies demonstrated what Henschen had often seen in autopsy—an abnormal auditory meatus (Fig. 5.7).

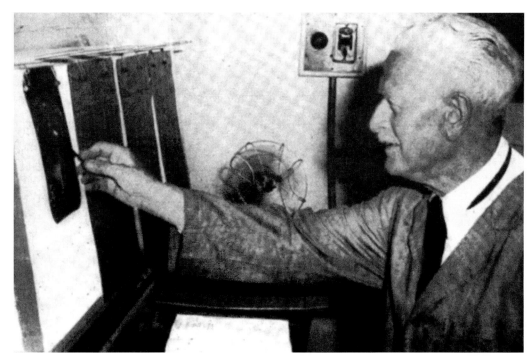

FIGURE 5.6. Arthur Schüller (1874–1957), in 1905, was the first to use the term *neuro-Röntgeno-logie.*

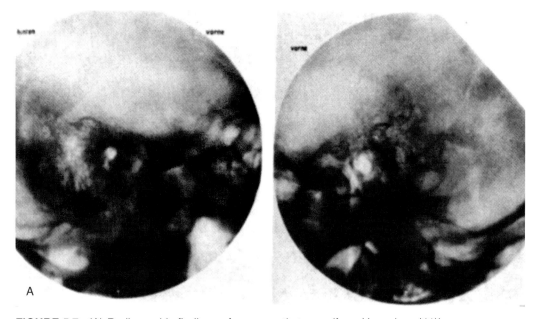

FIGURE 5.7. (A) Radiographic findings of an acoustic tumor (from Henschen (41)).

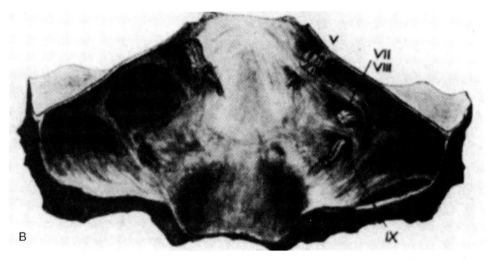

FIGURE 5.7. *Continued.* (B) An abnormal auditory meatus confirmed on autopsy. Henschen's original publication (from Henschen (41)).

The next month the patient died, and Henschen confirmed the radiographic findings in his autopsy suite (41,56). Such early radiographic studies could only demonstrate pathological bony changes or reveal abnormal sites of intracranial calcification. In 1921, Adolf Bingel (1879–1963) noted that these early studies were Röntgenology of the skull but not the brain (56). Clearly, something more would be needed to appreciate better the contents of the cranial vault. That something became contrast agents.

CONTRAST AGENTS

Less than a month after Röntgen's announcement, in January 1896, Lindenthal and Haschek produced a radiograph of the arteries of the hand of a corpse. The injection of Teichmann's mixture, which consisted of lime, cinnabar (mercury), and petroleum, via the brachial artery demonstrated the arteries in beautiful relief (Fig. 5.8) (30,39,50). The X ray photograph produced by injecting blood vessels suggested the possibility of visualizing other organs of the human body, such as the stomach, intestines, lungs, heart, esophagus, gallbladder, and brain. This was the first contrast-enhanced image. The search for the perfect contrast agent and dye to reveal organ function and pathology would ulti-

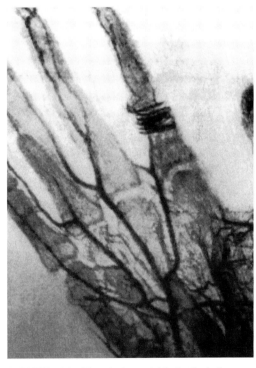

FIGURE 5.8. Haschek and Linderthal demonstrated the arterial tree in a cadaveric hand by injection of Teischmann's solution in 1896. Original paper (from Haschek and Linderthal (39)).

mately result in the development of neuroradiology.

Despite the numerous X ray images acquired
of the head during the first decade of the 20th
century, mischief-making intracranial gremlins
eluded the X rayer's photographic plates. It was
traumatic air in the head that "opened the door"
for better and more detailed neurodiagnostic images. On November 24, 1912, a confused young
machinist presented to the Harlem Hospital
emergency department with a laceration over his
right eyebrow and a suspected orbital fracture.
H. M. Luckett, the casualty surgeon on call, requested orbital X ray images (40,44,50). William
Stewart, a radiologist, confirmed the presence
of a bony abnormality consistent with a fracture
of the posterior wall of the frontal sinuses. The
patient improved with conservative therapy and
was discharged home. The machinist soon returned with severe headaches, vomiting, and
lethargy. The patient apparently sneezed and developed "a pain in my head and then a flow of a
large amount of clear fluid came from my nose"
(57,58). Repeat studies revealed never before
appreciated radiological shadows produced by
air (Fig. 5.9). Stewart reported, "(W)e were
dealing with a case of fracture of the skull complicated by distended cerebral ventricles (inflated) with air or gas." He called the condition
spontaneous pneumoencephalography (83). As
a result of these X ray images, the young machinist was taken to the operating theater. During surgery Luckett noted a gas bubbling from
the brain. The poor man died only 3 days after
surgery. At autopsy, the fracture in the posterior
wall of the frontal sinus was confirmed and part
of the skull was found to be depressed. The brain
was removed in toto and submerged in a bath
of water. Air escaped through a laceration in
the frontal lobe. This laceration was found to
communicate with the anterior horn of the ventricle. Luckett reported that the machinist succumbed to "pneumocephalus" (57,58).

One of the most important diagnostic procedures introduced in the 20th century was pneumoencephalography. It was the imagination of
a brilliant young 32-year-old Johns Hopkins'
Hospital resident surgeon Walter Edward Dandy
(1886–1946) who recognized air as a splendid
contrast medium (Fig. 5.10). Dandy stated, "It
is largely due to the frequent comment by Dr.

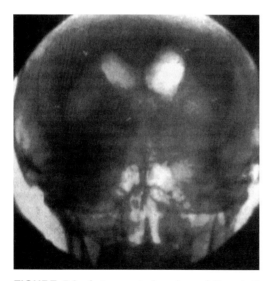

FIGURE 5.9. Anteroposterior view of the skull
films in Luckett's original report in 1913 (57,58)

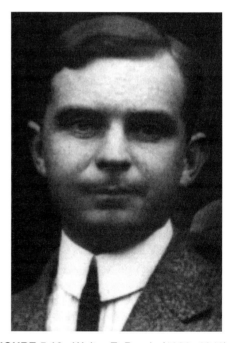

FIGURE 5.10. Walter E. Dandy (1886–1946) at
the age of 31 years.

Halsted on the remarkable power of intestinal gasses to perforate the bone that my attention was drawn to its practical possibilities in the brain, that is of injecting air into the ventricles.'' (20) Another case that allowed Dandy to appreciate air as a contrast agent occurred in 1917. While Dandy was examining the X ray image of a patient with a history of intestinal bleeding, he was able appreciate that the liver was separated from the diaphragm by a gaseous collection. Dandy later noted that it was this X ray image of the pneumoperitoneum that suggested to him that the injection of air would be useful for diagnosing cerebral lesions (20).

Dandy injected air into the ventricles through an open fontanelle or a small craniotomy (Fig. 5.11) (21). Turning the patient and relying on gravity was a means by which the location of the air was controlled. One year later, Dandy noted that air injected into the lateral ventricles was present over the surface of the brain. In 1919, he concluded that for the injected air in the ventricles to reach the surface of the brain and the sulci (Fig. 5.12), it would have to follow the normal pathways of the cerebrospinal fluid circulation. Dandy (19) then surmised

It also seems probable that we shall be able to localize spinal cord tumors by means of intraspinous injections there. If the spinal canal is not obliterated by the tumor, the injected air will pass freely into the intracranial subarachnoid space—none being left in the spinal canal. This happened in one of our cases in which a spinal cord tumor was suspected.

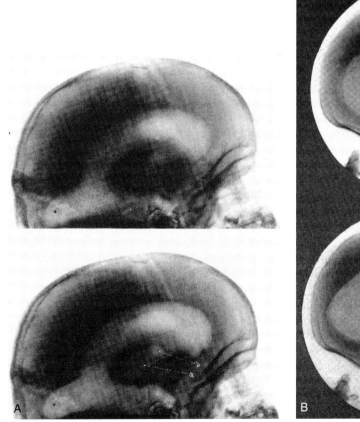
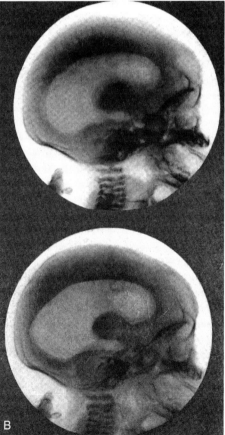

FIGURE 5.11. Air in the ventricles after injection through an open fontanelle (from Dandy (21)).

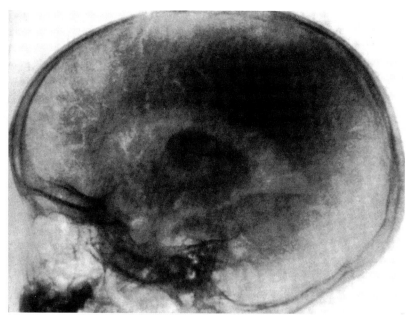

FIGURE 5.12. Air in the ventricles reaches the surface of the brain and the sulci (from Dandy (19)).

Dandy did not use the term *air myelogram* to describe visualization of the spinal cord; however, it is evident that air myelography had been performed. Dandy described his technique of pneumoencephalography via direct injection of air into the spinal canal. He described the disappearance of air, and he pointed out the anatomy of the cisterns. The Dandy techniques were used to diagnose atrophy of the brain, communicating and noncommunicating hydrocephalus, localization of cerebral and cerebellar masses, and spinal cord lesions (19–21). Unquestionably, Dandy's introduction and refinement of air encephalography, ventriculography, and air myelography advanced and changed forever the fields of neurology, neurosurgery, and neuroradiology. This technique was used for more than 50 years by radiologists and surgeons throughout the world. In 1933, Dandy was nominated for the Nobel Prize in physiology and medicine for his development of ventriculography and encephalography, and his studies on cerebrospinal fluid circulation. He did not receive the Nobel Prize in 1934; an honor well deserved but never given

(31). The final important development in pneumoencephalography occurred between 1963 and 1964, when Kurt Amplatz developed a special somersaulting device. This new chair allowed better management of air within the cranial cavity by rotating the patient as much as 360 degrees (Fig. 5.13). This allowed the examiner to direct air into the part of the ventricular system under study (72,84).

Walter Dandy was the first to describe clearly and publish the use of air for myelography; however, H. C. Jacobaeus (Fig. 5.14), from Stockholm, was the first to devote an entire paper to the subject in 1921 (46). In all the patients of Jacobaeus, the air was introduced specifically for the diagnosis of spinal cord tumors (46).

Four years after the introduction of air as a contrast agent into the central nervous system by Walter Dandy, Jan Athanase Sicard and Jacques Forestier (France) developed myelographic procedures using an iodized oil (Lipiodol) (44,50,80). Sicard was an early researcher in the cytology of cerebrospinal fluid. However, his greatest interest was the treatment of pain, par-

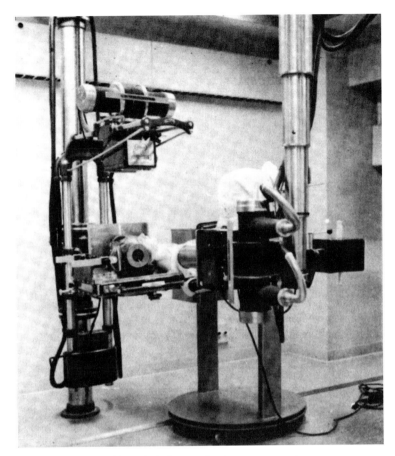

FIGURE 5.13. A new somersaulting chair for cerebral pneumography.

ticularly pain produced by sciatica. He become well-known for such pain therapy. He often used Lipiodol for treatment of this affliction. He became aware that Lipiodol was an excellent X ray contrast material, and was the founder of the use of positive contrast agents in neuroradiology. Sicard noticed under the fluorescent screen that Lipiodol tended to track along a nerve sheath. On one occasion, a student of Sicard's injected the recommended Lipiodol into a patient's lumbar musculature. On withdrawing the plunger of the syringe, cerebrospinal fluid was present. After concluding that the needle had coursed through the dura and into the subarachnoid space, the pupil notified his teacher. Sicard's response was a concern for the patient

(56). Under fluoroscopy it was observed that the contrast material dropped to the bottom of the subarachnoid space. Sicard and his student appreciated that raising or lowering the patient's head would allow the Lipiodol to move back and forth through the subarachnoid space (50,56,80). Lipiodol quickly replaced air as the agent of choice for myelography and for the study of spinal cord disease. This technique was quickly embraced in Europe; however, Lipiodol was not used in the United States until 1944 (36).

Many contrast materials were developed after Lipiodol. They included nonionic water-soluble agents and many water-soluble varieties. All of these agents relied on the difference in the specific gravity between the contrast agent and cere-

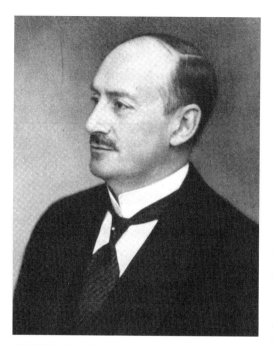

FIGURE 5.14. H. C. Jacobaeus.

brospinal fluid to position contrast material precisely over the targeted area. Pantopaque, an
organic iodine compound, proved more stable
than Lipiodol and produced excellent radiological studies. The use of myelography soon expanded beyond the visualization of spinal cord
tumors. As afflictions of the spine, and degenerative diseases in particular, became better appreciated, radiographic studies became more important.

In 1934, William Mixter and Joseph Barr (64)
presented their paper on ''Rupture of the Intervertebral Disc'' to the New England Medical
Society. Their paper ushered in a new era of
neurosurgery and spinal surgery (64). They used
Lipiodol myelography to assist in the diagnosis
of a ruptured intervertebral disc. Iodized contrast
agents became the standard material for myelography for several decades. Water-soluble materials became preferred because of their better imaging qualities and their ability to fill out the
nerve root sleeves. The first nonionic water solu-
ble contrast material was Metrizamide. Metrizamide was quickly accepted after its formal in-

troduction in radiology in 1975 by Skalpe and
Amundsen (81).

ANGIOGRAPHY

Although pneumoencephalography was a
giant leap forward for visualization of lesions of
the central nervous system, it could not be used
on every occasion in which an intracranial lesion
was suspected. It was soon appreciated that use
of air intracranially could not be used on patients
with increased intracranial pressure. António
Caetano de Abred Freire Egas Moniz, a Portu-
guese neuro-ophthalmologist, politician, psychi-
atrist, and neurologist, described the brain as
being ''mute to X-rays'' (33). Therefore, he
turned his experimental efforts toward a better
visualization of the central nervous system. In
1922, Sicard and Forestier tried using their Lipiodol to demonstrate the cerebral arteries of animals; unfortunately, all of the animals died (80).
Any oil-based agent such as Lipiodol was an
inappropriate agent to use because of oil embolism. The search for nontoxic agents for injection into the vascular system to appreciate better
intracranial anatomy and pathology became a
major area of investigation. Egas Moniz surmised that if cerebral vessels could be visualized
by radiographic means, a more precise localization of intracranial pathology, particularly tumors, could be appreciated. He postulated that
tumors would distort normal cerebrovascular
patterns. The technique of intra-arterial injection
was developed and used by von Knauer for the
injection of Neo-salvarsan into the carotid artery
percutaneously in 1919 for the treatment of general paralysis of the insane, syphilis (6,30).
Knowledge of this procedure provided Moniz
with the needed information to begin in vitro
studies in animals (Fig. 5.15). He used sodium
bromide and sodium iodine. Strontium bromide
was thought to be somewhat less toxic and,
therefore, was the first agent to be injected into
a living patient (37). The patient died from the
injection of strontium bromide. Moniz then tried
a 25% solution of sodium iodide. Unfortunately,
Moniz was plagued with severe gout in his hand
and was unable to perform the surgical procedures required to place needles into the vascular

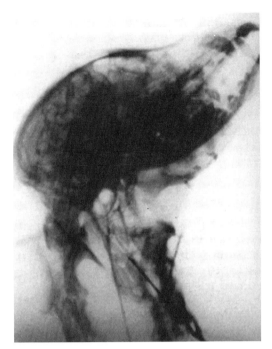

FIGURE 5.15. Angiogram obtained in a dog in 1926 using strontium bromide. Study performed by Egas Moniz.

nique proved safe, neurologists would be grateful for the discovery that would enable them to localize intracranial tumors, the site of which is often difficult to determine (4). Moniz soon replaced sodium iodine with thorium dioxide, a radioactive compound that was better known by its trade name Thorotrast (53). In 1931, Moniz's work resulted in his now classic book on angiography, *Diagnostic des tumeurs cerebrales et epreuve de l'encephalographie arterielle* (65).

Thorotrast was used by radiologists throughout the 1950s; however, it proved to be a very unwelcome agent in the human body. The particles in Thorotrast were insoluble in water and were eventually deposited in the liver and spleen, leading to cellular injury. José Pereira Caldas (10), a colleague of Moniz, developed a special carousel that permitted exposure of six films in a very rapid sequence to allow better visualization of the arterial, capillary, and venous phases (66). The ability to appreciate these vascular phases became an area of study, particularly with various vascular anomalies, lesions, and neoplasms of the brain. In 1930, stereoscopic viewing was added to angiographic systems (Fig 5.18). This allowed the surgeon to appreciate lesions better and to develop a plan of attack (84). Norman M. Dott, professor of neurosurgery at the University of Edinburgh, was the first to perform a carotid arteriogram to confirm the clinical diagnosis of a cerebral aneurysm. He communicated his experience in a paper published in 1937:

elements. Therefore he called on Almeida Lima, a young neurosurgical colleague, to assist (Fig. 5.16). Lima would cut down onto the internal carotid artery and perform a direct injection of the sodium iodine. After a sixth patient died, they switched from a 70% strontium bromide to a 25% sodium iodine; however, radiological studies were poor. The ninth contrast injection was administered to a 24-year-old blind man who presented with severe headaches and vomiting. The radiological studies revealed a pituitary tumor. Moniz was ecstatic about their findings and, after reviewing the displacement of the anterior cerebral arteries, Moniz declared the study to be a success. Moniz wasted no time in sharing his findings with his colleagues. In 1927, Moniz traveled to Paris and presented his work to the Neurological Society of Paris (Fig. 5.17) (65). Attending this society meeting were noted men of the field, such as Babinski and Sicard. After Moniz's presentation of his study demonstrating the pituitary lesion, Babinski said that if the tech-

> Arterial radiology has now come to our aid. By this means an intracranial aneurysm can be seen, together with the cerebral arteries, perfectly outlined on the X ray film. Its size, connection, and relations can be seen as clearly as if it were exposed. Our earliest attempts at cerebral arterial radiography were made in 1927, when we used sodium iodide as the opaque medium. This method, then, has put into our hands a means of defining whether a basal intracranial tumor is an aneurysm or some other swelling. Similarly, in a case of suspected aneurysm giving signs of spontaneous subarachnoid hemorrhage, an aneurysm may be detected and located accurately, and treatment planned accordingly. (28)

Krayenbühl and Yaşargil (52) demonstrated complex vascular anatomic variations in both ar-

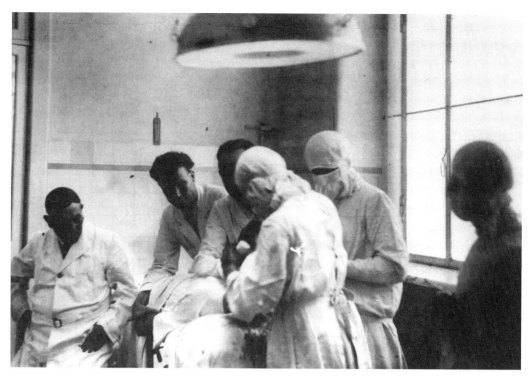

FIGURE 5.16. Egas Moniz (1874–1955) and Almeida Lima (1903–1985). (Courtesy of the Museum of Portugal)

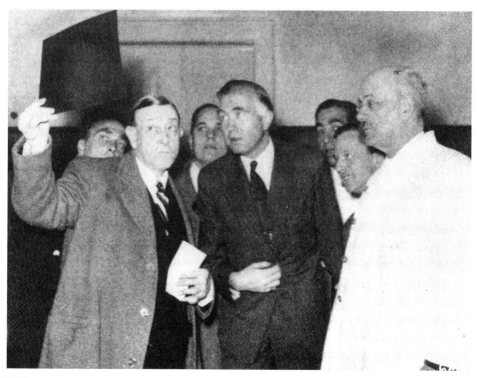

FIGURE 5.17. Egas Moniz (1874–1955) examining an angiograph as requested by a British physician. (Courtesy of the Museum of Portugal)

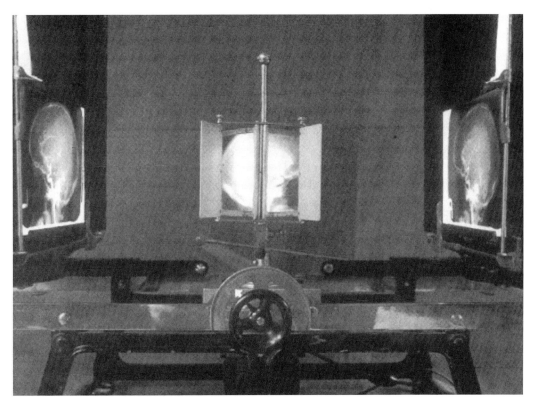

FIGURE 5.18. In 1930, stereoscopic viewing was added to angiographic systems. (From Yaşargil (86); reprinted with permission.)

teries and veins. They performed some 10,000 angiograms (M. G. Yaşargil, personal communication, September 1999). Angiography became and remains an important diagnostic tool in neuroradiology.

Early contrast agents used in cerebral angiography brought about great concerns regarding serious complications. Early agents produced seizure activity, transient and permanent hemiplegia, and even death. In 1928, Thorotrast was introduced for opacification of the liver and spleen. Shortly thereafter, Moniz adapted it to angiography. This became the agent of choice for European physicians; however, in the United States, concern about the radioactivity of Thorotrast prevented its widespread use (9). Until 1936, angiography required surgical exposure of the carotid arteries. In this year, Loman and Myerson performed a direct percutaneous puncture of the carotid artery (9). In 1937, the

use of Thorotrast continued to trouble the medical community. Evidence of risk continued to mount, and after 1940 it became evident that Thorotrast could cause problems such as cirrhosis of the liver and even the development of neoplasms. Both of these complications were related to Thorotrast's low-level radioactivity (9). Other contrast agents were sought for use in cerebral angiography. In 1939, Diodrast was introduced for use in angiography (30). Because of continued problems with contrast agents, angiography was undertaken with great caution. In 1941, Cornelius Dyke expressed his concerns about angiography. He stated, "Its main indication, in my opinion, is to determine whether or not an aneurysm or an arterial venous angioma exists" (29). Dyke (Fig. 5.19) later became the first full-time American neuroradiologist (9). Even with the use of percutaneous carotid puncture techniques, cerebral angiography was not greatly embraced

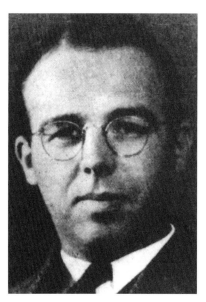

FIGURE 5.19. Cornelius Dyke (1900–1943), the first full-time American neuroradiologist, worked at the Neurological Institute of Columbia–Presbyterian Medical Center, New York (from Bull (9)).

by physicians until safer water-soluble contrast materials could be identified and tested. Diatrizoate sodium (Hypaque) eventually became the superior contrast agent and virtually replaced all other contrast materials for cerebral angiography (9).

In 1951, Seldinger developed a technique of using a guide wire—the next major advancement for cerebral angiography. The guide wire was passed through the puncture needle site, the needle was removed over the wire, and then the catheter was placed over the wire and into the artery. This eliminated the need for a cut-down when catheters were used during angiography (78). Amplatz, in 1963, introduced the use of femorocerebral catheterization. His technique has become the standard by which cerebral angiography is performed (2,3).

RADIOACTIVE ISOTOPES

Despite the enlightenment brought about by cerebral angiography, other methods of visualizing pathological processes of the brain continued. George Moore, a general surgeon, is given credit for the first use of isotopes in the detection of pathological processes. His early work concentrated on the thyroid gland. However, after noting that the use of fluorescein detected abdominal masses, Moore (67) extended his work to include brain tumors. In 1948, Moore and his team theorized that if the blood–brain barrier was altered, dyes could penetrate and disclose certain lesions. They first used fluorescein because even at low concentrations it was detected under ultraviolet light. They changed to sodium diodofluorescein labeled with I-131 for preoperative localization of brain tumors. A Geiger–Muller counter was used to detect any sites of dye uptake (67,68). Radioactive isotopes were considered to offer great possibilities in neuroradiology.

In 1953, G. L. Brownell and William H. Sweet measured the radioactivity of radioactive iodine with an external probe over the brain. Three years later, they refined their technique, which led to the development of radionuclide encephalography, which became a valuable tool in the diagnosis of brain pathology. Their technique was based on the use of positron emitters,

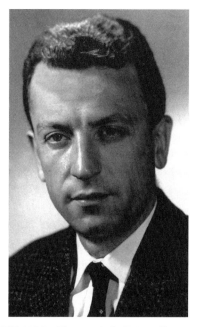

FIGURE 5.20. Giovanni di Chiro. (Courtesy of Mrs. Barbara di Chiro)

such as Mn-52, Cu-64, As-74, and counting methods with collimated detectors (7). The most commonly used radioactive substances were gamma-emitting radioiodinated serum albumin (I-131 tagged human serum albumin) and Hg-203 neohydrin.

In 1964, Giovanni di Chiro (Fig. 5.20) used I-131 serum albumin to study the flow of human cerebrospinal fluid. His radioiodinated serum albumin cisternography techniques increased the understanding of cerebrospinal fluid circulation and laid the groundwork for subsequent studies of hydrocephalus, cerebral atrophy, and rhinorrhea (24,25) (Fig. 5.21). In 1961, di Chiro published his now classic *An Atlas of Detailed Normal Pneumoencephalographic Anatomy* (22) and a companion volume of pathology in 1967 (23). When computed tomography CT was introduced, di Chiro's atlases were used to under-stand better the cross-sectional images. Radionuclide encephalography became a very important noninvasive diagnostic tool for the evaluation of pathology of the brain. Its decline was brought about by the introduction of CT in 1973.

COMPUTED TOMOGRAPHY

The development of CT was a quantum leap forward in neurological radiology. The history of the development of CT is almost as complex as the machine itself. William Oldendorf, a neurologist who performed his own pneumoencephalographic and angiographic studies, was not satisfied with brain imaging for his patients (50,70). In 1958, he was inspired to look for a better way to image the human brain. Oldendorf entered into a discussion with an engineer who had been asked by an orange-growing coopera-

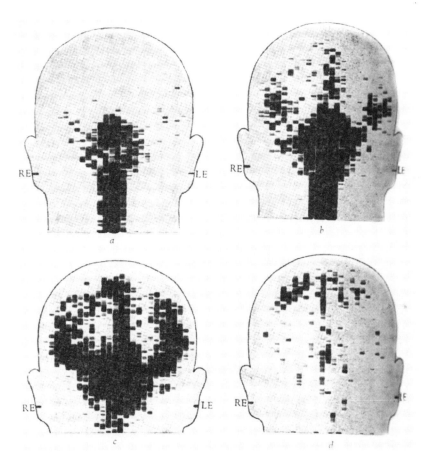

FIGURE 5.21. Movement of cerebrospinal fluid in human beings (from di Chiro (24)).

tive to develop a machine that could distinguish frostbitten oranges from good, marketable oranges. The engineer described the problem to his medical colleague. The problem involved sorting the bad oranges from the good oranges because they all look the same on the outside. Looking on the inside without cutting the orange was indeed a problem. This reminded Oldendorf of the human skull shielding the brain. The orange engineer thought that perhaps a kind of X ray would be helpful. The problem intrigued Oldendorf and he began researching it. His initial machine, developed between 1959 and 1960, consisted of 41 identical iron nails, one aluminum nail, and a plastic block (with holes for the nails) seated on a half original-gauge train flatbed and track. He used a gamma ray source within a lead shield rather than X rays. The gamma ray source sent a collimated beam of high-energy particles through a plane in the phantom head. Its goal was to locate the iron and the aluminum nails at the center of the block when the other 40 iron nails were ringed around

them (Fig. 5.22). The particles emerged, struck a photon detector or counter, and the recognizable dural pattern was then displayed as a two-dimensional image (50). Oldendorf received a patent for his machine in 1963. He approached several radiological manufacturers only to be turned down. One major corporation dismissed him by saying, ''Even if it could be made to work as you suggest, we cannot imagine a significant market for such an expensive apparatus that would do nothing but make radiographic cross-sections of the head'' (50). Oldendorf gave up on a commercial application of his CT scanning machine (70).

The research of Alan Cormack, a nuclear physicist, centered on mapping the body using X rays and the new computer language, Fortran. He developed an experimental scanner, but his clinical application of this device failed when he tried to develop a collaboration with physicians from Massachusetts General Hospital (50). William Sweet thought that perhaps Cormack's methodology would be a help in treating certain

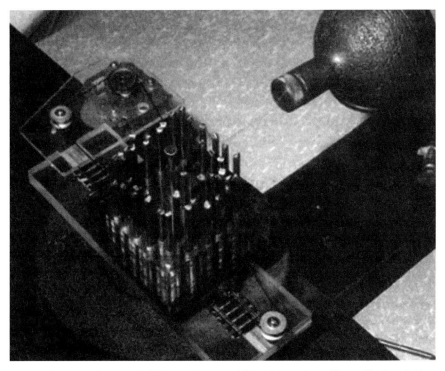

FIGURE 5.22. Oldendorf's model CT scanning machine, June 1960. (From Kevles (50); reprinted with permission.)

conditions, particularly the pituitary gland (50). Cormack, like Oldendorf, tried to find financial support for the development of his machine. He too failed, and his interest turned to other challenges (50). David Kuhl, a radiologist, was the next player to come to bat for computed imaging. While testing the effect of gravitational forces on the blood in Navy astronauts' lungs, a technetium compound was injected. A cross-sectional image of the lungs was obtained to define the site of the radioactivity (50). In 1966, Kuhl published the results of his Navy experimentation. This became the first cross-sectional image ever made by sending radioactive beams through a living subject (53). According to Kevles (50), Kuhl had the technical capacity to continue his cross-sectional imaging studies into computed scanning. All of the pieces of the puzzle were there; however, they were never brought together.

The commercialization of CT came about in the early 1970s as a result of the financial involvement of the London-based Electrical and Musical Industries, Ltd. (EMI). Sir Godfrey Newbold Hounsfield was the man behind the CT project. Hounsfield had a long-standing interest in pattern recognition. EMI developed its medical machine surrounded by a great deal of secrecy (45,50). EMI was founded in 1898 as the Gramophone Company. Through the years, the company became involved in numerous commercial projects. These projects, particularly in the 1950s, involved work in transistors and early computers. In the 1960s, EMI was best known for its involvement with the famous recording artists The Beatles. In fact, during its relationship with The Beatles, more than half the company's considerable earnings came from this recording group. Electronics accounted for less than one-quarter of sales, and medical instruments were nonexistent. It was at this time that Hounsfield began his relationship with EMI. Hounsfield's earlier experience with computers allowed him to understand that computers were able to store retrievable pictures. He became aware that a CT scan would provide more information than an ordinary X ray image. Hounsfield's laboratory demonstrated that cross-sectional scanning would provide an image much more accurate than any present-day conventional method. He and his team soon realized that the viewing of soft-tissue pictures would now be possible with CT. The powers-that-be at EMI needed proof that this machine would indeed be profitable. It was Len Broadway, director of research for EMI and Hounsfield's boss, who provided the needed clinical data to support additional research efforts (50). The Department of Health and Social Security (DHSS) of London was approached. Hounsfield told DHSS officials that this new machine may offer the opportunity to see inside the head and to image the living human brain (50). More than 50 years earlier, the newspaper tycoon, Hearst, challenged Thomas Edison to acquire an X ray image of the brain. The prospect of seeing a living human brain, again, brought about excitement.

In 1967, Hounsfield was introduced to James Ambrose, a British neuroradiologist. For the next 2 years Hounsfield devoted his time to imaging phantom subjects using gamma rays. It took more than 9 days to scan the subject and another 2.5 hours to process the data on the early computer. Soon he replaced the gamma rays with X rays, which immediately reduced the scanning time to 9 hours. His research progressed from using artificial subjects to animals (pig), then to the human brain itself. The initial funding came from EMI and the Medical Research Council of the DHSS. The initial machine was intended only to view the human brain. This project was undertaken with great secrecy. On October 1, 1971, Ambrose and Hounsfield placed their first patient into the newly developed machine. The patient was a 41-year-old woman who presented with symptoms suggesting an intracranial lesion, a brain tumor in the frontal lobe. A dark circular cyst was evident in the frontal lobe (Fig. 5.23). Ambrose (1) recognized this as a tumor that could be addressed surgically (50). It was immediately apparent that many other pathological lesions of the brain could be identified. The living human brain had now been imaged and opened for the entire world to see.

Eventually, numerous other imaging companies became involved in visualizing the human brain. Soon faster and more accurate scanners became available. The CT scan changed and continues to change the lives of patients through-

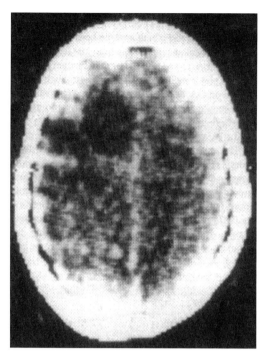

FIGURE 5.23. First clinical CT image obtained from the EMI prototype unit in 1972. In a woman with a suspected brain lesion, the scan clearly shows a dark, circular cyst. (From Kevles (50); reprinted with permission.)

imaging. The CT scan not only changed the evaluation of trauma patients in the emergency room, but it also changed the workup for demyelinating diseases and congenital anomalies in children. Hydrocephalus became readily apparent. In fact, recognizing the value of the CT scan in the pediatric population fueled the development of pediatric neuroradiology. The development of high-resolution scanners capable of obtaining sections as thin as 1 mm and having a wide range of gantry angles expanded imaging of not only the brain, but also the spine, orbital sinuses, temporomandibular joint, soft tissues of the neck, and skull base. Soon the CT scan had a great impact on diseases of the spinal cord, and stand-alone myelography diminished.

In the late 1970s, with the introduction of nonionic contrast materials for myelography, the postmyelographic CT scan became the optimal examination for diagnosing degenerative disc disease, syringomyelia, dysraphism, epidural soft tissues, and a host of other plagues. The CT scan became involved in the dreaded failed-back syndrome. The use of intravenously administered contrast materials distinguished recurrent disc/residual disc from the enhancing scar tissue. The use of stable xenon inhalation followed by sequential scanning has now provided the means for the measurement of cerebral blood flow. Today the CT scan is a major contributor to any part of a hospital's daily activities. It is difficult for most of us to ever imagine a hospital without a CT scanner.

In 1973, Dr. Hounsfield stated, "It is possible that this technique may open up a new chapter in X ray diagnosis" (45). Not only did it open up a new chapter, but it changed forever X ray diagnosis.

out the world by giving physicians the ability to look inside the body. In 1975, the Nobel Prize Committee for Medicine awarded the prestigious Prize to Godfrey Hounsfield and Allen Cormack (Fig. 5.24).

The CT scanner soon began to appear throughout the world. As this happened, the number of pneumoencephalograms fell to virtually zero. The medical literature became filled with papers and presentations about computed

Allan M.Cormack
(1924-1998)

USA

Tufts University
Medford,MA

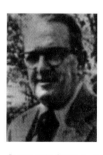

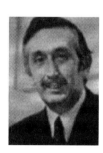

Sir Godfrey N.Hounsfield
(1919-   )

Great Britain

Central Research Labs, EMI
London

FIGURE 5.24. Allan M. Cormack (1924–1998) and Sir Godfrey N. Hounsfield (1919–).

MAGNETIC RESONANCE IMAGING

The introduction of magnetic resonance imaging (MRI) to neuroradiology was a natural event. The medical community was ready. CT had demonstrated that clinical tools could come from industry. Wolfgang Pauli, in 1924, suggested that protons and/or neutrons inside atomic nuclei would, under certain conditions, move with angular momentum or spin and become magnetic. Pauli went on to receive the Nobel Prize in 1945 for his work on atomic fusion (16,50). Dr. Isador Rabi, in the fall of 1937, demonstrated that the nuclear resonance signal was a physical reality. He coined the phrase *nuclear magnetic resonance* or *NMR*. In 1944, Dr. Rabi received the Nobel Prize for his method of measuring NMR (16,50). In 1946, Purcell, Torrey, and Pound (72) achieved the first nuclear resonance in bulk matter, a block of paraffin. Felix Block attained the same achievement in a sample of ordinary water. Block provided the mathematical characterizations of the nuclear resonance that MRI clinicians depend on today. The Block equations include the two rate constants, T1 and T2, that govern the rate of decay of the nuclear signal that are central to the formation of an MR image (16,50). The demonstrations of the behavior of certain nuclei in certain conditions initiated the new scientific discipline of NMR. Chemists immediately saw this as an excellent tool for chemical analysis. It would take, however, some 25 years before the medical applications of NMR would be recognized. In 1949, Edward Erwin Hahn discovered a second nuclear resonance signal, the spin echo. This was a major advance for imaging. By adjusting the echo timing one could now produce two pictures from the nuclear signal instead of one (16,50). The first NMR machines were quite unruly devices; they were cumbersome and used magnets, transmitters, and receivers that were all connected to a unit that recorded spectra. The study of organic compounds became the focus of most NMR research. In 1959, J. Singer studied blood flow in mice with an NMR machine. This was a major advance toward clinical imaging in that this technique could now be used successfully to study living creatures without harming them (16,50). It was now becoming evident that NMR spectroscopy may have a place in the field of medical imaging.

In 1947, Nicolaas Bloembergen characterized the relaxation times of nuclear response signals in more detail. He demonstrated that their values depended on the sample itself. Therefore, he concluded that these relaxation times varied with sample viscosity (16,50).

Raymond V. Damadian, a young physician and researcher, decided in the late 1960s to analyze water in different types of tumors using NMR. In 1970, tumor-burdened rat brains were evaluated at an NMR facility outside of Pittsburgh, Pennsylvania. As predicted, the tumor differed from healthy brain (18,50). Damadian recognized that relaxation times possessed the necessary discerning power in tissues to make NMR scanning a reality in clinical medicine. He began work on developing a new machine, an NMR machine that was capable of imaging the entire human body for the presence of abnormalities. His idea to develop such a machine was not accepted by the entire community (50). In the summer of 1977, Damadian and his research team introduced to the world his NMR imaging machine, which he called ''Indomitable'' (50). On March 17, 1972, Damadian filed for a United States patent for an apparatus and method of detecting cancer in tissue (Fig. 5.25) (16,17,50). The patent was granted in 1974. In 1973, Paul Lauterbur, a chemist, improved the NMR situation. He developed a technique he called *zeugmatography*, from the Greek for ''joining together.'' He answered the question of how to get from the one-dimensional spatial representation of a single gradient to a complete two-dimensional scan. He joined the gradient magnetic field and the radio frequency that corresponded to it in a single image (16,50). In 1973, his paper on image formation was published in *Nature* (55). His first scan was on two 1-mm test tubes of water (55). Unfortunately he was not able to file a patent on his discovery (50). Lauterbur's paper brought about a great deal of attention. Dr. Richard R. Earnst provided the next step in the development and refinement of MRI. Earnst had earlier pioneered the application of the Fourier transform to chemical spectroscopy as a means for obtaining chemical spectra of repulsed signals rather than from continuous-wave signals. Dr. Earnst and his colleagues, Dr. Anil Kumar and Deieter Welti, introduced a new

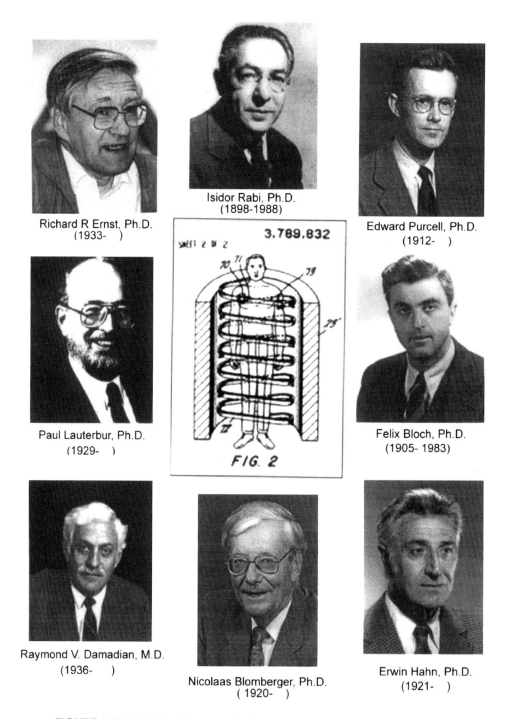

Richard R Ernst, Ph.D.
(1933-   )

Isidor Rabi, Ph.D.
(1898-1988)

Edward Purcell, Ph.D.
(1912-   )

Paul Lauterbur, Ph.D.
(1929-   )

Felix Bloch, Ph.D.
(1905- 1983)

Raymond V. Damadian, M.D.
(1936-   )

Nicolaas Blomberger, Ph.D.
(1920-   )

Erwin Hahn, Ph.D.
(1921-   )

FIGURE 5.25. MRI development. In the center is Damadian's patent picture.

technique of forming two- or three-dimensional images of a microscopic sample by means of NMR (16,50). Their technique provided a way of quickly receiving digital information. Peter Mansfield, a physicist at the University of Nottingham, focused his efforts on the ability to image solids with NMR. In March 1974, he imaged an entire mouse (62). In fact, the image was so sharp that it actually revealed a fracture of the animal's neck. He quickly applied for a Medical Research Council grant (50). The clinical expectations of MRI began to develop throughout the medical community. In the 1970s, physicians began to expect better radiological imaging of the nervous system. It soon became appreciated that NMR had the potential for becoming a major part of radiology, particularly neuroradiology. However, NMR was not a term that would be readily accepted by the medical world, much less by the lay population. NMR was a chemical research tool, and the word "nuclear" provoked negative feelings. Therefore, NMR was changed in the clinical environment to MRI. By the early 1980s, MRI had arrived. There is no doubt that MRI is a major part of any neuroradiology suite.

In 1872, James Da Costa, a noted physician at Jefferson Medical College, addressed an audience regarding medical progress. He stated,

> Let us take a glimpse into the future. Madam is in her boudoir, reclining on the sofa, in expectation of her medical attendance, when a team of four arrive: one to get a history and volumetric reading of every fluid in her body; a second to record her pulse and muscle contractions; a third uses an improved ophthalmoscope "to take photographs of her eyes," and finally, Dr. Magnet who gets the equivalent of an X ray. (15)

Dr. Da Costa's look into the future has become a reality, and Dr. Magnet is here. Although MRI began in the radiology suite, it is beginning to migrate to the operating theater (Fig. 5.26).

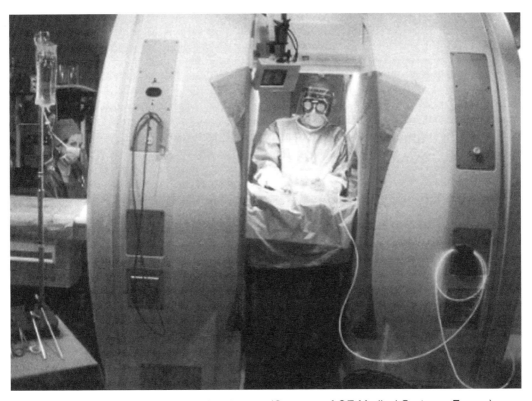

FIGURE 5.26. MRI in the operating theater. (Courtesy of GE Medical Systems, Europe)

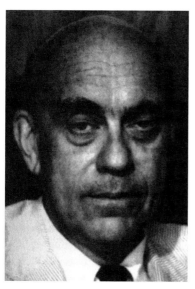

FIGURE 5.27. Alfred J. Luessenhop (1926–).

INTERVENTIONAL NEURORADIOLOGY

The concept of interventional neuroradiology is ascribed to Alfred Luessenhop (Fig. 5.27), a neurosurgeon at Georgetown University. His first effort was directed toward large arteriovenous malformations of the brain, which he embolized (59–61). Subsequently, percutaneous embolization of spinal cord angiomas was performed by Newton and Adams (69), and Doppman, di Chiro, and Ommaya (27) based on the existing techniques for spinal angiography (40).

Soon, there was new work in the development of magnetically guided catheters, and the development of balloon catheter techniques (40,43). Placement of detachable balloons in carotid cavernous fistulas by Serbinenko (79), a neurosurgeon from Moscow, served as a stimulus for physicians and surgeons. Interventional neuroradiology moved rapidly ahead (40). In 1975, Kerber, Bank, and Cromwell (48) developed an important technique using the "calibrated leak balloon" (40). Using this technique, a balloon catheter was passed into the intracranial arteries. When the balloon was inflated with the contrast medium, it obstructed antegrade arterial flow. At a prescribed degree of dilatation of the balloon, its contents were discharged into the artery distal to the obstruction. This was a significant advance. Soon a liquid embolization material, isobutyl cyanoacrylate, which forms a polymerized cast of the malformation on contact with ions in blood, began to be used with the calibrated leak balloon (40). Other embolization materials included polyvinyl alcohol, plastic spheres, coils, and detachable balloons made of latex and other materials. All interventionalist investigators owe a debt to René Djindjian et al. (26) of Paris, who, with his trainees, brought exquisite, superselective studies to the world's attention (40). Moret, Manelfe, Theron, Merland, Lasjaunias, Picard, and others carried the work forward after Djindjian's untimely death (40,63).

POSITRON EMISSION TOMOGRAPHY (PET)

PET is an inside–outside procedure in that it involves injecting a radioactive substance into a patient and then tracking the position of that substance on the inside from the outside. Emission tomography images a source that emits radiation, unlike CT and MRI, which are transmission techniques. The development of the PET machine involved the combining of two technologies: the first was the creation and then the safe application of biologically useful tracers, and the next was the construction of refined instrumentation that would be able to detect radioactive sources emitted from the body (50). Hevesy, a Hungarian physicist, devoted his life to working with naturally occurring radioisotopes. In 1935, Hevesy fed radioisotopes to his laboratory animals and then, on autopsy, he discovered that in each particular case the isotopes had migrated to a particular organ. This finding brought about the surge for new radiopharmaceuticals. Hevesy would later win the Nobel Prize for chemistry in 1943 for his work with radioactive substances.

After World War II, the Atomic Energy Commission provided isotopes for research endeavors. Select hospitals around the country were now provided with such material to begin their investigations (8,50). In 1951, Benedict Cassen, of the University of California at Los Angeles, brought about the next major step in the development of a PET machine for clinical use. He recognized that a newly developed photomultiplier tube (image intensifier) may be of use for isotopic readings. The photomultiplier tube allowed cameras to capture moving pictures of fluoroscopic images from a scintillating screen (49,50). This new device—the scintiscanner—allowed the reproduction of a crude picture of a spatial representation (50). Three years later the scintiscanner was replaced by the photoscan. In 1954, David Kuhl was able to record an image by sending the alpha rays from the photomultiplier tube directly onto a moving beam of light and then onto a sheet of photographic paper (50). In 1957, Sokoloff began experimenting with 2-deoxyglucose. He suggested that perhaps 2-deoxyglucose could be used to study cerebral blood flow. Almost 20 years later, Kuhl, Wolf, and Fowler attached radioactive fluorine to 2-deoxyglucose. This radioactive chemical, FDG, was well received and became an often-used radiopharmaceutical (50). In 1968, single photon emission computed tomography (SPECT) was developed. This was Kuhl's first system for mapping emissions from radioactive substances. Kuhl added a computer to the system. Niels Lassen, in 1972, used SPECT to track cerebral blood flow to correlate with function. Soon he introduced the use of color in the computer-reconstructed image (54). The use of color in computed imaging was received with mixed blessings. The color acceptors argued that color would delineate one kind of tissue from another. Opponents stated that the color merely exaggerated tissue differences and was only of use to help with public relations and subsequent investors (50). New generations of PET scanners soon became available. This imaging tool proved itself to be worthwhile, particularly in treating malignancies such as brain tumors. This imaging modality looks inside into the regional chemistry of a tumor and can often detect changes before structural signs are evident. The PET scanner and its offspring have provided oncologists with the means of evaluating the effectiveness of treatment (12). PET scanning has now provided physicians a means to evaluate brain dysfunction from numerous etiologies; however, a PET scan is not inexpensive, and the cost of operating such a machine often precludes its use. Currently, a functional MRI performs functional imaging. What was once a monopoly of the PET scanners is being taken over by a machine that is already operating in most hospitals. The ability of PET to demonstrate some degree of functioning of the brain has brought about an entirely new level in the world of neuroimaging. One can be most assured that, in this new millennium, emission tomography will play just as great a part in imaging as transmission studies.

TOMORROW

Neuroradiology was conceived in the 19th century but was born in the 20th century. It grew from the commitments of many dedicated individuals from numerous disciplines and countless brave patients. Only a few of those special individuals were named in this brief communication. They came from the ranks of clinicians (neurologists, surgeons, neurosurgeons, radiologists, and internists), engineers, physicists, chemists, mathematicians, nurses, technologists, and others. In 1896, William Randolph Hearst challenged Thomas Edison to produce a picture of the living brain. The challenge was met; however, it took some 71 years. The ability to see the pathology brought about new and better forms of therapy, both surgical and medical. Today the central nervous system is better imaged than at any other time in history. The ability to see the nervous system is limited only by our imaginations.

ACKNOWLEDGMENTS

The authors thank Betty Patterson for her patience, editing talents, and ability to find the owner of old pictures. We are also grateful to Ron Tribell, Chief Medical Illustrator, for ensuring that the figures and photographs were produced in a professional fashion.

REFERENCES

1. Ambrose J. Computed transverse axial scanning (tomography) pt. 2: Clinical applications. *Br J Radiol* 46: 1023–1047, 1973.

2. Amplatz K. An improved chair for pneumoencephalography and autotomography. *AJR Am J Roentgenol* 90: 184–188, 1963.

3. Amplatz K, Resch J, Hilal S. A catheter approach for cerebral angiography. *Radiology* 81:576–583, 1963.

4. Antunes JL. Egas Moniz and cerebral angiography. *J Neurosurg* 40:427–432, 1974.

5. Beclère A. La radiographie du crâne et le diagnostic de l'acromegalia. *Bull Mem Soc Med Hôp (Paris)* Dec. 5, 1902.

6. Brooks B. Intra-arterial injection of sodium iodine: Preliminary report. *JAMA* 82:1016–1019, 1924.

7. Brownell GL, Sweet WH. Scanning of positron-emitting isotopes in diagnosis of intracranial and other lesions. *Acta Radiol* 46:425–434, 1956.

8. Brucer M. Nuclear medicine begins with a boa constrictor. *J Nucl Med* 19:581–598, 1978.

9. Bull JWD. History of neuroradiology. *Br J Radiol* 34: 63–84, 1961.

10. Caldas JP. Arteriographie en série avec l'appareil radio-carrousel. *J Radiol Elect* 18:34–39, 1934.

11. Church A. Cerebellar tumor; recognized clinically, demonstrated by the X ray, and proved by autopsy. *Am J Med Sci* 117:126–130,1899.

12. Conti PS. Introduction to imaging brain tumor metabolism with positron emission tomography (PET). *Cancer Invest* 13:244–259, 1995.

13. Cushing H. Haematomyelia from gunshot wound of the cervical spine. *Bull Johns Hopkins Hosp* 8:195–197, 1897.

14. Cushing H. Haematolomyelia from gunshot wounds of the spine. A report of two cases, with recovery following symptoms of hemilesion of the cord. *Am J Med Sci* 115: 654–683, 1898.

15. Da Costa J. Modern medicine. Philadelphia, JB Lippincott, 1872, p 18.

16. Damadian RV. The History of MRI. Presented at the High Care '97 International Congress, Bochum, Germany, January 31–February 3, 1997.

17. Damadian RV. Tumor detection by nuclear magnetic resonance. *Science* 171:1151–1153, 1971.

18. Damadian R, Zaner K, Hor D, et al. Human tumors by NMR. *Physiol Chem Phys* 5:381–402, 1973.

19. Dandy WE. Röntgenography of the brain after the injection of air into the spinal canal. *Ann Surg* 70:397–403, 1919.

20. Dandy WE. Pneumoperitoneum: A method of detecting intestinal perforation—an aid in abdominal diagnosis. *Ann Surg* 70:379, 1919.

21. Dandy WE. Ventriculography following the injection of air into the cerebral ventricles. *Ann Surg* 68:6, 1918.

22. di Chiro G. An atlas of detailed normal pneumoencephalographic anatomy. Springfield, IL, Charles C Thomas, 1961.

23. di Chiro. An atlas of pathologic pneumoencephalographic anatomy. Springfield, IL, Charles C Thomas, 1967.

24. di Chiro G. Movement of the cerebral spinal fluid in human beings. *Nature* 204:290–291, 1964.

25. di Chiro G. Observations on the circulation of the cerebrospinal fluid. *Acta Radiol (Diagn)* 5:125–143, 1964.

26. Djindjian R, Cophignon J, Theron J, et al. Embolization by superselective arteriography from the femoral route in neuroradiology: Review of 60 cases. 1. Technique,

indications, complications. *Neuroradiology* 6:20–26, 1973.

27. Doppman JL, di Chiro G, Ommaya A. Obliteration of spinal-cord arteriovenous malformation by percutaneous embolisation. *Lancet* 1:477, 1968.

28. Dott NM. Intracranial aneurysms: Cerebral arterio-radiography. Surgical treatment. 40:219–234, 1933.

29. Dyke CG. Indirect signs of brain tumor as noted in routine roentgen examinations. Displacement of the pineal shadow. (A survey of 3000 consecutive skull examinations.) *AJR Am J Roentgenol* 23:598–606, 1930.

30. Fischgold H, Bull J. A short history neuroradiology. Presented at the VIIth Symposium Neuroradiologicum, Paris, France, September 1967.

31. Fox WL. Dandy of Johns Hopkins. Baltimore, Williams & Wilkins, 1984, pp 80, 175.

32. Fuchs A. Edison and roentgenology. *AJR Am J Roentgenol* 57:146–152, 1947.

33. Gawler J, et al. Computerized axial tomography with EMI-scanner, in Krayenbühl H (ed): *Advances and Technical Standards in Neurosurgery.* New York, Springer-Verlag, Wien, 1975, pp 3–32.

34. Glasser O. Dr. W. C. Röntgen. 2nd ed. Springfield, IL, Charles C Thomas, 1971.

35. Glasser O. Wilhelm Conrad Roentgen and the Early History of the Roentgen Rays. Springfield, IL, Charles C Thomas, 1934.

36. Gobo OJ. Localization techniques: Neuroimaging and electroencephalography, in Greenblatt SH, Dagi TF, Epstein MH (eds): *A History of Neurosurgery.* Park Ridge, IL, AANS, 1997, pp 223–246.

37. Gross SW. Cerebral angiography by means of a rapidly excreted organic iodide. *Arch Neurol Psychiatry* 44: 217–222, 1940.

38. Gutierrez C. The birth and growth of neuroradiology in the USA. *Neuroradiology* 21:227–237, 1981.

39. Haschek E, Linderthal OT. Ein beitrag zur pmmischen verwethung der photographie nach Röntgen. *Wien Klin Wochenschr* 9:63–64, 1896.

40. Heinz ER. History of neuroradiology, in Wilkins RH, Rengachary SS (eds): *Neurosurgery.* 2nd ed., New York, McGraw Hill, 1996, pp 11–23.

41. Henschen F. Die Akustikustumoren, eine neve Gruppe radiographisch darstellbarer Hirntumoren. *Fortschr Roentgenstr* 18:207–216, 1912.

42. Henschen SE. Die Röntgen–Strahlen im Dienste der Hirnchirurgie, Comptes rendus du XII Congrès International de Médecine, Moscow, 1897.

43. Hilal SK, Michelsen J, Driller J, et al. Magnetically guided devices for the vascular exploration: Potentials and limitations. Presented at the IX Symposium Neuroradiologicum, Gothenburg, Sweden, 1970.

44. Hockman MS, Stewart DA. Neuroradiology, in Gagliardi RA, McClennan BL, Knight N (eds): *A History of the Radiological Sciences.* Reston, VA, 1984.

45. Hounsfield GN. Computed medical imaging. Nobel lecture. *J Comput Assist Tomogr* 4:665–674, 1980.

46. Jacobaeus HC. On insufflation of air into the spinal canal for diagnostic purposes in cases of tumors of the spinal canal. *Acta Med Scand* 55:555–564, 1921.

47. Keen WW. The clinical application of the Roentgen rays. II in surgical diagnosis. *Proc Coll Phys Phil* (3rd ser.) 18:104–110, 1896.

48. Kerber CW, Bank WO, Cromwell LD. Calibrated leak balloon–microcatheter: A device for arterial exploration

and occlusive therapy. *AJR Am J Roentgenol* 132: 207–212, 1979.

49. Kereiakes JG. The history and development of medical physics instrumentation: Nuclear medicine. *Med Phys* 14:146–155, 1987.

50. Kevles BH. *Naked to the Bone: Medical Imaging in the Twentieth Century.* Reading, MA, Addison–Wesley, 1997.

51. Krause F (trans). Surgery of the brain and spinal cord based on personal experiences. 3 Vols., New York, Rebman Co., 1909–1912.

52. Krayunbühl H, Yaşargil MG. Die zerebrale Angiographie. Stuttgart, Thieme, 1964.

53. Kuhl D. Transmission scanning. *Radiology* 87: 278–289, 1966.

54. Lassen N. On the history of measurement of cerebral blood flow in man by radioactive isotopes, in Costa DC, Morgan CF, Lassen N (eds): *New Trends in Nuclear Neurology and Psychiatry.* London, John Libbey and Company, 1993, pp 3–13.

55. Lauterber PC. Image formation by induced local interactions: Examples employing nuclear magnetic resonance. *Nature* 242:190–191, 1973.

56. Lindgren E. A history of neuroradiology, in Newton TH, Potts DG (eds): *Radiology of the Skull and Brain. The Skull, Volume 1, Book 1.* St. Louis, CV Mosby, 1971, pp 1–25.

57. Luckett WH. Air in the ventricles of the brain following a fracture of the skull. *J Nerv Ment Dis* 40:326–328, 1913.

58. Luckett WH. Air in the ventricles of the brain following a fracture of the skull. Report of a case. *Surg Gynecol Obstet* 17:237–240, 1913.

59. Luessenhop AJ. Artificial embolization for cerebral arteriovenous malformations. *Prog Neurol Surg* 3: 320–362, 1969.

60. Luessenhop AJ, Spence WT. Artificial embolization of cerebral arteries: Report of use in a case of arteriovenous malformation. *JAMA* 172:1153–1155, 1960.

61. Luessenhop AJ, Valesquez AC. Observations on the tolerance of the intracranial arteries to catheterization. *J Neurosurg* 21:85–91, 1964.

62. Mansfield P. Proton spin imaging by nuclear magnetic resonance. *Contemp Phys* 17:553–576, 1976.

63. Merland JJ, Riche MC, Chiras J, et al. Therapeutic angiography in neuroradiology. Classical data, recent advances and perspectives. *Neuroradiology* 21:111–121, 1981.

64. Mixter WJ, Barr J. Rupture of the intervertebral disc with involvement of the spinal canal. *N Engl J Med* 211: 210–215, 1934.

65. Moniz E. L'angiographie cérébrale. Ses applications et résultats en anatomie, physiologie et clinique. Paris, Masson, 1934.

66. Moniz E. L'encéphalographie artérielle, son importance dans la localization des tumeurs cérébrales. *Rev Neurol* 2:72–90, 1927.

67. Moore GE. Use of radioactive diodofluorescein in the diagnosis and localization of brain tumors. *Science* 107: 569–571, 1948.

68. Moore GE, Kohl DA, Marvin JF, et al. Biophysical studies of methods utilizing fluorescein and its derivatives to diagnosis brain tumors. *Radiology* 55:344–362, 1950.

69. Newton TH, Adams JE. Angiographic demonstration and nonsurgical embolization of spinal cord angioma. *Radiology* 91:873–876, 1968.

70. Oldendorf WH. The quest for an image of the brain. New York, Raven Press, 1980.

71. Pfahler GE. Cerebral akiagraphy. *Trans Am Roentgen Ray Soc* 5:175–181, 1905.

72. Potts OG, Taveras JM. A new somersaulting chair for pneumoencephalography. *AJR Am J Roentgenol* 91: 1144–1149, 1964.

73. Purcell EM, Torrey HC, Pound RF. Resonance absorption by nuclear magnetic moments in a solid. *Physiol Rev* 69:37–38, 1946.

74. Röntgen WC. On a new kind of ray. Sitzgsber Physik-Med Ges Würzburg, 1895, CXXXVII. Ann Physik Chem, N.F. 64:1, 1898.

75. Schüller A. Archiv und Atlas der normalen und pathologischen Anatomie in typischen Röentgenbildern. Die Schädelbasis im Röentgenbilde. Hamburg, Gräfe & Sillem, 1905.

76. Schüller A. Röntgenologie in ihren Beziehungen zur Neurologie. *Dtsch Z Nervenheilkd* 50:188–202, 1914.

77. Schuster NH. Early days of Roentgen photography in Britain. *BMJ* 2:1164–1166, 1962.

78. Seldinger SI. Catheter replacement of the needle in percutaneous arteriography: A new technique. *Acta Radiol* 39:368–376, 1953.

79. Serbinenko FA. Balloon catheterization and occlusion of major cerebral vessels. *J Neurosurg* 41:125–145, 1974.

80. Sicard JA, Forestier J. Methode générale d'exploration radiologique par l'huile iodeé (Lipiodol). *Bull Mem Soc Med Hôp (Paris)* 46:463–469, 1922.

81. Skalpe IO, Amundsen P. Lumbar radiculography and metrizamide: A nonionic water-soluble contrast medium. *Radiology* 115:91–95, 1975.

82. Steinhansen TG, Dungan CE, Furst JB, et al. Iodinated organic compounds as contrast media for radiographic diagnoses. III. Experimental and clinical myelography with ethyliopophenylundecylate (Pantopaque). *Radiology* 43:230–234, 1944.

83. Stewart WH. Fracture of the skull with air in the ventricles. *AJR Am J Roentgenol* 1:83–87, 1913.

84. Taveras JM. Neuroradiology: Past, present, future. *Radiology* 175:593–602, 1990.

85. Tondreau RL. The retrospectoscope: Egas Moniz 1874–1955. *Radiographics* 5:994–997, 1985.

86. Yaşargil MG. Microneurosurgery: Microneurosurgery of CNS tumors. Vol. IVB., Stuttgart, Thiem, 1996.

6

The History of Optical Instruments and Microneurosurgery

M. Gazi Yasargil, MD

On November 3, 1999, in Boston, I was asked to deliver a chapter concerning the history of microneurosurgery. I accepted this challenging invitation with reservations, being aware that I lacked an academic background in history. However, because of my experience in the fields of neuroradiology, stereotactic neurosurgery, neurosurgery, and microneurosurgery for a period of 50 years, and through the many worldwide relationships in neuroscience that I have had the privilege to develop, it can be presumed I have actually "lived" the history of neurosurgery for half a century, and therefore qualify to reflect on historical events and circumstances. My aim in writing this contribution is to relay reliable information that will guide medical historians of the future in their research.

A review of the comparatively short but ongoing history of microneurosurgery reveals several aspects, including the technological evolution relating to the production of optical instruments in general and to the operating microscope in particular, and the scientific and technological developments incorporated in the art of neurosurgery and microneurosurgery.

TECHNOLOGICAL EVOLUTION OF OPTICAL INSTRUMENTS

A great number of inspiring publications are devoted to the history of the optical instruments such as crystal and glass lenses, which had already been manufactured 4000 years ago, spectacles in the 14th century, simple microscopes and telescopes in the 16th century, compound microscopes and telescopes in the 17th century, stereoscopic binocular microscopes in the 19th century, and operating microscopes in the 20th century.

The publications of historians offer us detailed descriptions of the technological and scientific evolution since the 17th century, but there is a remarkable uncertainty in definition and interpretation of the facts before the 17th century. Reading the informative books of Carpenter–Dallinger, Clay-Court, Bradbury, Hansen et al., Turner, Rosenthal, and Manguel, I consider the introductory remarks of Bradbury to be of great significance and value. I have, therefore, borrowed the following sentences from his publication:

> People are naturally curious about their surroundings. Their bodies need detailed information about the world around them in order that they may adapt smoothly to the demands and processes of living. More important, in human beings the search for information is carried much further than the bare requirements for existence in order to satisfy our innate desire to understand the world in which we live. We are provided with various receptive mechanisms or senses to help gather such informa-

tion: of all these senses, the most important by far is that of sight.

It seems natural, therefore, that when we want detailed information about some part of our surroundings we first take a very close look at it. Such visual examinations are normally perfectly adequate for the day to day processes of living, but we must remember that the visual gathering of detailed information relating to our surroundings, and the classification and study of such knowledge forms a large part of the discipline known as "natural science." For such purposes the human eye often proves to be a very inadequate tool indeed, excellent though it may be for the normal needs of existing in our world; this is because the amount of detail which it can reveal to us is very limited.

In "natural sciences," studies of both objects at great distances such as the stars, and very minute objects and structural details of larger objects were limited by the capabilities of the human eye. As more and more scientists took up such studies the need for supplementing the human eye became apparent; when the method of combining lenses to obtain an enlarged image was discovered at the end of the sixteenth century its possibilities were rapidly realized. The needs of the scientists stimulated rapid progress in microscopy and this, in its turn, gave immense benefits and impetus to the work of the scientists.

Probably the world's original lens was a clear pebble taken from the stream bed. After being tumbled by the water, it acted as a magnifying glass. In the graves of antique time periods, glass and crystal lenses have been found, dating to 2000 BC (Knossos, Cyprus, Ephesus, Troy, and Mesopotamia), and a lead eye shield was found in northwestern China (Uygur) and was dated to the 8th century AD, where paper was also invented in 200 AD. The art of glass melting and glass grinding has been practiced for a long time. Generations of people who polished quartz certainly observed its optical properties, in particular its magnifying effect. Remarkable also is that the *Old Testament* mentions mirrors, cutting of precious stones, and preparation of glass, but nowhere does it mention spectacles. The same is true for the *Talmud,* although it also mentions artificial teeth. However, the evolution of optical aids remained slow despite the fact that a great number of people had inborn or acquired weakness of their visual acuity. The fate of the poor-

sighted people remained unchanged until the 14th century, and for the most of them until the 16th century.

Nothing is known with certainty about the invention of spectacles. On February 23, 1306, from the pulpit of the Church of Santa Maria Novella in Florence, Giordano da Rivalto of Pisa reminded his flock of the invention of eye glasses, but he did not mention the name of the inventor. A manuscript from the ministry of St. Catherina of Pisa commemorating a death in 1313 says, "Brother Alexander della Spina . . . made spectacles which had been previously made by no one" (Rosenthal). A. A. Disney, in 1928, gave credit to Armati. An inscription in the Church of Maria Maggiore in Florence reads, "There lives Salvino d'Aramento degli Armato of Florence, inventor of spectacles. May God pardon his sins. MCCXVII." His sins were that he kept the secret of the manufacture of spectacles (Clay-Court).

The earliest known depiction of eye glasses is in a 1352 portrait of Cardinal Hugo de St. Cher, in Provence, by Tomasso de Modena. There is a unique portrait of Pope Leo X, painted by Raffael (1513–1520), with a magnifying glass in his hand, evidently intended to examine carefully the pages of a book open before him. The picture of Cardinal Guevera (Spain), painted by El Greco (1596–1600), shows him wearing spectacles.

It took another 300 years until eye glasses became generally available because "glasses" were shaped out of precious stone, either quartz or beryl, and there was substantial difficulty in polishing them. Moreover, the correction of visual defects must have been approximate, given the small amount of information known about optics and optometry at the time.

> The spectacles were expensive and few people needed them, since books themselves were in the possession of few people. After the invention of the printing press and relative popularization of the books, the demands for eyeglasses increased. (Manguel)

Besides the socioeconomic factors, the evolution of the technology needed for optical instruments required additional advances in science, particularly in mathematics.

Probably the first real appreciation of the action of a lens, in particular the ability of a convex form to produce a magnified image of an object, is attributed to the Arabian mathematician and astronomer Ibn Al-Haitham (926–1038), more commonly known by the Latin form of his name Alhazen (Bradbury). In his book *Optics*, he says, "If an object placed in a dense spherical medium of which the curved surface is turned to the eye and is between the eye and the center of the sphere, the object will appear magnified." Alhazen analyzed experimentally and theoretically the optic system, and he was the first to analyze the principle of the camera obscura, but no practical application of his observation was recorded (Bradbury, Lindberg).

Robert Grosseteste (1168–1253), Bishop of Lincoln and teacher of Roger Bacon, was interested in optics, and used Alhazen's book as his guide. He experimented with mirrors and with lenses (Manguel).

Roger Bacon (1220–1292) was obviously well versed in the theoretical and experimental studies of his predecessors, including Alhazen, for Bacon applied this knowledge of optics to such practical ends as the design of burning glasses and devising paraboloidal mirrors to concentrate the sun's rays to a point for the same purpose (Bradbury). He wrote a full account of his investigation in *Opus Majus*. In the year 1268, he wrote

> If one looks at letters or other minute things through the medium of crystal or glass or other lens put over the letters, and if it is the smaller portion of the sphere of which the convexity is towards the eye, and the eye in the air, he will see the letters much better and they will appear larger to him . . . Therefore this instrument is useful to the aged and to those with weak eyes . . . So we may even make the sun, moon, and stars descend lower in appearance. (Clay-Court)

Bacon clearly understood the principle of using a planoconvex lens as a magnifier, but he did not construct a single magnifier, as far as we know—the last 14 years of his life he was imprisoned.

In 1250, Vitellio, a Polish scientist, wrote a treatise on optics and compiled accurate tables of the angles of incidence and refraction of light at the surface of water and glass.

Leonardo da Vinci had been greatly interested in anatomy and physiology of the eye in the 1490s. He performed numerous physical and physiological experiments concerning vision. He devised complicated systems of light transmission using lenses, glass balls, or mirrors to simulate the structure and function of the eye. There is a unique drawing by Leonardo da Vinci that shows human faces wearing spectacles. In 1492, Leonardo da Vinci invented theoretically a telescope without a concave lens, and in 1508 he developed a telescope with a concave lens. In *Codex Arundel* (Atlanticus, Fol. 396 Verso-f), a drawing shows a concave mirror with a focus of 60.0 m for a gigantic telescope, which was planned to be erected in the Belvedere Garden in Rome (1513–1517). This plan was not realized because Leonardo da Vinci went to Amboise on the Loire River, France, where he spent the last year of his life at the Royal Manor of Cloux. He wrote about his ideas and experiments in code in voluminous notebooks that were not published until the 19th century (1892–1916).

In 1530, another great Italian scientist, Geralomo Fracastoro (1483–1553), made reference to a compound lens system. Gian Battista della Porta (1543–1615) provides, in one of his books entitled *Of Strange Glasses,* clear evidence of the practical use to which lenses had been applied in the 16th century for the correction of visual defects (Bradbury). Porta claimed to have invented a telescope in 1585.

There are conflicting opinions among historians concerning the contribution of China to the evolution of optic instruments. Needham accords credit to the Chinese instrument makers and scientists Po Yue and Sun Yuen Chiu, who manufactured optical instruments from 1620 to 1630. Telescopes were available for use in artillery battles in 1635. In 1638, Yuen Chiu wrote a book describing "strange instruments" such as the magnifying loupe, microscope, barometer, thermometer, and lanterna magica, which were manufactured by Huang Lue-Chuang. Needham said that the transmission of technology to China from the West was rapid, but that the Chinese already had magnifying glasses in use for reading, and dark glasses made of smooth quartz to be worn as protection against bright light. This synchronous evolution of advances in science and technology that was taking place in both the eastern and western regions of the world at the beginning of the 17th century is an interesting phenomenon worthy of note.

THE INVENTION OF THE MICROSCOPE AND THE TELESCOPE

The manufacturing methods for spectacles began to spread throughout Europe during the 15th century and led, apparently incidentally, to inventions of the microscope and telescope at the end of the 16th century (Clay-Court). Interestingly, there are controversial opinions among historians concerning the first inventor of the microscope and telescope. Thomas Diggest wrote in his book *Pantometria,* in 1571, that his father Leonard Diggest invented a telescope with a convex lens and a concave mirror in 1580. This remark is confirmed by William Bourne in a manuscript that is kept in the British Museum (Clay-Court). Pierre Borel (Borelius) gives in his treatise ''De Vero Telescopii Inventor,'' published in 1655, credit to Hans and Zacharias Jansen of Middelburg, Holland, who manufactured the first microscope and telescope in 1890. Van Swindon found in the library at Leyden, among manuscripts of Huygens, an original copy of a petition dated 1608, and sent by Jacob Adriaanzoon (also called James Metius, a native of Alkmaar, Holland) to the state general, in which he asked for the exclusive rights of selling an instrument he had invented by which distant objects appeared larger and more distinct. Descartes refers to Metius in his *Dioptics.* Among the government papers at the Hague, Van Swindon also found documents that showed that on October 2, 1608, the state Assembly considered the petition of John Lipperhey, a spectacle maker, born in Wessel but living in Middlebury, inventor of an instrument for seeing at a distance. Because the invention was known, they did not give him the exclusive right of manufacture. A. N. de Rheita supports, in his *Oculus Enoch et Eliae,* the claims of John Lipperhey and Jacob Metius (Clay-Court).

The importance of optical instruments for the promotion of advances in science became evident, and a flurry of inventions in Western Europe (Holland, Italy, England, Germany, and France) ensued. Not only opticians and instrument makers were involved, intent on improving the optical and mechanical quality of the microscope and telescope, but also mathematicians, astronomers, philosophers, scientists, and physicians, such as Galilei (1609), Kepler (1611), Fontano (1618), Drebbel (1621), Descartes (1637), Campani (1664), Divini (1665), Hooke (1665), Cock (1665), Newton (1672; reflecting microscope), van Leeuwenhoeck (1673), D'Orleans (1671; binocular stereoscopic microscope), Hugens (1678), Yarwell (1683), Bonanni (1691), Marshall (1693), van Musschenbroek (1695), Culpepper (1725), More Hall (1730; achromatic lens), Martin (1738), Cuff (1742), Adams (1746), Bass (1750), Dollond (1759), Euler (1762), Amici (1813; reflecting microscope), Lister (1830; spherical aberration), Wheatstone (stereoscope), Smith (1838), Becks (1840), Powel (1843), Leeland (1862), the Quekett brothers (1848), von Helmholtz (1851; ophthalmoscope and ophthalmometer), Nobert (1852), Riddel (1854), Spencer (1855), Ross (1857), Abbe (1877; angular aperture, binocular), Zeiss (1880; apochromatic lenses), and Otto Schott (1886; high-quality Jena glass).

Galilei used the term *occhiale* or *occhialino* for the microscope and telescope. In a letter to Cesi on April 13, 1625, Johannes Faber, a member of the academy of Lynx, founded by Cesi, proposed the name *microscope:* ''As I mention his (Galilei's) occhiale to look at small things and call it microscope.'' The Academia had also created the name *telescope.* Earlier, the word *perspicillium* (spyglass) had been used to designate both the telescope and the microscope. To interested colleagues, I recommend the following monographs: those by Hughes, Malies, Bradbury, Hansen et al., Turner, and Rosenthal.

Of the previously listed inventors, Giuseppe Campani (1635–1715), of Bologna, Italy, is of particular interest to surgeons. Campani was an outstanding scientist, mathematician, and inventor. He pioneered the development of the microscope and telescope as well as the pendulum clock, and in 1655, with his brother, designed

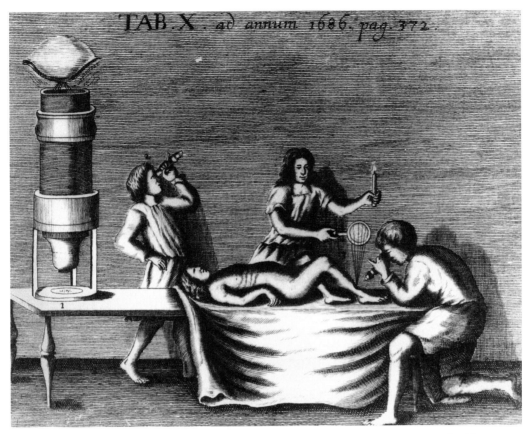

FIGURE 6.1. Illustration of the first clinical application of a microscope as a concept by Giusseppe Campani. *from.* (Courtesy of the National Library of Medicine, Bethesda, Maryland)

and built an ingenious "silent night clock." Campani invented the screw barrel type of optical viewing system. Two plates form the base of the microscope—an arrangement that enabled the user to hold the instrument up to the sky or to a candle flame to examine a specimen by the light thus transmitted (Fig. 6.1). Alternatively, the microscope could be placed over an opaque object to study its surface. In his publication *Descriptio Novi Microscopii,* a plate shows the instrument in use both for the examination of transparent specimens and for observing an opaque object. In a letter dated June 15, 1686, now archived in the Vatican Library, Campani, referring to his drawing wrote, "the illustration shows the application of the microscope to the examination of the wound of the leg." This incident can be declared the first practical use of a microscope in medicine and surgery. (A slide of

this unique picture was given to me 4 years ago by Dr. T. Glenn Pait in Little Rock, and I have often presented it in lectures.) During the course of researching this manuscript, I read the paper of Haden, "The Origin of the Microscope," which presents the illustration of Campani as Figure 11 and is probably the first English-language publication to include this picture.

The idea of Campani was sown in the 17th century, but the process of realizing Campani's vision would require additional advances in technology and science, a process that progressed successively for 235 years until the first operating microscope was applied to surgery in 1921 by Nylén, in Stockholm, Sweden.

The magnification offered by the first generation of optical instruments of the 17th century was most welcomed by astronomers and biologists who soon began to publish books of great interest, including Cesi, Stelluti, Kircher, Schott, Swammerdam (discovery of erythrocytes), Malphigi (capillaries), Hooke (definition of the cell), and van Leeuwenhoeck (discovery of protozoa and bacteria). Applying this simple microscope, spermatozoa were also discovered by van Leeuwnhoeck in 1679, thus influencing profound changes in embryological concepts and reasoning. The severe optical limitations of the microscope and consequent distrust of its capacities, however, hindered its routine application during the 18th century. The only outstanding scientist of this century to use the microscope was Wolff (1738–1796), founder of embryology. Otherwise microscopic investigation came to a perplexing standstill (Ackerknecht).

In 1744, Baker wrote a critical text analyzing the reasons and motives that caused rejection of the microscope, and rendered the following conclusion: secrecy, high price, technical difficulties, misuse as a toy, and lack of research ideas. The microscope was established less as a scientific tool and more as a recreational toy, owned and coveted by the upper class. A long span of almost 250 years bridged the interval between the birth of the microscope and the birth of microscopic pathology (Majno and Joris). Morgagni, for instance, had not used the microscope to research his famous monograph on pathology. Between the years 1770 and 1825, the industrial revolution took root, and within four decades, industrialization in England had reached its peak. Lister (father of Lord Joseph Lister) was successful in solving the problem of spherical aberration. Working with instrument maker Tulley, a high-quality microscope was designed and constructed in the mid 1830s. Industrialized technology and social dynamics created the fundamental conditions and stimulation for the proliferation of research in European laboratories, which culminated in an explosive development and advancement in science, particularly in microanatomy and microbiology subsequent to the pioneering work of Virchow, Henle, Purkinje, His, Golgi, Cajal, Pasteur, and Koch.

Ernst Abbe in Jena, Germany, finally succeeded in solving one more factor influencing the quality of the microscope—the angular aperture—which contributed greatly to improving its physical properties and practical functions. The Abbe formula, published in 1877, states, ''In order to achieve the maximum amount of resolution from a microscope, the objective lens must collect as large a cone of light as possible from the object.'' It was during the 1870s, while experimenting with water emission objective lenses that Abbe, working for Zeiss, elucidated his formula and brought Zeiss to the forefront in microscope technology. By the 1880s, using oil immersion objective lenses, a numerical aperture of 1.4 had finally been reached, allowing light microscopes to resolve two points only 0.2 μm apart. With the exception of some very unusual immersion fluids or ultraviolet light, this remains the limit today

MAGNIFYING LOUPES

From 1813 to 1825, English, French, and German opticians (Hudson, Lumiere, and Voigtlander) attempted to coordinate two monoculars into a single instrument and finally provided the modern binocular (opera glasses for the theater, field glasses for horse racing) (Rosenthal). Another improvement in opera glasses came with the invention of the binocular roof prism by Abbe and Zeiss circa 1870 to 1880. Such a prism binocular enables the user to achieve greater enlargement of the image without having to deal with the increased length of the optical tube.

Surprisingly, there are no comprehensive publications concerning the use of the magnifying loupe in medical settings. Donaghy gives credit to Schilling, who in 1833 studied intravascular clotting through a lens system. Donaghy also ascertained that Harrison used magnifying loupes for his research while operating on the spinal cord of animal embryos, and could therefore be acknowledged as the first microsurgeon. Barraquer credits Saemisch of Bonn with developing the first binocular magnifying device in 1876. T. C. Kriss and V. M. Kriss refer also to Landolt, who, it appears, collected data relevant to the use of loupes (Table 6.1).

In 1886, Westien of Rostock, Germany, an instrument maker, developed binocular loupes for Schulze, a zoologist in Berlin who was interested in performing more accurate dissections. In 1887, Westien designed and produced with

TABLE 6.1. *Development of optical instruments for surgery from a personal view*

Magnifying loupe		Operating microscope		
1823	Binocular opera glass	1921	Brinel-Leitz	Monocular
1876	Saemisch	1921	Nylén-Person	Monocular
c. 1880	E. Abbe/Zeiss	1922	Holmgren-Zeiss/Jenna	Binocular
1886	Westien and Schulze	1925	Hinselmann-Zeiss/Jena	Binocular, colposcope
1886	Westien and von Zehender	1938	Tullio-Zeiss/Jena	Binocular, floorstand
1899	Axenfeld	1953	OPMI 1	Binocular, floorstand
1910	Telescopic binocular loupe/Zeiss		Littman (Zeiss/Oberkochen):	(later ceiling
1911	von Hess		changeable magnification;	mounted)
1913	von Rohr and Stock		stereoscopic vision in sharp	
			focus through narrow surgical	
			corridors; coaxial light; beam-	
			splitter: observer tube, cameras	
1948	Riechert	1960	Littmann (Zeiss/Oberkochen)	Binocular diploscope
1951	Guiot	1972	Heller-Schattmaier-Yaşargil	Binocular, floorstand
1965	Drake		(Contraves-Zeiss):	
			counterbalanced stand; floating	
			movements; mouth switch to	
			release the brake system;	
			electrical eyepiece warmer	
		1992	Hensler-Yaşargil (modified	Binocular Zeiss
			Contraves stand attached to a	OPMI NCS NC32,
			Zeiss microscope)	floorstand

great care, binocular loupes for the ophthalmologist von Zehender. Later, Westien attempted to convert his stationary device into a surgical instrument that could be worn on the head. This offered a power of 5 to 6× magnification, but failed to achieve wide popularity because of its weight of 250 g (Harms and Machensen). In 1899, Axenfeld also developed an instrument with a headband that provided 5 to 6× magnification, which was also too heavy to wear.

In 1912, von Rohr of Jena constructed the first teleloupes, which had been advocated by Gullstrand of Sweden and were later manufactured commercially by Zeiss. These loupes were light in weight and had a magnification of 2×. They achieved great popularity with a large number of ophthalmologists (Harms et al., Barraquer). In 1948, Riechert, initially an ophthalmologist who later became a neurosurgeon in Freiburg, Germany, advocated the advantages of magnifying loupes for neurosurgical procedures. It is also well known that Charles Drake, the great master of conventional neurosurgery, who pioneered the surgery of acoustic neurinomas, intracranial aneurysms (particularly those of the vertebrobasilar system), and arteriovenous malformations, used magnifying loupes. The great French neurosurgeon Guiot, revived transsphe-

noidal pituitary surgery in 1957 using magnifying loupes and a headlight. For teaching purposes, he occasionally applied the operating microscope with an observing tube. In 1967, his pupil, Hardy, introduced the routine use of an operating microscope for the transsphenoidal approach. Undoubtedly, a great number of other neurosurgeons preferred the use of magnifying loupes but did not publish this fact.

OPERATING MICROSCOPE

In 1921, Carl Olof Nylén envisioned and pioneered microsurgery together with his teacher Holmgren. In his publication of 1954, Nylén describes the development as follows:

The idea of using a larger magnification than had previously been employed, occurred to me early in 1921 when I was experimenting with labyrinthine fistula operations on temporal bone preparations from human beings and in living animals. I found that the Brinell measuring microscope with an ocular micrometer with a magnification of 10–15×, when used in the operation cavity, was a much better aid than were loupes. The works of Ewald and more especially, of Maier and Lion, the latter of whom described the use of larger magnification in labyrinthine operations on living animals, convinced me of the practical value of using the microscope in various kinds of observations and operations on the ear of living persons.

In November 1921 I used the Brinell microscope for observations and operations in two cases of chronic otitis with labyrinthine fistulas, and in one case with bilateral pseudofistula symptoms. A few months later I took advantage of an opportunity to use an otomicroscope especially constructed by engineer N. Person and myself, as well as the Zeiss binocular microscope which had just been adapted for fenestration operation by Holmgren. The latter proved to be more suitable, and gave the best image. Holmgren subsequently took up, developed, and popularized the idea of operating under the microscope.

During the first experiments with aural operations on human subjects monocular microscopes were used. Before long, however, the binocular microscope proved to have such obvious advantages over the monocular one for the performance of the exquisitely delicate operation on the labyrinth, that the former was doubtless preferable. (pp 453–454)

In the very instructive Table 1 in Nylén's paper, 10 operating microscopes are listed according to the sequence of development of their optical and mechanical systems between 1921

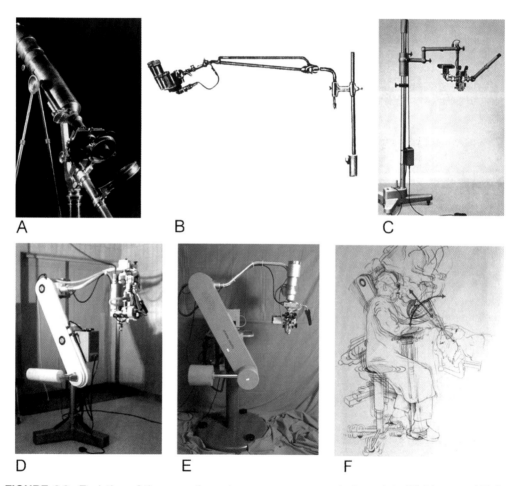

FIGURE 6.2. Evolution of the operating microscope, a personal viewpoint. (A) Lister and Tulley (1830), an excellent achromatic microscope. (B) Nylén and Holmgren (1922), first binocular operating microscope (Zeiss Jena). (C) Littman (Zeiss and Oberkochen) (1953), multiversatile operating microscope. (D) Heller, Schattmeier, and Yasargil (1972), counterbalanced Contraves Stand attached to a Zeiss microscope. (E) Hensler and Yasargil (1992), modified Contraves Stand attached to a Zeiss microscope. (F) Range of a surgeon's mobility coordinated between the hydraulic chair, arm support, and the counterbalanced operating microscope with mouth switch.

and 1952. The monocular microscope that Nylén first used had to be fixed to the head of the patient. In 1922, Holmgren used for the first time a Zeiss binocular microscope, which had to be attached to the operating table. The binocular operating microscope of Tullio and Zeiss, was, according to Table 1 of Nylén, mounted on a floor stand. During the first 30 years since Nylén's initial interest in the operating microscope, progress in the field of microsurgery was slow to develop; only a few otological surgeons displayed an interest.

The operating microscope attracted the attention of ophthalmological surgeons at a comparatively late date (Perrit, Barraquer, Harms and Machenson). The reason for this delay was presumably because the topography of the eye, being a superficial organ, offered favorable conditions for using binocular magnifying loupes.

The considerably delayed application of the operating microscope in general surgery can be related to the technical deficiencies of the microscope. The focal length (working distance) of 6 to 20 cm was too short, and the field of view (6–20 mm) was limiting. The microscope was unstable, immobile, and emitted insufficient illumination.

In 1952, Littmann (Zeiss–Oberkochen) succeeded in modifying the initial colposcope of Hinselmann to a sophisticated, maneuverable microscope for surgical requirements, and was known as the OPMI 1. The magnification could be changed without altering the focal length, and the object was always in sharp focus. The distance of 16 mm between the inner lenses enabled the surgeon to view the field stereoscopically through a narrow opening. The OPMI 1 was exhibited at the 5th International Congress of Otolaryngologists in Amsterdam, Holland, in 1953. This microscope, with a coaxial light system, was adaptable for various types of surgery, and therefore drew the attention not only of otological surgeons, but also ophthalmological surgeons and neurosurgeons (Fig. 6.2).

MICROSURGERY IN THE LABORATORY

It is well known that Lougheed and Toms in Toronto, and Echlin in New York studied sub-arachnoid hemorrhage in a laboratory setting, introducing blood into the subarachnoid space using the operating microscope. The microscope was also an advantage for Malis' laboratory experiments on the cerebral cortex of cats. Greenwood and Malis each developed a bipolar coagulation apparatus. This, in my opinion, was a revolutionary invention, not just for neurosurgery but for all surgical specialties.

Last year, Dwight Parkinson told me that he had used the operating microscope in the mid 1950s in the laboratory. No doubt other colleagues can claim to have conducted laboratory research using the microscope, but did not publish their use of the instrument.

In the mid 1950s, Ted Kurze, at the University of Southern California, observed a petrosal bone exploration by H. and W. House, and evolved the idea to explore small, medial acoustic tumors in a revolutionary way. After laboratory training to learn the detailed anatomy of the petrosal bone and the drilling technique, on August 1, 1957, he explored a tumor of the VIIth nerve through a subtemporal, epidural, transpetrosal approach on a 5-year-old child. This unique experience remained unpublished until 1962. Kurze presented this microsurgical technique and approach at the meeting of the Harvey Cushing Society in Chicago, Illinois, on April 30, 1962. In a publication with Doyle in the *Journal of Neurosurgery,* a statement reflects that Kurze performed microsurgical procedures together with W. House on 40 patients: progressive hearing loss in 8 patients and Menière's disease in 19 patients, VIIIth nerve tumors in 6 patients, neurinomas in 2 patients, epidermoid tumor in 1 patient, and VIIth nerve neuropathy in 3 patients. The concluding remarks of Kurze are elucidated with reserve, and indicate that additional clinical study and practical experience are necessary to elicit the value of this procedure in the therapy of acoustic neurinoma and Menière's disease. The potential advantages of microtechniques in many other surgical and neurosurgical areas are also expressed. This report was heeded by many neurosurgeons, but the question arose whether microtechniques could be applied to the removal of large tumors, particularly if they were attached to the pons.

The initial reaction of neurosurgeons was reluctance, but later they became more motivated to explore the possibilities of microtechniques. This trend of protracted development in microneurosurgery can be understood when reflecting on the history of modern neurosurgery, the various phases of which overlap and interlock with each other. Nevertheless, well-defined time periods of development can be distinguished: the pioneer phase, 1879 to 1919; the foundation phase, 1920 to 1955; and the subspecialization phase, 1955 to 2000.

The principles of neurosurgical diagnosis and treatment have been elaborated by the pioneering generation and strengthened by the foundation generation. During these two phases of neurosurgery, the diagnostic and surgical concepts, strategies, tactics, techniques, and tools remained generally unchanged. These phases are well documented in numerous monographs dedicated to the history of neurosurgery, and in publications documenting the Proceedings of the Congress of Neurological Surgeons, which began in 1952 with the first CNS honored guest, the outstanding Swedish neurosurgeon Herbert Olivecrona (unfortunately his lectures remain unpublished), followed by distinguished lecturers representative of our neurosurgical specialty. Historically, a remarkable publication is Volume 11, devoted to a great American neurosurgeon, James L. Poppen, who was the honored guest of the CNS in 1963 and who gave three outstanding lectures: ''Operative Techniques for Removal of Olfactory Groove Meningiomas and Saprasellar Meningiomas,'' ''Operative Treatment for Aneurysms,'' and ''Tricks of the Trade.'' Twelve other flawless lectures by prominent neurosurgeons frame these incomparable contributions from Poppen: Charles Drake discussed ''Diagnosis and Treatment of Lesions of the Brachial Plexus,'' Paul Bucy discussed ''Stereotactic Surgery: Philosophical Considerations,'' W. B. Hamby presented ''Carotid Cavernous Fistulas,'' and Lyle French described ''Cerebrovascular Malformations.''

In the midst of these symphonic, scientific articles, the genuine message of Kurze surfaces, ''Microtechniques in Neurological Surgery.'' This comprehensive vision is presented concisely and with modesty, void of any pretense.

Undoubtedly, Kurze was predicting an entirely new neurosurgical technique that posed many seemingly unresolvable challenges, because it was difficult to imagine how to surgically explore large lesions under the operating microscope and how to cope should an aneurysm or arteriovenous malformation rupture during exploration. Clearly, microtechniques offered advantages and the chance to improve on present methods. There seemed to be general, unspoken agreement that microtechniques should be applied for at least some neurosurgical procedures. However, the need to perfect systematically the procedural methodology, in particular the control of central nervous system vasculature and hemodynamics, would eventually lead to the development of new concepts in planning and performing neurosurgical procedures and resulted in a hesitation and reluctance to pursue neurosurgery in an arena dominated by the operating microscope. Specially designed magnification loupes for neurosurgery were readily available and comparatively inexpensive. They improved the neurosurgeon's vision, and he could adapt himself to performing delicate surgical maneuvers within a relatively short period of time. On the other hand, performing surgical procedures with the operating microscope demanded a long, time-consuming learning phase in the laboratory, not only to perfect operative techniques but also to acquire confidence in manipulating the microscope.

As the initial phase of microsurgery was emerging in California in the late 1950s, 3000 miles east of Los Angeles in the small university town of Burlington, Vermont, a synchronous development—another pillar representing microsurgery—was beginning to arise. In 1958, J. H. Jacobson, newly appointed director of surgical research at the University of Vermont, had been asked by the department of pharmacology to help with a project in which department members were trying to denervate the canine carotid artery. Jacobson found that the only way to denervate the artery effectively was to divide and reanastomose it. The patency rate of this procedure was approximately 70%. In analyzing the situation further, it became apparent that the major defect in technique was the inability of the eye to see, rather than the hand to do (Jacobson). With a borrowed microscope from the ear, nose, and throat department, Jacobson and Suarez attained superb results with microvascular vessel anastomosis.

In the latter years of the 1950s, five competing techniques had been investigated and were available for constructive and reconstructive vascular surgery: staples, adhesives, microlaser, electrocoaptation, and suturing. The principles of suturing techniques for macro- and mesovascular surgery were pioneered by Alexis Carrel. Jacobson and Suarez transferred Carrel's techniques to microvascular surgery (vessel diameter of less than 3.0 mm). This achievement in particular drew the attention of plastic, reconstructive, and vascular surgeons Buncke, Smith, Cobbet, Krizek, Fisher, and Lee, and a few neurosurgeons such as Donaghy, Lougheed, and his assistant Khodadad.

Embolectomy and thrombectomy of the middle cerebral artery had been attempted sporadically without using microtechniques. Scheibert, Driesen, and Chou observed successful results, whereas Welch, and Shillito failed to succeed. Donaghy, stimulated by Jacobson, began experimenting with microsurgery on small arteries of the extremities in rabbits and canines. On August 4, 1960, together with Jacobson, he performed an endarterectomy of the middle cerebral artery on a patient under the operating microscope. An additional eight patients with occlusive disease of the middle cerebral artery were also explored. The arteries could be reconstructed but the patency results were discouraging. Between 1960 and 1966, the operating microscope had been used for the removal of a few cases of schwannoma (Kurze and Doyle, Rand and Kurze) and chordoma (Stevenson et al.), and several aneurysms had been clipped (Adams and Witt, Pool and Colton, and Rand and Jannetta).

Retrospectively, these first, sporadic attempts to apply the operating microscope to the microsurgical treatment of central nervous system lesions can be viewed as courageous, because of the fact they were premature performances, executed before the development and adaptation of concepts and techniques suitable for operating under the microscope. The principles of tissue dissection and microvascular repair extracranially could not be transferred directly to techniques in craniospinal surgery for the elimination of tumors and various vascular lesions. The complex anatomy and physiology of the central nervous system, with its unique heterogeneous and heteromorphous parenchymal architecture closely intertwined with the cerebrospinal fluid, vascular, and endocrine systems, imposed the requirement to proceed with developing experimental animal models in the laboratory, and perfecting methods and techniques, as a basic preliminary to embarking on microneurosurgery in humans. This was my project in Burlington, Vermont, and this aim was accomplished in 1966 in the same laboratory where Jacobson and Suarez had pioneered peripheral microvascular surgery.

After acquiring the basic microtechniques to deal with small extracranial vessels in canines, I began, despite great skepticism, to explore the arteries of the brain within the cisternal–arachnoidal (aquatic) bed, which required evolving an entirely different dissection technique to maintain the surgical field continuously clean and clear. This venture challenged me to collate all my knowledge and experience. During the course of 2 months it seemed hopeless to achieve this goal, and I was beginning to feel justified in abandoning the task. In February 1966, however, a bipolar coagulation apparatus (which cost only $120) was purchased. This equipment proved to be an excellent tool and became instrumental in realizing the much-needed breakthrough to advance microneurosurgery. This gentle coagulation technology preserved surrounding normal tissue and permitted the surgeon to explore and dissect in narrow, cisternal (submarine) corridors, maintaining constant clean and clear conditions among the arachnoid spaces. By applying bipolar coagulation using fine -tip jewelers' forceps, it was possible to achieve point-to-point coagulation without heating or spasm effect to arteries. Consequently, the planned reconstructive surgery on small cortical arteries, and on the middle cerebral and basilar arteries, as well as extra- and intracranial bypass procedures, could be accomplished successfully. The application of microtechniques to the entire field of neurosurgery, employing delicate, atraumatic exploration along the cisternal pathways became a perceptible vision and viable methodology. Accurate exploration of intracranial and intraspinal structures along the subarachnoid pathways became a feasible concept, a cisternal navigation accomplished with minimal or no retraction of adjacent structures.

Numerous research papers had been published since 1960 dealing with the experiences and outcome of experimental procedures on extracranial small vessels in animals using sutures, microstaples, and adhesive substances. After 6 months of laboratory work in Burlington, I developed a curiosity to explore the current stage of laboratory and clinical work in other centers. Corresponding with authors who had published articles in this particular field, I organized a schedule to undertake a round-trip in the summer of 1966 to visit laboratories and institutions of general, vascular, and plastic surgery, as well as neurosurgery. I had the opportunity to visit one or several institutions in the following cities of the United States and Canada: Montreal, Ottawa, Toronto, Detroit, Chicago, San Francisco, Redding, Palo Alto, Los Angeles, Houston, Memphis, St. Louis, Cincinnati, Cleveland, Baltimore, New York, and Boston. It was an exciting trip in terms of geographical, cultural, and scientific aspects. I met leading surgeons in their fields and basic scientists. I toured their laboratories, examined their ongoing research, and realized that nowhere was any attempt being made to perform experimental surgery on brain arteries. For my part, I gave lectures based on slides and color movie film (16 mm) that recorded my laboratory experiences in microvascular surgery on brain arteries. At each institution I emphasized the importance and effectiveness of bipolar coagulation technique for microsurgery of brain arteries within the cisternal–arachnoidal bed. I observed associated but divergent, and often disruptive, concepts for the treatment of small vessels, such as the microstapler, adhesives, electrocoagulation, laser application, and suturing techniques. During my trip across the United States I became convinced that a conference devoted to the topic of microvascular surgery would gather all interested colleagues and pres-

ent the opportunity to exchange our experiences and ideas in open discussion. Thanks to the endeavors of Drs. Donaghy and Slater, and Mrs. Esther Roberts, the conference was planned and organized efficiently, and took place on October 6 and 7, 1966, at the University of Vermont, Burlington (Figs. 6.3 and 6.4).

This first conference on microvascular surgery can be considered a complete success, and it declared the beginning of a new era in surgery. The problems encountered in microvascular surgery provided a catalyst to unify 60 surgeons from four specialties: vascular, plastic, reconstructive, and neurosurgery. Otological and ophthalmological surgeons were absent because this topic failed to attract their interest at that time. Fisch, in Zurich, was the first otological surgeon, who, in 1967, began to appreciate the importance of bipolar coagulation. He initiated this technique in his department and advocated its use among all his colleagues.

The quintessential factor emerging from this now historic conference in Burlington, was the consensus among participants that extra- and intracranial small vessels could be resected and reconstructed successfully using suturing techniques. An important adjunct to this statement reads: Applying bipolar coagulation technique, a high patency rate following reconstruction of extra- and intracranial small vessels can be achieved. This meeting also revealed that each surgical specialty was engaged in resolving the problems posed by its own particular anatomic, physiological, and pathological context, which led to individual surgical specialties following differing paths of development and adjustment. The resulting consequences of this diverse evolution influenced the design of the optical and mechanical systems of operating microscopes and the various modifications to surgical instruments. In 1967, the papers of the contributors were published in a monograph.

The positive atmosphere of the conference in Burlington stimulated us (Donaghy, Malis, Rand, Jannetta, and myself) to arrange a meeting for neurosurgical colleagues only, to present the latest developments in microsurgery and to give instruction in new techniques, including the availability of bipolar coagulation technology.

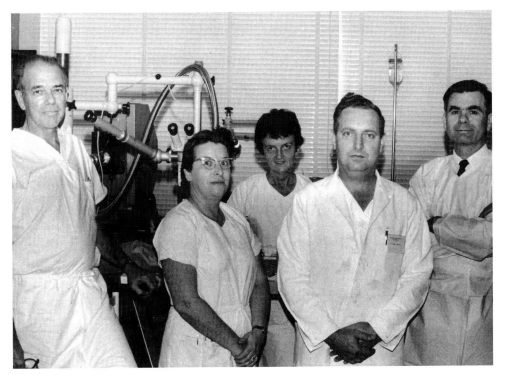

FIGURE 6.3. Microsurgical team of 1966 visiting the new laboratory, Mary Fletcher Hospital, University of Vermont, Burlington, in 1969. From left to right: Donaghy, Levin, Roberts, Comeau, and Yaşargil.

A decision was reached to arrange the first microsurgical meeting from April 13 to 15, 1967, at the University of California at Los Angeles, where in 1966 I had demonstrated to Rand and Jannetta the application of bipolar coagulation technique for the removal of a spinal juxtamedullary arteriovenous malformation. Buncke, Smith (leading microsurgeons in plastic and reconstructive surgery), Hardy, Jannetta, Khodadad, Kurze, Rand, engineer Jack Urban, and myself gave lectures. Donaghy and Malis were unfortunately absent from the program. The papers of contributors were published in a monograph edited by Rand, which generated great interest among young neurosurgeons, although an attitude of reluctance to accept new techniques persisted among others.

Hugo Krayenbühl, founder and chairman of the neurosurgical department in Zurich (1937–1973), had participated in the conference in Burlington on October 6, 1966, and gave an excellent lecture recalling his experience in the treatment of carotid–cavernous sinus fistula. He observed microsurgical procedures on brain arteries, and the use of bipolar coagulation in the laboratory, and was convinced that microtechniques should be applied routinely in neurosurgery. Krayenbühl did not use magnifying loupes for his operations and was not inclined to learn the microtechniques, but he was the most farsighted neurosurgeon of his generation, and he supported me wholeheartedly after my return to Zurich in December 1966.

The routine clinical application of microtechniques began in Zurich on January 18, 1967, with surgery on a patient for removal of a left middle frontal gyrus glioma and clipping of an aneurysm at the bifurcation of the middle cerebral artery, all in the same session. During the first 2 years of my return to Zurich, more than 200 patients were operated using microtechniques. Their lesions included aneurysms,

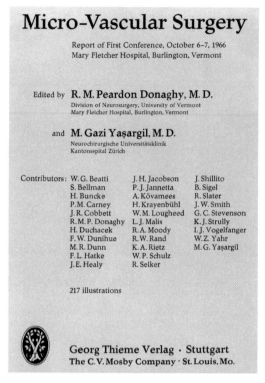

FIGURE 6.4. (A) The monograph of collected lectures from the historical conference of microvascular surgery, October 6 to 7, 1966, in Mary Fletcher Hospital, Burlington, Vermont. (B) The monography of collected lectures of the microsurgical meeting and the first hands-on course, Nov. 16–20, 1968, Zürich, Switzerland.

cranial and spinal arteriovenous malformations, tumors, and occluded cerebral arteries. Microsurgical procedures were observed by visiting colleagues from all over the world, the first year via an observation tube mounted on the microscope optic, and the next year via a black-and-white TV system. During the course of discussion with colleagues, and in particular as a result of the stimulation of Dr. H. G. McClintock of Denver, Colorado, who in 1965 had translated our monograph "Cerebral Angiography," the decision was reached to hold a microneurosurgery course in Zurich.

The second microneurosurgical conference and the first hands-on microsurgical course were held in the pathology department of University Hospital, Zurich, on November 19 and 20, 1968. We expected 20 to 40 participants, and had borrowed 10 operating microscopes from the Zeiss Company and bought some jewelers' instru-

ments for the course. It was a great surprise to me and my only secretary, Ms. M. Traber, to experience the arrival of 186 neurosurgeons from Europe, Canada, and the United States—a great number of them chairmen of neurosurgery departments.

The motto "No beverage but plenty of brain food" rescued me partially from social duties. Lectures were given by Krayenbühl, Donaghy, Fisch, Hardy, Jannetta, Malis, Pool, and Peerless, and engineers Borer, Littman, and Voelmy. The latter, a director of the Contraves Company, was involved in devising a counterbalanced operating microscope stand. I presented color movie films (16 mm), made in the laboratory in Burlington, Vermont, to demonstrate the surgery on brain arteries of dogs, and black-and-white videos of clinical microsurgery on aneurysms, arteriovenous malformations (cranial and spinal), acoustic neurinomas, craniopharyngiomas, and large pituitary adenomas. The basic elements involved in handling and manipulating the operating microscope (Zeiss OPMI 1) and surgical instruments, and the technique of bipolar coagulation, were demonstrated in the laboratory of the pathology department, where each participant could gain their initial experience in microsurgical dissection and suturing of carotid arteries on rats. A black-and-white camera was mounted on the teaching microscope to allow each participant to follow the sequence of each technique, and to observe exactly the principles of dissection and suturing manipulations. The lectures were published in a monograph in 1969. The names and addresses of the medical instrument companies were included, with the purpose of assisting those colleagues who may have had an interest in entering the field of microneurosurgery. The message relayed by this conference and all subsequent meetings comprised of the repeated emphasis on teaching participating colleagues in preliminary exercises at the hands-on course, and on encouraging continued practice at a home laboratory for a long period of time until competence in application of microtechniques had been reached, before performing surgery on patients. During the ensuing years, I participated as a teacher at numerous microneurosurgical meetings with hands-on courses (Burlington, New York, Cincinnati, Chicago, St. Louis, San Francisco, Tokyo, Kyoto, Brasilia), and, as visiting professor, I operated on patients (St. Louis, Los Angeles, Boston, New York, Barcelona, Madrid, Sevilla, Cape Town, Mexico City) and demonstrated the principles of the operating microscope and bipolar coagulation technique to explore lesions through the narrow surgical corridors of cisternal pathways.

The laboratory of the neurosurgical department, in Zurich, permanently offered courses that were attended by approximately 3000 colleagues from various disciplines for a period of 30 years: neurosurgeons, and ophthalmological, plastic and reconstructive, vascular, and orthopedic surgeons; as well as physiologists, neurophysiologists, and biochemists. Similar regular or periodic courses were also available in numerous laboratories throughout the world. By 1970, microtechniques had been accepted in the majority of surgical disciplines and research laboratories. Microsurgical models had been developed for surgical experiments as well as for physiological studies. Since 1973, satellite symposia devoted to microtechniques had become a regular event on national and international levels. Later they were incorporated into programs of the CNS (Table 6.2).

TABLE 6.2. *Data related to the development of microneurosurgery*

1953	*Multiversatile Operating Microscope* (OPMI 1) H. Littman (Zeiss-Jena)
1955	*Operating Microscope in Neurosurgical Labortories* W. R. Lougheed and M. Tom (1955) D. Parkinson (1955) T. Kurze (1956) FR. A. Echlin (1960) L. I. Malis (1955), bipolar coagulation technique
1958	*Microvascular Surgery of the Extracranial Small Arteries in Laboratory* Jacobson and Suarez (1958), Donaghy (1960), Lougheed and Khodadad (1965), Buncke (1965), Smith (1966), Cobbett (1967), Krizek et al. (1965), Fisher and Lee (1965) *Microvascular Surgery of Intracranial Arteries* M. G. Yaşargil (1966): cisternal exploration and microsurgical reconstruction of brain arteries applying bipolar coagulation technique
1966	*Microsurgical Conferences and Hands-on Courses* First Conference of Microvascular Surgery, October 6, 1966, Burlington, VT Microneurosurgical Symposium, April 13–15, 1967, UCLA, Los Angeles Microsurgical meeting and hands-on course, November 16–20, 1968, Zurich, Switzerland Microsurgical meeting and hands-on course, September 29–October 3, 1969, Burlington, VT Microsurgical meeting and hands-on course, November 11–14, 1970, Tokyo, Japan
Since 1971	Annual Courses in New York and Cincinnati Permanent courses in Zurich; Gainesville, Florida; St. Louis; and São Paulo, Brazil
1973	The First international symposium on microneurosurgical anostomosis for cerebral ischemia, in Loma Linda, CA, followed by symposium in Chicago, (1974), in Munich (1976), London-Ontario (1978), Vienna (1980), and Kyoto (1982)
1967	*Routine Clinical Application of Microtechniques in Neurosurgery* (Zürich)

Publication activities in the microsurgical field are enormous. Within the past 30 years, 60 monographs from microneurosurgeons and 75 monographs from microsurgeons in many different specialties have been published. The number of papers is overwhelming. In 1985, Ballantyne et al. published ''Organized Bibliography of the Microsurgical Literature,'' which, after 15 years, requires a new, up-to-date edition. The *Journal of Microsurgery* has been available since 1979, and offers articles of common interest to a variety of surgical disciplines.

As a natural and predictable sequel, each discipline in microsurgery developed its own modified versions of the operating microscope, tools, and instruments related to the needs of the specific anatomy, physiology, and pathology of each surgical specialty (Table 6.3).

TABLE 6.3. *Instrumental innovations in microneurosurgery*

Counterweight balanced binocular operating microscope can be attached to a monoscope, diploscope, triploscope, 2-D or 3-D videoscope monitor
Bipolar coagulation apparatus
Electrically powered perforator and craniotome
Double-pronged hook for scalp and muscle flap
Flexible dura dissector
Self-retaining retractor (Semisoft-Spatula)
Ultrasound suction apparatus and ultrasound detectors
Neurostimulator
Microinstruments
  Spring loaded bayonet bipolar coagulation forceps in seven different lengths (20–135 mm working length) and four different tip sizes (0.3–1.3 mm)
  Three-ring tipped tumor or aneurysm grasping forceps with or without teeth
  Three bipolar forceps with various curved and angled tips
  Bayonet-shaped scissors in four different lengths (50–135 mm working length) with straight or curved tips
  Rongeurs in two different lengths and six different jaw sizes
  Micro-Rongeur with malleable shaft
  Tumor-grasping forks in four different tip sizes and forked forceps
  Suction tips: four lengths (50–150 mm) and five diameters (1.5–4.5 mm)
  Regulator for suction pressure
  Dissectors: 20 various shapes and sizes
  Clips: 180 aneurysm clips, various shapes and sizes, hemoclips, temporary clips, microclips
  Microsuture
  Mobile tip mirrors (5.0–7.0 mm)
Hydraulic surgeon's chair
Hydraulic arm support
Hydraulic instrument table for scrub nurse

THE SPECIALTY OF MICRONEUROSURGERY

In the 1960s, approximately 10 neurosurgeons were interested in microtechniques. Ten years later, 30 to 40 pioneers were involved in microtechnical developments. It is beyond the limits of this chapter to enumerate the particular contributions of the numerous pioneering microneurosurgeons of succeeding generations in the fields of vascular and neoplastic lesions of the central nervous system, skull base, and spine, and central and peripheral nerve, microsurgery. Since 1967, tremendous advances have been established in the microneurosurgical treatment of skull base and brain base lesions, as well as in the targeting and navigation through aquatic cisternal corridors for surgical treatment of lesions in various compartments of the central nervous system, or for the decompression of cranial nerves and brainstem (Fig. 6.5).

Reconstructive neurovascular surgery is now applied routinely. Extra- and intracranial as well as intra- and intracranial bypass procedures are accomplished in cases of giant aneurysm, arteriovenous malformation, and skull base tumor (Figs. 6.6 and 6.7).

Sustained application of endeavors resulted in mastering of combined approaches—for instance, transsphenoidal–transsylvian and transsylvian–transcallosal explorations in one session, and numerous approaches through the skull base such as pure transsphenoidal or extended frontal transbasal, fronto- orbitozygomatic, infratemporal partial or total petrosal, pre- and retrosigmoidal, transcondylar, extreme lateral transretrocondylar, transmaxillary, transoral, and transpharyngeal clival approaches. There is an excellent literature review of the transcondylar approach in Table 1 in the paper of Alleyne and Spetzler.

It is also beyond the limits of this paper to mention all the second- and third-generation pioneers of microneurosurgery, and the leading schools by name. In the coming decades, a number of them will surely reflect on and document their own experiences and concepts. These publications will supplement and enhance our archives and prove to be a valuable resource for those professional historians who choose to evaluate the evolution of neurosurgery. There

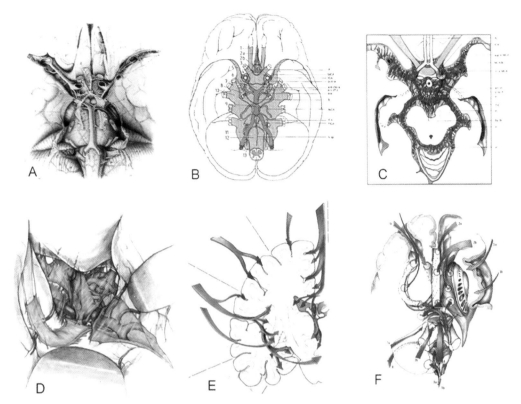

FIGURE 6.5. A series of illustrations emphasizing the importance of being thoroughly acquainted with the cisternal anatomy of the brain relative to the particular concept of microsurgical approaches. (A) The basal cisternal comparments dissected by Key and Retzius in 1875. (B) Microsurgical view of the basal cisternal compartments and their relationship to the brain nerves and main brain arteries. (C) Schematic representation of the basal cisterns. (D) Parachiasmatic cisterns revealed during the course of a pterional transsylvian approach. (E) Schematic illustration of the fissural and sulcal microsurgical explorations. (F) Schematic drawing of fissural approaches to deeply located lesions.

are a great number of well-established and equipped microneurosurgical units throughout the world, where daily, excellent microsurgical treatments of patients are exercised. Those lesions declared inoperable during the first half of the 20th century are today explored routinely. The mortality and morbidity of microneurosurgical procedures have been remarkably reduced within the last 30 years, which is certainly a result of multiple factors but is definitely also attributable to the advantages of microneurosurgery. Today, every lesion of the central nervous system can be well accessed by applying expert microsurgical techniques, and can be completely eliminated, with an acceptable surgical outcome for the patient.

SUBSPECIALIZATION IN NEUROSURGERY

Interestingly, microtechnology and microtechniques arrived on the scene in the mid 1950s during the inaugural phase of neurosurgical subspecialization: functional, epilepsy, pediatric, and spine neurosurgery. The continuous innovations in technology together with the invention of sophisticated diagnostic and therapeutic methods is an ongoing dynamic process that further influenced subspecialization (e.g., the sectors of neurovascular and neoplastic surgery). In Table 6.4, the subspecialties of neurosurgery are listed on the left and the available, appropriate therapeutic modalities are listed on the right. The crucial factor derived from analyzing this devel-

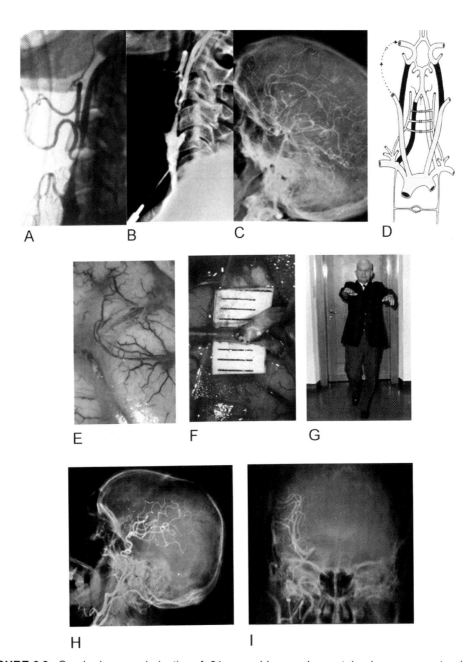

FIGURE 6.6. Cerebral revascularization. A 61-year-old man who sustained syncope on turning his head to the right side, and the subsequent development of temporary left-side hemiparesis and visual field defect. Angiographic studies revealed the following: (A) Right internal carotid artery occlusion. (B) Left internal carotid artery occlusion (the right vertebral artery was also occluded). (C) Left vertebral angiogram visualized both infra- and supratentorial arteries. (D) Diagram depicting the extent of the arterial occlusion in the case described. Blackened vessels indicate occluded segments. Dotted line indicates extra-/intracranial anastomoses performed on November 7, 1967. (E) An exposed cortical artery (1.0 mm in diameter) within its cisternal bed on the anterior part of the right superior temporal gyrus. (F) End-to-side anastomosis between the right superficial temporal artery and a temporal branch of the middle cerebral artery. (G) The patient, after surgery, fully recovered, experienced no more transient ischemia attacks, and died 14 years later from a cardiovascular insult. (H) Postoperative angiography 6 months later showing excellent filling of the middle cerebral artery and its branches. (I) Anteroposterior view of the right external carotid angiogram. *from* Yaşargil MG. Microsurgery applied to neurosurgery., Thieme, 1969, pp. 110–111.

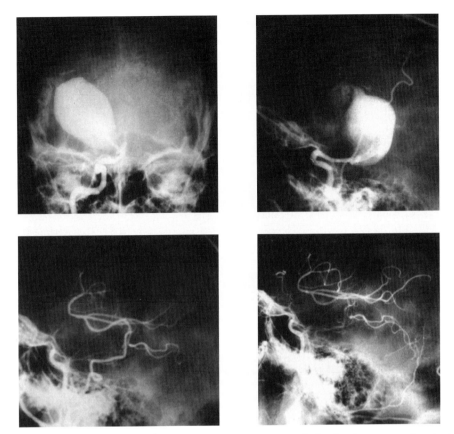

FIGURE 6.7. On December 18, 1968, the first cerebral revascularization in a case of a giant aneurysm of the right internal carotid artery was performed on a 19-year-old woman who presented with focal epilepsy and progressive weakness of her left arm. (A) Right-side carotid angiogram (anteroposterior view) shows a giant aneurysm at the bifurcation of the internal carotid artery. (B) Lateral angiogram displays no collaterals from the left carotid and right posterior communicating arteries (*from* Yasargil MG. Microsurgery applied to neurosurgery. Stuttgart, Thieme, 1969, pp. 112–117.). (C, D) Uneventful postoperative course. Immediate recovery of preoperative left arm weakness. Postoperative angiography 3 months later showing well-established hemodynamics of the right middle cerebral artery and its branches. The patient married, had two children, and is doing very well 32 years after surgery.

opment seems to be the necessity to induce and initiate additional improvements in surgical treatment (Table 6.5). A sequence of dynamic events and developments have influenced and guided microneurosurgery and benefited patients. However, an avenue of concern can be detected (see Tables 6.4 and 6.5).

The excellence of modern magnifying loupes is unquestioned, but surgery with loupes cannot be judged equal to microneurosurgery. The quality of loupe surgery is dependent on the magnifying factor, which is sufficient for the treatment of lesions on the surface. The operating microscope, on the other hand, offers, besides magnification, other very essential qualities: sharp, stereoscopic, well-illuminated depth perception through narrow cisternal corridors, and real-time telecommunication, which enhances effective, perioperative team work and teaching, and permits documentation (Table 6.6).

The terms *microtechnique* and *microsurgery* initially gave the impression that only small structures with a diameter of less than 1.0 mm were intended to be the objects of microsurgical

TABLE 6.4. *Evolution in neurosurgery (1955–2000)*

Subspecialties	Treatment modalities
Functional neurosurgery	Conventional
Pediatric neurosurgery	neurosurgery
Spine neurosurgery	Microneurosurgery
Trauma neurosurgery	Endoscopic
Central and peripheral	neurosurgery
nerve surgery	Endoscopic +
Tumor surgery	microneurosurgery
Extrinsic tumors	Endovascular
Pituitary tumors	surgery
Craniopharyngiomas	Endovascular +
Meningiomas	microneurosurgery
Schwannomas	Stereotactic surgery
Dermoid-epidermoids	Image-guided
Chordoma-chondromas	stereotaxy
Pineal tumors	Image-guided
Intrinsic tumors	neuroendoscopy
Gliomas	Stereotactic
Embryonal tumors	radiosurgery
Germ cell tumors	linear accelerator
Lymphomas	Photoradiation
Vascular tumors	Thermotherapy
Metastatic tumors	Chemotherapy
Intraventricular tumors	Local
Vascular neurosurgery	Systemic
Occlusive arterial or	Gene therapy
venous diseases	Implantation
Aneurysms	Transplantation
Arteriovenous	Focused ultrasound
malformations	
Fistulas	
Cavernous	
Other angiomas	
Hematomas	
Infarcts	

TABLE 6.5. *Evolution in surgery and neurosurgery*

Problems	Goal
Pain	Pharmacology, anesthesiology
Infection	Asepsis, antisepsis, antibiotics
Immune reaction	Immune suppression
Immune weakness	Immune protection
Explorations	
Surface	Deep
Invasive	Noninvasive
Amputation	Reconstruction, transplantation
Ligature	Repair
Destructive	Reconstructive
Extirpation	Implantation
	Autotransplantation
	Allotransplantation
	Tissue and organ culture
Hemorrhage	Hemostasis
Systemic functions	Induced hypotension,
(blood pressure,	hypothermia, and cardiac
temperature)	arrest
Imbalanced	Balanced homeostasis
homeostasis	

exploration: It was believed, for instance, that the microtechnique in neurosurgery would be dealing only with the surgery of small vessels, and cranial and peripheral nerves. With regard to the pathomorphology and the predilection sites of central nervous system lesions, microneurosurgery can be applied not only to micro structures but also to meso and macro structures on the surface of the brain, and to those at variable depths reaching 10 cm or more (see Table 6.7). The size of the lesion to be explored is not considered a factor in determining the definition of microneurosurgery. On the contrary, the narrow, confined, and winding pathway followed by the surgeon, snaking his approach toward the lesion (regardless of its size), and applying precise and gentle manipulation piloted by the specialized optical system of the operating micro-

scope, comprise crucial factors that determine the true definition of microneurosurgery. The architecture of the brain cannot be compared with the homogeneous and compact structure of an apple, but rather with the construction of an orange, with compartments (slices) with well-defined membranous borders. The compartments of the brain reveal another unique organization consisting of intricate, winding convolutes with water inlets in between (similar to fjords) containing circulating cerebrospinal fluid (see Fig. 6.5).

As honored guest of the CNS in New Orleans in 1986, I had the opportunity to give three lectures: "Reflections of a Neurosurgeon," "Neurosurgical Horizons," and "Surgical Approaches to Inaccessible Brain Tumors." The complex anatomy of the brain requires our specific attention and study, particularly in connection with the ongoing developments in robotic surgery, which have been discussed in the following sentences:

The unique construction of the brain has been recognized and reproduced in literature and art since the early dawn of man's intellectual awakening. Its gross anatomical features have been described by anatomists for centuries and subsequently studied by all students of the nervous system. Although every neurosurgeon is

TABLE 6.6. *Visual dimensions of the operating microscope[a]*

Stereoscopic view: In sharp focus on surface and in changing depth through narrow surgical (cisternal) corridors, due to interlens distance of 16 mm (26 mm in some microscopes). The operating microscope in neurosurgery can be defined as a navigation tool.

Magnification: Actual magnification of 2.5X–10X, using 300 mm objective lens, 12X eye pieces, and f160 binocular tubes.

Coaxial illumination

High-quality color

Telecommunications: 2-D or 3-D video recording, 16 mm movie film, photographic slides.

  Real-time monitoring, real-space monitoring: Enhances team work; quintet or sextet of surgeon, anesthesiologist, assistant and nurses. Teaching observers. Transmitting to other areas, local or global.

  Remote time, remote space: Transmitting recorded material locally: self-teaching as well as student or colleagues teaching, and globally (presentation at congresses, etc.)

Counterbalanced stand: Improved mobility of microscope.

  Fundamentals

    Rotational movement and six translational movements

    Mouth switch—limited movement

    Warming system for eye pieces

HMD system and PIP connected to operating microscope elicits 3-D view from microscope and 2-D view from endoscope (Aesculap).

Future perspective: Videoscopic digital microsurgery incorporating high-resolution 3-D camera system coordinated with views from endoscope, fluoroscope, ultrasound, intraoperative MRI, MRA, MRV, angiography, spectroscopy, functional MRI, EEG, and laboratory data.

---

[a] 2-D, 3-D, two-dimensional, three-dimensional; HMD, head-mounted display; PIP, picture in picture; MRI, magnetic resonance imaging; MRA, magnetic resonance angiography; MRV, magnetic resonance venography; EEG, electroencephalogram.

well informed about gyral, sulcal, and fissural anatomy, the classical neurosurgical concepts partition the brain into supratentorial and infratentorial components each composed of hemispheres, lobes, and a connecting brainstem. The gyri and sulci have been excluded from a surgical perspective, as surgeons have not been able to perform manipulations without microtechniques in such small crevices.

The attitude among neurosurgeons, relative to gyral and sulcal anatomy, has been one of neglect because of the seemingly endless variations. Differences also exist between the two hemispheres. However, neurosurgeons are currently confronted with a similar situation that occurred almost 50 years ago with the advent of cerebral angiography. The recognition of all the arteries and veins and their numerous variations seemed overwhelming at that time. Further study and analysis, however, showed that there were basic structural patterns to the arterial and venous systems. This axiom holds true for gyral and sulcal anatomy. Up until now, neurophysiology and gross anatomic studies have shown the diversity and asymmetry of the brain, but the fissural, sulcal, and gyral morphologies, and their variations have not been studied precisely (see Ono et al.).

Microsurgical experiences necessitated the development of surgical concepts appropriate to the specific localizations of arteriovenous malformations and tumors. Lesions of the cerebrum and cerebellum have been divided into two groups: convex and central. This separation may initially seem arbitrary. However, after careful observation and scrutiny, the convex (neopallial) part of the hemispheres is related more to the anatomy of the gyral and sulcal systems, with their unique arrangement of arteries and veins within the sulci. The central areas (including ar-

TABLE 6.7. *Pathomorphologic aspects of central nervous system lesions*

Size	Location	Shape	Construction	Vascularity	Relation	Occurrence
Micro = <3.0 mm	Survace	Spheric	Homogeneous	Avascular	Circumscribed	Unicentric
Meso = 3.0–30.0 mm	Dorsal	Ellipsoid	Heterogeneous	Normal	Cleavaged	Multicentric
Macro = 30.0–60.0 mm	Basal	Pyramidal	Calcified	Hypervascular	Unattached	Unilateral
Giant = >60.0 mm	Fissural	Mushroom	Ossified	Fistulous	Adherent	Bilateral
	Sulcal	Dysmorphic	Cystic		Adhesive	Cerebrocerebellar
	Central				Infiltrative	Craniospinal
					Diffuse	

chi- and paleopallial limbic and paralimbic systems) are aligned more closely with the fissural system, especially the transverse fissure, and its special arterial and venous architectures.

To master the techniques of microsurgery, it is necessary to become familiar with the detailed anatomy of the cisternal, fissural, sulcal, and neurovascular systems. These systems provide natural pathways for the accurate exploration of the lesions, dissection of the adjacent vasculature, and preservation of the hemodynamics. For example, in the management of saccular aneurysms, which in 99% of cases are located within the basal subarachnoid cisterns, the precise anatomic knowledge of cisternal systems in relation to arteries and cranial nerves becomes quintessential.

Detailed anatomic knowledge of the skull base is also fundamental for the removal of some tumors at the base of the cranium and brain, and some basal arteriovenous malformations. The majority of these arteriovenous malformations and tumors, however, are localized within the hemispheres and brainstem. For this reason, knowledge of the sulcal and fissural microanatomy, the course and variation of arteries and veins, and the distinct architecture of gyral segments, as well as the connective fibers in neopallial, paleopallial, and central areas, becomes an indispensable asset for conducting a cohesive, refined surgical treatment. Knowledge of this new concept of neuroanatomy is but one element of microsurgery. Another component is the mastery of the microtechnique.

The microscope's function is not only the enlargement of structures in the operative field, but the sharp stereoscopic vision both on the surface and in deep areas through a narrow surgical corridor. The optical devices of the operating microscope reduce the interpupillary distance of the surgeon's eyes (generally approximately 60 mm) to 16 mm. This permits the surgeon to work in a field four times smaller, because the light reflected from an image can enter the surgical microscope through an opening of only 16 mm and can be perceived stereoscopically. This advantage of the operating microscope, combined with the use of specifically designed microinstruments and bipolar coagulation techniques,

makes it possible for the surgeon to reach and to treat deep lesions of the brain through narrow cisternal corridors. The factor of magnification is certainly very important, but more important is the capability of sharp stereoscopic focus in deep narrow surgical corridors with adequate illumination. Thus the operating microscope can be declared an optimal navigational tool to explore lesions on the surface as well as lesions in all locations at various levels of depth, through narrow surgical corridors along the cisternal–subarachnoidal pathways.

Microtechniques in neurosurgery enabled us to rediscover cisternal anatomy, which was studied precisely by Key and Retzius, and published in their monumental monograph in 1875. Microneurosurgery instigated the rediscovery of the gyral, sulcal, fissural, and vascular architecture of the central nervous system, which has contributed to more accurate surgical manipulation. Microneurosurgery rediscovered the segmental and compartmental architecture of the cranial base, spine, and central nervous system. Thus, the predilection sites of vascular, neoplastic, malformative, and degenerative lesions in these compartments can be defined precisely (Figs. 6.8 and 6.9). Microneurosurgery offers a more reliable method to approach each location, and practically every region of the skull base, spine, and central nervous system can now be explored. Microneurosurgery rediscovered the special architecture and variations of the arteries and their course within the cisternal cavities. Microneurosurgery allows us to recognize and identify the perforators, their variations, and courses. Microneurosurgery allows recognition of the real morphology of aneurysms, and their relation to the parent vessels, perforators, and surrounding structures. The architecture of arteriovenous malformations, cavernomas, and extrinsic and intrinsic lesions can now be defined accurately; and the transit and feeding arteries, and draining veins identified and preserved during exploration, dissection, and removal of the lesion. The goal of microsurgery is "pure lesionectomy" without causing damage to surrounding vital structures and systemic vital functions. The self-retaining retractor system was invented to eliminate the human error factor during application

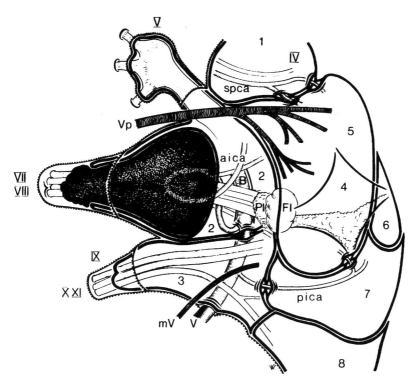

FIGURE 6.8. Diagrammatic representation of the cisterns in the cerebellopontine angle illustrating the growth pattern of a schwannoma (acoustic neuroma) in relation to the arachnoidal membranes, brain nerves, arteries, brainstem, and choroid plexus in the foramen of Luschka. This diagram was widely appreciated by my generation of neurosurgeons and contributed to the advancement in the removal of CPA lesions.

of a spatula. It was considered a protective instrument. However, observing the misuse of this tool in 1980, I began to operate by applying high-quality cotton balls in differing sizes (1.0 to 15 mm) to keep the fissure and sulci open, and to avoid any retraction of the brain and spinal cord.

The strategy, tactics, and techniques of microneurosurgery applied to the treatment of aneurysms, arteriovenous malformations, cavernomas, and extrinsic and intrinsic cranial tumors, and the surgical outcome in more than 7000 patients have been published. My surgical experiences with microsurgery of spinal lesions (arteriovenous malformations, cavernomas, angioblastomas, and extrinsic and intrinsic tumors), lumbar disc, as well as with selective amygdalohippocampectomy in patients with intractable seizures, have been published separately.

NEW EQUIPMENT AND SURGICAL CONCEPTS

Technological and scientific developments in the second half of the 20th century provided neurosurgery with new equipment and novel surgical concepts: computer-assisted frameless stereotactic targeting and navigation, stereotactically applied focused radiosurgery, image-guided stereotactic surgery, neuroendoscopy, and endovascular surgery. These new technologies are a sound, competitive force in neurosurgery, but also play an effective role in microneurosurgery by complementing certain features of this technique. Stereotactic targeting of a central nervous system lesion is appreciated since the reintroduction of this technique by Spiegel, Wycis, and others (Table 6.8). The targeting of a lesion is perfectly accomplished. The neuronavigation to the lesion is accurate. How-

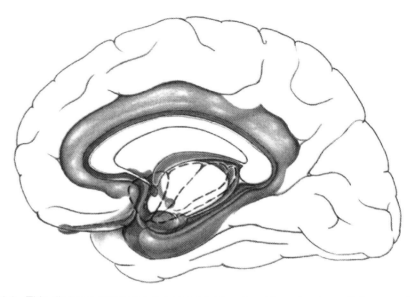

FIGURE 6.9. This diagram portraying the topography of archi- and paleopallial areas of the brain has value in the mental process of perceiving and appreciating sites of lesions in the compartments of the limbic and paralimbic systems.

TABLE 6.8. *Navigation technology for the treatment of central nervous system lesions*

Steeotactic navigation		Endocsopy		Neuroendoscopy		Endovascular		Radiation
1630	R. Descartes	1854	Garcia	1910	Lespinasse	1844	Claude, Bernard	Conventional radial
1880–1990	Cranio-,		(laryngoscope)	1923	Dandy	1860	Nelaton	Interstitial radiation
	Encephalometry	1876	Nitze	1924	Fay/Prant	1905	Bleicheroeder	Linear accelerator
	Kocher, Kroenlein		(cystoscope)	1925	Mixter	1911	Von Knauer	Focused radiosurge
1873	C. Ditmar	1878	Turke	1931	Purnam	1930	Brook	1949	Leksell
	D. Ludwig		(laryngoscope)		(myeloscope)	1968	Jaeger	1951	Tobial et .
1889	Zernow		Czermac	1960	Scarff	1969	Luessenhop	1971	Kjellberg
	Altukhov		(laryngoscope)		(spinoscope)	1970	Djindjian	1972	Steiner
1906	Clarke	1898	Killian	1938	Pool	1964	Dolce	1977	Norén
	Horsley		(bronchoscope)		(spinoscope)	1970	Serbinenko,	1982	Lundford
1909	E. Sachs	1911	Jacobus	1963	Guiot		Seljeskog,
1918	Mussen		(Thoracoscope,	1961	Fukushima		Shchegelov,
1947	Spiegel		Gastroscope)	1962	Griffith		Romadonov,
	Wycis	1976	Robinson HB	1963	Ogata		DiChiro,
1949	Talairach		(laparoscope)	1964	Ooi et al.		Doppman,
	Narabayashi	1922	Smith EW	1965	Prott		Kerber, Kikuchi,
	Riechert		(laparoscope)	1977	Apuzzo		Merland, Mullan,
1966	Walker			1978	Vries		Debrun,
1967	Alksne			1981	Oppel		Lasjaunias,
1975	Goodenough			1981	Loew et al.		Bernstein, Hilal,
1976	Bergstrom			1991	Hellwig/Bauer		Higashida,
	Greitz			1992	Caemert et al.		Hieshima, Fox,
1977	Kelly			1993	Cohen		Vinuella,
1980	Bocthius			1966	Huewel et al.		Valavanis
1982	Lundford			1987	Pernetzky et al.
1985	Kwoh et al.			1999	Manwaring
1991	Drake
1991	Watanube
1991	Kato
1992	Benabid et al.
1993	Apuzzo
1993	Pillay
1993	Koivukanga et al.
1996	Thomas et al.

ever, traveling to the lesion involves passing through the brain parenchyma. Neuronavigation cannot be compared with traversing an imaginary sea or ocean, for this method of stereotactic targeting and navigation is, in reality, a severing of the brain belonging to a patient (see Table 6.8).

Studying the history of medicine reveals that navigation (exploration) is not a new concept in medicine, surgery, or neurosurgery. During the phase of modern neurosurgery, six navigational (explorational) modalities have been developed:

1. Conventional: puncture, incision, transcerebral exploration
2. Stereotactic: transcerebral
3. Endoscopic: transcisternal, transcerebral
4. Endovascular
5. Focused neuroradiation: transcerebral
6. Microneurosurgery: cisternal exploration

Those neurosurgeons practicing in the pioneering and foundation phases began initially to explore lesions at the periphery and surface of the brain: pituitary and orbital tumors, meningiomas, gliomas, abscesses, foreign bodies resulting from trauma, pain surgery (trigeminal, glossopharyngeal), Menière's disease, and spinal lesions. Outstanding surgeons like Krause and Dandy were more courageous, and in addition successfully explored lesions localized deep in the brain.

At the end of the 19th and the beginning of the 20th centuries, neurosurgeons were well versed in the special anatomy of the brain; the convolutions and their gyral, sulcal, and fissural organization; the complexity of the connecting fibers; and the unique topography of the basal ganglia, central nuclei, compartments of the brainstem and spinal cord, ventricular system, and choroidal plexus. The lobar concept of describing the location of a lesion, defined by the neuroanatomists Gratiolet and Ecker, was accepted for neurosurgical procedures and is still in general use today. In the near future, neuroimaging technology will provide real-time stereoscopic visualization of the very detailed morphology and physiology of the central nervous system, and the pathomorphology, pathophysiology, and biochemistry of lesions and perilesio-

nal areas as well as the entire brain. The younger generation of neurosurgeons is already actively involved in learning and applying electronic technology: image-guided stereotaxy, stereotaxic neuroendoscopy, and intraoperative MRI. Currently, the ultrasonic device has proved to be an indispensable tool for the intraoperative topographic diagnosis of lesions and for measurement of hemodynamics. The ultrasonic invention for the suction of tumor tissue is very much appreciated. The high-field (1.5 -T) MR system (Sutherland-Saunders) has the potential to elicit excellent solutions for intraoperative controls.

FUTURE DEVELOPMENTS

With the introduction of the Zeiss OPMI 1 operating microscope in 1953, the era of microsurgery was inaugurated. The specific needs of the various surgical specialties as well as the individual disposition of surgeons incited continuous modification of the optic and mechanical systems of the microscope. The lack of free and effortless mobility inherent in the initial surgical microscope was improved with the introduction of a counterbalanced "floating" microscope, coupled with an electromagnetic braking system at various joints that provided absolute stability with good mobility. The addition of a mouth switch allowed effortless movement of the microscope (as well as focusing capability), and left the surgeon's hands free for surgical manipulations. An electrical warming cable around the eyepieces eliminated the annoying "fogging" of the ocular lenses. The present generation of this operating microscope, the NC32, has been available from the Zeiss Company since 1999. Other companies have imitated the counterbalanced system of this microscope with some modifications (see Table 6.1).

There are, however, still other negative factors hindering optimal use of current operating microscopes. I mentioned these in my New Orleans lecture in 1986:

> Looking through the narrow openings of the microscope's eyepieces and maintaining a relatively fixed posture of the head, neck, and body can be very tiring during a long and complex

procedure and may affect the surgeon's technical performance. A high-resolution stereoscopic color television monitor placed outside the operative field might provide more freedom and better mobility for the surgeon.

An ophthalmic microsurgeon in San Francisco, California, had already installed a monitor some 25 years earlier. Currently, the HMD System (head-mounted display) is available with a PIP System (three-dimensional microscopic view connected to a two-dimensional endoscopic view—a picture in a picture), but high-resolution, stereoscopic, color, three-dimensional TV monitors are not currently available. With this system, the cumbersome diploscope and triploscope can be discarded. If the surgeon prefers to operate with one or two assistants, or is involved in resident teaching, observing the course of surgery on an HMD monitor will equal or even surpass the quality of binocular observer tubes mounted on the microscope.

INTRAOPERATIVE IMAGINATION

The preoperative study of collected data, multidimensional graphic imagination, and planning in the brain of the surgeon, and extrapolation, exploration, and execution of a surgical procedure is known to be the most challenging part of an operation. Microsurgery offers the opportunity for accurate navigation along the cisternal corridors to the surface of a lesion, which is often only the tip of the iceberg. The surgeon contantly has to recollect and reflect on the preoperative films gained from highly appreciated modern neuroimaging studies, which, however, present merely serial visual information similar to serial photographs. The surgeon relies, in such a situation, on anatomic knowledge, accumulated surgical experiences, and a multidimensional graphic imagination to assess the true extent of the lesion and its relation to perilesional structures. These may be distorted and displaced in various degrees or may present as individual variations. The subjective task of surgery may in many cases prove to be perplexing. This is perfectly expressed by Al-Mefty in the following sentences:

Our knowledge of cerebral venous anatomy is gleaned from many sources: anatomists, radiologists, clinicians, and pathologists. Added to the wide range of normal variation, this makes the task of mastering the anatomy of the cerebral vasculature a formidable challenge. The surgeon, however, should have a clear conception of the topographical pattern of the cerebral vascular tree. This pattern eventually becomes as familiar to the surgeon as a frequently traveled road, and anatomical variation becomes a curious detour on this road. In tumor surgery, recognition of structures is more difficult because the surgeon works within a distorted vascular pattern. Consequently, all vessels should be regarded as vital branches until the surgeon is absolutely sure they are tumor feeders.

A large lesion can occasionally obscure the reference points for intraoperative orientation, which may give the surgeon the disconcerting feeling of being in a jungle without any prospects. Additional advances in science and technology will hopefully offer to the surgeon efficient intellectual support, with instantaneous and constant intraoperative three-dimensional pictures displaying the morphology and real-time parameters of the physiology and biochemistry of the central nervous system and other functional systems of the body. Furthermore, with modern technology it will hopefully be possible to transfer the images of the real-time measurements to a computer capable of converting it into a three-dimensional format and to project the images through the optic systems (microscope or videoscope) into the operating field.

This would depict the lesion in three dimensions, surrounded by normal structures such as ventricles, deep nuclei, cranial nerves, vessels, and so forth. The computer could also be programmed to reconstruct the image in any orientation, thereby permitting approaches from any desired angle. The use of color graphics could further enhance structural details. In addition, during surgery this stereoscopic image could be projected into the operative field, providing the surgeon a continuous spatial configuration of the lesion within the brain. Furthermore, in situations that require the use of laser or CUSA, the position of the laser beam or ultrasonic aspiration tip could be computer monitored in relation to the precise three-dimensional boundaries of the lesion. Such controlled maneuverability

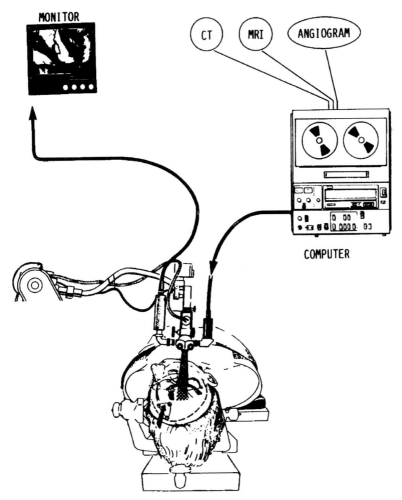

FIGURE 6.10. Schema illustrating videoscopic microsurgery, a futuristic model envisioned and proposed to the instrument companies in the 1980s. Three-dimensional computer-generated images from CT, MRI, ultrasound, and angiograms are projected into the operative field and are viewed concurrently with the microsurgical exploration on a three-dimensional monitor.

would permit easier, safer, and more efficient operative approaches for many types of lesions (Fig. 6.10).

It is interesting to note that the modern two-dimensional neuroendoscopes surpass the operating microscope in projecting a more detailed enhancement of the structures. The availability of a three-dimensional neuroendoscope attached to a high-resolution TV monitor will advance the possibility to perform more intricate microsurgical manipulations.

I remain optimistic that videoscopic micro-neurosurgery encompassing these ideals will be practiced in the new century. I greatly enjoyed reading the articles of Guthrie and Kikinis, who indicate the unswerving course being pursued by the technological evolution for improving the intraoperative morphological and functional transparency not only of the lesion, but also perilesional areas and the entire brain.

My philosophy and vision for microneurosurgery remains unchanged. I will therefore conclude my reflections with an excerpt from a lecture given in 1986 in New Orleans:

The perfection of microtechnique requires end-less hours of practice in the laboratory in conjunction with progressively complex clinical exposure. It is conceivable that a 3D imaging system could also be used for instructional purposes. The computer could simulate a lesion such as an angioma or tumor with its anatomical surroundings on a stereoscopic monitor. The young neurosurgeon, using an electronic system, could attempt to dissect the mass under variable circumstances which could be preadjusted. The experience of the surgeon would dictate the speed of dissection, complexity of the lesion, etc., and expected difficulties encountered (such as bleeding from an arteriovenous malformation) could be simulated. Exposure of this kind would greatly improve the 3D graphic imagination ability of young neurosurgeons before clinical exposure.

Despite our considerable advances in operative approaches to the brain, the imagination of the neurosurgeon must never cease to reach for even better means of providing more precise visualization of the lesion both before as well as during operation. The tools of the neurosurgeon must be constantly improved and advanced. Only by continual reassessment and development beyond our present boundaries can we hope to make our intrusions into the brain not just possible but safe for all our patients. The transition to new ideas is achieved by integrating the past and present knowledge with our imagination to form a bridge to new developments of the future.

It was most encouraging and a great pleasure to read the article of Deia Loferdo, ''In the New Millennium,'' and the remarks of Keith L. Black: ''Fluorescent ligand binding specifically to tumor cells, will illuminate malignant cells during surgery and, much to the pleasure of many surgeons the surgical microscope will be replaced by digital optics worn like eyeglasses.''

Undoubtedly, the development of new diagnostic capabilities and their integration with surgical innovations will simultaneously advance and perpetuate each other to the benefit of our patients.

THE HISTORY OF THE MICROSCOPE

1. Abbe E. On Stephenson's system of homogeneous immersion for microscope objectives. *J R Microsc Soc* 279, 1879.
2. Abbe E. The new microscope. *S Ber Jena Ges Med* 2: 107–108, 1886.
3. Abbe E. On improvements of the microscope with the aid of new kinds of optical glass. *J R Microsc Soc* 20, 1887.
4. Ahlstrom O. Chinese spectacles. *Optician (XIX)* 3076: 201–208, 1950.
5. Allen RM. The microscope. New York, Van Nostrand, 1940.
6. Baker H. Employment for the microscope. London, 1753, p 434.
7. Bedini SA. Giuseppi Campani, pioneer optical inventor. Ithaca: 26VIII–2IX, 1962.
8. Bedini SA. Seventeenth century Italian compound microscopes. Physis, Rivista Storia Della Scienza. 1963, vol V, fasc 4.
9. Bodemer CN. The microscope in early embryological investigation. *Gynecol Invest* 4:188–209, 1973.
10. Borellus P. De vero telescopii inventore, cum brevi omnium conspicilorum historia . . . etiam centuria observanonum microscopicanum. The Hague. 1655.
11. Bradbury S. The evolution of the microscope. London, Pergamon Press, 1965.
12. Bradbury S, Turner GLE (eds): *Historical Aspect of Microscopy.* Cambridge, W. Heffner & Sons, 1962.
13. Carpenter WN, Dallinger WH. The microscope and its revelations. London, Churchill Livingstone, 1901.
14. Chevalier C. Des microscopes et de leur usage. Paris, 1839.
15. Clay RS, Court TH. History of the microscope. London, Charles Griffin, 1932.
16. Cruickshanks BR. Evolution of the wide field stereomicroscope for surgery. *Int Surg* 59:331–332, 1974.
17. Descartes R. La dioptrique. Leyden, 1637.
18. Disney AN, Hill CF, Watson Baker WE. The origin and development of the microscope. London, Royal Microscopical Society, 1928.
19. Gage SH. Microscopy in America (1830–1945), in Richards OW (ed): Trans Am Microsc Soc 83(4 Suppl), 1964.
20. Galileo G. Sidereus nuucius. Venice, 1610, p 10.
21. Haden RL. The origin of the microscope. *Ann Med Hist* 1:30–66, 1939.
22. Hansen JL, Schrader NA, Cowau WR. The Billings microscope collection. Washington, DC, Armed Forces Institute of Pathology, 1974.
23. Harting P. Das Mikroskop. Braunschweig, 1886.
24. Highmore NI. The history of generation. Martin, Lundor, 1651.
25. Hooke R. Micrographia. London, 1665.
26. Hughes A. Studies in the history of microscopy I. The influence of achromatism. *J R Microsc Soc* 75:1, 1955.
27. Hughes A. Studies in the history of microscopy II. The later history of the achromatic microscope. *J R Microsc Soc* 76:47, 1955.
28. Kircher A. Ans magna lucis et umbrae. 1646, p 834.
29. Lister JJ. On some properties in achromatic object glassed applicable to the improvement of the microscope. *Philos Trans* 130:187.
30. Majno G, Joris I. The microscope—the history of pathology. *Virchow Arch A Pathol Anat* 360:273–286, 1973.
31. Malies HM. The microscope during the last hundred years. *Microscope* 10:113–149, 1955.
32. Malis LI. New trend in microsurgery and applied technology, in Pluchino F, Broggi G (eds): *Advanced Technology in Neurosurgery.* Springer, 1987, pp 1–10.

33. Manguel A. *A History of Reading.* Canada, Knopf, 1996.

34. Needham J. Wissenschaft und Zivilisation in China. Herbster R (trans). Frankfurt, Suhrkampf, 1978, p 328.

35. Needham J. The grand titration. Science and Society in East and West. London, G Allen and Unwin, 1979, 78–80.

36. Needham J. Wissenschaftlicher Universilasmus. Frankfurt, Suhrkampf, 1993, pp 124–125.

37. Needham J, Gwei–Djen L. The optic artists of Chiangsu, in Bradbury S, Turner GLE (eds): Cambridge, 1967.

38. Nobert FA. Ueber die Prüfung und Vollkommenheit unserer jetzipen mikroscope. *Ann Phys Chem* 67:173–185, 1852.

39. Otto L. Vergleiche zur optischen Leistung historischer microscope. *Microskopie* 20:189–195, 1965.

40. Otto L. Zur Kenntnis der zusammen gesetztem Mikroscope des Giuseppe Campani (1635–1715). *Rom Mikroscope* 21:306–313, 1966.

41. Porta JB. Natural magic. London, Young X Speed, 1658.

42. Rosenthal JW. Spectacles and other vision aids. St. Francis, Norman Publishing, 1996.

43. Turner GLE. The history of optical instruments. A brief survey of sources and modern studies. History of science. An annual review of literature, research, and teaching. 1969, vol 8.

44. Turner GLE. The study of the history of the microscope. *Proc P Micro Soc* 7(2):121–149, 1972.

45. Turner GLE. Essays on the history of the microscope. Oxford, Senecio Publishing, 1980.

46. Turner GLE. The microscope as a technical frontier in science, in Turner GLE (ed): *Essays on the History of the Microscope.* Oxford, Senecio Press, 1980.

47. Zahn J. Oculus artificialis, etc. Nuremberg, 1702, ed 2.

THE HISTORY OF THE OPERATING MICROSCOPE

1. Ackerknecht EH. A short history of medicine. New York, Ronald Press, 1955.

2. Axenfeld TH. Eine neue Westien'sche binokulare Hand–loupe (Brillenloupe) zum Präparieren und für klinische Zwecke, mit veränderlicher Pupillendistanz und verstellbarem Kopfhalter. *Klin Mbl Augenheilk* 38:20–25, 1900.

3. Barraquer JI. The microscope in ocular surgery. *Am J Ophthalmol* 42:916–918, 1956.

4. Barraquer JI. The history of the microscope in ocular surgery. *J Microsurg* 1:288–299, 1980.

5. Becker B. The Zeiss operating microscope. *Am J Ophthalmol* 42:302–303, 1956.

6. Browli Smith A. Operating microscope. *Br Med S* 1:776, 1992.

7. Dekking HM. Use of binocular microscope in eye operations. *Arch Ophthalmol* 55:114–117, 1956.

8. Dekking HM. Microsurgery of the eye: The present and the future. *Arch Ophthalmol* 71:881–883, 1964.

9. Dohlman GF. Carl Olof Nylen and the birth of the otomicroscope and microsurgery. *Arch Otolaryngol* 90:161–165, 1969.

10. Donaghy RM. The history of microsurgery in neurosurgery. Clin Neurosurg Vol. 26, chap. 27, 5, 1978.

11. Donaghy RMP. The history of microsurgery in neurosurgery. *Clin Neurosurg* 26:619–625, 1979.

12. Donaghy RM. History of microneurosurgery, in Wilkins RH, Renfachary SS (eds): *Neurosurgery.* 1996, ed 2, vol I, pp 37–42.

13. Ecker A. The cerebral convolutions of man (English translation). New York, D. Appleton & Co. 1973.

14. Gibson WPR. The operating microscope and the development of ear surgery. *J R Soc Med* 73:52–55, 1980.

15. Gould JS. Raymond Madiford Peardon Donaghy, MD, in tribute. *Microsurgery* 13:109–110, 1992.

16. Gratiolet LP. Les plis cérébraux de l'homme et des primates. Paris, 1854.

17. Grünberger V, Ulm R. Diagnostische Methode, in *Geburtshilfe, Gynakologie.* Stuttgart, Thieme, 1968.

18. Harms H. Augenoperationen unter dem binocularen Mikroskop. *Ber Dtsch Ophth Gesellsch* 58:119–122, 1953.

19. Harms H, Mackensen G. Augenoperationen unter dem Mikroskope. Stuttgart, Thieme, 1966.

20. Harms H, Mackensen G. Ocular surgery under the microscope. Chicago, Year Book Medical Publishers, 1967.

21. Heller R. Das Binocular—Stative (oder die ''Brille'' des chirurgen). *Zeiss Inform* 5:7–9, 1972.

22. Hess C. Pathologie und Therapie des Linsensystems, in Graefe A, Saemisch T (eds): *Handbuch der gesamten Augenheilkunde.* 3. Aufl., Kap. IX 2. Leipzig, Engelmann, 1911.

23. Hinselmann. Quoted by Grünberger und Ulm (1968).

24. Hoerenz P. Magnification: Loupes and the operating microscope. *Clin Obstet Gynecol* 23 (4):1151–1162, 1980.

25. Hoerenz P. The operating microscope. I. Optical principles, illumination systems, and support systems. *J Microsurg* 1:364–369, 1980.

26. Hoerenz P. The operating microscope. II. Individual parts, handling, assembling, focusing, and balancing. *J Microsurg* 1:419–427, 1980.

27. Hoerenz P. The operating microscope. III. Accessories. *J Microsurg* 2:22–26, 1980.

28. Hoerenz P. The operating microscope. IV. Documentation. *J Microsurg* 2:126–139, 1980.

29. Hoerenz P. The operating microscope. V. Maintenance and cleaning. *J Microsurg* 2:179–182, 1981.

30. Holmgren G. Opération sur temporal a l'aide de la loupe et du microscope. *Acta Otolaryngol* 4:386, 1922.

31. Jannetta PJ. The surgical binocular microscope in neurological surgery. *Am Surg* 34:31, 1968.

32. Kennerdell JS, Maroon JC, Rehkopk P. Why use the operating microscope in orbital surgery? *Ophthalmology (Rochester)* 86:2040–2047, 1979.

33. Kriss TC, Kriss VM. History of the microscope from magnifying glass to microneurosurgery. *Neurosurgery* 42:899–908, 1998.

34. Lim ASM. Ophthalmic microsurgery: Adjustment problems. *Aust N Z J Surg* 50:335–338, 1980.

35. Littmann H. Ein neues Operations–Mikroskop. *Klin Mbl Augenheilk* 124:473–476, 1954.

36. McGrouther DA. The operating microscope: A necessity or a luxury? *Br J Plast Surg* 33:453–460, 1980.

37. Nylen CO. The microscope in aural surgery, its first use and later development. *Acta Otolaryngol* 116:226–240, 1954.

38. Nylen CO. The otomicroscope and microsurgery. *Acta Otolaryngol* 73:453–454, 1972.

39. O'Brien B. The triploscope—a triple operating microscope. *Plast Reconstr Surg* 45:279–281, 1970.

40. O'Brien B. A modified triploscope. *Br J Plast Surg* 26: 301–303, 1973.
41. Owen ER. Practical microsurgery. I. A choice of optical aids for fine work. *Med J Aust* 1:244–246, 1971.
42. Owen E. The operating microscope isn't everything—a warning and a prediction. J Bone Joint Surg Br 58B: 397–398, 1976.
43. Perrit RA. Recent advances in corneal surgery. *Arch Ophthalmol Otol* 288: 1950.
44. Perritt RA. Micro-ophthalmic surgery. XVIII. Belgica, Concil Ophthal, 1958.
45. Rand RW, Urban JC. The surgical microscope: Its use and care, in Rand RW (ed): *Microneurosurgery.* CV Mosby, 1969.
46. Rice JC. The microsurgical revolution in otolaryngology. *Med J Aust* 2:1011–1014, 1972.
47. Riechert T. Die Operationen an der WS und am Rückenmark, in *Chirurgische Operationslehre.* Leipzig, 1948, vol 2, p 753. Hrsg. Bier, Braun und Kümmel, Vol. 2, 7. Aufl., Barth,
48. Rohr M, Stock W. Über eine achromatische Brillenlupe schwacher Vergröberung. *Klin Mbl Augenheilk* 51: 206–210, 1913.
49. Roper–Hall MJ. Microsurgery in ophthalmology. *Br J Ophthalmol* 51:408–414, 1967.
50. Shambaugh GE. Surgery for otosclerosis. Indications, techniques and results. *Fortschr Hals-Nas-Ohrenheilk* 8:367–428, 1961.
51. Silber J. Microsurgery. Williams & Wilkins, 1979.
52. Simpson JF. An operating microscope for the fenestration operation. *Proc R Soc Med* 60:320, 1946.
53. *Trans Am Ophthalmol Soc* 63:335–348, 1965.
54. Troutman RC. The operating microscope in ophthalmic surgery.
55. Troutman RC. The operating microscope: Past, present and future. *Trans Ophthalmol Soc UK* 87:205–218, 1967.
56. Tullio P. Die mikrochirurgie d. Ohres v. Anwendung d. binocularen Stereoskop. *Mikroscope Arch ONK* 145: 382, 1938.
57. Urban JC. The surgical microscope: Its use and care, in Rand RW (ed): *Microsurgery.* St. Louis, CV Mosby, 1961, pp 9–20.
58. Van Zuylen J. The microscopes of Antoni van Leeuwenhoek. *J Microsc* 121:309–328, 1981.
59. Virchow R. Die cellular pathology. A. Hirschwald, 1858.
60. Wullstein H. Technik und bisherige Ergebnnisse d. *Tympanoplastik* 87:308, 1953.
61. Yaşargil MC. Die Anwendung des Operationsmikroscopes in der Neurochirurgie. *Zeiss Inform* 16:129–131, 1968.
62. Yaşargil MG. Microsurgery applied to neurosurgery. Stuttgart, Thieme, 1969.
63. Yaşargil MG. History of microneurosurgery, in Spetzler RF, Carter LP, et al. (eds): *Cerebral Revascularization.* Stuttgart, Thieme, 1985, pp 28–33.
64. Yaşargil MG. The operating microscope (weight counterbalanced), in Yaşargil MG: *Microneurosurgery.* Vol. IVB, Thieme, 1996, pp 7–10.
65. Zehender W. Beschreibung der binocularen Cornealoupe. *Klin Mbl Augenheilk* 25:496–499, 1887.
66. Zeki S. A vision of the brain. Oxford, Blackwell, 1993.
67. Zingg R. Aus der Entwicklung sgeshichte des microscopes. 33:26–32, 1969.
68. Zöllner F. Mikroskopstativ für operation. *Laryngol Rhinol Otol* 28:209, 1949.

MICROSURGERY IN LABORATORY RESEARCH

1. Acland R. Prevention of thrombosis in microvascular surgery by the use magnesium sulphate. *Br J Plast Surg* 25:292–304, 1972.
2. Acland R. Signs of patency in small vessels anastomoses. *Surgery* 72:744, 1972.
3. Ballantyne DL, Rosenberg BB. Organized bibliography of the microsurgical literature. Rockville, MD, Aspen System Corporation, 1985.
4. Buncke HJ. Microsurgery—retrospective. *Clin Plast Surg* 13:315–318, 1986.
5. Buncke HJ. Forty years of microsurgery: What's next? J Hand Surg (Am) 20A:S35–S45, 1995.
6. Buncke HJ, Cobbett JR, Smith JW, et al. Techniques of microsurgery. Sommerville, Ethicon, 1967.
7. Buncke HJ Jr, Daniller AI, Schulz WP, et al. The fate of autogenous whole joints transplanted by microvascular anastomoses. *Plast Reconstr Surg* 39:333, 1967.
8. Buncke HJ Jr, Schulz WP. Experimental digital amputation and reimplantation. *Plast Reconstr Surg* 36:62, 1965.
9. Carrel A, Guthrie CC. Uniterminal and biterminal venous transplantations. *Surg Gynecol Obstet* 2:266, 1906.
10. Chase N, Schwartz SI. Consistent patency of 1.5mm arterial anastomoses. *Surg Forum* 13:220–222, 1962.
11. Cobbett JR. Microvascular surgery. *Surg Clin North Am* 47:92, 1967.
12. Collins RE, Douglass FM. Small vein anastomosis with and without operative microscope. A comparative study. *Arch Surg Chicago* 88:740, 1964.
13. Crowell RM, Yaşargil MG. End-to-side anastomosis of superficial temporal artery to middle cerebral artery branch in the dog. *Neurochirurgia* 16:73–77, 1973.
14. Daniel RK. Microsurgery: Through the looking glass. *N Engl J Med* 300:1251–1257, 1979.
15. Daniel RK, Taylor GI. Distant transfer of an island flap by microvascular anastomoses. A clinical technique. *Plast Reconstr Surg* 52:111, 1973.
16. Diaz FG, Mastri AR, Ausman JI, et al. Acute cerebral revascularization after regional cerebral ischemia in the dog. *J Neurosurg* 51:644–653, 1979.
17. Donaghy RMP. Patch and by-pass in microangeional surgery, in Donaghy RMP, Yaşargil MG (eds): *Micro-Vascular Surgery.* St. Louis, CV Mosby, Thieme, 1967.
18. Donaghy RMP, Yaşargil MG. Microvascular surgery. St. Louis, CV Mosby, Thieme, 1967.
19. Echlin FRA. Spasm of basilar and vertebral arteries caused by experimental subarachnoid hemorrhage. *J Neurosurg* 23:1–11, 1965.
20. Fisher B, Lee S. Microvascular surgical technique in research, with special reference to renal transplantation in the rat. *Surgery* 58:904, 1965.
21. Jacobson JH. Introduction, in: Silver SJ (ed): *Microsurgery.* Williams & Wilkins, 1979, pp XV–XVII.
22. Jacobson JH II, Suarez EI. Microsurgery in anastomosis of small vessels. *Surg Forum* 11:243–245, 1960.
23. Jacobson JH II, Suarez EI. Microvascular surgery. *Dis Chest* 4:220–224, 1962.

24. Khodadad G. Microvascular surgery, in Rand RW (ed): *Microneurosurgery.* St. Louis, CV Mosby, 1969, pp 170–182.

25. Khodadad G. Extracranial–intracranial by-pass graft. *J Neurol Neurosurg Psychiatry* 35:522–526, 1972.

26. Khodadad G. Sublingual and lingula–basilar artery anastomoses and carotid–basilar bypass grafts. *Surg Neurol* 1:175–177, 1973.

27. Khodadad G. Eight-year follow-up of experimental carotid–middle cerebral and carotid–basilar arterial bypass grafts and anastomoses. *Neurosurgery* 2:246–251, 1978.

28. Khodadad G, Lougheed WM. Repair and replacement of small arteries, microsuture technique. *J Neurosurg* 24:61–69, 1966.

29. Khodadad G, Lougheed WM. Stapling technique in segmental vein autografts and end-to-end anastomosis of small vessels in dogs. Utilization of the operating microscope. *J Neurosurg* 24:855–864, 1966.

30. Kobayashi T, Houkin K, Ho F, et al. Transverse cervical artery bypass. *Neurosurgery* 45:299–302, 1999.

31. Kosse KH, Suarez EL, Fagan WT, et al. Microsurgery in ureteral reconstruction. *J Urol* 87:48, 1962.

32. Krizek IJ, Tani T, Desprez JD, et al. Experimental transplantation of composite grafts by microsurgical vascular anastomoses. *Plast Reconstr Surg* 36:538, 1965.

33. Lougheed WM, Tom M. A method of introducing blood into the subarachnoid space in the region of the circle of Willis in dogs. *Can J Surg* 4:329–337, 1961.

34. Millesi H. Erfahrungen wit der microchirurgie peripherer nerveu chir. *Plast Reconstr* 3:47–55, 1967.

35. Millesi H. Microsurgery of peripheral nerves. *Hand* 5: 157–160, 1973.

36. Millesi H. Looking back on nerve surgery. *Int J Microsurg* 2:143–158, 1980.

37. O'Brien B. Symposium in microsurgery. St. Louis, CV Mosby, 1976.

38. O'Brien B. Microvascular reconstructive surgery. London, Churchill Livingstone, 1978.

39. O'Brien B, Henderson P, Bennet R, et al. Microvascular surgical technique. *Med J Aust* 1:722–725, 1970.

40. Peerless SJ. Techniques of cerebral revascularization. *Clin Neurosurg* 23:258–269, 1976.

41. Reichman OH. Experimental lingual–basilar arterial microanastomosis. *J Neurosurg* 34:500–505, 1971.

42. Samii M. Die operative Wiederherstellung verletzler Nerven. *Langenbecks Arch Chir* 332:355–362, 1972.

43. Samii M. Modern aspect of peripheral and cranial nerve surgery. *Adv Tech Stand Neurosurg* 2:33–106, 1975.

44. Samii M, Wallenborn R. Tierexperimentelle Untersuchungen über den Einfluss der Spannung auf den Regenerationserfolg nach Nervennaht. *Acta Neurochir (Wien)* 27:87–110, 1972.

45. Samii R, Willebrand H. The technique of and indications for autologous interfascicular nerve transplantation. *Excep Med Int Congress Ser* 217:39, 1970.

46. Sandvoss G, Smith RD, Yaşargil MG. Experimentelle, microchirurgische Freilegung Hirnnerven III, IV und VI beider Katze. *Neurochirurgia* 27:179–132, 1984.

47. Schulz MR. Beitrag zur Nahttechnik am Sinus sagittalis superior (Vorläufige Mitteilung) (Suture technique for the superior sagittal sinus—preliminary results). *Z Exp Chir Transplant Künstliche Organe* 16:120–124, 1983.

48. Shields CB, Donaghy RM. Arterial venous graft for cerebral revascularization. *Surg Forum* 28:463–464, 1977.

49. Silver SJ. Microsurgical technique, in Silver SJ (ed): *Microsurgery.* Baltimore, Williams & Wilkins, 1979, pp 1–29.

50. Smith JW. Microsurgery of peripheral nerves. *Plast Reconstr Surg* 33:317–329, 1964.

51. Smith JW. Microsurgery: Review of the literature and discussion of microtechniques. *Plast Reconstr Surg* 37: 227–245, 1966.

52. Stahl WM, Katsumura T. Reconstruction of small arteries. A study of methods. *Arch Surg* 88:384, 1964.

53. Terzis JK, Strauch B. Microsurgery of the peripheral nerve: A physiological approach. *Clin Orthop* 133: 39–48, 1978.

54. Torrens M, Al-Mefty O, Kobayashi (eds): *Operative Skull Base Surgery.* Edinburgh, Churchill Livingstone, 1997.

55. Urschel HC Jr, Roth EJ. Small arterial anastomoses: I. Nonsuture. *Ann Surg* 153:599, 1961.

56. Urschel HC Jr, Roth EJ. Small arterial anastomoses: II. Suture. *Ann Surg* 153:610, 1961.

57. Villegas LD. Technique for end-to-end anastomoses between artificial grafts and arteries with minimal interruption of the circulation. *Surgery* 40:1035, 1956.

58. Weiss EW, Lam CR. Tantalum tubes in the nonsuture method of blood vessel anastomosis. *Am J Surg* 80:452, 1950.

59. Woringer E, Kunlin J. Anastomose entre le carotide primitive et la carotide intra-cranienne ou la sylvienne par greffon selon la technique da la suture suspendue. *Neurochirurgie* 9:181–188, 1963.

60. Yaşargil MG. Experimental small vessel surgery in the dog including patching and grafting of cerebral vessels and the formation of functional extra–intracranial shunts, in Donaghy RMP, Yaşargil MG (eds): *Micro-Vascular Surgery.* St. Louis, CV Mosby, 1967, pp 87–126.

61. Yaşargil MG. History of microsurgery, in Spetzler RR, Carter LP, (eds): *Cerebral Revascularization.* Thieme–Stratton, 1985, pp 28–33.

62. Yaşargil MG, Yonekawa Y, Denton I, et al. Experimental intracranial transplantation of autogenic omentum majus. *J Neurosurg* 40:213–217, 1974.

63. Yonekawa Y, et al. Laboratory training in microsurgical technique and microvascular anastomosis. *Op Tech Neurosurg* 2:149–158, 1999.

64. Young PH, Yaşargil MG. Experimental carotid artery aneurysms in rats: A new model for microsurgical practice. *J Microsurg* 3:135–146, 1982.

CLINICAL MICRONEUROSURGERY

1. Abdulrauf SI, Al-Mefty O. The petrosal approach. *Op Tech Neurosurg* 2:58–64, 1999.

2. Alexander MS, Vishteh AG, Spetzler RF. By-pass surgery in the management of complex aneurysm. *Op Tech Neurosurg* 2:123–141, 1999.

3. Alleyne CA, Spetzler RF. The transcondylar approach. *Op Tech Neurosurg* 2:74–86, 1999.

4. Al-Mefty O. Surgery of the cranial mass. Kluver Academic Press, 1989.

5. Al-Mefty O (ed): *Meningiomas.* New York, Raven Press, 1991.

6. Al-Mefty O. The cranio-orbitozygomatic approach for intracranial lesions. *Contemp Neurosurg* 14:1–6, 1992.

7. Al-Mefty O. Operative atlas of meningiomas. Philadelphia, Lippincott–Raven, 1998.

8. Al-Mefty O, Holoubi A, Rifai A, et al. Microsurgical removal of suprasellar meningiomas. *Neurosurgery* 16:364–372, 1985.

9. Al-Mefty O, Origitano TC, Harkey HL (eds): *Controversies in Neurosurgery*. New York, Thieme, 1996.

10. Al-Mefty O, Smith RR. Surgery of tumors invading the cavernous sinus. *Surg Neurol* 30:370–381, 1988.

11. Arnautovic KI, Al-Mefty O. Giant and large paraclinoid aneurysms, in Eisenberg MB, Al-Mefty O (eds): *The Cavernous Sinus*. Baltimore, Lippincott, Williams & Wilkins, 1999, pp 177–190.

12. Ausman JI, Moore J, Chou SN. Spontaneous cerebral revascularization in a patient with STA–MCA anastomosis. *J Neurosurg* 44:84–87, 1976.

13. Barrow DL, Tindall GT, Tindall SC. Combined simultaneous transsphenoidal operative approach to selected sellar tumors. *Perspect Neurol Surg* 3:49–57, 1992.

14. Bertalanffy H, Seeger W. The dorsolateral, suboccipital, transcondylar approach to the lower clivus and anterior portion of craniocervical junction. *Neurosurgery* 29:815–821, 1991.

15. Chater N, Spetzler R, Tonnemacher K, et al. Microvascular bypass surgery. *J Neurosurg* 44:712–714, 1976.

16. Chater N, Spetzler R, Tonnemacher K, et al. Microvascular bypass surgery. Part 1: Anatomical studies. *J Neurosurg* 44:712–714, 1976.

17. Chou SN. Embolectomy of the middle cerebral artery: Report of a case. *J Neurosurg* 20:161–163, 1963.

18. Ciric I, Mikhael M, Stafford T, et al. Transsphenoidal microsurgery of pituitary macroadenomas with long-term follow-up results. *J Neurosurg* 59:395–401, 1983.

19. Ciric IS, Tarkington J. Transsphenoidal microsurgery. *Surg Neurol* 2:207–213, 1974.

20. Conforti P, Tomasello T, Albanese V. Cerebral revascularization. Padua, Piccifi Nuova Librario, 1984.

21. David CA, Vishteh AG, Spetzler RF, et al. Late angiographic follow-up review of typically treated aneurysms. *J Neurosurg* 91:396–401, 1999.

22. Day JD, Fukushima T, Giannotta SL. Microanatomical study of the extradural middle fossa approach to the petroclival and posterior rhomboid construct. *Neurosurgery* 34:1009–1016, 1994.

23. Day JD, Giannotta SL, Fukushima T. Extradural temporopolar approach to lesions of the upper basilar artery and infrachiasmatic region. *J Neurosurg* 81:230–235, 1994.

24. Derome PJ. Surgical management of tumors invading the skull base. *Can J Neurol Sci* 12:345–347, 1985.

25. Dolenc V. Microsurgical removal of large sphenoidal bone meningiomas. *Acta Neurochir (Wien)* 28:391–396, 1979.

26. Dolenc VV (ed): *The Cavernous Sinus*. New York, Springer, 1982.

27. Dolenc VV, et al. Treatment of tumors invading the cavernous sinus, in Dolenc VV (ed): *The Cavernous Sinus*. New York, Springer, 1987, pp 377–391.

28. Donaghy RM. The history of microsurgery in neurosurgery. *Clin Neurosurg* 26:619–625, 1979.

29. Donaghy RMP, Jacobson JH III, Wallman LJ, et al. Microsurgery: A neurological aid. No. 36, Excerpta Medica International Congress Series, Washington, DC, Second International Congress of Neurological Surgeons, 1961, pp E175–E176.

30. Donaghy RM, Upton PD, Collier J, et al. Experimental study of intravascular fat. *Am J Surg* 117(4):595–598, 1969.

31. Donaghy RM, Wallman LJ, Flanagan MJ, et al. Sagittal sinus repair. Technical note. *J Neurosurg* 38(2):244–248, 1973.

32. Donaghy RMP, Yaşargil MG. Microvascular surgery. Thieme, 1967.

33. Donaghy RMP, Yaşargil MG. Extraintracranial blood flow diversion. Presented at the American Association of Neurological Surgeons, Chicago, IL, April 11, 1968.

34. Donaghy RM, Yaşargil G. Microangeional surgery and its techniques. *Prog Brain Res* 30:263–267, 1968.

35. Drake CG. Total removal of large acoustic neuromas. A modification of the McKenzie operation with special emphasis on saving the facial nerve. *J Neurosurg* 26:554–561, 1967.

36. Eisenberg MB, Al-Mefty OA. The cavernous sinus. Lippincott, Williams & Wilkins, 1999.

37. Fein JN, Flamm ES. Cerebrovascular surgery. New York, Springer, 1985, vol I-6.

38. Ferguson GG, Drake CG, Peerless SS. Extracranial–intracranial arterial bypass in the treatment of giant intracranial aneurysm. *Stroke* 8:11, 1977.

39. Fisch U. Otoneurosurgical approach to acoustic neuromas. Springer Neurol Surg 9:318–336, 1978.

40. Fisch U. Infratemporal fossa approach for glomus tumors of the temporal bone. *Laryngoscope* 93:36–44, 1983.

41. Fisch U, Mattox D. Microsurgery of the skull base. Thieme, 1988.

42. Fisch U, Pillsbury HC. Infratemporal fossa approach to lesions in the temporal bone and base of the skull. *Arch Otolaryngol* 105:99–107, 1979.

43. Fischer G, Mercier P, Sindou M. Microsurgery in neurosurgery. *Int Surg* 65:491–494, 1980.

44. Flamm ES. History of neurovascular surgery, in Greenblatt SH (ed): *History of Neurosurgery*. Park Ridge, AANS, 1997, pp 259–288.

45. Fox JL. Intracranial aneurysms. Springer, 1983, 3 vols.

46. Gilsbach J, Eppert HR. Transoral operations for craniospinal malfunctions. *Neurosurg Rev* 6:199–209, 1983.

47. Gionnatta SL, Maceri DR. Retrolabyrinthine transsigmoid approach to basilar trunk and vertebrobasilar junction aneurysms. *J Neurosurg* 69:461–466, 1988.

48. Hakuba A. Total removal of cerebellopontine angle tumor with a combined transpetrosal–transtentorial approach (in Japanese). *No Shinkei Geka* 6:347–354, 1978.

49. Hakuba A (ed): *Surgery of the Intracranial Venous System*. Springer, 1996.

50. Hakuba A, Hashi K, Fujitani K, et al. Jugular foramen neurinomas. *Surg Neurol* 11:83–94, 1979.

51. Hakuba A, Lie SS, Nishimura S. The orbitozygomatic infratemporal approach: A new surgical technique. *Surg Neurol* 26:271–276, 1986.

52. Hakuba A, Ogata K, Baba M. Surgical anatomy of the skull base. Tokyo, Miwa Shoten, 1996.

53. Handa H (ed): *Microneurosurgery*. Tokyo, Gaku Shoin, Ltd., 1973.

54. Hardy J. Exerese de adenomes hypophysaires par voi transsphenoidale. *Ann Med Can* 91:933–945, 1962.

55. Hardy J. Transsphenoidal microsurgery of the normal and pathological pituitary. *Clin Neurosurg* 16:185–216, 1969.

56. Hardy J. Transsphenoidal hypophysectomy. *J Neurosurg* 34:582–594, 1971.

57. Hardy J. Subnasal transsphenoidal approach to the pituitary, in Rand RW (ed): *Microneurosurgery*. St. Louis, CV Mosby, 1978, ed 2, pp 105–130.

58. Hardy J. Transsphenoidal microsurgery of prolactinomas: Report on 355 cases, in Tolis G, Stefanis C, Mountokalakis T (eds): *Prolactin and Prolactinomas*. New York, Raven Press, 1983, pp 431–440.

59. Hardy J. Microneurosurgery of the hypophysis, in Rand RW (ed): *Microneurosurgery*. St. Louis, CV Mosby, 1989, pp 87–103.

60. Hitzelberger WE, House WF. A combined approach to the cerebellopontine angle. *Arch Otolaryngol* 84:267–285, 1966.

61. House WF. Surgical exposure of the internal auditory canal. *Laryngoscope* 71:1363–1385, 1961.

62. House WF (ed): *Acoustic Neuromas Otolaryngol* 88:76–715, 1968.

63. House HP, House WF. Historical review and problem of acoustic neuroma. *Arch Otolaryngol* 80:599–604, 1964.

64. House H, House W, Hildyard KV. Congenital stapes footplate fixation. *Trans Am Laryngol Rhinol Soc* 139–152, 1958.

65. Housepian EN. Intraorbital tumors, in Schmiedek NH, Sweet WH (eds): *Operative Neurosurgical Techniques.*, Grune/Stratton, 1988, Vol 1, pp 235–244.

66. Jack CR Jr, Sundt TM Jr, Fode NC, et al. Superficial temporal–middle cerebral artery bypass: Clinical pre- and postoperative angiographic correlation. *J Neurosurg* 69(1):46–51, 1988.

67. Jacobson JH, Wallman LJ, Schumacher GA, et al. Microsurgery as an aid to middle cerebral artery endarterectomy. *J Neurosurg* 19:108–115, 1962.

68. Jannetta PJ. Microsurgery of cranial nerve. *Clin Neurosurg* 20:607–618, 1978.

69. Jannetta PJ. Operative techniques and clinicopathologic correlation in the surgical treatment of cranial rhizopathies (honored guest lecture). *Clin Neurosurg* 44:181–195, 1997.

70. Jannetta PJ. Vestibular neurilemomas (honored guest lecture). *Clin Neurosurg* 44:529–548, 1997.

71. Jannetta PJ, et al. Microvascular decompression. *Neurosurgery* 43:1–9, 1998.

72. Jannetta PJ, Levy EI, Clyde B, et al. Medullary compression and hypertension. *J Neurosurg* 89(1):169–70, 1998 (letter, comment).

73. Jannetta PJ, Rand RW. Trigeminal neuralgia. Microsurgical technique. *Bull Los Angeles Neurol Soc* 31:93–99, 1966.

74. Jannetta PJ, Rand RW. Vascular compression of the trigeminal nerve at the pons in patients with trigeminal neuralgia, in Donaghy RMP, Yaşargil MG (eds): *Micro–Vascular Surgery*. St. Louis, CV Mosby, Stuttgart, Thieme, 1967, p 150.

75. Jannetta PJ, Rand RW. Transtentorial retrogasserian rhizotomy in trigeminal neuralgia. St. Louis, CV Mosby, 1969, pp 156–169.

76. Kline DG. Macroscopic and microscopic concomitants of nerve repair. *Clin Neurosurg* 26:487–606, 1978.

77. Kobayashi T, Nakane T, Kageyawa N. Combined transsphenoidal and intracranial surgery of craniopharyngioma. *Prog Exp Tumor Res* 30:341–349, 1987.

78. Konovalov AN, Makhmudov UB. Methodology and results of total acoustic neurinoma using microsurgical techniques (in Russian)). *Zh Vopr Neirokhir* 2:3–10, 1981.

79. Koos NT, Spetzler RF, Lang J. Color atlas of microneurosurgery. Stuttgart, Thieme, 1993, vol 1, 1997, vol 2.

80. Koos NT, Spetzler RF, Pendl G, et al. Color atlas of microneurosurgery. Stuttgart, Thieme, 1985.

81. Kurze T. Microtechniques in neurological surgery. *Clin Neurosurg* 11:128–137, 1964.

82. Kurze T. A neurosurgical conspectus of otology. *Clin Neurosurg* 13:238–51, 1965.

83. Kurze T. Approaches to the incisura. *Clin Neurosurg* 25:700–716, 1978.

84. Kurze T. Microsurgery of the posterior fossa. *Clin Neurosurg* 26:463–478, 1979.

85. Kurze T, Doyle JB. Extradural intracranial (middle fossa) approach to the internal auditory canal. *J Neurosurg* 19:1033–1037, 1962.

86. Laws ER Jr. Transsphenoidal tumor surgery for intrasellar pathology. *Clin Neurosurg* 26:391–397, 1979.

87. Laws ER Jr. Transsphenoidal microsurgery in the management of craniopharyngioma. *J Neurosurg* 52:661–666, 1980.

88. Laws ER Jr. Transsphenoidal surgery for tumors of the clivus. *Head Neck Surg* 92:100–1101, 1984.

89. Laws ER. Schools of neurosurgery, in Greenblatt SH (ed): *Their Development and Evolution in a History of Neurosurgery*. Park Ridge, AANS, 1997.

89. Laws ER Jr, Piepgras DG, Randall RV, et al. Neurosurgical management of acromegaly. Results in 82 patients treated between 1972 and 1977. *J Neurosurg* 50:454–461, 1979.

90. Lougheed WM. Surgery of intracranial vascular occlusion, in Donaghy RMP, Yaşargil MG (eds): *Micro–Vascular Surgery*. St. Louis, CV Mosby, Stuttgart, Thieme, 1967, pp 142–147.

91. Lougheed WM. Selection, timing, and technique of aneurysm surgery of the anterior circle of Willis. *Clin Neurosurg* 16:95–113, 1969.

92. Lougheed WM, Elgie RG, Barnett HJ. The results of surgical management of extracranial internal carotid artery occlusion and stenosis. *CMAJ* 95(25):1279–1298, 1966.

93. Lougheed WM, Gunton RW, Barnett JM. Embolectomy of internal carotid, middle and anterior cerebral arteries. *J Neurosurg* 22:607, 1965.

94. Lougheed WM, Gunton RW, Barnett HJ. Embolectomy of internal carotid, middle, and anterior cerebral arteries. Report of a case. *J Neurosurg* 22(6):607–609, 1965.

95. Lougheed WM, Marshall BM. The diploscope in intracranial aneurysm surgery: Results in 40 patients. *Can J Surg* 12(1):75–82, 1969.

96. Lougheed WM, Marshall BM, Hunter M, et al. Common carotid to intracranial internal carotid bypass venous graft: Technical note. *J Neurosurg* 34:114–118, 1971.

97. Lougheed WM, Tom M. A method of introducing blood into the subarachnoid space in the region of the circle of Willis in dogs. *Can J Surg* 4:329–337, 1961.

98. Malis LI. Tumors of the parasellar region. *Adv Neurol* 15:281–299, 1976.

99. Malis LI. Intramedullary spinal cord tumors. *Clin Neurosurg* 25:512–539, 1978.

100. Malis LI. Microsurgery for spinal cord arteriovenous malformation. *Clin Neurosurg* 26:543–555, 1979.

101. Malis LI. Neurosurgical photography through the microscope. *Clin Neurosurg* 28:233–245, 1981.

102. Malis LI. The petrosal approach. *Clin Neurosurg* 37: 528–540, 1991.

103. Malis LI. Transpetrosal approach and sinus division. *J Neurosurg* 86(6):1072–1073, 1997 (letter, comment).

104. Malis LI. Acoustic neuroma. Elsevier, 1998.

105. Malis LI, Decker RE. Microvascular clips. *J Neurosurg* 32(2):266, 1970.

106. Malmros R. Experiences in embolectomy (7 cases with embolectomy of MCA), in Fusek, Kunc (eds): *Present Limits of Neurosurgery.* 1972, p 395.

107. Maroon JC, Kennerdell JS. Microsurgical approach to orbital tumors. *Clin Neurosurg* 26:479–489, 1978.

108. Maroon JC, Kennerdell JS. Surgical approaches to the orbit. *J Neurosurg* 60:1226–1235, 1984.

109. Maroon JC, Roberts E, Numoto M, et al. Microvascular surgery: Simplified instrumentation. Technical note. *J Neurosurg* 38(1):119–126, 1973.

110. McLaughlin MR, Jannetta PJ, Clyde BL, et al. Microvascular decompression of cranial nerves: Lessons learned after 4400 operations. *J Neurosurg* 90(1):1–8, 1999.

111. Ogata M. An anatomical and technical note for surgery of clivus. *No Shinkei Geka* 11:463–971, 1983.

112. Ono M, Kubik ST, Abernaty CD. Atlas of cerebral sulci. Stuttgart, Thieme, 1990.

113. Parkinson D. Carotid cavernous fistula: Direct repair with preservation of the carotid artery. Technical note. *J Neurosurg* 38:99–106, 1973.

114. Parkinson D. Carotid cavernous fistula. History and anatomy, in Dolenc VV (ed): *The Cavernous Sinus.* New York, Springer, 1982, pp 3–29.

115. Pasztor E, Vajda S, et al. Transoral surgery for craniocervical space occupying process. *Neurosurgery* 60: 278–281, 1984.

116. Pieper DR, Al-Mefty O. Total petrosectomy. Approach of lesions of the skull base, in Robertson JT et al. (eds): *Cranial Base Surgery.* London, Churchill Livingstone, 2000, pp 449–472.

117. Pool JL, Colton RP. The dissecting microscope for intracranial vascular surgery. *J Neurosurg* 25: 315–318, 1966.

118. Poppen JL. Tricks of the trade. *Clin Neurosurg* 11: 14–20, 1964.

119. Rand RW. Micro-neurosurgery. St. Louis: CV Mosby, 1969.

120. Rand RW. Suboccipital transmeatal microneurosurgical resection of acoustic tumors. *Ann Surg* 174(4): 663–671, 1971.

121. Rand RW, Jannetta PJ. Micro-neurosurgery for aneurysms of the vertebral–basilar artery system. *J Neurosurg* 27(4):330–335, 1967.

122. Rand RW, Jannetta PJ. Microneurosurgery: Application of the binocular surgical microscope in brain tumors, intracranial aneurysms, spinal cord disease, and nerve reconstruction. *Clin Neurosurg* 15:319–342, 1968.

123. Rand RW, Jannetta PJ. Microneurosurgery in brain tumors, intracranial aneurysms, spinal canal disease, and nerve reconstruction. *Clin Neurosurg* 75:319–391, 1968.

124. Rand RW, Kurze TL. Micro-neurosurgery in acoustic tumors (suboccipital transmeatal approach). *Trans Am Acad Ophthalmol Otolaryngol* 71(4):682–694, 1967.

125. Rand RW, Kurze T. Preservation of vestibular, cochlear, and facial nerves during microsurgical removal of acoustic tumors. Report of two cases. *J Neurosurg* 28:158–161, 1968.

126. Rhoton AL Jr. Microsurgery of the internal acoustic meatus. *Surg Neurol* 2:311–318, 1974.

127. Rhoton AL Jr. Microsurgical removal of acoustic neuromas. *Surg Neurol* 6:211–210, 1976.

128. Rhoton AL Jr. Microsurgical anatomy of the internal acoustic meatus and facial nerve, in Rand RW (ed): *Microneurosurgery.* St. Louis, CV Mosby, 1978, ed 2, pp 162–181.

129. Rhoton AL Jr. Microsurgical anatomy of the posterior fossa cranial nerves. *Clin Neurosurg* 26:398–462, 1979.

130. Rhoton AL Jr. Transcranial microsurgical approaches to the sellar region, in Tindall GT, Collins WF (eds): *Clinical Management of Pituitary Disorders.* New York, Raven Press, 1979, pp 353–372.

131. Rhoton AL Jr, Buza R. Microsurgical anatomy of the jugular foramen. *J Neurosurg* 42:541–550, 1975.

132. Rhoton AL Jr, Hardy DG. Microsurgical anatomy of the sphenoid bone, cavernous sinus, and sellar region, in Tindall GT, Collins WF (eds): *Clinical Management of Pituitary Disorders.* New York, Raven Press, 1979, pp 1–73.

133. Rhoton AL Jr, Hardy DG, Chamber SM. Microsurgical anatomy and dissection of the sphenoid bone, cavernous sinus and sellar region. *Surg Neurol* 12:63–104, 1979.

134. Rhoton AL Jr, Renn WH, Harris FS. Microsurgical anatomy of the sellar region and cavernous sinus, in Rand RW (ed): *Microneurosurgery.* St. Louis, CV Mosby, 1978, ed 2, pp 71–92.

135. Rhoton AL Jr, Saeki N, Perlmutter D. Microsurgical anatomy of the circle of Willis, in Rand RW (ed): *Microneurosurgery.* St. Louis, CV Mosby, 1978, ed 2, pp 278–310.

136. Rhoton AL Jr, Saeki N, Perlmutter D, et al. Microsurgical anatomy of common aneurysm sites. *Clin Neurosurg* 26:248–306, 1979.

137. Robertson JT, Ranier JK. Transsphenoidal microsurgery of pituitary tumors. *J Tenn Med Assoc* 75: 253–255, 1982.

138. Samii M (ed): *Surgery In and Around the Brain Stem and the Third Ventricle.* Stuttgart, Thieme, 1986.

139. Samii M, Ammirati M. Surgery of skull bone meningiomas. Berlin, Springer, 1992.

140. Samii M, Jannetta P (eds): *The Cranial Nerves.* New York, Springer, 1981.

141. Samii M, Mathies C. Management of 1000 vestibular schwannomas (acoustic neuromas): Hearing function in 1000 tumor resections. *Neurosurgery* 40:248–262, 1997.

142. Samii M, Mathies C. Management of 1000 vestibular schwannomas (acoustic neuromas): The facial nerve—preservation and restitution. *Neurosurgery* 40: 684–695, 1997.

143. Samii M, Mathies C. Management of 1000 vestibular

schwannomas: Complications. *Neurosurgery* 40: 11–23, 1997.

144. Samson DS, Boones L. Extra–intracranial arterial by-pass; past performance and current concepts. *Neurosurgery* 3:79–86, 1998.

145. Schmiedek P, Gratzl O, Spetzler R, et al. Selection of patients for extra–intracranial arterial by-pass surgery based on rCBF measurements. *J Neurosurg* 44: 303–321, 1976.

146. Seeger W. Atlas of topographical anatomy of the brain and surrounding structures. Vienna, Springer, 1978.

147. Seeger W. Microsurgery of the brain. Wien, Springer, 1980, vol 1–2.

148. Seeger W. Anatomical dissections for use in neurosurgery. Wien, Springer, 1987, vol 1.

149. Sekhar LN, de Oliveira E. Cranial neurosurgery. Stuttgart, Thieme, 1999.

150. Sekhar LN, Estonillo R. Transtemporal approach to the skull base. An anatomical study. *Neurosurgery* 19: 799–808, 1986.

151. Sekhar LN, Jannetta PJ. Cerebellopontine angle meningiomas. Microsurgical excision and follow-up results. *J Neurosurg* 60:500–505, 1984.

152. Sekhar LN, Kalakonda C. Saphenous vein and radial artery grafts in the management of skull base tumors and aneurysms. *Op Tech Neurosurg* 2:129–141, 1999.

153. Sekhar LN, Lanzino G, Sen CN, et al. Reconstruction of the third through sixth cranial nerves during cavernous sinus surgery. *J Neurosurg* 76:935–943, 1992.

154. Sen CN, Sekhar LN. Direct vein graft reconstruction of the cavernous, petrous, and upper cervical internal carotid artery; lessons learned from 30 cases. *Neurosurgery* 30:732–743, 1992.

155. Sen CN, Sekhar LN, Schramm LV, et al. Chordoma and chondrosarcoma of the cranial base. *Neurosurgery* 25:931–941, 1989.

156. Sengupta RP, McAllister VL. Subarachnoidal hemorrhage. Berlin, Springer, 1986.

157. Shillito J. Intracranial arteriotomy in three children and three adults, in Donaghy RMP, Yaşargil MG (eds): *Micro-Vascular Surgery.* St. Louis, CV Mosby, Stuttgart, Thieme, 1967, pp 138–142.

158. Smith JW. Facial nerve paralysis and microsurgery, in Daniller AI, Strauch B (eds): *Symposium on Microsurgery.* St. Louis, CV Mosby, 1976, pp 172–176.

159. Spetzler RF, Carter LP. Revascularization and aneurysm surgery: Current status. *Neurosurgery* 16: 111–116, 1985.

160. Spetzler RF, Chater N. Occipital artery–middle cerebral anastomosis for cerebral artery occlusive disease. *Surg Neurol* 2:235–238, 1976.

161. Spetzler RF, Chater NL. Microvascular bypass surgery. Part 2: Physiological studies. *J Neurosurg* 53: 22–77, 1980.

162. Spetzler RF, Daspit CP, Pappas CTE. The combined supra- and infratentorial approach for lesions of the petrous and clival regions: Experience with 46 cases. *J Neurosurg* 76:588–599, 1992.

163. Stein BM. Surgical treatment of orbital tumors. *Clin Neurosurg* 26:490–512, 1978.

164. Stevenson GC. Trans-clival exposure of the basilar artery: A case presentation of basilar artery embolectomy in man, in Donaghy RMP, Yaşargil MG (eds): *Micro-Vascular Surgery.* St. Louis, CV Mosby, Stuttgart, Thieme, 1967, pp 148–149.

165. Stevenson GC, Stoney RJ, Perkins RK, et al. A trans-cervical transclival approach to the ventral surface of the brain stem for removal of a clivus chordoma. *J Neurosurg* 24:544, 1966.

166. Sugita K. Microneurosurgical atlas. Stuttgart, Thieme, 1985.

167. Sugita K, Kobayashi S, Mutsuga N, et al. Microsurgery for acoustic neurinoma—lateral position and preservation of facial and cochlear nerves. *Neurol Med Chir (Tokyo)* 19:637–641, 1979.

168. Sundt TM Jr. Neurovascular microsurgery. *World J Surg* 3(1):53–65, 127, 1979.

169. Sundt TM Jr. Was the international randomized trial of extracranial–intracranial arterial bypass representative of the population at risk? *N Engl J Med* 316(13): 814–816, 1987.

170. Sundt TM Jr, Fode NC, Jack CR Jr. The past, present, and future of extracranial to intracranial bypass surgery. *Clin Neurosurg* 34:134–153, 1988.

171. Sundt TM Jr, Grant WC, Garcia JH. Restoration of middle cerebral artery flow in experimental infarction. *J Neurosurg* 31(3):311–321, 1969.

172. Sundt TM Jr, Kees G Jr. Miniclips and microclips for surgical hemostasis. Technical note. *J Neurosurg* 64(5):824–825, 1986.

173. Sundt TM Jr, Kobayashi S, Fode NC, et al. Results and complications of surgical management of 809 intracranial aneurysms in 722 cases. Related and unrelated to grade of patient, type of aneurysm, and timing of surgery. *J Neurosurg* 56(6):753–765, 1982.

174. Sundt TM Jr, Kobayashi S, Fode NC, et al. Results, complications, and follow-up of 415 bypass operations for occlusive disease of the carotid system. *Mayo Clin Proc* 60(4):230–240, 1985.

175. Sundt TM Jr, Murphy F. Clip-grafts for aneurysm and small vessel surgery. 3. Clinical experience in intracranial internal carotid artery aneurysms. *J Neurosurg* 31(1):59–71, 1969.

176. Sundt TM Jr, Nichols DA, Piepgras DG, et al. Strategies, techniques, and approaches for dural arteriovenous malformation of the posterior dural sinuses. *Clin Neurosurg* 37:155–170, 1991.

177. Sundt TM Jr, Piepgras DG. Occipital to posterior inferior cerebellar artery bypass surgery. *J Neurosurg* 48(6):916–928, 1978.

178. Sundt TM Jr, Piepgras DG. Surgical approach to giant intracranial aneurysms. Operative experience with 80 cases. *J Neurosurg* 51(6):731–742, 1979.

179. Sundt TM Jr, Piepgras DG, Fode NC, et al. Giant intracranial aneurysms. *Clin Neurosurg* 37:116–154, 1991.

180. Sundt TM Jr, Piepgras DG, Stevens LN. Surgery for supratentorial arteriovenous malformations. *Clin Neurosurg* 37:49–115, 1991.

181. Sundt TM III, Sundt TM Jr. Principles of preparation of vein bypass grafts to maximize patency. *J Neurosurg* 66(2):172–180, 1987.

182. Takahashi T, Kuwayama A, Kobayashi T, et al. Transsphenoidal microsurgery of sellar–parasellar chordomas (in Japanese). *Neurol Med Chir (Tokyo)* 22: 141–146.

183. Tew JR, Tobler WD. The laser: History, biophysics, and neurosurgical applications. *Clin Neurosurg* 31: 506–549, 1983.

184. Tew JR, van Loveren HR. Atlas of operative microneurosurgery. WB Saunders, 1994.

185. Tindall GT, McLanahan CS, Christy JH. Transsphenoidal microsurgery for pituitary tumors associated with hyperprolactinemia. *J Neurosurg* 48:849–869, 1978.

186. Tulleken CAF, et al. High flow excimer laser- assisted extra–intra and intra–intracranial bypass. *Op Tech Neurosurg* 2:142–148, 1999.

187. Umansky F, Elidan J, Valarezo A. Dorello's canal: A microanatomical study. *J Neurosurg* 75:294–298, 1991.

188. Vajkoczy P, Horn P, Schmiedek P. Standard superficial temporal artery–middle cerebral artery bypass surgery in hemodynamic cerebral ischemia: Indication and technique. *Op Tech Neurosurg* 2:106–115, 1999.

189. Wilson CB, Dempsey LC. Transsphenoidal microsurgical removal of 250 pituitary adenomas. *J Neurosurg* 48:13–22, 1978.

190. Yaşargil MG. Microsurgery applied to neurosurgery. Stuttgart, Thieme, 1969.

191. Yaşargil MG. Microneurosurgery. Clinical considerations, surgery of the intracranial aneurysms and results. Stuttgart, Thieme, 1984, vol II.

192. Yaşargil MG. Microsurgical anatomy of the basal cisterns and vessels of the brain, diagnostic studies, general operative techniques and pathological considerations of the intracranial aneurysms. Stuttgart, Thieme, 1984, vol I.

193. Yaşargil MG. Neurosurgical horizons. *Clin Neurosurg* 34:22–41, 1986.

194. Yaşargil MG. Microneurosurgery. AVM of the brain. Stuttgart, Thieme, 1987, vol IIIA.

195. Yaşargil MG. Microneurosurgery. AVM of the brain. Stuttgart, Thieme, 1988, vol IIIA.

196. Yaşargil MG. Microneurosurgery. CNS tumors. Stuttgart, Thieme, 1994, vol IVA.

197. Yaşargil MG. Microneurosurgery. CNS tumors. Stuttgart, Thieme, 1996, vol. IVB.

198. Yaşargil MG. A legacy of microneurosurgery. *Neurosurgery* 45:1025–1093, 1999.

199. Yaşargil MG, Cravens GF, Roth P. Surgical approaches to "inaccessible" brain tumors. *Clin Neurosurg* 34:42–110, 1986.

200. Yaşargil MG, Yonekawa Y. Results of microsurgical extra–intracranial arterial bypass in the treatment of cerebral ischemia. *Neurosurgery* 1:11–24, 1977.

201. Yonekawa Y, Yaşargil MG. Extra–intracranial arterial anastomosis: Clinical and technical aspects. *Adv Tech Stand Neurosurg* 3:47–78, 1976.

SPINAL MICROSURGERY

1. Abernathey CD, Yaşargil MG. Technique of microsurgery, in Watkins RG, Williams RW, McCullock JA, Young PH (eds): *Microsurgery of the Lumbar Spine*. Rockville, MD, Aspen Publishers, 1990, pp 87–93.

2. Arnautovic KI, Al-Mefty O. Giant and large paraclinoid aneurysms, in Eisenberg MB, Al-Mefty O (eds): *The Cavernous Sinus*. Philadelphia, Lippincott, Williams & Wilkins, 1999, pp 177–190.

3. Avman N, Ozkal E, Erdogan A. Microsurgical removal of anterolateral spinal lesions. *J Microsurg* 3:176–179, 1982.

4. Caspar W, Loew F. Die mikrochirurgische Operation

des lumbalen Bandscheibenvorfalls. *Dtsch Aerztebl* 13: 863–868, 1977.

5. Eisenberg MB, Al-Mefty O. The cavernous sinus. Philadelphia: Lippincott, Williams & Wilkins, 1999.

6. Fischer G, Mercier P, Sindou M. Microsurgery in neurosurgery. *Int Surg* 65:491–494, 1980.

7. Hoff JT, Wilson CB. Microsurgical approaches to the anterior cervical spine and spinal cord. *Clin Neurosurg* 26:513–528, 1978.

8. Malis LI. Intramedullary spinal cord tumors. *Clin Neurosurg* 25:512–539, 1978.

9. Rand RW. Experiences with microneurosurgery in spinal cord tumors and vascular malformations, in Rand RW (ed): *Microneurosurgery*. St. Louis, CV Mosby, 1969, pp 210–220.

10. Seeger W. Microsurgery of the spinal cord and surrounding structures: Anatomical and technical principles. Wien, Springer, 1982.

11. Stein BN. Surgery of intramedullary spinal cord tumors. *Clin Neurosurg* 26:529–542, 1978.

12. Tulleken CAF, et al. High flow excimer laser-assisted extra–intra and intra–intracranial bypass. *Op Tech Neurosurg* 2:142–148, 1999.

13. Vajkoczy P, Horn P, Schmiedek P. Standard superficial temporal artery–middle cerebral artery bypass surgery in hemodynamic cerebral ischemia: Indication and technique. *Op Tech Neurosurg* 2:106–115, 1999.

14. Watkins RG, Williams RW, McCulloch JA, et al. Microsurgery of the lumbar spine. Rockville, MD, Aspen Publishers, 1990, p 271.

15. Williams RW. Microlumbar discectomy. A conservative surgical approach to the virgin herniated disc. *Spine* 3:175–182, 1978.

16. Yaşargil MG. Surgery of vascular malformations of the spinal cord with the microsurgical technique. *Clin Neurosurg* 18:257–265, 1969.

17. Yaşargil MG. Microsurgical operation for herniated lumbar disc, in *Advances in Neurosurgery*. Berlin, Springer, 1977, vol 4, p 81.

18. Yaşargil MG, DeLong WB, Guarnaschelli JJ. Complete microsurgical excisions of cervical extra- and intramedullary malformation. *Surg Neurol* 4:211–229, 1975.

19. Yaşargil MG, Perneczky A. Operative Behandlung der intramedullären spinalen Tumoren, in Schiefer W, Wieck HH (eds): *Spinale raumfordernde Prozesse*. Erlangen, Verlag Peri Med, pp 299–312.

20. Yaşargil MG, Symon L, Teddy P. Arteriovenous malformations of the spinal cord. *Adv Tech Stand Neurosurg* 11:61–102, 1984.

21. Yaşargil MG, Tranmer, BI, Adamson T. Unilateral partial hemilaminectomy for the removal of spinal-cord intramedullary tumors and AVM's. *Adv Tech Stand Neurosurg* 18:113–130, 1991.

TECHNOLOGY IN MICRONEUROSURGERY

1. Alexander E III, Maciumas RJ. Advanced neurosurgical navigation. New York, Thieme, 1999.

2. Alexander E, Nashold BS. A history of neurosurgical navigation, in Alexander E, Maciumas RJ (eds): *Advanced Neurosurgical Navigation*. New York, Thieme, 1999, pp 3–14.

3. Apuzzo ML, Heifetz MD, Weiss MH, et al. Neurosurgical endoscopy using side-viewing telescope. *J Neurosurg* 46:398–400, 1977.

4. Benabid AL, et al. Is there any future for robots in neurosurgery? *Adv Tech Stand Neurosurg* 18:4–45, 1991.

5. Cappabianca P, de Divitiis E, et al. Instruments for endoscopic endonasal transsphenoidal surgery. *Neurosurgery* 45:392–396, 1999.

6. Cesarini KRG, Hardemark HG, Persson L. Improved survival after aneurysmal subarachnoid hemorrhage. *J Neurosurg* 90:664–672, 1999.

7. Chandler WF, et al. Intraoperative use of real-time ultrasonography in neurosurgery. 57:157–163, 1982.

8. Cohen A. Ventriculoscopic surgery. *Clin Neurosurg* 41:546–562, 1994.

9. Dandy WE. Cerebral ventriculoscopy. *Bull Johns Hopkins Hosp* 57:157–163, 1982.

10. Dolce G. Ueber eine neue methode. Der Arterien-katheterismus des Gehims. *Psychopharmacologia* 5:313–316, 1964.

11. Drake JM. Ventriculostomy for treatment of hydrocephalus. *Neurosurg Clin North Am* 4:657–666, 1993.

12. Eguchi T, Tamaki N, Durata H. Endoscopy of the spinal cord. Cadaveric study and clinical experience. *Minim Invasive Neurosurg* 42:146–151, 1999.

13. Flamm ES, Ransohoff J, et al. Preliminary experience with ultrasound aspiration in neurosurgery. *Neurosurgery* 2:240–295, 1978.

14. Fukushima T, et al. Ventriculofiberscope. A new technique for endoscopic diagnosis and operation. *J Neurosurg* 38:251–256, 1974.

15. Greenblatt SH, Dagi TF, Epstein MH. A history of neurosurgery. Park Ridge, AANS, 1997.

16. Greenwood J Jr. Two point coagulation. A new principle and instrument for applying coagulation current in neurosurgery. *Am J Surg* 50:267–270, 1940.

17. Griffith HB. Endoneurosurgery. *Adv Tech Stand Neurosurg* 14:2–24, 1986.

18. Guglielmi G. The interventional neuroradiologic treatment of intracranial aneurysms. *Adv Tech Stand Neurosurg* 24:216–255, 1998.

19. Guthrie BL. The medical videoscope. Neurosurgery in the 21st century. *Microsurgery* 15:547–554, 1994.

20. Guthrie BL, Adler JR. Frameless stereotaxy, in Barrow DL (ed): *Perfectives in Neurological Surgery*. St. Louis, Quality Medical Publishing, 1991, vol 2, pp 1–19.

21. Guthrie BL, Adler JR. Computer-assisted preoperative planning, interactive surgery and frameless stereotaxy. *Clin Neurosurg* 38:112–131, 1992.

22. Heilbrun RP. Stereotactic neurosurgery. Williams & Wilkins, 1988.

23. Hirschberg H, Samset E. Intraoperative image directed dye-marking of tumor margins. *Minim Invasive Neurosurg* 42:123–127, 1999.

24. Houkin S, Kuroda. Digital recording in microsurgery. Technical no. 6. *J Neurosurg* 92:176–180, 2000.

25. Housepian EM, Unger WH, Scharff TB, et al. Experience with videotape monitoring of microscopic neurosurgical procedures. *J Neurosurg* 42:204–208, 1975.

26. John ER, Prichep LS, Ransohoff J. Intraoperative monitoring with evoked potentials, in Pluchino FR, Broggi G (eds): *Advanced Technology in Neurosurgery*. New York, Springer, 1985, pp 64–84.

27. Kelly PJ. Volumetric stereotactic surgical resection of intra-axial brain mass lesions. *Mayo Clin Proc* 63:1186–1198, 1988.

28. Kelly PJ. Tumor stereotaxis. Philadelphia. WB Saunders, 1991.

29. Kelly PJ, Alker GL Jr. A stereotactic approach to deep-seated central nervous system neoplasms using the carbon dioxide laser. *Neurology* 15:331–334, 1981.

30. Kelly PJ, Alker GJ Jr, Goerss S. Computer-assisted stereotactic microsurgery for the treatment of intracranial neoplasms. *Neurosurgery* 10:324–331, 1982.

31. Kelly PJ, Kall BA, Goerss S, et al. Present and future developments of stereotactic technology. *Appl Neurophysiol* 6:223–229, 1986.

32. Kikinis R, Shelton W. Image guided surgery in OR. Surgical Product pp. 17–18, Dec. 1999.

33. Kikuchi T, Strother CM, Royer M. New catheter for endovascular interventional procedures. *Radiology* 165:870–871, 1987.

34. Kosugi Y, et al. An articulated neurosurgical navigation system using MRI and CT images. *IEEE Trans Biomed Eng* 35:147–152, 1988.

35. Kurze T, Dyck P, Barrow HS. Neurosurgical evaluation of ultrasonic encephalograph. *J Neurosurg* 22(5):437–440, 1965.

36. Lake NC. The use of suction in surgery. *Lancet* 1:1166–1168, 1924.

37. Laws ER, Warren RE, Anderson RP. The treatment of brain tumors by photoradiation, in Pluchino FR, Broggi G (eds): *Advanced Technology in Neurosurgery*. Berlin, Springer, 1985, pp 46–61.

38. Lawton MT, et al. The state of art of neuronavigation with frameless stereotaxy. *Op Tech Neurosurg* 1:27–38, 1998.

39. L'Espinasse VL. in Davis (ed): *Neurological Surgery*. Philadelphia, Lea and Febiger, 1943, ed 2, p 442.

40. Lüdecki DK, Triege W. Pressure–irrigation–suction system. Technical note. *Acta Neurochir (Wien)* 66:123–126, 1982.

41. Luessenhop JJ, Spence WT. Artificial embolization of cerebral arteries. Report of use in a case of arteriovenous malformation. *JAMA* 172:1153, 1960.

42. Lunsford LD. A dedicated CT system for the stereotactic operating room. *Appl Neurophysiol* 45:376–378, 1982.

43. Lunsford LD, Kondziolka D, Bissonette DJ. Intraoperative imaging of the brain. *Stereotact Funct Neurosurg* 66:58–64, 1996.

44. Malis LI. Bipolar coagulation in microsurgery, in Donaghy RMP, Yaşargil MG (eds): *Microvascular Surgery*. St. Louis, CV Mosby, Stuttgart, Thieme, 1967, 126–130.

45. Malis LI. Instrumentation and techniques in microsurgery. *Clin Neurosurg* 26:626–636, 1979.

46. Malis LI. New trends in microsurgery and applied technology, in Pluchino FR, Broggi G (eds): *Advanced Technology in Neurosurgery*. Berlin, Springer, 1985, pp 4–16.

47. Malis LI. Electrosurgery. *J Neurosurg* 85:970–975, 1996.

48. Manwaring K, Crone KR (eds): *Neuroendoscopy*. New York, NA Liebert, 1992, vol 1.

49. Mixter WJ. Ventriculoscopy and puncture of the third ventricle. *Boston Med Surg J* 22:1373–1376, 1923.

50. Pait TG, Dennis NW, Laws ER, et al. The history of the neurosurgical engine. *Neurosurgery* 28:111–129, 1991.

51. Perneczky A, Tschabitscher N, Resch KDM. Endoscopic history of neurosurgery. Stuttgart, Thieme, 1993.
52. Putnam T. Treatment of hydrocephalus by endoscopic coagulation of the choroid plexus. *N Engl J Med* 22: 1373–1376, 1934.
54. Rischer J, Mustafa H. Endoscopic-guided clipping of cerebral aneurysms. *Br J Neurosurg* 8:559–565, 1994.
55. Scarff JE. Non-obstructive hydrocephalus. Treatment by endoscopic cauterization of the choroid plexus. *J Neurosurg* 9:164–176, 1952.
56. Scarff JE. Fifty years of neurosurgery. *Int Abst Surg* 101:417–513, 1955.
57. Steiner L, Lindquist C, Adler JR, et al. Clinical outcome of radiosurgery for cerebral arteriovenous malformations. *J Neurosurg* 77:1–8, 1991.
58. Tamigu M, et al. Application of a rigid endoscope to the microsurgical management of 54 cerebral aneurysms. Results in 48 patients. *J Neurosurg* 91:231–237, 1999.
59. Teo C, Rothman S, Boop FA, et al. Complications of endoscopic neurosurgery. *Child Nerv Syst* 12:248–253, 1997.
60. Valavanis A, Yaşargil MG. The endovascular treatment of brain arteriovenous malformations. *Adv Tech Stand Neurosurg* 24:132–204, 1998.
61. Yaşargil MG, Krayenbuhl HA, Jacobson JH. Microsurgical arterial reconstruction. *Surgery* 67:221–233, 1970.
62. Zamorano L, Vinas FC, Jiang Z, et al. Use of surgical wands in neurosurgery. *Adv Tech Stand Neurosurg* 24: 78–128, 1998.

7

A History of Cerebrovascular Surgery

Sunghoon Lee, MD, Louis Marroti, BS, Isaam A. Awad, MD, MsC, FACS

The history of cerebrovascular surgery during the first 50 years of the Congress of Neurological Surgeons (1951–2000) was characterized by a splendid symphony of technical advances and scientific maturation. The interplay between scientific inquiry at the clinical and basic mechanistic levels and an explosion of technologic possibilities continues to characterize this subspecialty of neurological surgery. Long recognized as possibly the field with utmost technical challenge and precision in all of medicine, neurovascular surgery has also come of age as a scientific discipline that defines questions about epidemiology, natural history, and pathophysiology, and struggles to improve the outcome of patients with cerebrovascular disease.

The field was braced for a leap at the threshold of the second half of the 20th century, building upon the evolution of general neurosurgical techniques and progress in vascular diagnosis and surgery, and the contributions of early pioneers of the school of neurosurgery. These pioneers would barely tackle neurovascular pathology themselves, but their methods enabled their pupils to take advantage of a confluence of advances in various fields. These methods included epidemiology, imaging and diagnosis, anesthesiology and critical care, and the evolving tools of neurosurgical technique. During the next 50 years, these pupils would develop and propagate intracranial microsurgery, including cisternal dissection, microvascular reconstruction, and skull base approaches, would refine bipolar electrocautery, clips, and microsurgical tools, and would integrate anatomic, vascular, and functional imaging. They would tackle questions of natural history, scientific assessment of therapy, outcomes science, and the molecular basis of cerebrovascular disease. They would remain at the forefront of research in stroke and brain protection, and would succeed at the integration of endovascular, radiosurgical, and pharmacologic tools into a truly multidisciplinary armamentarium.

INTRACRANIAL ANEURYSMS

State of the Art in 1951: The Dawn of an Era—Possibilities of Treatment and Diagnosis

As early as the 19th century, therapeutic carotid ligation became popularized and gained a

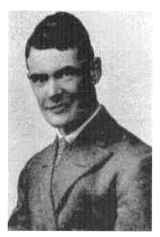

Norman Dott (1897–1973)
The first intracranial approach to the therapy of intracranial aneurysms was performed by Dr. Norman Dott in 1931.

wide spectrum of applications. It was attempted in the treatment of seizures, trigeminal neuralgia, and psychosis, in addition to its application in the therapy of carotid injury and aneurysms (148). Sir Victor Horsley was the first to apply carotid ligation to an intracranial aneurysm that he discovered during a surgical exploration (71).

The first planned direct intracranial attack or an aneurysm was performed by Norman Dott (1897–1973). In 1931, Dott successfully wrapped an intracranial aneurysm that had bled on three separate occasions. The patient was noted to have done well and remained active until he succumbed to a myocardial infarction 12 years later (71,176). Dott continued to be an innovator in aneurysm surgery. In 1941, he reported the opening of a large, ruptured MCA aneurysm, following occlusion of the proximal feeding vessel (58,71,176). The principle of aneurysm clip obliteration and preservation of the parent artery was introduced and established by Walter Dandy (1886–1946). In 1937, Dandy applied a silver clip to the neck of a posterior communicating artery aneurysm in a 43-year-old man presenting with a third nerve palsy (71). Dandy collected a series of cases of intracranial aneurysms and published the first monograph on aneurysm surgery in 1944 (71). Henry Schwartz reported the first surgical trapping of a vertebrobasilar aneurysm in 1948 (71).

The evolving understanding of intracranial aneurysms benefited greatly from concurrent advances in diagnostic imaging. Preoperative visualization of cerebral aneurysms was made possible by the development of cerebral angiography by Egas Moniz of Portugal (111). Moniz experimented with a variety of contrast agents in animal and human subjects with varying toxicity. In 1931, he published a monograph on successful angiograms that visualized both arterial and venous flow using the contrast agent thorotrast. In the subsequent years, Moniz published a series of monographs that detailed the angiographic characteristics of neurovascular pathology, including aneurysms, large vessel occlusive diseases, and arteriovenous malformations (AVMs) (111).

However, there remained a hesitancy regarding the wide application of angiography partially due to the fact that the procedure required a surgical exposure of the carotid artery. Although Loman and Myerson devised methods of percutaneous carotid access, angiography would not flourish until the development of safer contrast agents. The 1950s saw the introduction of diatrizoate sodium (Hypaque) which became regarded as an agent with superior safety and radiopacity. Angiography became the standard in the evaluation of intracranial aneurysms, and was further refined and automated by transfemoral access, and more recently, digital and subtraction imaging.

Angiography allowed precise preoperative evaluation of the aneurysm, its exact location, its architecture, and its association with surrounding vessels. It allowed the neurosurgeon, for the first time, to devise a meaningful preoperative surgical strategy. With the advent of cerebral angiography and the initial surgical ventures in the treatment of this formidable pathology, neurosurgery in 1951 lacked only the final element, operative microscopy, before its exponential growth in the latter half of the century.

The 1950s and 1960s: Strategies and Techniques—Hunterian Versus Direct Treatment, the First Cooperative Study, Improved Clips and the Emergence of Microsurgery

Throughout the 1950s and early 1960s, scattered series reflected the increasing experience with direct approaches to intracranial aneurysms with the aim of ligation or clipping (59). However, many neurosurgeons still favored the apparently safer technique of extracranial ligation of the internal or common carotid arteries for treatment of intracranial aneurysms (59). The first Cooperative Study was an ambitious multidisciplinary undertaking which chronicled the natural history of subarachnoid hemorrhage and the outcome of current treatment approaches (154). This undertaking was not designed to answer a specific question with sufficient statistical power (hypothesis driven), but was rather a registry with little control on enrollment, treatment, or outcome assessment. Still, it was the vanguard of multi-institutional clinical research collaborations aimed at overcoming limitations of smaller series reported by individual surgeons.

A seminal advance during this era of aneurysm surgery was the evolution of the aneurysm clip. Dandy's first aneurysm clipping was performed with a Cushing–Mckenzie type of clip that could not be reopened once it was applied. Herbert Olivecrona recognized this limitation and developed a new aneurysm clip that could be reopened and adjusted after its application (71), Scoville developed a spring clip, Schwartz deviced a crossover clip and a box type applier, and further developments were made by Mayfield, who introduced different shapes and sizes of aneurysm clips suitable for different surgical situations. Later, Yaşargil, Sundt, and Sugita would introduce a series of clips made of noncorrosive alloys and with predictable closing pressures, thus setting the modern standard.

Numerous other technical advances were destined to favor direct surgical approaches to intracranial aneurysms. The era of monopolar cautery gave way to bipolar coagulation. With the contributions of technical pioneers, such as James Greenwood and Leonard Malis, bipolar cautery became the standard in most neurosurgical procedures, including the surgery for intracranial aneurysms (118). The development of the bipolar cautery system allowed a more efficient method of hemostasis, which resulted in faster coagulation with decreased damage to the surrounding brain.

Artificial hypothermia as an adjunct to aneurysm surgery was also introduced in this era by

Lougheed and Bottrell in Toronto in 1956 (22). The technique allowed surgeons to avoid ischemic complications from temporary arterial occlusion. Although this technique generated wide interest in its earlier years, it was found not to be necessary in most situations (59). Deep hypothermia with medically induced cardiac arrest and bypass was tried in the early 1960s, but was found to be associated with coagulopathy and other complications; the technique was abandoned by most surgeons in the 1960s in favor of adjunctive hypotension during aneurysm dissection and clipping (59). Hamby had reported on the use of nitroprusside as an excellent agent for induced hypotension.

Prior to the championing of loupe magnification by Charles Drake in the late 1960s most aneurysms were clipped, ligated, or wrapped without magnification of vision.

The next giant leap in the evolution of surgical therapy for intracranial aneurysms would await the advent of microscopic surgery. For the first time, aneurysm surgeons could visualize, with improved illumination and magnification, the complex vascular structures and the association of vital perforators with the aneurysm. The earliest use of an operating microscope for the surgical therapy of intracranial aneurysms was reported in 1966 by Pool (142). In 1969, Lougheed and Marshall published their experience with the microscope in intracranial aneurysm surgery (113).

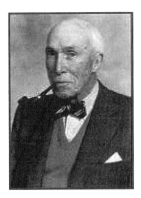

J. Lawrence Pool (b. 1906)
Pioneer of microneurosurgery and the first to apply the binocular microscope to the intracranial surgical therapy of aneurysms.

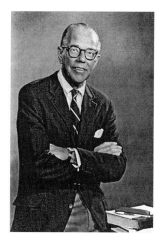

R. Peardon Donaghy (1910–1991)
Dr. Donaghy introduced the operating microscope to neurosurgery in 1961 by using it to perform the first microsurgical middle cerebral endarterectomy. His most prominent trainee in microneurosurgery is Professor M. Gazi Yaşargil.

Central to the microsurgical revolution was the work of M. Gazi Yaşargil, a disciple of Hugo Krayenbuhl in the Department of Neurological Surgery in Zurich, Switzerland. Early in his career, Yaşargil contributed to the advancement of neuroangiography and was a pioneering force in its greater acceptance in the latter half of the 20th century. The careful neuroangiographical delineation of the cerebral vasculature demanded a new surgical philosophy with equal rigor. Yaşargil pursued this idea under the tutelage of "Pete" Donaghy in a microvascular laboratory in Burlington, Vermont. Later, from Zurich he introduced his newly learned microsurgical skills to the world's neurosurgeons. Yaşargil's contributions included a variety of technical innovations, including the floating microscope, microsurgical instrumentation, and ergonomic aneurysm clips and clip appliers that have revolutionized aneurysm surgery. Yaşargil's greatest contribution to aneurysm surgery may be in his conceptualization of cisternal dissections and operating bloodlessly within the subarachnoid spaces with microscopic guidance.

A central figure in the revolution in aneurysm surgery during this period was Charles Drake (1920–1998). Drake's greatest contribution was

in the advancement of the surgical therapy for posterior circulation aneurysms. In 1996, he published a monograph on the unprecedented and since unmatched series of 1,700 vertebrobasilar aneurysms (60), an astonishing experience amassed over a 40-year span. Direct operation on aneurysms of the vertebrobasilar system was slow in development secondary to their relative low incidence and the prevailing opinion that their difficult exposure precluded direct surgical obliteration. Drake's main contributions were in the development of the understanding of the complex anatomical considerations of posterior circulation aneurysms and the development of surgical windows to ablate them. Drake was widely respected for his unflinching honesty in reporting his most humbling complications.

The 1970s and 1980s: The Golden Era—Generalization of Microsurgical Technique, Cross Sectional Imaging, Endovascular Pioneers, the Shift to Early Surgery, and Fight Against Vasospasm

During this era, neurovascular surgeons strived to improve outcomes from open surgery with expanding expertise in microsurgical techniques, advances in neuroanesthesia, brain protection, and skull base exposure strategies. These advances were heralded by leading neurovascular surgeons of our generation, including Spetzler, Dolenc (52–54), Samson (155,156), Yaşargil (185,186,188), and others. Reports of larger and more impressive series documented improved outcome with a greater proportion of aneurysms. A pattern of travel by trainees to observe these masters and the subsequent launching of more formal fellowship training under Drake, and later Spetzler, created a cadre of young disciples destined to generalize (and at times enhance) the success of their mentors, insuring a widening impact of microsurgical advances beyond the early pioneering centers. For example, surgery for posterior circulation aneurysms and giant and complex lesions would routinely be attempted only at a handful of centers such as Zurich, London (Ontario), and the Mayo Clinic in the 1970s, but became widespread by the late 1980s.

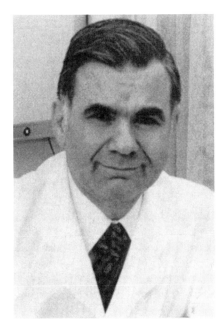

M. Gazi Yaşargil (b. 1925)
Critical figure in the transition to modern neurovascular surgery. One of the fathers of microneurosurgery, Dr. Yaşargil introduced the ideas of cisternal dissection for aneurysm exploration under microscopic guidance. Dr. Yaşargil innovated many neurosurgical instruments including the floating microscope, microsurgical instruments, and the ergonomic aneurysm clip and clip appliers.

This era was marked by parallel advancement in diagnostic modalities with the advent of cross-sectional imaging. The introduction of computed tomography (CT) scanning in the 1970s allowed the accurate diagnosis of subarachnoid hemorrhage. The first CT scan was developed by Godfrey Hounsfield in 1972. Although Hounsfield's EMI machine was limited in resolution, it was able to resolve basic neuroanatomical structures and could delineate the presence of altered radiodensities representative of neuropathology. The CT scan rapidly replaced pneumoencephalography and revolutionized diagnosis in neuroradiology. The radiographic identification and characterization of intracranial aneurysms would be enhanced by contrast enhancement, higher resolution scanning, and later, magnetic resonance imaging (MRI) (85).

At the same time, there was the early development of endovascular therapeutic approaches, as pioneered by Serbinenko, and followed by contributions from Debrun, Djindjian, Lasjaunias, Berenstein, Higashida, and others. This approach achieved secure endovascular navigation and occlusion of parent arteries, and attempted aneurysm obliteration with balloons (109).

Hunt and Hess reported a simple grading system that predicted a more dismal outcome in patients with more impaired level of consciousness (92). This scheme was widely applied to the surgical selection of cases likely associated with better outcome. Some patients who were initially in poor condition would improve and eventually undergo successful treatment. It was believed that others who would succumb to the sequelae of the initial hemorrhage, rebleeding, or vasospasm would not have fared better if earlier treatment, with higher morbidity, had been attempted. Early pioneers of aneurysm surgery advised against direct tackling of aneurysms in the setting of acute hemorrhage and brain edema. The approach to deeper aneurysms was felt to be particularly risky and generally ill-advised in the acute state. In the 1970s and early 1980s, neurosurgeons generally favored delayed surgery after aneurysmal rupture (58). Early rebleeding was widely recognized and feared, so patients were frequently kept in dark isolated rooms, often heavily sedated, until it was believed that brain edema subsided to allow direct surgery on the aneurysm. This practice was supported by prevalent anecdotal reports of severe morbidity and even frequent need to abort surgery in the setting of acute hemorrhage. It was also believed that antifibrinolytic agents could partially protect against early rebleeding.

However, on closer examination in the early 1980s, significant morbidity and mortality associated with delayed treatment of ruptured aneurysms became apparent. Drake, a champion of delayed surgery, himself documented that only 1/3 of patients with aneurysmal rupture ever survived to undergo an operation (57). Such "cherry-picking" of cases in good clinical condition and simpler aneurysms (now recognized in statistical terminology as selection bias) would surely enhance reported *treatment out-*

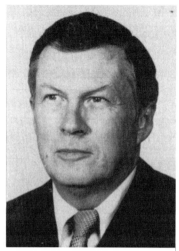

Charles Drake (1920–1998)
Pioneer in the surgical therapy of posterior circulation aneurysms. Dr. Drake performed surgery on unprecedented 2000 aneurysms of the
posterior circulation, and close to 4000 cases of
aneurysms. The reported outcomes from Dr.
Drake's series continues to remain the standard
by which modern therapies for aneurysms are
measured.

come by various groups, but there was concern
about the impact of such selection on overall
management outcome.

At the same time, reports from Japan and subsequent isolated reports from North America and
Europe reported feasibility of early surgery in a
selected, and increasing fraction of cases—first,
superficial aneurysms and good grade patients,
and later, all cases with subarachnoid hemorrhage. The second Collaborative Study aimed
specifically to compare management outcome
with early and late surgery (103,104). It was not
felt that surgeons would agree to randomize
cases, as each camp strongly believed that it was
not ethical to do other than what they knew was
best for their patients. Therefore, the outcomes
were monitored in a registry with adjudicated
outcome assessment. While the results of the
study in fact reported no advantage with delayed
surgery (103,104), a paradigm shift in clinical
practice had taken hold. The emerging generation of neurovascular surgeons was more facile
with cisternal dissection, ventricular drainage,

and with optimizing extradural exposure so as
to minimize brain retraction and injury during
early surgery. This and the lack of evidence of
truly worsened outcome with early surgery resulted in a dominant trend by the late 1980s toward early surgical intervention, except perhaps
in cases with highest grade or most difficult lesions.

At the same time, recognition of arterial vasospasm as a delayed sequel of subarachnoid
hemorrhage was recognized, and its clinical
and radiologic correlates were defined (59,106,
131,179). Because of its deadly nature, arterial
vasospasm became one of the focused areas of
research in neurosurgery. Wide application of
various vasoactive medications were tried in
order to alleviate vasospasm. One agent, nimodipine, was shown in a controlled prospective randomized double blinded trial to result in improved outcome after subarachnoid hemorrhage,
presumably (although not demonstrably) by
preventing vasospasm or brain tolerance to
its sequelae (106,131). Also in the 1980s, it
was suggested and later largely accepted that intravascular volume expansion and induced arterial hypertension can improve blood rheology
and effectively combat ischemic sequelae of arterial vasospasm (9). Early surgery would permit
more aggressive hypervolemia and hypertension
to combat ischemic sequelae of vasospasm without the risk of inducing aneurysm rupture. It also
was suggested that early surgery would allow
removal of blood products and hence lessen the
prevalence and severity of vasospasm.

The 1990s: The End of the
Beginning—Endosaccular Embolization,
Further Advances in Microsurgical
Techniques, Outcomes Assessment, and
Natural History Revisited

The therapy for intracranial aneurysms was
altered in the 1990s by the introduction of the
technique of endosaccular embolization using
detachable thrombogenic coils. Capitalizing on
advances in digital subtraction imaging, safer
contrast agents and ever improved microcatheter
design, Guglielmi, Vinuela, and others demonstrated the feasibility and safety of aneurysm

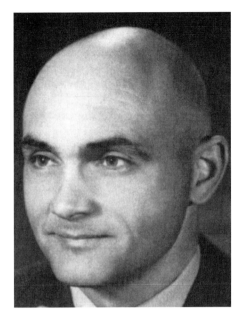

Thoralf Sundt

Dr. Sundt has been one of the seminal figures in the modern era in pioneering the surgical management of cerebro-occlusive disease with end-arterectomy and extracranial-intracranial bypass surgery. He has also had a central contribution to the surgical management of intracranial aneurysms and in defining the natural history of subarachnoid hemorrhage.

obliteration with parent artery preservation using the Guglielmi Detachable Coil (GDC) (79,177). It was now possible to occlude smaller aneurysms than with endosaccular balloons, and with apparently better safety and effectiveness. Approval of the GDC device in North America was specified for aneurysms where conventional microsurgical approach would pose higher risk due to aneurysm features or the patient's clinical condition (3). In effect, this definition was vague from the onset and subject to varying interpretations. The GDC coil has in fact been used in all types of aneurysms and in patients with any clinical condition. A decade of experience has allowed refining of indications based on initial reports of morbidity and effectiveness. GDC embolization is associated with comparable morbidity rates as in open surgery, but substantially lower rates of aneurysm obliteration. Larger aneurysms treated with GDC have a high

rate of recanalization, coil compaction, and growth. Large and giant aneurysms, those with broad necks or splaying and incorporation of parent vessel branches, cannot be treated satisfactorily with GDC. GDC embolization has emerged as an excellent option for smaller aneurysms of the posterior circulation, in paraclinoid location, or in patients in unstable medical or neurologic condition.

Endovascular therapy has also expanded the options of parent artery occlusion which is now applied both extradurally and intradurally in the management of complex aneurysms. Improved catheters, newer generation coils, and emerging stent technology hold the promise of continued enhancement of endovascular options for aneurysm treatment.

Open surgical techniques have continued to evolve in the 1990s, with popularization of radical skull base approaches for more difficult aneurysms, better options for brain protection during focal circulatory arrest (temporary clipping), the selective use of deep hypothermia and global circulatory arrest, and extracranial-intracranial bypass for selected cases. The introduction of intraoperative angiography with portable digital subtraction equipment has allowed prompt control and optimization of anatomic outcome of surgical clipping, and heralded the increasing use of endovascular adjuncts in open surgical treatment (e.g., proximal endovascular control and suction decompression for complex paraclinoid aneurysms). Leading neurovascular centers are approaching more complex aneurysms with planned multidisciplinary attack, taking advantage of both surgical and endovascular measures.

The general availability of noninvasive imaging has opened an unprecedented opportunity to screen asymptomatic high risk populations for unruptured intracranial aneurysms. These include patients with autosomal dominant polycystic kidney disease, and family members of patients with ruptured aneurysms. However, a large cooperative study with prospective follow-up of untreated unruptured aneurysms has questioned the long held views about their natural risk of rupture (and prophylactic treatment), especially small aneurysms (less than 1 cm) in

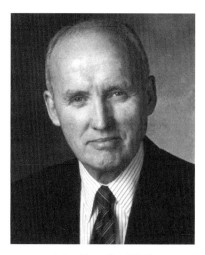

John Tew (b. 1936)
Dr. Tew has had a wide contribution in modern neurosurgery, including the surgical management of facial pain syndromes, hemifacial spasm, and acoustic neuromas. He has been a central figure in modern neurovascular surgery, especially in relation to supratentorial cerebral revascularization and the surgical management of intracranial aneurysms.

older patients without prior history of subarachnoid hemorrhage (81). Ongoing prospective studies using rigorous biostatistical tools and functional outcome instruments will likely clarify remaining questions about the natural history and treatment outcome of intracranial aneurysms.

VASCULAR MALFORMATIONS

State of the Art in 1951: Early Clinicopathologic Classification and Feasibility of Surgery

The history of the neurosurgical therapy for vascular malformations in the modern era must be reviewed in light of the essential contributions of neurosurgical pioneers in the first half of the 20th century. In 1928, Harvey Cushing and Percival Bailey published their classical monograph Tumors Arising from the Blood-Vessels of the Brain, a landmark publication that elaborated on contemporary experience regarding vascular malformations with a synthesis of the previous literature on the subject (43). In the same year, Cushing's former student at Johns Hopkins University, Walter Dandy, published his experience with eight cases of intracranial arteriovenous aneurysms (44) that likely represented "angioma arteriale" as described by Cushing and Bailey. Among Cushing and Bailey's series of 16 cases and Dandy's series of 8 cases, no lesions were successfully removed. In addition, their extensive review of the literature did not report any surgical success in previous cases. In the years following the publication of these two series (in 1928), other investigators continued to echo the pessimism of Cushing and Dandy.

Subsequently, a bolder attitude gradually emerged in the neurosurgical literature. An exception to the prevailing pessimism in the era of Cushing and Dandy is noted in reports by Bergstrand, Olivecrona, and Tonnis (20). Olivecrona reported the successful surgical resection of two vascular malformations related to cutaneous nevi in Sturge-Weber Syndrome, and three lesions noted as "arteriovenous malformations." Tonnis reported a successful surgical resection of an "angioma racemosum venosum." The authors exhibited a new confidence in the neurosurgical treatment of vascular malformations, stating that the attempt to radically resect these formidable lesions was not only preferable, but also necessary, as they found other palliative options to be generally inadequate.

In 1948, Olivecrona published his more comprehensive series of surgical successes in the "arteriovenous aneurysms of the brain" (134). Olivecrona and Riives reported their experience with 48 patients treated from 1935 to 1946 in the neurosurgical clinic in Stockholm, Sweden. Like their predecessors, they characterized the cardinal signs associated with vascular malformations, which consisted of "epileptic fits, subarachnoid hemorrhage, and hemiplegia." Importantly, Olivecrona and Riives recognized the propensity of vascular malformations to cause hemorrhage, and in attempting to quantify its frequency, accomplished the first steps toward understanding its natural history. The authors found that hemorrhage was observed in 22 of

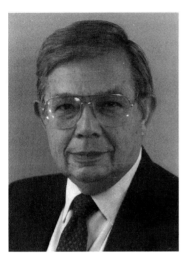

Leonard Malis (b. 1919)
Dr. Malis has had a central influence in neurovascular surgery with the development of the Malis bipolar forceps and the advancement of microneurosurgical techniques.

their 48 cases, and noted that several cases were marked by repeated hemorrhagic episodes. Furthermore they observed, that the hemorrhage could be both subarachnoid as well as intracerebral, often leaving the afflicted patients with contralateral hemiplegia.

The legacy of Olivecrona was in his vast and distinguished surgical experience which established an aura of optimism toward neurosurgical intervention for vascular malformations. Olivecrona and his co-workers came to the conclusion that "the choice lies between removing the lesion and leaving it alone" (134). Of their 43 reported cases of arteriovenous aneurysms, radical surgical resections were attempted in 24 patients, with 3 fatalities and a calculated rate of mortality of 13%. Olivecrona and Riives reported that 2/3 of the surviving patients were without additional postoperative deficit.

This advance in outcome was largely a reflection of improvements in operative technique. Olivecrona recognized that the principal difficulty in the removal of arteriovenous aneurysms is in obtaining adequate hemostasis. Olivecrona prepared intravenous infusions and blood transfusions in sufficient quantities and exposed the ipsilateral cervical carotid artery for potential temporary occlusion. He emphasized the technique of dividing the pia and the arachnoid close to the nidus of the aneurysm and developing this plane as a method of serially ligating the deep arterial feeders of the aneurysm. Olivecrona noted that when the last of the arterial feeders are ligated, "the aneurysm, formerly tense and pulsating, suddenly collapses," and the formerly arterialized venous drainage can then be safely ligated. Olivecrona advocated en block resection of arteriovenous aneurysms located in non-eloquent areas of the brain, simplifying the procedure in these instances. He also noted that early surgery, following an episode of hemorrhage, may facilitate the surgical resection of the lesion as "the clot leaves a large cavity," allowing a readily accessible surgical plane.

Progress in the 1950s and 1960s: Surgical Challenges and Modern Clinicopathologic Classification

Olivecrona's surgical successes had a significant impact on the contemporary neurosurgical community. In 1946, Cobb Pilcher, a neurosurgeon from Vanderbilt University, reported three cases of angiomatous malformations of the brain successfully removed without detrimental sequelae (140). Although his experience was limited in comparison to that of Olivecrona's, Pilcher's work also denoted significant technical advances. Pilcher, like Olivecrona, felt that the largest hurdle in the endeavor was in achieving hemostasis. He advocated advanced preparation for intravenous fluid and blood infusion, and the generous use of silver clips, fibrin foam (93), and gelatin sponges (141), which had become available by this time. Pilcher insisted on the availability of "electrosurgical" equipment (78), which was becoming a standard in neurosurgical care. The results of Olivecrona and Pilcher were soon reproduced by other teams in the 1950s and 1960s, with evolving nuances of techniques but also continued caution and skepticism in view of significant morbidity. Despite electrocautery, vascular clips for serial ligation of feeders, and various adjuncts for hemostasis, surgery for AVMs remained a formidable undertaking with frequent morbidity, and the not uncommon occurrences of intraoperative exsanguination or malignant brain swelling.

This technical evolution was complemented with progress in efforts to understand and rationally classify vascular malformations. While Dandy offered a scheme of classification, it was not convincingly predictive of the pathology, the pathogenesis, or the natural history. Dandy's classifications were largely phenomenological; he emphasized the careful observations that were made in the operating room when these lesions were uncovered. Cushing and Bailey's work revealed a more comprehensive scheme of classification based largely on case-by-case clinical-pathologic correlations in addition to intraoperative observations. With foresight ahead of his time, Cushing noted correctly the separations between arterial and venous angiomas. He recognized the entity of capillary telengiectasia and speculated regarding its potential to evolve into arterial or venous angioma. Although Cushing and Bailey's classification closely mirrors our modern scheme of understanding vascular malformations, the ensuing literature on the subject did not uniformly adopt their conceptualization.

In fact, confusion associated with complex and conflicting systems of classification persisted into the 1960s. Pathologists continued to be uncertain with regards to the relationship of vascular malformations to vascular neoplasms, although most, by the 1960s, had become convinced that AVMs represented true developmental malformations or vascular hamartomas with secondary flow-induced changes (122,130, 133,134,152,189). Zulch, however, noted that the distinction between vascular malformations and vascular neoplasms was difficult and might be ascertained only on the basis of clinical observations in the autonomous growth noted in the latter (189). Russell and Rubinstein noted that vascular malformations may not remain ''static'' and can ''inflict progressive destruction on the adjacent brain'' (152). Noran (130) echoed Cushing and Bailey's view that intervening brain parenchyma within the vascular nidus implies a malformation rather than a neoplasm. McCormick (122) noted, however, that the presence of intervening brain tissue does not hold

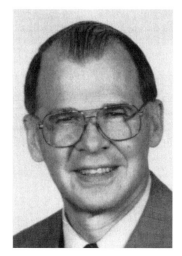

Robert Ojemann (b. 1931)
Dr. Ojemann has been an innovator in the modern era of the surgical management of intracranial aneurysms, vascular malformations, and occlusive cerebrovascular disease. He has played a pivotal role in the development of modern surgical techniques for the treatment of skull base lesions and the use of intraoperative auditory-evoked potentials to preserve hearing in surgery for acoustic neuroma.

true for all vascular malformations, ''most notably the cavernous angiomas.''

Reports of angiographically occult vascular malformations occurred largely in the reports of tumor series and in discussions of encapsulated brain hemorrhage (7). Dorothy S. Russell made further developments in reference to the improved pathologic understanding of the so-called ''cryptic'' or angiographically occult vascular malformations (151,152). In their monograph entitled ''Cryptic arteriovenous and venous hamartomas of the brain,'' Crawford and Russell presented a series of 20 cases of spontaneous cerebral hemorrhage where the etiology of the hemorrhage was ''cryptic'' in the sense that prior to the bleed, the lesion was either clinically silent or angiographically occult. The authors noted that ''some forms of vascular hamartomas are so small that they may pass undetected or even fail to visualize by angiogram'' (37). A thorough histopathologic classification of vascular malformations was later advanced when McCormick published ''The pathology of vascular ("arteriovenous") malformations" in 1966 (122).

Progress in the 1970s and 1980s: Microsurgical Techniques, Presurgical Embolization, Imaging and Grading of Lesions, and Emergence of Radiosurgery

The 1970s and 1980s were marked by technological advances and consequent improvements of therapeutic outcome. The early use of silver clips and monopolar cautery gave way to more efficient, safer, and more precise bipolar cautery (78). With the contributions of technical pioneers such as Leonard Malis, bipolar cautery became the standard in most neurosurgical procedures, including surgery for AVMs (32,119). Bipolar cautery has undergone further improvements in the modern age, including the addition of computerized power output and automated irrigation, which allows more precise coagulation and minimization of tissue adhesion (18,96,174). Malis's contributions were beyond innovations in surgical instruments. One of the pioneers of microneurosurgery, Malis described the technique of retracing the nidus of the AVM from its major venous outflow trunk.

The introduction of the microscope in the operating room allowed a finer optical resolution of the lesion and its vascular relationships, as well as a superior technical precision during excision. Yaşargil played a critical role in the evolution of microneurosurgery (184). His pioneering work in the microsurgical treatment of AVMs emphasized a comprehensive and exact selective angiography as a mandatory prerequisite to a careful microscopic approach in surgery. Yaşargil also noted that preoperative partial embolization may be an important adjunct to the microsurgical treatment. Wilson et al. reported their surgical series of 85 patients with vascular malformations. The authors attributed the outstanding surgical outcome to the technical contributions of bipolar coagulation and operative microscopy. Their oustanding surgical outcome allowed the extension of traditional indications for surgery to include favorably situated AVMs that had not bled and lesions situated in critical regions of the brain (182). Fox et al.

(72,73) presented a review of the application of microneurosurgery in neurovascular diseases. The authors emphasized the need for neurosurgeons dedicated to the treatment of vascular diseases "to acquire the special skills and instrumentation of microneurosurgery, to implement the 'team-of-experts' concept in the operating room, and to enlist the support of related disciplines."

During this period, Robert Spetzler, while a young resident working with Charles Wilson in San Francisco, advanced a compelling concept with some experimental support in an animal model. He proposed that sudden excision of a lesion with marked arteriovenous shunting would result in hyperemia in adjacent brain, and potential perfusion breakthrough edema and hemorrhage, even at normal pressure (167).

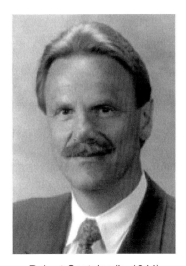

Robert Spetzler (b. 1944)
Dr. Spetzler has made prominent contributions in the development of surgical strategies for the treatment of AVMs and in the development of multimodal approaches for managing complex vascular malformations. He has been a leader in defining rational treatment paradigms for cerebrovascular diseases by studying the physiology of the disease process and defining the natural history of the disease. He has also made seminal contributions in the management of intracranial aneurysms, especially in regards to the surgical management of giant aneurysms and in the application of skull base approaches for improved surgical exposure.

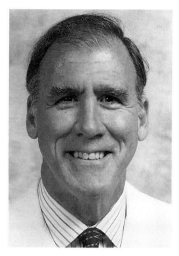

Roberto Heros (b. 1942)
Dr. Heros has helped advance the field of neurovascular surgery by contributing to the development and refinement of surgery for AVMs, aneurysms, and carotid disease.

Careful physiologic measurements have later questioned this concept and other studies demonstrated the potential role of venous occlusion or residual AVM in this phenomenon. Nevertheless, Spetzler popularized the strategy of staged embolization or feeder ligation prior to final excision of the AVM nidus. His published series included spectacular results with giant lesions previously considered inoperable (161,162,165, 168). Spetzler would use intraoperative embolization of larger feeders and staged serial occlusion of multiple feeders prior to tackling the lesion for final microsurgical excision. Safer and more facile extraoperative embolization would await the evolution of microcatheter and glue embolization techniques, as well as their wider application in the late 1980s and 1990s. Modern neurosurgical giants, including Stein (40,121, 170,171), Heros (87–89), and Day (45), have all contributed seminal perspectives to AVM surgery through careful documentation of patient selection, technical strategies, and outcome.

At the same time, imaging techniques, such as CT and then MRI began to emerge. They allowed a spacial definition of the nidus of vascular malformations in relation to adjacent brain. Features of lesion size, location, and pattern of vascular supply would be used to predict the risk of potential therapeutic intervention as a simple grading system conceptualized and validated by Spetzler and Martin (160). More accurate diagnosis became possible with all but rare lesions imaged with sensitivity and specificity by MRI. Incidental lesions and others associated with minor symptoms were increasingly discovered raising the relevance of ongoing discourse about natural history. A number of studies carefully documented prospective risk of hemorrhage from AVMs with and without prior bleeding. Jane et al. estimated an annualized rate of hemorrhage to be 3% (98). Ondra et al. (135) provided a comprehensive prospective study of 166 patients with intracerebral AVMs, and found an annualized rate of major hemorrhage to be 4% with an annualized rate of mortality of 1%. Careful clinical-radiologic-pathologic correlations allowed recognition and characterization of a large number of previously undetected occult or cryptic vascular malformations, including the first studies on prevalence and the natural history of cavernous malformations (147). These lesions moved from the domain of pathologist's interest to a genuine problem of clinical decision-making.

The era was also marked by the emergence of alternative modalities of therapy that have yielded definitive treatment in select cases and allowed multidisciplinary tackling of lesions previously considered inoperable. There have been anecdotal reports of successful treatment of AVMs with X-ray irradiation since the series of Cushing and Bailey (43). In spite of occasional successes, the method was considered largely ineffective and was abandoned in favor of direct surgical approaches (134). Lars Leksell (1907–1986) is credited with the implementation of stereotactic radiosurgery in the treatment of AVMs (110,172). Systemic application of stereotactic radiosurgery has led to the publication of large case studies that documented its efficacy in obliteration of selected AVMs (114,132). Lunsford et al. (114) heralded the emergence of modern stereotactic radiosurgery as an important treatment modality in North America by reporting their prospective study of 227 patients treated over a three year period. Curative obliteration of AVMs was achieved in a volume-depen-

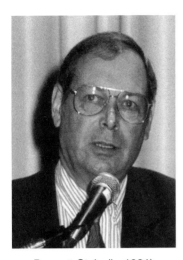

Bennett Stein (b. 1931)
Dr. Stein has made numerous contributions to the field of neurosurgery, notably in the advancement of surgical techniques for treating AVMs and tumors of the spinal cord and pineal gland.

dent fashion. The rationale for the potential application of radiosurgery for inoperable, symptomatic cavernous malformations has remained in evolution (2).

Progress in the 1990s: The Era of Multimodality Management and Themes of Molecular Pathogenesis

Attempts at angiographic embolization of vascular malformations were made as early as the 1930s, when Hamby and Gardner, in conjunction with direct arterial ligation, embolized a traumatic carotid cavernous fistula (83,100). Luessenhop introduced embolization with silicone spheres in the 1970s. Refinements were made in endovascular technique which allowed superselective catheterizations and feeder vessel embolizations (51). Recent observations have been made as to the acceptable safety and the efficacy of modern techniques of embolizations (127,138). With technical advancements, angiographic embolizations became an important adjunct to preoperative preparation for surgical management of AVMs (181,187). An increasing fraction of lesions would be largely devascularized preoperatively with more advanced nidal

embolization with acrylic, which in turn enhanced the safety of subsequent definitive cure by microsurgical excision.

Furthermore, along with direct surgery and radiosurgery, arterial embolization made possible the multimodal therapy of complex AVMs with improved outcome (50,77,86,108,127,136, 138,158). AVMs in exquisitely eloquent areas of the brain, such as the thalamus, brain stem, and the basal ganglia, have been treated successfully using individually tailored, multimodal treatment strategies (108). One such strategy may prescribe a staged treatment of embolization, which may allow a technically safer surgical resection of a largely devascularized lesion (136,158). Embolization has also been applied to decrease the size of the nidus as to allow radiosurgical targeting of larger lesions. Recent studies have suggested an acceptable rate of radiosurgical obliteration with such a treatment strategy, with a low rate of morbidity and mortality (77,86,158).

The availability of multiple treatment options and strategies has driven a parallel effort at better characterizing natural history and therapeutic outcome. In particular, the 1990s witnessed numerous careful reports of natural history of cavernous, venous, spinal, and dural vascular malformations that defined benign and more aggressive lesions and the range of expected outcome with available treatment modalities (6–8,14,97).

This decade witnessed the application of molecular techniques to the study of lesion biology, ultimately aiming to explain, predict, and modify mechanisms of clinical behavior. Molecular dissection has revealed unregulated angiogenesis activity in vascular malformations (149). Familial cases of AVM in association with hereditary hemorrhagic telangiectasia (Osler Weber Rendu Disease) were subjected to linkage and gene mapping studies, and defined two gene loci at chromosomes 9q and 12q (139). The genes for HHT1 and HHT2 have been identified: both proteins modulate receptor binding of transforming growth factor-beta, which is known to influence endothelial cell vascular matrix interactions during angiogenesis. Familial cases of cavernous malformation have been linked to

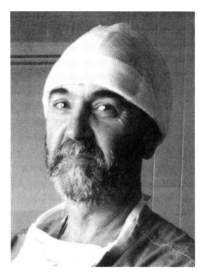

Duke Samson (b. 1943)
Dr. Samson has been a modern pioneer in the surgical management of occlusive cerebrovascular disease, vascular malformations, and intracranial aneurysms.

three potential gene foci at 7p, 7q, and 3q (80,81). The CCM1 gene has been found to be responsible for all cases of cavernous malformation in Hispanic Americans of Mexican descent, including apparent sporadic cases (81). More recently, the CCM1 gene has been identified as coding a previously little known protein, RIT-1, related to the Rap/Ras signaling pathway presumed to modulate cell differentiation (107, 153). Careful genotype-phenotype correlations are already underway, and future studies will aim to uncover mechanisms whereby these abnormal genes cause the genesis of a vascular malformation and other factors that influence lesion progression and clinical manifestations. The potential role of these mechanisms in the pathogenesis of more common sporadic lesions will be examined and hopefully yield strategies for better prognostication and potential modification of clinical lesion behavior.

INTRACEREBRAL HEMATOMAS

State-of-the-Art in 1951: Disease Pathophysiology and the Option of Hematoma Evacuation

Intracerebral hemorrhage is the underlying etiology in approximately 8–15% of all strokes in the United States and up to 20–30% of all strokes in China and Japan. It is a devastating disease with 30-day mortality rates approaching 50% and very poor functional outcomes (21,23). Although the last 50 years have chronicled significant advances in the surgical management of cerebrovascular occlusive disease, progress in the treatment of intracerebral hemorrhage has been less forthcoming. Hamilton and Zabramski (84) recently chronicled the history of surgery for intracerebral hematomas. The clinical literature of the 19th and early 20th centuries contains scattered reports of attempts at surgical hematoma evacuation, mostly involving severely ill patients. Working without the benefit of modern imaging technologies, early physicians had to infer information about the size and location of a hematoma on the basis of physical findings and patient symptoms. Not surprisingly, the results of surgical intervention under these circumstances were often quite variable, and the early literature contains great debates over the potential utility or advisability of surgical intervention for hemorrhage (36,84).

Cushing was one of the earliest surgeons to report the successful treatment of cerebral hemorrhage by open craniotomy and clot evacuation in 1903 (36,42). He also was the first to describe the response of systemic blood pressure to the increase in intracranial pressure following intracerebral hemorrhage (41) and showed that the reactive hypertension was reversed upon evacuation of the hematoma. In the early 1930s, Penfield described the use of ventriculography to localize a clot in a woman suffering headaches, vomiting, and seizures (36,132). Removal of the clot ameliorated the patient's symptoms, but she died suddenly six months later. Concurrent with these early surgical experiences, postmortem examinations and clinical-pathological correlations were beginning to provide valuable information on the underlying causes of hemorrhage and on the variables affecting clinical outcome (30,36,146). In 1932, Bagley reported that hemorrhages involving deep subcortical structures were more often associated with a depressed level of consciousness and poor prognosis (12). Two years later, Geiger made the observation that clinical symptoms and signs tended to vary with the size of the hemorrhage, and noted that

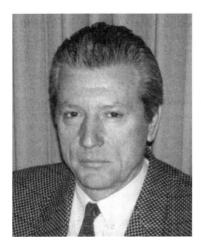

Vinko Dolenc (b. 1940)
Dr. Dolenc has made valuable contributions in microsurgery and the development of techniques for cavernous sinus exploration. His work has made it possible to extend surgical treatment to a wider anatomical range of vascular lesions.

last half-century was an ongoing evolution in surgical techniques and an emerging spectrum of opinions on indications for surgical intervention. Much of what has been learned about surgery for hemorrhage has come from anecdotal reports of experiences with individual patients or small patient series, with very little or no bias control influencing patient selection and the assessment of outcome. It was not until the early 1960s that surgical intervention was subjected to analysis by a clinical trial with randomized concurrent control. In 1961, McKissock reported the first prospective randomized trial that investigated the effectiveness of surgical hematoma evacuation (123). Although the study failed to demonstrate a statistical benefit of surgery in comparison to nonsurgical management, it is possible that the lack of accurate imaging may have influenced diagnostic accuracy and biased patient selection (65).

patients suffering coma and convulsions generally recovered poorly (36,76).

Progress in the 1950s and 1960s: Case Series and the First Clinical Trial

The past 50 years have witnessed an assimilation of knowledge from pathological and radiological studies that led to the formulation of a cohesive pathophysiologic framework for understanding intracerebral hemorrhage. Our knowledge of the spectrum of vascular anomalies underlying hemorrhage has been expanded to include previously unrecognized etiologies, such as cerebral amyloid angiopathy (29,69, 70,120). Postmortem studies have contributed reliable data on the anatomical predilection of intracerebral hemorrhage (74), and have revealed that most bleeds arise in deep brain structures, with a smaller proportion occurring in the cerebral lobes. In tandem with this, several natural history studies helped establish the impact of hematoma size and location, patient age, and baseline neurological status on the survival and functional outcome probabilities following cerebral hemorrhage (84,115).

Commensurate with the expansion in pathophysiologic knowledge that has occurred in the

Progress in the 1970s and 1980s: The Era of Imaging, Minimally Invasive Approaches, and Continued Therapeutic Controversies

The introduction of CT in the 1970s revolutionized the surgical treatment of cerebral hemorrhage. The increased diagnostic sensitivity offered by CT made it possible to extend surgical intervention to a broader spectrum of patients, including those with less severe hemorrhages. The CT also improved the ability to accurately localize hematomas, hence improving surgical planning. The advent of MRI and continued evolution of CT has made possible a more accurate assessment of potential etiologies underlying cerebral hemorrhage and more rational therapeutic planning in light of such etiologies. Nevertheless, the role of surgical evacuation of hematoma itself remained controversial in all but younger patients with lobar or cerebellar clots and impending herniation.

Two clinical trials were undertaken in this era to evaluate the effectiveness of hematoma evacuation (15,101) and produced inconclusive or negative results. The study by Batjer et al. was prematurely stopped after only 21 patients had been randomized due to poor recruitment and dismal outcome in all treatment arms. Both studies suffered from a lack of sufficient case numbers, which precluded any meaningful statistical analysis of patient subgroups.

In the late 1970s and early 1980s, advances in stereotactic instrumentation kindled interest in the application of minimally invasive techniques for the evacuation of intracerebral hemorrhage (11,128). These techniques often spared the patient the risks associated with major craniotomy and general anesthesia, and allowed access to deep clots without retraction or major disruption of unaffected brain tissue. In 1978 Backlund and Von Holst reported subtotal evacuation of cerebral hematoma by stereotactic aspiration and since that time, numerous reports of CT-guided stereotactic evacuations have appeared in the literature (128). One of the challenges for such procedures has been the ability to aspirate a sufficient portion of the hematoma without damaging the surrounding neural tissue or causing rebleeding. Endoscopic techniques offered the added advantage of direct visualization and control of hematoma evacuation. In 1989, Auer et al. published the results of what remains, to date, the only randomized controlled trial that demonstrates the benefit of hematoma evacuation (4). Operated patients had significantly lower mortality and better clinical outcomes than cases treated medically, although the benefit was limited to young patients and those with lobar hemorrhage. This study has been criticized since surgical patients were generally younger and had lower initial Glasgow coma scores, and the outcome assessment was not blinded; hence, the positive findings could have reflected an element of randomization or assessment bias (65).

Progress in the 1990s: Continued Search for Effective Therapy

In the 1990s, several large case series were performed (largely in Japan) and involved hundreds of patients with intracerebral hemorrhage treated with stereotactic hematoma evacuation using a variety of adjunctive techniques (102). Sufficient hematoma could be evacuated without significant risk of rebleeding or other therapeutic complications. These studies did not include randomization or stratification of treat-

ment, and the techniques were not standardized or compared in a controlled fashion. Outcome assessment was rarely blinded or adjudicated. Hence, despite large numbers of patients, this experience failed to provide reliable data on therapeutic indications or effectiveness.

The primary challenge of stereotactic hematoma evacuation has been to aspirate sufficient clot material, but the technique continues to be refined, integrating more facile image guidance and other adjuncts, such as the use of thrombolytic agents to liquefy clots for more effective evacuation (128,129). Recent results from several groups in Japan on the use of urokinase for intracavitary thrombolysis have been encouraging, and demonstrate satisfactory hematoma evacuation in most cases and very low procedure-related morbidity, including a low rate of rehemorrhage.

A pressing need exists for additional clinical trials to more thoroughly investigate potential benefits of surgery for cerebral hemorrhage, to identify specific subgroups of cases more likely to benefit from surgery, and to address questions regarding the optimal time window for surgical intervention and the choice of surgical technique. Other studies will investigate the role of adjunctive pharmacotherapy for brain protection and control of secondary damage from cerebral hemorrhage. The answers to these questions will determine what position surgery will occupy in the spectrum of treatments for cerebral hemorrhage in the future.

CEREBROVASCULAR OCCLUSIVE DISEASE

State of the Art in 1951: Conceptual and Technical Foundations

The neurologic manifestations of stroke have been appreciated for close to 3,000 years (5), but it is only within the last 50 years that surgical treatment strategies for the prevention of stroke have been put forth. The origins of surgery for stroke can be traced to the anatomical revolution that occurred after the Renaissance (66). Working on autopsy materials, early anatomists, such as Berengario da Carpi (1470–1530), Andreas Vesajius (1514–1564), Franciscus de la Boe (1614–1672), and William Harvey (1578–1657), made great strides towards accurately defining the arterial circulation of the brain (5,35,49,66). The formulation of an accurate cerebrovascular anatomical framework facilitated insights into the relationship between lesions of the extracranial vessels and impaired cerebral function. Johann Wepfer (1658–1724) (180) was the first to demonstrate a correlation between cerebral ischemic symptoms and extracranial carotid occlusion. Over the course of the last 400 years since his initial observations, numerous clinicopathological studies have appeared in the literature to support his results and strongly implicate extracranial carotid occlusion as an important cause of stroke (1,34,91,157).

In the early decades of this century, concepts and potential strategies of surgical revascularization for carotid occlusive disease began to emerge (26). Early experiments of vascular reconstructions in animal models by Jaboulay (94) and Carrel (26) suggested the feasibility of surgical revascularization, but the application of these techniques to humans awaited the development of an effective clinical diagnostic technique. This was realized in 1927, with the introduction of cerebral angiography by Moniz (125).

The early 1950s were a pivotal time in the history of surgery for stroke. In 1951, Fisher published what is considered a landmark clinico-pathologic study that helped to further establish the importance of extracranial carotid occlusion in stroke (68). He noted the frequent occurrence of atheromas at the carotid bifurcation in patients with symptoms of ischemia in the ipsilateral hemisphere, and pointed out that the distal internal carotid and its intracranial branches were usually patent. He went on to postulate that ''some day vascular surgery will find a way to bypass the occluded portion of the artery. . . . Anastomosis of the external carotid artery or one of its branches, with the internal carotid artery above the area of narrowing should be feasible'' (68).

Progress in the 1950s and 1960s: Feasibility of Surgery and Technical Evolution

After reading Fisher's article, Carrea et al. performed the first successful carotid reconstruction in Buenos Aires on October 20, 1951 (not reported until 1955) (25). Their patient had suffered a stroke and was found to have stenosis of the left internal carotid artery. The stenosed area was partially resected, and a direct anastomosis of the external and distal internal carotid arteries was performed with successful restoration of blood flow. In 1954, Eastcott et al. (61) of St. Mary's Hospital in London described another resection of an occluded carotid bifurcation, with end-to-end anastomosis, to restore blood flow in a woman suffering recurrent transient ischemic attacks. This operation was done under hypothermia to protect the brain during temporary clamping of the arteries. Also in 1954, Denman et al. (48) reported the use of a preserved homograft to reestablish cerebral blood flow following excision of an occluded left carotid bifurcation. Two years later, Lyons and Galbrieth (116) described the use of a subclavian-carotid bypass graft.

The procedure of peripheral arterial endarterectomy for the removal of atherosclerotic plaques obstructing flow in vessels supplying the lower extremities was first described by dos Santos in 1946 (56). The technique took advantage of the plane of cleavage that could be formed between the subintimal atheromatous plaque and the medial arterial layer. Wylie et al. (183) introduced endarterectomy into the United States in 1951, but this was not immediately applied to the carotid arteries. On January 28, 1953, Strully et al. (173) of the Montefiore Hospital in New York City, reported the first attempt at endarterectomy of the carotid artery in a patient with complete left internal carotid occlusion. Although they were successful in removing some clot material, retrograde flow could not be established and the artery was ligated. It was suggested, though, that successful endarterectomy should be possible in cases with patent distal runoff. In 1965, De Bakey (46) reported that their group performed the first successful thromboendarterectomy on August 7, 1953, on a patient who had suffered a frank stroke secondary to complete occlusion of the left internal carotid. Postoperative angiography demonstrated the patency of the operated vessel and the patient lived for 19 years with no further ischemic symptoms. This operation is regarded as the earliest *reported* successful carotid endarterectomy, but there is some disagreement over whether De Bakey was actually the first to successfully use endarterectomy to treat carotid occlusion (145). After review of hospital records, De Bakey's neurological colleague, W.S. Fields, has suggested that credit go to the late Dr. Stanley Crawford (145).

With increasing experience, the popularity of carotid reconstruction waned, and endarterectomy became the procedure of choice. Several reports of successful carotid endarterectomies appeared in the literature in the late 1950s and 1960s, and the technique was eventually applied to treating stenosis of the vertebral arteries (28,33,38,39,46,63,99,112,126,175). Numerous technical advances and innovations, such as the introduction of intravascular shunting by Cooley in 1956 (33), the development of intraoperative cerebral monitoring, and the use of new techniques in anesthesia, helped to improve the technical results and safety of carotid surgery.

Surgical methods for improving cerebral circulation in patients with occlusive lesions that are inaccessible or otherwise not amenable to conventional endarterectomy were also devised. The development of microvascular surgical techniques in the early 1960s, led by the contributions of Jacobson, provided the possibility of direct anastomosis of cerebral arteries (95). In 1968, Yaşargil (b. 1925) and Donaghy (1910–1991), working in Zurich and Burlington, respectively, simultaneously reported the first successful extracranial-to-intracranial (EC-IC) bypass revascularizations by direct anastomosis of the superficial temporal and middle cerebral arteries (55).

Progress in the 1970s and 1980s: Questions of Effectiveness and Surgical Accreditation by Clinical Trials

The continuing widespread use of endarterectomy for carotid stenosis engendered the need for organized studies to examine, in a controlled manner, the efficacy of the procedure in reducing the risk of stroke. To this end, the cooperative study of cerebrovascular insufficiency was initiated in 1959 (67); the results were published in 10 separate articles that appeared in the *Journal of the American Medical Association* from March 1968 through June 1976. The study provided valuable information on surgical and angiographic complication rates, identified contraindications to the operation, and defined methods of measuring stenosis of the common carotid, internal carotid, and vertebral arteries: However, it failed to demonstrate any definitive benefit of surgery in comparison to medical therapy. Endarterectomy continued to be used with great enthusiasm, but significant questions about the indications for surgery and the ratio of clinical benefit to surgical risk still remained. In addition, technological improvements in noninvasive diagnostic testing were causing an explosion in the number of patients diagnosed with carotid stenosis and raising new questions about the role of endarterectomy in patients with asymptomatic disease.

At the same time, the EC-IC bypass procedure gained popularity among the neurosurgeons eagerly applying emerging microsurgical techniques. TEC-IC was thought to provide a complementary option for cases with occlusive cerebrovascular lesions not amenable to conventional endarterectomy. By 1984, it was estimated that 5000–6000 patients worldwide had undergone EC-IC bypass (13). Improvements in cerebral perfusion were demonstrated by sophisticated imaging methods such as positron emission tomography (PET) and single photon emission computed tomography (SPECT), and anecdotal evidence of improvements in neurologic function and cessation of transient ischemic attacks abounded (169).

In the early 1980s, EC-IC bypass revascularization became the first neurovascular surgical procedure to be subjected to evaluation by a multi-institutional clinical trial, with the initiation of the Cooperative EC-IC Bypass Study (62). Concluded in 1985, the study demonstrated that there was no benefit to EC-IC bypass surgery, as compared to the best available medical therapy, in reducing the risk of stroke. The EC-IC bypass study was praised for its rigorous design and execution, but was also criticized for possibly including a majority of cases without ongoing symptoms whose clinical natural history was largely benign. Yet, these were the cases generally subjected to this operation. In light of results of this clinical trial, the use of the procedure for stroke prevention was effectively halted (178). It has been suggested that certain subgroups of patients, specifically those with progressive ischemia despite the best available medical therapy and those with clearly documented hemodynamic compromise, may not have been adequately studied and could potentially stand to benefit from the procedure (10). In addition, EC-IC bypass may still be of value in augmenting collateral reserve in patients undergoing therapeutic carotid occlusion for tumor or aneurysm.

The results of the EC-IC bypass study ushered in an era of greater doubt and skepticism about the potential effectiveness of the more commonly used carotid endarterectomy procedure. Numerous clinical trials were initiated in the 1980s, including the highly publicized North American Symptomatic Carotid Endarterectomy Trial (17), the Asymptomatic Carotid Atherosclerosis Study (64), and the Carotid Artery Stenosis with Asymptomatic Narrowing: Operation Versus Aspirin Study (24). Studies also were undertaken in Europe (143), the Mayo Clinic (144), and in Veterans Administration Hospitals of North America (90). These studies demonstrated a highly beneficial effect of surgery in reducing the risk of stroke in symptomatic patients with high-grade stenosis (70–99%). A statistical benefit in stroke risk reduction was also shown in patients with asymptomatic stenosis of >60%, provided perioperative morbidity and mortality was kept below 3%.

Progress in the 1990s: Renewed Enthusiasm for Surgery and the Emergence of Endovascular Techniques

In view of results of clinical trials, the 1990s has seen a renewed enthusiasm for carotid surgery, with an expansion of the number of procedures performed. An evolution toward benchmark outcomes defined by the clinical trials is the norm. Audits of surgical complications have become a standard of practice along with an awareness of variability of results among surgeons and communities. Length of hospital stay after the procedure has been dramatically reduced. While clinical trials have provided valuable information on the safety and efficacy of endarterectomy and helped refine indications for the procedure, serious concerns have been raised in regard to the generalization of the findings, the cost-effectiveness of surgery, and the need for patient subgroup analysis (13,27,31,82). Future studies addressing these issues, as well as questions of durability of the operation, indications for reoperation, and the impact of risk factor modification, are likely to follow in coming years (5).

At the same time, there has been an emergence of minimally invasive endovascular techniques for the treatment of vascular occlusive diseases. The successful application of percutaneous transluminal angioplasty and stenting of occlusive lesions of the coronary and peripheral arteries (19,124) has raised questions about the potential utility of similar techniques in the carotid arteries. However, each vascular system presents its own unique set of challenges and concerns, and several unresolved issues have thus far prevented the significant development of carotid angioplasty and stenting (117). Acute arterial occlusion (which can occur after angioplasty), brain embolization, decreased cerebral perfusion during the period of balloon inflation, and cardiac bradyarrhythmias secondary to carotid sinus manipulation are among the many potential complications of the procedure. Improvements in endovascular instrumentation and technical protocols are beginning to address some of these drawbacks.

Despite the many persisting challenges, several centers have reported impressive preliminary clinical results with carotid angioplasty (19,105,117). Clinicians have accepted this preliminary uncontrolled data with a mix of enthusiasm and skepticism. Widespread debate still exists over indications for carotid angioplasty, and many believe that controlled trials are necessary before this procedure can be accepted as a therapeutic option in comparison to existing proven therapies (16). In this regard, two clinical trials, the Carotid Revascularization Endarterectomy versus Stent Trial and the Carotid Artery Stenting versus Endarterectomy Trial, were recently initiated, and the results will likely play a substantial role in determining the future role of angioplasty in the treatment of cerebrovascular occlusive disease (145). As with surgery, these studies will also likely define benchmark outcome thresholds for clinical benefit and may discredit the procedure in at least some clinical scenarios.

Another potentially valuable therapy that has received growing attention in recent years is the use of intra-arterial thrombolytics for reperfusion in acute ischemic stroke (47,75,117). As with angioplasty, controlled studies are needed to evaluate the indications for thrombolysis, to determine optimum protocols for administration, and to elucidate potential clinical benefits in relation to the associated risks.

NEUROVASCULAR SURGERY: A SUBSPECIALTY WITH AN IDENTITY, METHOD, AND PURPOSE

We have reviewed the major advances in each of the neurovascular diseases where surgery has had a significant impact in the past 50 years. In such a broad overview of the field's evolution, numerous catalysts contributed closely to sharpening every detail of a most complex and evolving canvas. The authors apologize for mentioning some pioneers and giants of the field, but necessarily omitting many others in such a short treatise.

The subspecialty of neurovascular surgery remains most vibrant, with cerebrovascular papers accounting for the great majority in the neurosurgical literature and at professional meetings, while neurovascular diseases continue to lure the best and brightest of neurosurgery toward remaining challenges in an evolving frontier. As we enter the next millennium, one can envision continued technological improvements, possibly including the use of laser-guidance systems, surgical robotics, and biologic vector therapy, to augment existing therapies and further improve our ability to prevent and treat stroke (5,117). The field has achieved an identity of innovation and a commitment to the scientific method

which will allow it to take advantage of the ongoing explosion of technology, information, and biology. It is well positioned at a vibrant multidisciplinary interface, challenging the next generation of neurovascular surgeons to remain relevant and renewing its commitment to the core values and sense of purpose which fueled the birth and growth of the field in the past 50 years.

REFERENCES

1. Abercrombie J. *Pathological and Practical Researches on Diseases of Brain and Spinal Cord.* Edinburgh, Waugh and Innes, 1828.
2. Amin-Hanjani S, Ogilvy CS, Candia GJ, et al. Stereotactic radiosurgery for cavernous malformations: Kjellberg's experience with proton beam therapy in 98 cases at the Harvard Cyclotron. *Neurosurgery* 42: 1229–1236; discussion 1236–1238, 1998.
3. Anonymous. Guglielmi Detachable Coil (GDC): *U.S. Clinical Study Summary.* Fremont, CA: Target Therapeutics, 1995.
4. Auer LM, Deinsberger W, Niederkorn K, et al. Endoscopic surgery versus medical treatment for spontaneous intracerebral hematoma: A randomized study. *J Neurosurg* 70:530–535, 1989.
5. Awad IA. History of Neurovascular Surgery, II. Occlusive Disease, Cerebral Hemorrhage, and Vascular Malformations, in, G. S. et al. (ed): *History of Neurological Surgery.* Park Ridge, Ill., AANS Publishers, 1997.
6. Awad IA, Barrow DL. *Cavernous Malformations.* Park Ridge, IL: AANS Publishers, 1993.
7. Awad IA, Barrow DL. *Dural Arteriovenous Malformations.* Park Ridge, IL: AANS Publishers, 1993.
8. Awad IA, Barrow DL. *Giant Intracranial Aneurysms.* Park Ridge, IL: AANS Publishers, 1995.
9. Awad IA, Carter LP, Spetzler RF, et al. Clinical vasospasm after subarachnoid hemorrhage: Response to hypervolemic hemodilution and arterial hypertension. *Stroke* 18:365–372, 1987.
10. Awad IA, Spetzler RF. Extracranial-intracranial bypass surgery: A critical analysis in light of the international cooperative study. *Neurosurgery* 19:655–664, 1986.
11. Backlund E, von Holst H. Controlled subtotal evacuation of intracerebral hematomas by stereotactic technique. *Surg Neurol* 9:99–101, 1978.
12. Bagley C. Spontaneous cerebral hemorrhage: Discussion of four types, with surgical considerations. *Arch Neurol Psychiatry* 27:1133–1174, 1932.
13. Barnett HJM, Taylor DW. Clinical trials in stroke prevention: Persisting uncertainties, firm answers. *Neurology* 43:2163–2166, 1993.
14. Barrow DL, Awad IA. *Spinal Vascular Malformation.* Park Ridge, IL: AANS Publishers, 1999.
15. Batjer HH, Reisch JS, Allen BC, et al. Failure of surgery to improve outcome in hypertensive putaminal hemorrhage: A prospective randomized trial. *Arch Neurol* 47:1103–1106, 1990.
16. Beebe HG, Archie JP, Baker WH, et al. Concern about

the safety of carotid angioplasty. *Stroke* 27:197–198, 1996.

17. Beneficial effect of carotid endarterectomy in symptomatic patients with high-grade carotid stenosis. North American Symptomatic Carotid Endarterectomy Trial Collaborators. *N Engl J Med* 325:445–453, 1991.

18. Bergdahl B, Vallfors B. Studies on coagulation and the development of an automatic computerized bipolar coagulator: Technical note. *J Neurosurg* 75:148–151, 1991.

19. Bergeron P, Pinot JJ, Poyen V, et al. Long term results with the Palmaz stent in the superficial femoral artery. *J Endovasc Surg* 2:161–167, 1995.

20. Bergstrand H, Olivecrona H, Tonnis W. *Fefassmissbildungen und Gefassgeschwulste des Gehirns.* Leipzig: George Thieme, 1936.

21. Boonyakarnkul S, Dennis M, Sandercock P, et al. Primary intracerebral hemorrhage in the Oxfordshire Community Stroke Project: 1. Incidence, clinical features and causes. *Cerebrovasc Dis* 3:343–349, 1993.

22. Bottrell EH, Lougheed WM, Scott JW, et al. Hypothermia and interruption of carotid, or carotid and vertebral circulation in the surgical management of intracranial aneurysms. *J Neurosurg* 13:1–42, 1956.

23. Broderick JP, Brott T, Tomsick T, et al. Intracerebral hemorrhage more than twice as common as subarachnoid hemorrhage. *J Neurosurg* 78:188–191, 1993.

24. Carotid surgery versus medical therapy in aymptomatic carotid stenosis. The CASANOVA Study Group. *Stroke* 22:1229–1235, 1991.

25. Carrea RME, Molins M, Murphy G. Surgical treatment of spontaneous thrombosis of the internal carotid artery in the neck, carotid-carotideal anastomosis: Report of a case. *Acta Neurol Lationam* 1:71–78, 1955.

26. Carrel A. Results of the transplantation of blood vessels, organs, and limbs. *JAMA* 51:1662–1667, 1908.

27. Castaldo J. Is carotid endarterectomy appropriate for asymptomatic stenosis? Yes. *Arch Neurol* 56:877–879, 1999.

28. Cate WR Jr, SHJ. Cerebral ischemia of central origin: Relief by subclavian-vertebral artery thromboendarterectomy. *Surgery* 45:19–30, 1959.

29. Challa VR, Moody DM, Bell MA. The Charcot-Bouchard aneurysm controversy: Impact of a new histologic technique. *J Neuropath Exp Neurol* 51:264–271, 1992.

30. Charcot JM, Bouchard C. Nouvelles recherches sur la pathogenie de l'hemorrhagie cerebrale. *Arch Physiol Norm Pathol* 1:110–127, 643–665, 725–734, 1868.

31. Chaturvedi S. Is carotid endarterectomy appropriate for asymptomatic stenosis? No. *Arch Neurol* 56:879–880, 1999.

32. Chehrazi B, Collins WF Jr. A comparison of effects of bipolar and monopolar electrocoagulation in brain. *J Neurosurg* 54:197–203, 1981.

33. Cooley DA, Al-Naaman YD, Carton CA. Surgical treatment of arteriosclerotic occlusion of common carotid artery. *J Neurosurg* 13:500–506, 1956.

34. Cooper A. A case of aneurysm of the carotid artery. *Med Chir Trans* 1:1–15, 1809.

35. Corner G. *Anatomy. Clio Medica. A Series of Primers on the History of Medicine.* New York: Paul B. Hoeber, 1930.

36. Craig WM, Adson AW. Spontaneous intracerebral hemorrhage: Etiology and surgical treatment, with a report of nine cases. *Arch Neurol Psychiatry* 35:701–716, 1936.

37. Crawford JV, Russell DS. Cryptic arteriovenous and venous hamartomas of the brain. *J Neurol Neurosurg Psychiatry* 19:1–11, 1956.

38. Crawford ES, DBM, Fields WS. Roentgenographic diagnosis and surgical treatment of basilar artery insufficiency. *JAMA* 168:509–514, 1958.

39. Crawford ES, DBM, Garrett HE, et al. Surgical treatment of occlusive cerebrovascular disease. *Surg Clin N Am* 46:873–884, 1966.

40. Cunhae Sa MJ, Stein BM, Solomon RA. The treatment of associated intracranial aneurysms and arteriovenous malformations. *J Neurosurg* 77:853–9, 1992.

41. Cushing H. The blood pressure reaction of acute cerebral compression, illustrated by cases of intracranial hemorrhage. *Am J Med Sci* 125:1017–1044, 1903.

42. Cushing H. The blood pressure reaction of acute cerebral compression. *Am J Med Sci* 125:1017, 1903.

43. Cushing H, Bailey P. *Tumours Arising from the Blood-Vessels of the Brain. Angiomatous Malformations and Hemangioblastomas.* London: Balliere, Tindall and Cox, 1928.

44. Dandy W. Arteriovenous aneurysms of the brain. *Arch Surg* 17:190–243, 1928.

45. Day AL, Friedman WA, Sypert GW. Successful treatment of the normal perfusion pressure breakthrough syndrome. *Neurosurgery* 11:625–630, 1982.

46. De Bakey ME, Morris GC Jr, Jordan GL Jr, et al. Segmental thrombo-obliterative disease of branches of aortic arch: Successful surgical treatment. *JAMA* 166:998–1003, 1958.

47. del Zoppo GJ, Higashida RT, Furlan AJ, et al. PROACT: A phase II randomized trial of recombinant pro-urokinase by direct arterial delivery in acute middle cerebral artery stroke. PROACT Investigators. Prolyse in Acute Cerebral Thromboembolism [see comments]. *Stroke* 29:4–11, 1998.

48. Denman FR, Ehnl G, Duty WS. Insidious thrombotic occlusion of cervical carotid arteries, treated by arterial graft. *Surgery* 38:569–577, 1955.

49. DeReuck J. Historical anatomical aspects of stroke. *J Hist Neurosci* 3:103–107, 1994.

50. Deveikis JP. Endovascular therapy of intracranial arteriovenous malformations: Materials and techniques. *Neuroimaging Clin N Am* 8:401–424, 1998.

51. Djindjian R. Superselective internal carotid artery arteriography and embolization. *Neuroradiology* 9:145–156, 1975.

52. Dolenc V. Direct microsurgical repair of intracavernous vascular lesions. *J. Neurosurg* 58:824–831, 1983.

53. Dolenc VV. A combined epi- and subdural direct approach to carotid-ophthalmic artery aneurysms. *J Neurosurg* 62:667–672, 1985.

54. Dolenc VV, Skrap M, Sustersic J, et al. A transcavernous-transsellar approach to the basilar tip aneurysms. *Br J Neurosurg* 1:251–259, 1987.

55. Donaghy RMP, Yaşdargil MG. Extra-intracranial bloodflow diversion. *Presented at the American Association of Neurological Surgery Annual Meeting, Chicago, Illinois,* 1968.

56. dos Santos J. Sur la desobstruction des thromboses arterielles anciennes. *Mem Acad Chir* 73:409–411, 1947.

57. Drake CG. 1981. Progress in cerebrovascular disease:

Management of cerebral aneurysm. *Stroke* 12: 273–283, 1981.

58. Drake CG. Gordon Murray lecture: Evolution of intracranial aneurysm surgery. *Can J Surg* 27:549–555, 1984.

59. Drake CG. Earlier times in aneurysm surgery. *Clin Neurosurg* 32:41–50, 1985.

60. Drake CG, Peerless SJ, Hernesniemi J. *Surgery of the Vertebrobasilar Aneurysms: London Ontario Experience on 1767 Patients.* Vienna: Springer, 1996.

61. Eastcott HHG, Pickering G, Rob CG. Reconstruction of internal carotid artery in a patient with intermittent attacks of hemiplegia. *Lancet* 2:994–996, 1954.

62. EC/IC Bypass Study Group, et al. Failure of extracranial-intracranial arterial bypass to reduce the risk of ischemic stroke. *N Engl J Med* 313:1191–1200, 1985.

63. Ennix CL Jr, LG, Morris GC Jr. Improved results of carotid endarterectomy in patients with symptomatic coronary disease: An analysis of 1546 consecutive carotid operations. *Stroke* 10:122–125, 1979.

64. Endarterectomy for asymptomatic carotid artery stenosis. Executive Committee for the Asymptomatic Carotid Atherosclerosis Study. *JAMA* 273:1421–1428, 1995.

65. Fayad PB, Awad IA. Surgery for intracerebral hemorrhage. *Neurology* 51:S69–S73, 1998.

66. Fein J. *A History of Cerebrovascular Disease and its Surgical Management.* New York: Raven Press, 1984.

67. Fields WS, et al. Joint study of extracranial arterial occlusion as a cause of stroke. 1. Organization of study and survey of patient population. *JAMA* 203:955–960, 1968.

68. Fisher C. Occlusion of the internal carotid artery. *Arch Neurol* 65:346–377, 1951.

69. Fisher CM. Pathological observations in hypertensive cerebral hemorrhage. *J Neuropathol Exp Neurol* 30: 536–550, 1971.

70. Fisher CM. Cerebral miliary aneurysms in hypertension. *Am J Pathol* 66:313–324, 1972.

71. Flamm ES. History of Neurovascular Surgery: I. Cerebral Aneurysms and Subarachnoid Hemorrhage in Greenblatt S et al. (eds): *History of Neurological Surgery.* Park Ridge, IL: AANS Publishers, 1997.

72. Fox JL, Albin MS, Bader DC, et al. Microsurgical treatment of neurovascular disease. Part I. Personnel, equipment, extracranial-intracranial anastomosis. *Neurosurgery* 3:285–304, 1978.

73. Fox JL, Albin MS, Bader DC, et al. Microsurgical treatment of vascular disease. Part II. Intracranial aneurysms, intracranial and intraspinal arteriovenous malformations. *Neurosurgery* 3:305–320, 1978.

74. Freytag E. Fatal hypertensive intracerebral haematomas: A survey of the pathologic anatomy of 393 cases. *Neurol Neurosurg Psychiatry* 31:616–620, 1968.

75. Furlan A, Higashida R, Wechsler L, et al. Intra-arterial prourokinase for acute ischemic stroke. The PROACT II study: A randomized controlled trial. Prolyse in Acute Cerebral Thromboembolism [see comment]. *JAMA* 282:2003–2011, 1999.

76. Geiger A. Purpura haemorrhagica with cerebrospinal hemorrhage: Report of two cases. *JAMA* 102:1000, 1934.

77. Gobin YP, Laurent A, Merienne L, et al. Treatment of brain arteriovenous malformations by embolization

and radiosurgery [see comments]. *J Neurosurg* 85: 19–28, 1996.

78. Greenwood J Jr. Two point coagulation: A new principle and instrument for applying coagulation current in neurosurgery. *Am J Surg* 50:267–270, 1940.

79. Guglielmi G. Endovascular treatment of intracranial aneurysms. *Neuroimaging Clin N Am* 2:269–278, 1992.

80. Gunel M, Awad IA, Anson J. Mapping a gene causing cerebral cavernous malformation to 7q11.2-q21. *PNAS* 92:6620–6624, 1995.

81. Gunel M, Awad IA, Finberg K, et al. A founder mutation as a cause of cerebral cavernous malformation in Hispanic Americans. *N Engl J Med* 334:946–951, 1996.

82. Hachinski V. Carotid endarterectomy for asymptomatic stenosis. *Arch Neurol* 56:881, 1999.

83. Hamby WB, Gardner WJ. Treatment of pulsating exopthalmos with report of two cases. *Arch Surg* 27: 676–685, 1933.

84. Hamilton MG, Zabramski JM. Intracerebral hematomas, in, Carter P, Spetzler R, Hamilton MG, (eds): *Neurovascular Surgery.* New York, NY: McGraw-Hill, 1995, pp 477–496.

85. Heinz ER. History of neuroradiology, in, Rengachary WA, (ed): *Neurosurgery,* Vol. 1. New York, NY: McGraw Hill, 1996, pp 11–23.

86. Henkes H, Nahser HC, Berg-Dammer E, et al. Endovascular therapy of brain AVMs prior to radiosurgery [In Process Citation]. *Neurol Res* 20:479–492, 1998.

87. Heros RC. Arteriovenous malformations of the medial temporal lobe: Surgical approach and neuroradiological characterization. *J Neurosurg* 56:44–52, 1982.

88. Heros RC, Tu YK. Is surgical therapy needed for unruptured arteriovenous malformations? *Neurology* 37: 279–286, 1986.

89. Heros RC, Debrun GM, Ojemann RG, et al. Direct spinal arteriovenous fistula: A new type of spinal AVM. Case report. *J Neurosurg* 64:134–139, 1986.

90. Hobson RW II, Weiss DG, Fields WS, et al. Efficacy of carotid endarterectomy for asymptomatic carotid stenosis. *N Engl J Med* 328:221–227, 1993.

91. Hunt J. The role of the carotid arteries, in the causation of vascular lesions of the brain, with remarks on certain special features of the symptomatology. *Am J Med Sci* 147:704–713, 1914.

92. Hunt WE, Hess RM. Surgical risk as related to time of intervention in the repair of intracranial aneurysms. *J Neurosurg* 28:14–20, p 1968.

93. Ingraham FD, Bailey OT. Clinical use of human plasma fractionation. III. The use of products and fibrinogen and thrombin in surgery. *JAMA* 126:680, 1944.

94. Jaboulay M. Chirurgie des arteres, ses applications a quelques lesions de l'artere femorale. *Semin Med* 22: 405–406, 1902.

95. Jacobson JH, Suarez EL. Microsurgery in anastomosis of small vessels. *Surg Forum* 11:243, 1960.

96. Jacques S, Bullara LA, Pudenz RH. Microvascular bipolar coagulator: Technical note. *J Neurosurg* 44: 523–524, 1976.

97. Jafar JJ, Awad IA, Rosenwasser RH. *Vascular Malformations of the Central Nervous System.* Philadelphia, PA: Lippincott, Williams & Wilkins, 1999.

98. Jane JA, Kassell NF, Torner JC, et al: The natural his-

tory of aneurysms and arteriovenous malformations. *J Neurosurg* 62:321–323, 1985.

99. Javid H, Julian OC. Prevention of stroke by carotid and vertebral surgery. *Med Clin N Am* 51:113–122, 1967.

100. Johnson HC. Surgery of cerebral vascular anomalies, in, AE Walker, (ed): *A History of Neurological Surgery.* Baltimore: Williams & Wilkins, 1951, pp 250–269.

101. Juvela S, Heiskanen O, Poranen A. The treatment of spontaneous intracerebral hemorrhage: A prospective randomized trial of surgical and conservative treatment. *J Neurosurg* 70:755–758, 1989.

102. Kanaya H, Kuroda K. Development in neurosurgical approaches to hypertensive intracerebral hemorrhage in Japan, in, Kaufman HH (ed): *Intracerebral Hematomas.* New York, Raven Press, 1992, pp 197–209.

103. Kassell NF, Torner JC, Haley EC Jr, et al. The International Cooperative Study on the Timing of Aneurysm Surgery. Part 1: Overall management results. *J Neurosurg* 73:18–36, 1990.

104. Kassell NF, Torner JC, Jane JA, et al. The International Cooperative Study on the Timing of Aneurysm Surgery. Part 2: Surgical results. *J Neurosurg* 73:37–47, 1990.

105. Katzen BT, Becker GJ. Intravascular stents: Status of development and clinical application. *Endovasc Surg* 72:941–957, 1992.

106. Krueger C, Weir B, Nosko M. Nimodipine and chronic vasospasm in monkeys: Part 2. Pharmacological studies of vessels in spasm. *Neurosurgery* 16:137–40, 1985.

107. Laberge-le Couteulx S, Jung HH, Labauge P, et al. Truncating mutations in CCM1, encoding KRIT1, cause hereditary cavernous angiomas. *Nat Genet* 23: 189–193, 1999.

108. Lawton MT, Hamilton MG, Spetzler RF. Multimodality treatment of deep arteriovenous malformations: Thalamus, basal ganglia, and brain stem. *Neurosurgery* 37:29–35; discussion 35–36, 1995.

109. Lee SH, Huddle DO, Awad IA. Which aneurysms should be referred for endovascular therapy? Proceedings of Annual CNS Meetings (Boston, 1999). *Clinical Neurosurg* 102:316–319, 2000.

110. Leksell L. The stereotaxic method. *Acta Chir Scand* 102, 1951.

111. Ligon BL. The mystery of angiography and the "unawarded" Nobel Prize: Egas Moniz and Hans Christian Jacobaeus. *Neurosurgery* 43:602–611, 1998.

112. Lin PM, Javid H, Doyle EJ. Partial internal carotid artery occlusion treated by primary resection and vein graft: Report of a case. *J Neurosurg* 13:650–655, 1956.

113. Lougheed WM, Marshall BM. The diploscope in intracranial aneurysm surgery: Results in 40 patients. *Can J Surg* 12:75–82, 1969.

114. Lunsford LD, Kondziolka D, Flickinger JC, et al. Stereotactic radiosurgery for arteriovenous malformations. *J Neurosurg* 75:512–524, 1991.

115. Luyendijk W. Intracerebral haematoma, in, Vinken PJ, Bruyn GW, (eds): *Handbook of Clinical Neurology. Vol II: Vascular Diseases of the Nervous System, Part I.* New York, Elsevier, 1972, pp 660–719.

116. Lyons C, Galbrieth G. Surgical treatment of atherosclerotic occlusion of the internal carotid artery. *Ann Surg* 146:487–498, 1957.

117. Mackay B. Endovascular thrombolysis and angioplasty, in, I. Awad (ed): *Cerebrovascular Occlusive Disease and Brain Ischemia.* Park Ridge, IL, American Association of Neurological Surgeons, 1992.

118. Malis LI. Instrumentation and techniques in microsurgery. *Clin Neurosurg* 26:626–636, 1979.

119. Malis LI. Electrosurgery: Technical note. *J Neurosurg* 85:970–975, 1996.

120. Mandybur T. Cerebral amyloid angiopathy: The vascular pathology and complications. *J Neuropathol Exp Neurol* 45:79–90, 1986.

121. Mawad ME, Hilal SK, Michelsen WJ. Occlusive vascular disease associated with cerebral arteriovenous malformations. *Radiology* 153:401–408, 1984.

122. McCormick WF. The pathology of vascular ("arteriovenous malformations") malformations. *J Neurosurg* 24:807–816, 1966.

123. McKissock W, Richardson A, Taylor J. Primary intracerebral hemorrhage: A controlled trial of surgical and conservative treatment in 180 unselected cases. *Lancet* 2:221–226, 1961.

124. Meier B. Long-term results of coronary balloon angioplasty. *Ann Rev Med* 42:47–60, 1991.

125. Moniz E, Dias A, Lima A. La radio-arteriographie et la topagraphie cranio. *J Radiologie* 12:72–83, 1928.

126. Murphey F, Maccubbin MD. Carotid endarterectomy: A long-term follow-up study. *J Neurosurg* 23: 156–168, 1965.

127. Nakstad PH, Nornes H. Superselective angiography, embolisation and surgery in treatment of arteriovenous malformations of the brain. *Neuroradiology* 36: 410–413, 1994.

128. Nguyen J-P, Decq P, Brugieres P, et al. A technique for stereotactic aspiration of deep intracerebral hematomas under computed tomographic control using a new device. *Neurosurgery* 31:330–335, 1992.

129. Niizuma H, Shimizu Y, Yonemitsu T. Results of stereotactic aspiration in 175 cases of putaminal hemorrhage. *Neurosurgery* 24:814–819, 1989.

130. Noran HH. Intracranial vascular tumors and malformations. *Arch Pathol* 39:393–416, 1945.

131. Nosko M, Weir B, Krueger C. Nimodipine and chronic vasospasm in monkeys: Part 1. Clinical and radiological findings. *Neurosurgery* 16:129–136, 1985.

132. Ogilvy CS. Radiation therapy for arteriovenous malformations: A review [see comments]. *Neurosurgery* 26:725–735, 1990.

133. Olivecrona H, Landenheim J. *Congenital Arteriovenous Aneurysms of Carotid and Vertebral Arterial Systems.* Berlin: Springer-Velag, 1957.

134. Olivecrona M, Riieves J. Arteriovenous aneurysms of the brain: Their diagnosis and treatment. *Arch Neurol Psychiatry* 59:567–602, 1948.

135. Ondra SL, Troupp H, George ED, et al. The natural history of symptomatic arteriovenous malformations of the brain: A 24-year follow-up assessment [see comments]. *J Neurosurg* 73:387–391, 1990.

136. Pasqualin A, Scienza R, Cioffi F. Treatment of cerebral arteriovenous malformations with a combination of preoperative embolization and surgery. *Neurosurgery* 29:358–368, 1991.

137. Penfield W. The operative treatment of spontaneous intracerebral hemorrhage. *Can Med Assoc J* 28:369, 1933.

138. Perini S, Zampieri P, Rosta L, et al. Endovascular treat-

ment of pial AVMs: Technical options, indications and limits in pediatric age patients. *J Neurosurg Sci* 41: 325–330, 1997.

139. Piantanida M, Buscarini E, Dellavecchia C, et al. Hereditary haemorrhagic telangiectasia with extensive liver involvement is not caused by either HHT1 or HHT2. *J Med Genet* 33:441–443, 1996.

140. Pilcher C. Angiomatous malformations of the brain: Successful extirpation in three cases. *Ann Surg* 123: 766–784, 1946.

141. Pilcher C, Meacham WF. Absorbable gelatin sponge and thrombin for hemostasis in enurosurgery. *Surg Gynecol Obstet* 81:365, 1945.

142. Pool JL, Colton RP. The dissecting microscope for intracranial aneurysm surgery. *J Neurosurg* 25: 315–318, 1966.

143. Randomised trial of endarterectomy for recently symptomatic carotid stenosis: Final results of the MRC European Carotid Surgery Trial (ECST). *Lancet* 351: 1379–1387, 1998.

144. Results of a randomized controlled trial of carotid endarterectomy for asymptomatic carotid stenosis. Mayo Asymptomatic Carotid Endarterectomy Study Group. *Mayo Clin Proc* 67:513–518, 1992.

145. Robertson J. Carotid endarterectomy: A saga of clinical science, personalities, and evolving technology. *Stroke* 29:2435–2441, 1998.

146. Robinson GW. Encapsulated brain hemorrhages: A study of their frequency and pathology. *Arch Neurol Psychiatry* 27:1441–1444, 1932.

147. Robinson JR, Awad IA, Little JR. Natural history of the cavernous angioma. *J Neurosurg* 75:709–714, 1991.

148. Roski R, Spetzler RF. Carotid ligation in the treatment of cerebral aneurysms, in, L Hopkins, Long DM, (ed): *Clinical Management of Intracranial Aneurysms.* New York, Raven Press, 1982, pp 11–19.

149. Rothbart D, Awad IA, Lee J, et al. Expression of angiogenic factors and structural proteins in central nervous system vascular malformations. *Neurosurgery* 38:915–924; discussion 924–925, 1996.

150. Russell DS. Discussion: The pathology of spontaneous intracranial haemorrhage. *Proc R Soc Med* 47: 689–693, 1954.

151. Russell DS. The patholgy of spontaneous intracranial hemmorhage. *Proc R Soc Med* 47:689–693, 1954.

152. Russell DS, Rubinstein LJ, Lumsden CE. Tumours and hamartomas of blood vessels, in, Russell DS, Rubinstein LJ, (ed): *Pathology of Tumours of the Nervous System.* London, Edward Arnold, 1959, pp 72–92.

153. Sahoo T, Johnson EW, Thomas JW, et al. Mutations in the gene encoding KRIT1, a Krev-1/rap 1a binding protein, cause cerebral cavernous malformations (CCM1). *Hum Mol Genet* 8:2325–2333, 1999.

154. Sahs A, Perret GE, Locksley HB, et al. *Intracranial Aneurysms and Subarachnoid Hemorrhage: A Cooperative Study.* Philadelphia, J.B. Lippincott, 1969.

155. Samson DS, Hodosh RM, Clark WK. Microsurgical evaluation of the pterional approach to aneurysms of the distal basilar circulation. *Neurosurgery* 3:135–141, 1978.

156. Samson DS, Neuwelt EA, Beyer CW, et al. Failure of extracranial-intracranial arterial bypass in acute middle cerebral artery occlusion: Case report. *Neurosurgery* 6:185–188, 1980.

157. Savory W. Obliteration of the main arteries of the upper extremities and left side of the neck. *Medicochirurgical Trans (London)* 39:205–219, 1856.

158. Smith KA, Shetter A, Speiser B, et al. Angiographic follow-up in 37 patients after radiosurgery for cerebral arteriovenous malformations as part of a multimodality treatment approach [In Process Citation]. *Stereotact Funct Neurosurg* 69:136–142, 1997.

159. Spetzler RF, Carter LP. Revascularization and aneurysm surgery: Current status. *Neurosurgery* 16: 111–116, 1985.

160. Spetzler RF, Martin NA. A proposed grading system for arteriovenous malformations. *J Neurosurg* 65: 476–483, 1986.

161. Spetzler RF, Zabramski JM. Surgical management of large AVMs. *Acta Neurochir Suppl (Wien)* 42:93–97, 1988.

162. Spetzler RF, Zabramski JM. Grading and staged resection of cerebral arteriovenous malformations. *Clin Neurosurg* 36:318–337, 1990.

163. Spetzler RF, Hadley MN, Martin NA, et al. Vertebrobasilar insufficiency. Part 1: Microsurgical treatment of extracranial vertebrobasilar disease. *J Neurosurg* 66: 648–661, 1987.

164. Spetzler RF, Hadley MN, Rigamonti D, et al. Aneurysms of the basilar artery treated with circulatory arrest, hypothermia, and barbiturate cerebral protection [see comments]. *J Neurosurg* 68:868–879, 1988.

165. Spetzler RF, Martin NA, Carter LP, et al. Surgical management of large AVM's by staged embolization and operative excision. *J Neurosurg* 67:17–28, 1987.

166. Spetzler RF, Selman W, Carter LP. Elective EC-IC bypass for unclippable intracranial aneurysms. *Neurol Res* 6:64–68, 1984.

167. Spetzler RF, Wilson CB, Weinstein P, et al. Normal perfusion pressure breakthrough theory. *Clin Neurosurg* 25:651–672, 1978.

168. Spetzler RF, Zabramski JM, Flom RA. Management of juvenile spinal AVM's by embolization and operative excision: Case report. *J Neurosurg* 70:628–632, 1989.

169. Spetzler RF, Carter LP, Selman WR, et al. *Cerebral Revascularization for Stroke.* New York, NY: Thieme-Stratton, 1985.

170. Stein BM. Arteriovenous malformations of the medial cerebral hemisphere and the limbic system. *J Neurosurg* 60:23–31, 1984.

171. Stein BM, Wolpert SM. Arteriovenous malformations of the brain. II. Current concepts and treatment. *Arch Neurol* 37:69–75, 1980.

172. Steiner L, Leksell L, Greitz T. Stereotaxic radiosurgery for cerebral arteriovenous malformations. *Acta Chir Scand* 138:459–464, 1972.

173. Strully KJ, Hurwitt E, Blankenberg HW. Thromboendarterectomy for thrombosis of the internal carotid artery in the neck. *J Neurosurg* 10:474–482, 1953.

174. Sugita K, Tsugane R. Bipolar coagulator with automatic thermocontrol: Technical note. *J Neurosurg* 41: 777–779, 1974.

175. Sundt TM, Sandok B, Whisnant JP. Carotid endarterectomy: Complications and preoperative assessment of risk. *Mayo Clin Proc* 50:301–306, 1975.

176. Todd NV, Howie JE, Miller JD. Norman Dott's contribution to aneurysm surgery. *J Neurol Neurosurg Psychiatry* 53:455–458, 1990.

177. Vinuela F, Duckwiler G, Mawad M. Guglielmi detachable coil embolization of acute intracranial aneurysm:

Perioperative anatomical and clinical outcome in 403 patients. *J Neurosurg* 86:475–482, 1997.

178. Walker P. Symposium: The current management of carotid artery disease. 1. Carotid surgery: A historic perspective. 15th Annual Meeting of the *Canadian Society for Vascular Surgery,* Vancouver, BC, 1994.

179. Weir B. The history of cerebral vasospasm. *Neurosurg Clin N Am* 1:265–276, 1990.

180. Wepfer J. *Treatise on Apoplexy.* Schauffhausen: JD Suter, 1658.

181. Wilson C, Stein BM. *Intracranial Arteriovenous Malformations.* Baltimore, MD: William and Wilkins, 1984.

182. Wilson CB, Hoi Sang, U, Domingue J. Microsurgical treatment of intracranial vascular malformations. *J Neurosurg* 51:446–454, 1979.

183. Wylie EJ, KE, Davies O. Experimental and clinical experiences with use of fascia lata applied as a graft about major arteries after thrombo-endarterectomy and aneurysmorrhaphy. *Surg Gynecol Obstet* 93:257–272, 1951.

184. Yaşargil MG. Intracranial microsurgery. *Clin Neurosurg* 17:250–256, 1970.

185. Yaşargil MG, Fox JL. The microsurgical approach to intracranial aneurysms. *Surg Neurol* 3:7–14, 1975.

186. Yaşargil MG, Antic J, Laciga R, et al. Microsurgical pterional approach to aneurysms of the basilar bifurcation. *Surg Neurol* 6:83–91, 1976.

187. Yaşargil MG, Symon L, Teddy PJ. Arteriovenous malformations of the spinal cord. *Adv Tech Stand Neurosurg* 11:61–102, 1984.

188. Yaşargil MG, Vise WM, Bader DC. Technical adjuncts in neurosurgery. *Surg Neurol* 8:331–336, 1977.

189. Zulch KJ. *Brain Tumors: Their Biology and Pathology.* New York, Springer, 1957.

8

The Development of Neuro-Oncology in the Second Half of the 20th Century

Edward R. Laws, MD, FACS

INTRODUCTION

The development of neuro-oncology in the second half of the 20th century is a fascinating story. It combines technological advances with conceptual progress and provides a strong base for anticipated breakthroughs in the 21st century in our ability to manage effectively malignant primary tumors of the brain. This discussion will consider the concepts underlying the evolution of neuro-oncology and how they developed over time, the diagnostic methods utilized for brain tumors and how they have improved, the adjunctive forms of management and therapy for primary brain tumors, and the march of discoveries in basic science that have allowed for translational advances to occur in our clinical practice.

PRE-1951

Brain tumors and their management have long been the focus of intense activity on the part of neurosurgeons and provided the initial impetus for the development of neuro-oncology. By 1951, the concept of the glioblastoma was fairly well developed. In 1926, Bailey and Cushing published a histogenetic classification of gliomas of the brain, which was widely adopted. Subsequent efforts by Kernohan and Ringertz led to schemes of grading of gliomas of the brain. Scherer provided a series of experimental observations that showed that the incidence of gliomas was proportional to the area of brain at risk. He also contributed a detailed description of the invasion and spread of many gliomas as they were studied in whole mount sections. These concepts were confirmed by Dandy's observations that even a hemispherectomy was incapable of curing a glioblastoma and Maxwell's observations of spread through the corpus callosum of certain malignant gliomas.

Before 1951, the diagnosis of brain tumor was made primarily on the basis of clinical analysis and neurologic signs. These were supplemented by air contrast studies, mainly in the form of ventriculography and occasionally, pneumoencephalography. Dandy introduced ventriculography in 1919, and by the early 1950s, it was widely used in diagnosis by most neurosurgeons (Cushing remained reluctant to use ventriculography throughout his career). Electroencephalography had been applied since the mid 1930s to the diagnosis of many types of brain disorders; in fact, Penfield made some significant contributions regarding the utility of the EEG in the diagnosis of brain tumors. Angiography had been introduced by Moniz, but still was not widely applied by the time the Congress of Neurological Surgeons was founded in 1951.

Radiation therapy was used on some patients with brain tumors, and in 1942, Dyke and Davidoff produced a monograph with regard to their experience with radiation treatment for brain tumors. However, the majority of physicians treating malignant brain tumors did not consider this therapy particularly effective.

Technical aspects of brain tumor surgery prior to 1951 depended upon techniques devised by Dandy, Cushing, and other pioneering neurosurgeons. The use of osteoplastic flaps with concealed incisions had become a standard. Electrocautery had been introduced by Bovie and Cushing, and was widely utilized. In addition, Dandy reported on ventriculoscopy for dealing with intraventricular pathology.

Because of the lack of precision with which brain tumors were localized, this was an era of large exposures. If a tumor was not visualized on the surface of the brain, the brain was carefully probed or palpated with the finger and surgical excision usually consisted of a biopsy or an ''internal decompression'' for most malignant gliomas. The prognosis was poor and careful closure of the wound was advocated for fear of a ''cerebral fungus'' as the tumor enlarged in the postoperative period.

With regard to the basic science of brain tumors, the primary observation regarding aerobic glycolysis that had been made by Warburg and the pertubation of normal glucose metabolism that occurs in brain tumors had been established. A few attempts were made at tissue culture and cell culture of human brain tumors, while initial efforts were made to develop experimental brain tumor models in animals. The first brain tumor model in animals was produced by Seligman, who implanted methyl-cholanthrene crystals subdurally in rodents.

DEVELOPMENTS IN THE 1950s

A number of significant advances were made during the 1950s as a result of experiences and surgeries performed by neurosurgeons during World War II. Penfield analyzed epilepsy associated with brain tumors (long known to be a fairly common association) by providing some localizing information. The development of cortisone by Kendall and Hench allowed for effective use of steroid compounds for replacement therapy in patients undergoing surgery for pituitary tumors and craniopharyngiomas. This subsequently led to the critical observation of Galicich and French that steroids were effective in treating the brain edema associated with malignant gliomas.

Metastatic endocrine cancer from the prostate and the breast was a focus of investigation. The concept of hypophysectomy for the treatment of these endocrine malignancies, as reported by Luft and Olivecrona, Walker, and Ray and Patterson, gave neurosurgeons a large new area of endeavor.

Diagnostic methods improved significantly in the 1950s with the introduction of the first nuclear brain scans and with Sweet's initial attempts at using positrons for brain scanning. French introduced the use of echoencephalography, and steady improvements in the technical aspects of angiography continued with the emphasis being on the indirect effects of tumors on the vasculature of the brain.

The 1950s saw the first attempts at chemotherapy of brain tumors, initially using nitrogen mustard and bioactive amines as reported by French and Woodhall. Radiation therapy became more generally applied to the treatment of brain tumors, and at the end of the decade, Sweet introduced the concept of boron neutron capture therapy.

Basic science efforts in neuro-oncology consisted of the development of the newer and more reliable forms of tissue culture, and reports of brain tumor growth and brain tumor vasculature when tumors were transplanted to the anterior chamber of the eye of the guinea pig. Some initial attempts at vaccination therapy for brain tumors were made at this time, as were early studies of the use of fluorescent methods of brain tumor detection intraoperatively.

THE 1960s

The 1960s saw the gradual introduction and spread of microneurosurgery, with reports from Kurze, Rand and Jannetta, Pool, Yasargil, and Malis. Leksell introduced stereotactic radiosurgery, and Hardy and Guiot reintroduced transsphenoidal surgery for pituitary tumors.

A major advance was the development of bipolar cautery, which became an essential part of microsurgical technique. The instruments developed by Greenwood and Malis provided a major advance in the handling of blood vessels in brain and tumor tissue. Neuroanesthesia began to be developed as a subspeciality within anesthesia, and mannitol began to replace urea as the ideal osmotic agent for decreasing intracranial pressure. From the standpoint of tumor analysis in the operating room, the introduction of cytologic smears occurred in the 1960s with the work of Jane and Yashon.

In the study of gliomas, perhaps the most influential paper of the decade was that of Jelsma and Bucy, who clearly showed improved prognosis in malignant gliomas with radical resection of the lesion. The multicentricity of some gliomas was established by Batzdorf.

With regard to improved diagnosis, the 1960s saw the development of the catheter-based angiography, which provided excellent detail for anatomic diagnosis and depiction of malignant tumor vessels.

Also during this decade, radiotherapy became generally accepted as an effective form of treatment, and dose response analyses became available so that the tolerances of normal brain became better understood. Nuclear particle therapy enjoyed some emphasis during the 1960s as well, and brain tumors were treated with protons, neutrons, alpha particles, and neon beams; unfortunately, none of these treatments proved particularly effective. Additional attempts at immunotherapy under the leadership of Mahaley continued, as did the evolution of the use of antimetabolites and alkylating agents for chemotherapy.

Experimental techniques available during the 1960s included histochemistry and cytochemistry, and fluorometric analysis with the ability to characterize enzymatic reactions. Adenosine 5'triphosphate (ATP) was recognized as the major source of brain energetics, and the dependence upon glucose metabolism was an obvious area of focus. Electron microscopy was applied to the analysis of brain tumors, and the structure and function of the blood brain barrier was intensively investigated.

THE 1970s

The development of microsurgery continued in the 1970s with major emphasis on microsurgi-

cal anatomy, as led by Rhoton. Ransohoff was an outspoken advocate of radical resection of gliomas. The first clinical trials of combination treatment for brain tumors were accomplished under the auspices of the Brain Tumor Study Group. This nationwide clinical trial suggested that BCNU, in addition to radiation therapy, provided a more effective form of adjunctive management of malignant gliomas.

The revival of the transsphenoidal approach to pituitary tumors led to an explosion in knowledge with regard to neuroendocrinology, with many neurosurgeons participating in these developments. From the neuropathological point of view, new entities were described, including the primitive neuroectodermal tumors (PNET) and the pleomorphic xanthoastrocytoma (PXA).

By the 1970s, neuroanesthesia was effective and reliable. The use of nitrous-narcotic techniques became widespread, with marked improvement in control of intracranial pressure. The influences of hyperventilation and autoregulatory phenomena in the cerebral circulation were carefully investigated.

From the diagnostic standpoint, the great breakthrough of the 1970s was the development of computed tomography (CT) scanning, which became available in the United States in 1973. Improved localization of brain tumors, improved microsurgical methods, and improved neuroanesthesia led to the beginning of a whole new paradigm for the treatment of all brain tumors. Later in this decade, intraoperative ultrasound was introduced, as were the ultrasonic aspirator, lasers for neurosurgery, and reasonably sophisticated electrophysiological monitoring.

Adjunctive treatment in the 1970s consisted of radiation therapy as a primary postoperative treatment modality, with the use of chemotherapy in some cases. Walker et al. presented the results of the original clinical trials of combination therapy and embarked on additional trials using other agents. Radiosensitizers had been developed and were tested in clinical trials. Innovative forms of therapy, such as hyperthermia and photodynamic therapy, were introduced but never widely adopted. In addition, experimental work on the role of viruses in the production of brain tumors began in the 1970s. It also became possible, through the use of cytogenetic methodologies, to karyotype brain tumors.

A major conceptual change in the 1970s was the understanding of tumor cell kinetics, a scientific effort led by Hoshino and Wilson. This investigation of tumor cell kinetics led to a rational basis for subsequent treatment and what Sano called "integrative therapy." Efforts in immunotherapy continued with the use of potentiators of the immune response.

THE 1980s

The introduction and development of a variety of skull base approaches to neoplasms of the brain began in the 1980s. This proved to be an intense area of interest for neurosurgeons and led to significant technical advances in the management of many types of brain tumors. Studies characterizing the biology and prognosis of low grade gliomas were made and correlated with prior epidemiologic studies that had attempted to determine the actual incidence of various types of brain tumors. The first such contribution was by Zulch, who in 1959 published a large pathologic series. Other epidemiologic studies attempted to characterize brain tumors on a population based analysis and included work by Walker, Percy et al., Schoenberg et al., and Mahaley et al. More recent efforts included using the various tumor registries in the United States that provided approximate information with regard to brain tumor incidence. New types of gliomas were described in the 1980s, and included the central neurocytoma, the dysembryoplastic neuroepithelial tumor (DNET) and the DIG. A new classification system, called the Ste. Anne-Mayo grading system, was put forth by Daumas-Duport.

One of the most important aspects of the 1980s was the introduction by Kelly of the concept of stereotactic volumetric resection of brain tumors. Initially, these studies were based on CT imaging information, but ultimately became more precise with the introduction of magnetic resonance imaging (MRI), and actually provided the basis for the image-guided surgery that is so prevalent today.

The 1980s led to significant improvements in brain tumor diagnosis with the development and widespread use of MRI. Positron emission tomography (PET) scanning was introduced in the

1980s as well, and has been useful in studying the metabolism and epiphenomena of brain tumors. Finally, magnetoencephalography was introduced in the 1980s and is a technique that is still under investigation.

In the operating room, use of evoked potentials for localization of "eloquent" brain was widespread, intraoperative angiography became a practical reality, and neuronavigation and image-guided surgery provided significant technical advances. The accepted combinations of radiation therapy and chemotherapy were expanded to include more in the way of immunotherapy. Multi-agent chemotherapy became the rule, particularly when it became evident that oligodendrogliomas responded to a combination of procarbazine, vincristine, and CCNU (PCV). During this decade there was a significant interest in the stereotactic implantation of radioactive sources, so-called interstitial radiotherapy or brachytherapy, but enthusiasm for these methods has faded. Interferons became the subject of clinical investigation in the 1980s and were part of the immunotherapeutic armamentarium.

On the basic science front, the 1980s saw the development of major understanding of tumor genetics with isolation of oncogenes and tumor suppressor genes. Monoclonal antibodies were developed and showed promise both in diagnosis and in therapy. Studies of experimental tumors in the nude mouse were accomplished and important studies of the phenomenon of tumor cell invasion were reported. Technical advances included the widespread use of immunohistochemical analysis of brain tumors and flow cytometry for the analysis of DNA and ploidy.

THE 1990s

The 1990s are characterized by an unparalleled series of advances in science and technology that have impacted neurosurgery and neuro-oncology in many ways. From the standpoint of concepts, a dominant theme has been the development of minimally invasive approaches. This has led to the expansion of neuroendoscopy, to many different varieties of image-guided surgery and biopsy, and to the increasing use of radiosurgery in the treatment of a variety of different types of tumors affecting the central nervous system. Intraoperative monitoring has expanded so that tumors located near or in eloquent areas of cerebral cortex may be removed with minimal risk of damage.

The use of a variety of evolving diagnostic methods has also contributed to the efficacy and safety of tumor resection. Functional MRI and magnetic source imaging have assisted in documenting the displacement of cerebral function produced by brain tumors. MR spectroscopy has some promise in allowing for an imaging diagnosis of specific types of brain tumors, and intraoperative MRI studies allow for confirmation of completeness of resection and real-time correction for shifting of the brain.

Operative adjuncts that are being evaluated are the use of polymer implants impregnated with chemotherapeutic agents for the treatment of malignant tumors, and as previously mentioned, the use of intraoperative MRI to control the surgical aspects of brain tumor therapy.

Adjuncts to surgery in the management of gliomas of the brain have included several attempts at gene therapy, with a number of different strategies being employed. These include inactivation of oncogenes, insertion of tumor suppressor genes, insertion of genes to produce differentiation of tumors, and insertion of "suicide" genes. Progress has been made in the engineering of monoclonal antibodies to couple with immunotoxins and radioisotopes. Interleukins, tumor-specific lymphocytes, and natural killer cells have all been used for brain tumor treatment, often by direct infusion. The development of convection-enhanced catheter infusion is also under evaluation for delivery of both immunotherapeutic and chemotherapeutic agents.

Underlying these advances are numerous developments in basic science. The 1990s have seen sophisticated quantitative methods of analyzing DNA, RNA, and protein products of genes using Northern, Southern and Western blots, comparative genomic hybridization, and DNA microarrays. Initial work done with restriction fragment lengthy polymorphism (RFLP) hybridization has led to the development of a number of hybridomas and to the insertion and deletion of genes in transgenic animals. It has become evident that although some malignant gliomas may begin as monoclonal tumors,

they rapidly undergo polyclonal expansion, which presents a major problem for chemotherapeutic approaches.

Pathologic evaluation of brain tumors has benefited from techniques such as in-situ hybridization and targeted fluorescent and immunocytochemical antibodies.

TABLE 8.1. *Concepts in neuro-oncology*

Pre-1951
  Histogenetic Glioma Classification—Bailey & Cushing, 1926
  Tumor Metabolism—Warburg, 1933
  Grading of Gliomas—Kernohan, 1949; Ringertz, 1940
  Structure, Origin and Spread of Gliomas—Scherer, 1938, 1940
  Spread Across Corpus Callosum—Maxwell, 1949
  Failure of Hemispherectomy to Cure—Dandy
  Stereotaxis in Humans—Spiegel & Wycis, 1947
1950s
  Steroids for Brain Edema from Gliomas—Galicich & French
  Epilepsy and Brain Tumors—Penfield
  Hypophysectomy for Endocrine Malignancies—Luft & Olivecrona, Walker, Ray & Patterson
  Stereotactic Radiosurgery—Leksell
  Steroids for Replacement in Pituitary Tumors & Craniopharyngiomas
1960s
  Microneurosurgery—Kurze, Rand & Jannetta, Pool, Yasargil, Malis
  Revival of Transsphenoidal Surgery—Hardy, Guiot
  Multicentricity of Some Gliomas—Batzdorf
  Improved Prognosis with Radical Resection—Jelsma & Bucy
1970s
  Neuroendocrinology
  Craniofacial Approaches to Tumors—Derome
  Microsurgical Anatomy—Rhoton
  Radical Resection—Ransohoff
  Clinical Trials—BTSG
  Description of PXA
  Description of PNET
  Neuroanesthesia, Autoregulation
1980s
  Skull Base Approaches
  Invasiveness of Gliomas
  Stereotactic Volumetric Resection—Kelly
  Description of: DNET, DIG, Central Neurocytomas, Li-Fraumeni syndrome
  Ste. Anne-Mayo Grading System—Daumas-Duport
1990s
  Radiosurgery
  Image-Guided Resection
  Intra-Operative Monitoring
  Minimally Invasive Approaches
  WHO Classification of Brain Tumors

BTSG = Brain Tumor Study Group; PXA = pilocytic xanthoastrocytoma; PNET = primitive neuroectodermal tumors; DNET = dysembryoblastic neuroepithelial tumor; WHO = World Health Organization.

TABLE 8.2. *Diagnostic methods in neuro-oncology*

Pre-1951
  Ventriculography & Pneumoencephalography—Dandy, 1919
  Electroencephalography—Berger, 1933
  Angiography—Moniz
1950s
  Nuclear Brain Scan
  Positron Scan
  Echoencephalography
1960s
  Catheter Angiography
1970s
  CT Scan
  Intraoperative Ultrasound
1980s
  MRI Scan
  PET Scan
  Magnetoencephalography and Magnetic Source Imaging
1990s
  Functional MRI
  MR Spectroscopy
  Intraoperative MRI

TABLE 8.3. *Operative adjuncts in neuro-oncology*

Pre-1951
  Electrocautery—Bovie & Cushing
  Ventriculoscopy—Dandy
1950s
  Steroids for Brain Tumors—Galicich & French
  Urea for ICP—Javid
1960s
  Bipolar Cautery—Greenwood, Malis
  Mannitol
  Neuroanesthesia
  Cytologic Smears—Jane & Yashon
1970s
  Electrophysiological Monitoring
  Intraoperative Ultrasound
  Lasers
  Ultrasonic Aspirator
  Stereotactic Biopsy
1980s
  Evoked Potentials
  Neuronavigation, Image-guided Surgery
  Intraoperative Angiography, Embolization of Tumors
1990s
  Intraoperative MRI
  Chemotherapy—Polymer Implants

TABLE 8.4. *Adjuncts to surgery in the management of gliomas*

Pre-1951
  Radiation Therapy—Dyke & Davidoff, 1942
1950s
  Chemotherapy (Nitrogen Mustard, amines)—French, Woodhall
  Radiation Therapy—Taveras
  Boron Neutron Capture Therapy—Sweet
1960s
  Immunotherapy—Mahaley
  Radiotherapy—Wara & Sheline, Bouchard, Kramer
  Nuclear Particle Therapy—protons, neutrons, alpha particles, neon beam
1970s
  Radiation & Chemotherapy—Walker
  Intra-arterial Chemotherapy
  Hyperthermia—Selker
  Radiosensitizers
  Photodynamic Therapy
1980s
  Radiotherapy & Chemotherapy & Immunotherapy
  Combination Chemotherapy (PCV)—Cairncross)
  Interstitial Radiotherapy—Brachytherapy
  Interferons
  Blood-Brain Barrier Disruption—Neuwelt
1990s
  Gene Therapy
  Immunotoxins
  Interleukins, Lymphocyte and NK Cell Infusions
  Chemotherapy Polymer Implants
  Convection Enhanced Infusions
  Anti-angiogenesis Agents
  Protease Inhibitors

As the human genome project continues and as more and more evidence suggest that the genesis of malignant brain tumors is from a ''multiple hit'' progression of genetic events, we can be hopeful that gene sequencing techniques will allow us to identify the genomic structure of specific brain tumors and to design truly effective therapy that will provide the curative strategy that eluded us during the 20th century.

The text and tables in this chapter can only provide highlights of an historical analysis of this complex subject, neuro-oncology. The author apologizes to those whose work may not have been adequately emphasized and for what may be perceived as errors in the assignation of various advances to specific decades. One is impressed as how progress is made both incrementally, from the work of many dedicated clinicians and scientists, and also dramatically by the introduction of paradigm—shifting ideas and techniques.

TABLE 8.5. *Basic science advances in neuro-oncology*

Pre-1951
 Hanging Drop Tumor Culture
 Cell Culture—Tissue Culture
 Experimental Brain Tumors—Methyl-Cholanthrene
1950s
 Tissue Culture, Anterior Chamber Guinea Pig Eye
 Vaccination
 Fluorescence Detection
1960s
 Electron Microscopy
 Immunologic Principles
 Anti-metabolites and Alkylating Agents
 Histochemistry and Cytochemistry
 Autoradiography
 Scintillation Detection
1970s
 Viruses and Brain Tumors
 Tumor Kinetics—Hoshino & Wilson
 Cytogenetics & Karyotyping
 ELISA
 Improved Immune Response in Brain Tumor Patients
1980s
 Tumor Genetics—Oncogenes and Tumor Suppressor Genes
 Lymphoma and EBV—Hochberg
 AIDS and Brain Tumors—Rosenblum
 Monoclonal Antibodies
 Nude Mouse Models
 Tumor Cell Invasion
 Immunohistochemistry
 Flow Cytometry
 Tissue Culture Spheroids
 Genetics of Drug Resistance
 Apoptosis
1990s
 DNA and RNA Analysis (Northern, Southern, Western blots, CGH, Microarrays) (RFLP hybridization)
 Role of Upregulated EGFR and VEGFR
 Transgenic Mice
 Multiple Hit Therapy of Tumor Genetics
 Polyclonal Expansion in Malignant Gliomas
 Gene Sequencing (Neurofibromatosis, VHC, MEN-1)
 In-situ Hybridization
 Anti-sense and Mis-sense Oligonucleotides
 Antiangiogenesis

ELISA = enzyme-linked immunosorbent assay; EBV = Epstein-Barr Virus; AIDS = acquired immunodeficiency syndrome; RFLP = restriction fragment length polymorphism; EGFR = epidermal growth factor receptor; VEGFR = vascular endothelial growth factor receptor.

ACKNOWLEDGMENT

The author is grateful to Ms. Pamela Leake for her expert assistance in the preparation of this submission.

SUGGESTED READINGS

1. Bailey P, Cushing H. *A Classification of the Tumors of the Glioma Group on a Histogenetic Basis with a Correlated Study of Prognosis.* Philadelphia: JB Lippincott, 1926 (also New York: Argosy-Antiquarian, 1971).

2. Batzdorf U, Malamud N. The problem of multicentric gliomas. *J Neurosurg* 20:122–136, 1963.

3. Berens ME, Rutka JT, Rosenblum ML. Brain tumor epidemiology, growth, and invasion. *Neurosurg Clin N Am* 1:18–, 1990.

4. Bernstein JJ, Goldberg W, Laws ER Jr. Human malignant astrocytoma xenografts migrate in rat brain: A model for central nervous system cancer research. *J Neurosci Res* 22:134–144, 1989.

5. Bigner DD, Swenberg JA. *Jänisch and Schreiber's Experimental Tumors of the Central Nervous System.* Kalamazoo, Michigan: Upjohn, 1977.

6. Bigner SH, Humphrey PA, Wong AJ, Volgestein B, et al. Characterization of epidermal growth factor receptor in human glioma cell lines and xenografts. *Cancer Res* 50:8017–8022, 1990.

7. Bjerkvig R, Tonnesen A, Laerum OD, et al. Multicellular tumor spheroids from human gliomas maintained in organ culture. *J Neurosurgery* 72:463–475, 1990.

8. Bogler O, Huang HJ, Kleihues P, Cavenee WK. The P53 gene and its role in human brain tumors. *Glia* 15:308–327, 1995.

9. Bonnin JM, Rubinstein LJ. Immunohistochemistry of central nervous system tumors: Its contributions to neurosurgical diagnosis. *J Neurosurg* 60:1121–1133. 1984.

10. Bouchard J. Radiation therapy in the management of primary brain tumors. *Ann NY Acad Sci* 159:563–570, 1969.

11. Brem H, Mahaley MS Jr, Vick NA, et al. Interstitial chemotherapy with drug polymer implants for the treatment of recurrent gliomas. *J Neurosurg* 74:441–446, 1991.

12. Bressler J, Smith BH, Kornblith PL. Tissue culture techniques in the study of human gliomas, in Wilkins RH, Rengachary SS (eds): *Neurosurgery.* New York: McGraw-Hill, 1985, pp 542–548.

13. Brooks WH, Netsky MG, Levin JE. Immunity and tumors of the nervous system. *Surg Neurol* 3:184–186, 1975.

14. Bullard DE, Bigner DD. Applications of monoclonal antibodies in the diagnosis and treatment of primary brain tumors. *J Neurosurg* 63:2–16, 1985.

15. Bullard D, Schold S, Bigner S, Bigner DD. Growth and chemotherapeutic response in athymic mice of tumors arising from human glioma-derived cell lines. *Expl Neurol* 40:410–427, 1981.

16. Burger PC, Dubois PJ, Schold SC Jr, et al. Computerized tomographic and pathologic studies of the untreated, quiescent, and recurrent glioblastoma multiforme. *J Neurosurg* 58:159–169, 1983.

17. Burger PC, Mahaley MS, Dudka L, Vogel FS: The morphological effects of radiation administered therapeutically for intracranial gliomas: A post-mortem study of 25 cases. *Cancer* 44:1256–1272, 1979.

18. Cairncross JG, Macdonald DR. Successful chemotherapy for recurrent malignant oligodendroglioma. *Ann Neurol* 23:360–364, 1988.

19. Cheng SY, Huang HJ, Nagane M, Ji XD, et al. Suppression of glioblastoma angiogenicity and tumorigenicity

by inhibition of endogenous expression of vascular endothelial growth factor. *Proc Natl Acad Sci* 93: 8502–8507, 1996.

20. Choucair AK, Levin VA, Gutin PH, et al. Development of multiple lesions during radiation therapy and chemotherapy in patients with gliomas. *J Neurosurg* 65: 654–658, 1986.

21. Ciric I, Vick NA, Mikhael MA, et al. Aggressive surgery for malignant supratentorial gliomas. *Clin Neurosurg* 36:375–383, 1990.

22. Collins VP, Loeffler RK, Tivey H. Observations on growth rates of human tumors. *AJR* 76:988–1000, 1956.

23. Cravioto HM, Weiss JF, Goebel HH, et al. Preferential induction of central or peripheral nervous system tumors in rats by nitrosourea derivatives. *J Neuropathol Exp Neurol* 33:595–615, 1974.

24. Daumas-Duport C, Scheithauer BW, Chodkiewicz JP, et al. Dysembryoplastic neuroepithelial tumor: A surgically curable tumor of young patients with intractable partial seizures. Report of thirty-nine cases. *Neurosurgery* 23:545–556, 1988.

25. Daumas-Duport C, Scheithauer B, O'Fallon J, Kelly P. Grading of astrocytomas: A simple and reproducible method. *Cancer* 62:2152–2165, 1988.

26. de Tribolet N, Frank E, Mach JP. Monoclonal antibodies: Their application in the diagnosis and management of CNS tumors. *Clin Neurosurg* 34:446–456, 1988.

27. Ekstrand AJ, James CD, Cavanee WK, et al. Genes for epidermal growth factor receptor, transforming growth factor alpha, and epidermal growth factor and their expression in human gliomas in vivo. *Cancer Res* 51: 2164–2172, 1991.

28. Elvidge AR. Long-term survival in the astrocytoma series. *J Neurosurg* 28:399–404, 1968.

29. Fewer D, Wilson CB, Levin VA. *Brain Tumor Chemotherapy.* Springfield, Illinois: Charles C Thomas, 1976.

30. Galicich JH, French L, Melby JC. Use of dexamethasone in treatment of cerebral edema associated with brain tumors. *Lancet* 81:46–53, 1961.

31. Goldberg W, Laws ER, Bernstein JJ. Individual C6 glioma cells migrate in adult rat brain after neural homografting. *Int J Dev Neurosci* 9:427–436, 1991.

32. Gomez JG, Garcia JH, Colon LE. A variant of cerebral glioma called pleomorphic xanthoastrocytoma: Case report. *Neurosurgery* 16:703–706, 1985.

33. Grossi-Paoletti E, Paoletti P, Pezzotta S, et al. Tumors of the nervous system induced by ethyl-nitrosourea administered either intracerebrally or subcutaneously to newborn rats: Morphological and biochemical characteristics. *J Neurosurg* 37:580–590, 1972.

34. Gutin PH, Phillips TL, Wara WM, et al. Brachytherapy of recurrent malignant brain tumors with removable high-activity iodine-125 sources. *J Neurosurg* 60: 61–68, 1984.

35. Hart NM, Earl KM. Primitive neurectodermal tumours in children. *Cancer* 32:172–188, 1973.

36. Hassoun J, Gambarelli D, Grisoli F, et al. Central neurocytoma: An electron-microscopic study of two cases. *Acta Neuropathol (Berl)* 56:151–156, 1982.

37. Hochberg FH, Miller G, Schooley RT, et al. Central-nervous-system lymphoma related to Epstein-Barr virus. *N Engl J Med* 309:745–748, 1983.

38. Hoshino T, Wilson CB. Review of basic concepts of cell kinetics as applied to brain tumors. *J Neurosurg* 42: 123–131, 1975.

39. Hoshino T, Wilson CB, Rosenblum ML, et al. Chemotherapeutic implications of growth fraction and cell cycle time in glioblastoma. *J Neurosurg* 43:127–135, 1975.

40. Jane J, Yashon D. *Cytology of Tumors Affecting the Nervous System.* Springfield, Illinois: Charles C Thomas, 1969.

41. Jelsma R, Bucy PC. Glioblastoma multiforme: Its treatment and some factors affecting survival. *Arch Neurol* 20:161–171, 1969.

42. Kapp J, Vance R, Parker JL, et al. Limitations of high dose intra-arterial 1, 3-Bis (2-choloroethyl)—1-nitrosourea (BCNU) chemotherapy for malignant gliomas. *Neurosurgery* 10:715–719, 1982.

43. Kelly PJ. Stereotactic biopsy and resection of thalamic astrocytomas. *Neurosurgery* 25:185–195, 1989.

44. Kelly PJ, Daumas-Duport C, Kispert DB, et al. Image-based stereotaxic serial biopsies in untreated intracranial glial neoplasms. *J Neurosurg* 66:865–874, 1987.

45. Kelly PJ, Kall BA, Goerss S, et al. Computer-assisted stereotaxic laser resection of intra-axial brain neoplasm. *J Neurosurg* 64:427–439, 1986.

46. Kepes JJ, Rubinstein LJ, Eng LF. Pleomorphic xanthoastrocytoma: A distinctive meningeal glioma of young subjects with relatively favorable prognosis. A study of 12 cases. *Cancer* 44:1839–1842 1979.

47. Kernohan JW, Mabon RF, Svien HJ, et al. A simplified classification of the gliomas. *Proc Staff Meet Mayo Clin* 24:71–75, 1949.

48. Kessinger A: High dose chemotherapy with autologous bone marrow rescue for high-grade gliomas of the brain: A potential for improvement in therapeutic results. *Neurosurgery* 15:747–750, 1984.

49. Kleihues P, Burger PC, Scheithauer BW. The new WHO classification of brain tumors. *Brain Pathol* 3:255–268, 1993.

50. Kornblith PL, Walker M. Chemotherapy for malignant gliomas. *J Neurosurg* 68:1–17, 1988.

51. Kramer S. Radiation therapy in the management of brain tumors in children. *Ann N Y Acad Sci* 159:571–584, 1969.

52. Latif F, Tory K, Gnarra J, Yao M, et al. Identification of the von Hippel-Lindau disease tumor suppressor gene. *Science* 260:1317–1320, 1993.

53. Laws ER Jr., Cortese DA, Kinsey JH, et al. Photoradiation therapy in the treatment of malignant brain tumors: A phase I (feasibility) study. *Neurosurgery* 9:672–673, 1984.

54. Laws ER Jr., Goldberg WJ, Bernstein JJ. Migration of human malignant astrocytoma cells in the mammalian brain: Scherer Revisited. *Int J Dev Neurosci* 5:691–697, 1993.

55. Leibel SA, Sheline GE. Radiation therapy for neoplasms of the brain. *J Neurosurg* 66:1–22, 1987.

56. Leibel SA, Sheline GE, Wara WM, et al. The role of radiation therapy in the treatment of astrocytomas. *Cancer* 35:1551–1557, 1975.

57. Leksell L. The stereotactic method and radiosurgery of the brain. *Acta Chir Scand* 102:316–319, 1951.

58. Levy RM, Pons VG, Rosenblum ML. Central nervous system mass lesions in the acquired immunodeficiency syndrome (AIDS). *J Neurosurg* 61:9–16, 1984.

59. Li FP, Fraumeni JF, Jr, Mulvihill JJ, Blattner WA, et al. A cancer family syndrome in twenty-four kindreds. *Cancer Res* 48:5358–5362, 1988.

60. Lindgren M: On tolerance of brain tissue and sensitivity of brain tumors to irradiation. *Acta Radiol (Suppl)* 170: 1–73, 1958.

61. Louis DN, Ramesh V, Gusella JF. Neuropathology and molecular genetics of neurofibromatosis 2 and related tumors. *Brain Pathol* 5:163–172, 1995.

62. Mahaley MS Jr, Mettlin C, Natarajan N, et al. National survey of patterns of care for brain-tumor patients. *J Neurosurg* 71:826–836, 1989.

63. Martuza RL. Genetics in neuro-oncology. *Clin Neurosurg* 31:417–440, 1984.

64. Miescher S, Whiteside TL, de Tribolet N, et al. In situ characterization, clonogenic potential, and antitumor cytolytic activity of T lymphocytes infiltrating human brain cancers. *J Neurosurg* 68:438–448, 1988.

65. Neuwelt EA, Frenkel EP, Diehl J, et al. Reversible osmotic blood-brain barrier disruption in humans: Implications for the chemotherapy of malignant brain tumors. *Neurosurgery* 7:44–52, 1980.

66. Nishizaki T, Orita T, Furutani Y, et al. Flow-cytometric DNA analysis and immunohistochemical measurements of Ki-67 and BudR labeling indices in human brain tumors. *J Neurosurg* 70:379–384, 1989.

67. Ommaya AK. Immunotherapy of gliomas: A review. *Adv Neurol* 15:337–359, 1976.

68. Percy AK, Elveback LR, Okazaki H, Kurland LT. Neoplasms of the central nervous system: Epidemiologic considerations. *Neurology* 22:40–48, 1972.

69. Perese DM, Moore GE. Methods of induction and histogenesis of experimental brain tumors. *J Neurosurg* 17: 677–698, 1960.

70. Ramsey RG, Brand WN. Radiotherapy of glioblastoma multiforme. *J Neurosurg* 39:197–202, 1973.

71. Ringertz J. Grading of gliomas. *Acta Pathol Microbiol Scand* 27:51–64, 1950.

72. Roberts M, German J. A long-term study of patients with oligodendrogliomas: (Follow-up of 50 cases, including Dr. Harvey Cushing's series). *J Neurosurg* 24: 697–700, 1966.

73. Rouleau GA, Merel P, Lutchman M, Sanson M, et al. Alteration in a new gene encoding a putative membrane-organizing protein causes neurofibromatosis type 2. *Nature* 353:5115–521, 1993.

74. Russell DS, Rubenstein LJ. *Pathology of Tumors of the Nervous System, 5th ed.* Williams & Wilkins: Baltimore, 1992.

75. Saez RJ, Campbell RJ, Laws ER. Chemotherapeutic trials on human malignant astrocytomas in organ culture. *J Neurosurg* 46:320–327, 1977.

76. Salcman M, Samaras GM. Hyperthermia for brain tumors: Biophysical rationale. *Neurosurgery* 9:327–335, 1981.

77. Sano K. Integrative treatment of gliomas. *Clin Neurosurg* 30:93–124, 1983.

78. Scherer H: Structural development in gliomas. *Am J Cancer* 34:333–351, 1938.

79. Scherer H. A critical review: the pathology of cerebral gliomas. *J Neurol Psychiatry* 3:147–177, 1940.

80. Scherer H: Cerebral astrocytomas and their derivatives. *Am J Cancer* 40:159–197, 1940.

81. Scherer HJ: The forms of growth in gliomas and their practical significance. *Brain* 63:1–35, 1940.

82. Shapiro WR, Green SB, Burger PC, Mahaley MS, et al. Randomized trial of three chemotherapy regimens and two radiotherapy regimens in postoperative treatment of malignant glioma: Brain Tumor Cooperative Group Trial 8001. *J Neurosurg* 71:1–9, 1989.

83. Sheline G. Radiation therapy of brain tumors. *Cancer* 39:873–881, 1977.

84. Taratuto AL, Monges J, Lylyk P, Leiguarda R. Superficial astrocytoma attached to dura: Report of six cases in infants. *Cancer* 54:2505–2512, 1984.

85. VandenBerg S. Desmoplastic infantile ganglioglioma and desmoplastic cerebral astrocytoma of infancy. *Brain Pathol* 3:275–281, 1993.

86. von Deimling A, Louis DN, von Ammon K, et al. Association of epidermal growth factor receptor gene amplification with loss of chromosome 10 in human glioblastoma multiforme. *J Neurosurg* 77:295–301,1992.

87. Walker AE, Robins M, Weinfeld FD. Epidemiology of brain tumors: The national survey of intracranial neoplasms. *Neurology* 35:219–226, 1985.

88. Walker MD, Alexander E Jr, Hunt WE, et al. Evaluation of BCNU and/or radiotherapy in the treatment of anaplastic gliomas: A cooperative clinical trial. *J Neurosurg* 49:333–343, 1978.

89. Walker MD, Green SB, Byar DP, et al. Randomized comparisons of radiotherapy and nitrosoureas for the treatment of malignant glioma after surgery. *N Engl J Med* 303:1323–1329, 1980.

90. Weir B, Elvidge AR. Oligodendrogliomas. *J Neurosurg* 29:500–505, 1968.

91. Westphal M, Herrmann HD. Growth factor biology and oncogene activation in human gliomas and their implications for specific therapeutic concepts. *Neurosurgery* 25:681–694, 1989.

92. Young HF, Sakalas R, Kaplan AM. Inhibition of cell-mediated immunity in patients with brain tumors. *Surg Neurol* 5:19–23, 1976.

93. Zimmerman HM. The nature of experimental gliomas. *Clin Neurosurg* 7:247–258, 1959.

94. Zulch KJ. *Brain Tumors: Their Biology and Pathology, 3rd Edition.* Heidelberg: Springer, 1986.

9

Head Trauma and Intensive Care in 1951

T. Forcht Dagi, MD, FACS, FCCM, Christina Spetzler, Mark Preul, MD

INTRODUCTION

In its preface to Volume I of Clinical Neurosurgery in 1955, the editorial committee, made up of Drs. Raymond K. Thompson, Ira J. Jackson, Lee A. Christoferson, Gordon J. Strewler, and Edgar N. Weaver, defined a two-fold purpose: ''First, to honor one or more scientists in the field of the neurological sciences and to have him present some of his original studies. Secondly, to record for the future and for those not members of the Society the valuable ideas of those men who have contributed to the success of the program.'' This volume, the first comprehensive offering published by the Congress of Neurological Surgeons (CNS), saw the light of day four years after the foundation of the Congress. It articulated a premise that was no less valid then it would have been in 1951, nor at any other point in the history of neurosurgery, including the present: progress in neurological surgery is a function of individuals and of their valuable ideas, which require publication and dissemination for maximum impact.

This chapter addresses the problem of head trauma and neurological intensive care in a particular historical context: the way they were seen in 1951, the year the CNS was founded, and how they came to be seen that way. The year 1951

was the seventh anniversary of the founding of the Journal of Neurosurgery. It came about eight years after antibiotics had entered neurosurgical practice, six years after the end of World War Two, and four years after the publication of the highly influential War Surgery Supplement of the British Journal of Surgery, which summarized the approach to penetrating head trauma evolved under the leadership of Brigadier Sir Hugh Cairns and his colleagues in Great Britain.

Many physicians returned from the war with an interest in neurological surgery. Some had interrupted their training to serve. Others had received partial training, or had joined or been assigned to medical units built around the most famous teaching hospitals, where remarkably excellent surgery was carried out under variable circumstances. Training programs were full and increasing in number. Neurosurgery was seen, arguably, as the most prestigious of the specialties, thrilling not only for its technical challenges, but also for the very fact of its dedication to the nervous system and the opportunity to explore its science.[1] The CNS

---

[1] Sir Geoffrey Jefferson, for example, offered the following remarks at the end of the third annual meeting of the CNS in New Orleans, in 1954: ''I do want to say one last thing, and that is that I can never forget that we are the surgeons of the master system of the human body. Every-

TABLE 9.1. *The four phases of neurosurgery: Changes in diagnostic and surgical focus*[43]

	Phase I	Phase II	Phase III	Phase IV
Diagnostic Means				
Inspection	***	**	*	*
Palpation	***	**	*	*
Surgical Exploration	***	**	*	*
Neurological Examination	*	****	***	***
Plain Films	n/a	***	***	*
Ventriculography	n/a	n/a	***	
Arteriography	n/a	n/a	***	*
Cisternography, Polytomography, Others	n/a	n/a	**	*
Sectional Imaging	n/a	n/a	n/a	****
Diagnostic Purpose				
Fracture	****	**	*	*
Neurological Deficit	*	***	****	**
Fragments	***	****	**	
Extra-axial collections	*	**	***	****
Intra-axial lesions		*	**	
Contusion			**	
Increased ICP		**	***	****
CSF leak			**	***
Surgical Purpose				
Verify Diagnosis, Extradural Exploration	****	***	**	*
Elevation of depressed fracture	****	***	**	**
Verify Diagnosis, Subdural Exploration		**	***	
Decompression for ICP		***	****	**
Drainage of Extra-axial Collection		*	***	****
Debride Penetrating Wound Track	**	****	****	**
Dural Closure and Anatomical Restoration			**	****

[43] Higher number of asterisks reflects greater importance. Four maximum. N/A means technology not available. Lack of entry (blank space) implies absence of historical importance.

was dedicated to the mission of educating young neurosurgeons.

This was also the second year of the Korean War. Despite general agreement on the way head trauma should be managed, the new generation of young neurosurgeons sought to refine its understanding from both a surgical and a non-surgical perspective, and from both a clinical and a basic science approach. The Korean War would eventually be construed as a turning point in the management of head trauma because it led to outcome studies that demonstrated the impor-

tance of the timing of intervention to survival. These were not the first outcome studies in neurosurgery, but they were probably the best as of that point.

So how does one go about reconstructing a sense of head trauma and intensive care half a century past? This interval is long enough to allow historical perspective, and short enough to be just within the reach of accurate memory for many neurosurgeons still in practice.

One good approach is to examine the literature of the time. In the United States, articles of neurosurgical interest were published in the surgical, neurological, and the neurosurgical literature. From the time of the founding of the *Journal of Neurosurgery* in 1944, however, any matter of interest or consequence was alluded to in some way in the *Journal*. To get a sense of the time, we reviewed the contents of the *Journal* for the first ten years, and categorized and analyzed the literature on trauma according to several topics.

Table 9.2 shows the relative proportion of

thing else that exists, all the rest of our body exists, as something to maintain and to move about and increase the opportunity of our nervous system of doing its functions. And all people who deal with stomach, lungs, heart or gall-bladder are the kind of maintenance engineers full able to deal with the thing that makes us men and women. Some people at some times said to me, some of my more malicious friends, 'Of course you know that really the glamour has gone out of neurosurgery. You boys aren't where you were. The heart people have stolen it from you.' Well, my answer to that is that if any other branch of surgery is doing work which is in any way comparable to our own, we welcome their development. We have grown up, and in time they will do so too.'' (225)

TABLE 9.2. Publications on trauma in the Journal of Neurosurgery the first 10 years, 1944–1954

Year	1944	1945	1946	1947	1948	1949	1950	1951	1952	1953	1954	Total
Number of papers on trauma	8	12	11	2	5	6	5	2	6	7	3	67
Total number of papers	46	58	68	64	48	72	89	84	77	90	83	779
% related to trauma	17.4%	20.7%	16.2%	3.1%	10.4%	8.3%	5.6%	2.4%	7.8%	7.8%	3.6%	8.6%

publications dedicated to trauma between 1944 and 1954. Sixty-seven articles were published, constituting less than 9% of the whole.

Table 9.3 shows the major issues that were emphasized in these 67 publications by year. The three most important concerns by number of publication were penetrating head injury, extra-axial hemorrhage and clinical diagnosis. Laboratory work was not highly emphasized.

Table 9.4 is a bibliography of trauma in the first 10 years of the Journal of Neurosurgery, annotated to show authors, main concerns, and types of studies performed.

The surgical tools and techniques relied upon by neurosurgeons have changed less than one might expect, but the ideas and concepts associated with these tools and techniques have changed more, and more times, than one might imagine. Surgery for head trauma in 1951, for example, was both diagnostic and therapeutic. Today, it is only very rarely diagnostic. Surgery for head trauma in 1951 was extended to almost every case of unconsciousness. Surgery today is far more reserved. Intensive care in 1951 was essentially nonexistent. Intensive care today is at the center of the management of head trauma and research about head trauma. Physiological monitoring in 1951 was rudimentary. It is paradigmatic today. In 1951, the neurosurgeon did it all. Today, the management of head trauma often involves the cooperation of several specialties.

TABLE 9.3. Primary subject matter in 67 publications on head trauma Journal of Neurosurgery, 1944–1954

Year	1944	1945	1946	1947	1948	1949	1950	1951	1952	1953	1954	Total
Arachnoidal cysts	1									1		2
Cerebellar hemorrhage										1		1
Cerebral edema				1								1
Clinical diagnosis	2		1						2	1		6
Closed head injury	1								1		1	3
Complications		1	1						2			4
Cranioplasty					1				2			3
Electroencephalography		1	1									2
Experimental animal studies	1	2	2									5
Extra-axial fluid collections					1							1
Extra-axial hemorrhages	1				3	2	2	1	1			10
Fungus cerebri		1										1
Infections		1	2									3
Intracranial hemorrhage								1				1
Medical management				1			1				1	3
Pathophysiology	2	1	1				1					5
Penetrating head injury		3	3		1		1			2	1	11
Sequelae						1						1
Skull fraccture		1			1							2
Subdural hemorrhage					1							1
Surgical technique		1										1
TOTAL	8	12	11	2	6	5	5	2	6	7	3	67

TABLE 9.4. *Analysis of articles on trauma in the Journal of Neurosurgery 1944–1955: Bibliography, central issues, and study design[44]*

Year	Authors	Title	Volume: Pages	Main subject	Secondary subject	Other issues of interest	Study design
1944	Walker A, Kollros J, Case T:	The physiological bases of concussion	1: 103–116	Closed head injury	Experimental animal study	Pathophysiology	bench research
1944	Kaplan A:	Traumatic pneumocephalus with spontaneous ventriculograms; report of a case	1: 166–170	Clinical diagnosis	Skull fracture		case report
1944	Falconer M, Russell D:	Experimental traumatic cerebral cysts in the rabbit	1: 182–189	Arachnoidal cysts	Experimental animal study		bench research
1944	Holbourn A:	The mechanics of trauma with special reference to herniation of cerebral tissue	1: 190–200	Pathophysiology	Intracranial pressure		conceptual, review paper
1944	Evans J, Scheinker M:	Histologic studies of the brain following head trauma; IV. Late changes: atrophic sclerosis of the white matter	1: 306–320	Pathophysiology	Sequelae		*small series
1944	Turnbull F:	Extradural cerebellar hematoma; a case report	1: 321–324	Extra-axial hemorrhage			single case
1944	Brenner C, Friedman A, Merritt H, Denny-Brown D:	Post-traumatic headache	1: 379–391	Clinical diagnosis	Complications		large series
1944	Gurdjian E, Lissner H:	Head injury as studied by the cathode ray oscilloscope preliminary report	1: 393–399	Experimental animal study	Pathophysiology	Closed head injury	bench research
1945	Groat R, Windle W, Magoun H:	Functional and structural changes in the monkey's brain during and after concussion	2: 26–35	Experimental animal study	Closed head injury	Pathophysiology	bench research

Year	Author	Title	Citation	Topic 1	Topic 2	Topic 3	Series
1945	Glaser M, Shafer F:	Depressed fractures of the skull; their surgery, sequelae and disability	2: 140–153	Skull fracture	Sequelae		large series
1945	Dow R, Ulett G, Raaf J	Electroencephalographic studies in head injuries	2: 154–169	Electroencephalography	Clinical diagnosis		large series
1945	Evans J, Scheinker M:	Histologic studies of the brain following head trauma: I. Post-traumatic cerebral swelling and edema	2:306–314	Pathophysiology	Cerebral edema	Autopsy studies	small series
1945	Friedman A, Brenner C, Denny-Brown D:	Post-traumatic vertigo and dizziness	2:364–366	Complications	Clinical diagnosis		large series and literature review
1945	Butler E, Puckett W, Harvey E, McMillen J	Experiments on head wounding by high velocity missiles	2: 358–363	Experimental animal study	Penetrating head injury		bench research
1945	Haynes W:	Penetrating brain wounds; analysis of 342 cases	2: 365–378	Penetrating head injury	Surgical technique and medical management	Sequelae	very large series
1945	Carmichael F:	The reduction of hernia cerebri by tantalum cranioplasty; a preliminary report	2: 379–383	Fungus cerebri	Surgical technique	Cranioplasty	small series
1945	Ecker A:	Tight dural closure with pedicled graft in wounds of the brain	2: 384–390	Surgical technique	Dural closure		small series
1945	Rowe S, Turner O:	Observations on infection in penetrating wounds of the head	2: 391–401	Infections			small series
1945	Haynes W:	Transventricular wounds of the brain	2: 463–468	Penetrating head injury	Surgical technique		very large series
1945	Haynes W:	Extensive brain wounds; analysis of 159 cases occurring in a series of 342 penetrating war wounds of the brain	2: 469–478	Penetrating head injury	Surgical technique	Sequelae	large series

(Continued)

TABLE 9.4. *Continued.*

Year	Authors	Title	Volume: Pages	Main subject	Secondary subject	Other issues of interest	Study design
1946	Ecker A:	A bacteriologic study of penetration wounds of the brain, from the surgical point of view	3: 1–6	Infections	Medical management	Antibiotics	medium series
1946	Webster J, Schneider R, Lofstorm J:	Observations on early type of brain abscess following penetrating wounds of the brain	3: 7–14	Infections	Surgical technique and medical management	Antibiotics	medium series
1946	Matson D, Wolkin J:	Hematomas associated with penetrating wounds of the brain	3: 46–53	Penetrating head injury	Cerebral hematomas	Surgical technique	very large series
1946	Martin J, Campbell E	Complications following penetrating wounds of the skull	3: 58–73	Complications	Surgical technique and medical management	Infections	very large series
1946	Evans J, Scheinker M:	Histologic studies of the brain following head trauma; II Post-traumatic petechial and massive intracerebral hemorrhage	3: 101–113	Pathophysiology	Autopsy studies		small series
1946	Weaver TA, Fishman AJ:	Treatment of craniocerebral wounds	3: 149–156	Clinical diagnosis	Sequelae	Surgical technique and medical management	large series
1946	Windle W, Rambach W, Arellano M, Groat R, Becker R:	Water content of the brain after concussion and its noncontributory relation to the histopathology of concussion	3: 157–164	Experimental animal study	Cerebral edema		bench research
1946	Maltby G:	Evaluation of the late results in a group of 200 consecutive penetrating cranial war wounds	3: 239–249	Penetrating head injury	Sequelae		very large series

184

Year	Authors	Title	Reference	Category			Series type
1946	Webster J, Schneider R, Lofstorm J:	Observations upon the management of orbito-cranial wounds	3: 329–336	Penetrating head injury	Surgical technique		medium series
1946	Troland C, Baxter D, Schatzki R:	Observation on encephalographic findings in cerebral trauma	3: 390–398	Electroencephalography	Clinical diagnosis		large series
1946	Pudenz R, Shelden C:	The lucite calvarium - a method for direct observation of the brain	3: 487–505	Experimental animal study	Intracranial pressure		bench research
1947	Aita J:	Modern considerations of the man with brain injury	4: 240–254	Medical management	Sequelae		small series
1947	Scheinker M:	Cerebral swelling: histopathology, classification and clinical significance of brain edema	4: 255–275	Cerebral edema			large series
1948	Grantham E:	Cranioplasty and the post-traumatic syndrome	5: 19–22	Cranioplasty	Sequelae		large series
1948	MacCarty S, Horning D, Weaver E:	Bilateral extradural hematoma; report of case	5: 88–90	Extra-axial hemorrhage			single case
1948	Dickinson E, Pastor B:	Two cases of acute subdural hygroma simulating massive intracranial hemorrhage	5: 98–101	Extra-axial fluid collections	Intracranial pressure		two cases
1948	Gorky P:	Case report and technical notes; extradural hemorrhage of the anterior and posterior fossae	5: 294–298	Extra-axial hemorrhage	Sequelae	Clinical diagnosis	two cases
1948	Gross S:	Pneumocephalus secondary to a penetrating wound of the brain	5: 405–406	Penetrating head injury	Clinical diagnosis		single case

(Continued)

TABLE 9.4. *Continued.*

Year	Authors	Title	Volume: pages	Main subject	Secondary subject	Other issues of interest	Study design
1949	Bacon A:	Cerebellar extradural hematoma; report of a case	6: 78–81	Extra-axial hemorrhage	Clinical diagnosis		single case
1949	Guthkelch A:	Extradural hemorrhage as a cause of cortical blindness	6: 180–182	Extra-axial hemorrhage	Clinical diagnosis	Sequelae	single case
1949	Anderson F:	Extradural cerebellar hemorrhage; review of the subject and report of a case	6: 191–196	Extra-axial hemorrhage	Surgical technique and medical management		small series
1949	Echlim F:	Traumatic subdural hematoma - acute, subacute and chronic; an analysis of seventy operated cases	6: 294–303	Subdural hemorrhage	Clinical diagnosis		medium series
1949	Raney A, Raney R, Hunter C:	Chronic post-traumatic headache; and the syndrome of cervical disc lesion following head trauma	6: 458–465	Sequelae	Clinical diagnosis		conceptual review paper
1949	Storey W, Love W:	Traumatic bilateral abducent and facial paralysis with good restoration of function; a case report	6: 539–542	Skull fracture	Sequelae		single case
1950	Gurdjian E, Webster J, Lissner H:	The mechanism of skull fracture	7: 106–114	Pathophysiology	Skull fracture		retrospective review
1950	Greenwood J Jr:	Removal of foreign body (bullet) from the third ventricle	7: 169–172	Penetrating head injury	Surgical technique		single case
1950	Smith G, Mosberg W, Pfeil E, Oster R:	The electroencephalogram in subdural hematoma; with a review of the literature and the presentation of seven cases	7: 207–218	Extra-axial hemorrhage	Diagnosis	Electroencephalography	small series
1950	Ward A. Jr:	Atropine in the treatment of closed head injury	7: 398–402	Medical management			small prospective series

Year	Author	Title	Citation				Series
1950	Jackson I, Speakman T:	Chronic extradural hematoma	7: 444–447	Extra-axial hemorrhage	Clinical diagnosis		single case
1951	Webster J, Dawson R, Gurdjian E:	The diagnosis of traumatic intracranial hemorrhage by angiography	8: 368–376	Intracranial hemorrhage	Diagnosis	Angiography	medium series
1951	Meredith J:	Chronic or subacute subdural hematoma due to indirect head trauma	8: 444–447	Extra-axial hemorrhage	Closed head injury		two cases
1952	Schneider R:	Fat embolism: a problem in the differential diagnosis of craniocerebral trauma	9: 1–13	Clinical diagnosis	Medical management		three cases
1952	Turner O:	Tantalum cranioplasty and repeated trauma	9: 100–103	Cranioplasty	Materials		single case
1952	Lemmen L, Schneider R:	Extradural hematomas of the posterior fossa	9: 245–253	Extra-axial hemorrhage	Diagnosis	Exploratory burr holes	three cases
1952	Lockhart W. Jr, Van Den Noort G, Kimsey W, Groff R:	A comparison of polyethylene and tantalum for cranioplasty	9: 254–257	Cranioplasty			medium series
1952	Beller A, Peyser E:	Extradural cerebellar hematoma	9: 291–298	Extra-axial hemorrhage			three cases
1952	Dodge P, Meirowsky A:	Tangential wounds of scalp and skull	9: 472–483	Closed head injury			medium series
1952	Schneider R, Lemmen L:	Traumatic internal carotid artery thrombosis secondary to non-penetrating injuries to the neck	9: 495–507	Clinical diagnosis	Extracranial vascular injury	Angiography	two cases
1953	Schneider R, Lemmen L, Bagchi B:	The syndrome of traumatic intracerebellar hematoma: with contrecoup supratentorial complications	10: 122–137	Cerebellar hemorrhage	Clinical diagnosis		small series

(Continued)

187

TABLE 9.4. *Continued.*

Year	Authors	Title	Volume: pages	Main subject	Secondary subject	Other issues of interest	Study design
1953	Taveras J, Ransohoff J:	Leptomeningeal cysts of the brain following trauma with erosion of the skull	10: 233–241	Complications	Skull fracture		seven cases
1953	Verbiest H:	Post-traumatic pulsating exophthalmos; cause by perforation of an eroded orbital roof by a hydrocephalic brain	10: 264–271	Complications			two cases
1953	Clayton RS, Barnett LB, Nobles MW:	Removal of bullet from the brain by gravity	10: 434–436	Penetrating head injury	Surgical technique		single case
1953	Meirowsky A:	Wounds of dural sinuses	10: 496–514	Penetrating head injury	Venous sinus injury	Surgical technique	large series
1953	Nichols P, Manganiello J:	Case reports and technical notes; traumatic arachnoidal cyst simulating acoustic neurinoma	10: 538–539	Arachnoidal cysts	Complications		single case
1953	Stortebecker T:	Post-traumatic oculocardiac syndrome from a neurosurgical point of view	10: 682–685	Clinical diagnosis			single case
1954	Ruge D:	The use of cholinergic blocking agents in the treatment of cranio-cerebral injuries	11: 77–83	Medical management	Experimental animal study		bench research
1954	Wannamaker G:	Transventricular wounds of the brain	11: 151–160	Penetrating head injury	Surgical technique and medical management		large retrospective series
1954	Carrie A, Jaffe F:	Thrombosis of superior sagittal sinus caused by trauma without penetrating injury	11: 173–182	Closed head injury	Venous sinus injury	Autopsy studies	two cases

[44] Definitions: Small study: <35 patients. Medium study: 36–99 patients; Large study: 100–250 patients; Very large study: >251 patients.

188

Some have argued that the history of neurosurgery parallels the history of the management of head trauma. Others believe the reverse obtains. This argument cannot be resolved very easily. There can be no question the two are inextricably linked: the principles and techniques that were initially developed to open and close the calvaria, to reduce fractures, to drain clots, or to decompress injured brain served eventually as the basis for sophisticated neurosurgical approaches to intracranial infection, brain tumors, cerebrovascular disease, and even craniofacial reconstruction. Head injury was, historically, the leading category of neurological pathology from which even the first, rudimentary concepts of cerebral localization evolved. Advances in neural protection, control of intracranial pressure (ICP), determination of cerebral blood flow (CBF) and neurosurgical outcome assessment have emerged from the study and the treatment of head injured patients.

The founding of the CNS was, from an historical perspective, an event of great historical significance in the evolution of American neurosurgery. But in addition, its founding also signaled a critical inflection point for the specialty. The ideas behind this change, which are reflected in the management of head trauma in 1951, will emerge as the unifying theme of this chapter.

AN OVERVIEW OF THE HISTORY OF HEAD INJURY

The history of the management of head injury is very rich, and lends itself to a number of organizational models. The chronological approach lists important events in the order they occurred. The great man approach focuses on leadership in the field. An integrated approach arrays this history against a broader backdrop of history of the neurosciences. This chapter looks at a fourth model, a model of critical ideas, defined as ideas that successfully challenged the received wisdom of the profession, and those that resulted in new or changing clinical and research paradigms.

Four Phases in the History of Head Injury

From the standpoint of critical ideas, there are four phases as shown in Table 9.1. The first ex-

tended from antiquity to the mid-nineteenth century, and was characterized equally by a preference for description rather than intervention, and profound pessimism. This is the pre-modern era.

The second phase spans the introduction of anesthesia; of antisepsis and, later, of asepsis; of the development of effective wound treatment; of radiography; and of modern principles of cranial surgery. It extends from shortly after the close of the American Civil War to the end of the First World War. During this phase, early neurosurgeons established the specialty and demonstrated that proper technique could improve outcome after head injury. Textbooks were developed, as well as schools and standards of practice.

The third phase was characterized by a focus on technique, and by the introduction of medications, such as antibiotics and anticonvulsants, that facilitated the overall management of the patient. As neurodiagnostic techniques proliferated, debates over the relative merits of ventriculography, pneumoencephalography, arteriography, and, eventually, electroencephalography, dotted the literature. There were no really significant changes in surgical approach during the interbellum, even though instruments such as the Bovie electrocautery proved their enduring value. During the Second World War, however, the importance of early evacuation, early surgery, and primary dural closure were made clear. The third phase can be said to have closed in the late 1960s or early 1970s, after the Korean War and towards the end of the Vietnam conflict. This phase was characterized by intellectual and technical consolidation. Neurosurgeons were fairly confident that the basic parameters for managing penetrating head injury had been well established and were looking to refine their understanding of the mechanisms of injury and recovery. This is the phase during which the CNS was founded.

We are now in the fourth phase. The fourth phase began with the introduction of sectional imaging studies in the early 1970s,[2] and a shift

---

[2] The term "sectional imaging studies" is used generically in this paper to refer to both computerized tomography (CT) and magnetic resonance imaging (MRI).

in focus from open or penetrating injury to closed head trauma. New research paradigms include the epidemiology of head injury, the biochemistry and molecular biology of head injury, monitoring techniques, neuro-intensive care, prevention, neural salvage, and outcomes. This chapter will not discuss the fourth phase at all, except to suggest that the fourth phase appears to be proceeding upon a course of conceptual reassessment and reformulation.

To the extent historically appropriate, this chapter will address both the surgical and the non-surgical management of the problem.

PHASE I: THE PRE-MODERN ERA

Overview

Head trauma was treated long before the advent of modern neurosurgery. The birth of modern neurosurgery can be reasonably ascribed to Europe between 1870 and 1885. This is the period during which Lister's work on asepsis was applied to cranial surgery, when the principles of cerebral localization first directed surgical exploration, and when surgeons began to think in terms of operating on the brain rather than just its coverings.

One of the most important trends in the development of modern neurosurgery is the overall reduction in variation amongst various therapeutic approaches. The majority of approaches reflect a relatively small number of scientifically derived principles. New approaches, to the extent that they increase the variance, must be justified by an appeal to a new interpretation of existing principles, or newly discovered principles. This turns out to be a critical idea, equally applicable in 1951, and equally pertinent. We shall return to it.

The historical perspective on neurosurgery requires that the pre-modern principles of head trauma be reviewed as well.

Pre-modern Principles of Head Trauma Management

The Classical Physician: Diagnosis, Prognosis, and Therapy

The classical, European pre-modern physician was required to demonstrate proficiency in three domains: diagnosis, prognosis, and therapy. Diagnosis either followed obviously from doctrines of symptoms, signs and methods, (the same conditions might be diagnosed very differently by the Hippocratic and by the Ayurvedic physician), or it was impenetrably veiled. The vast majority of conditions were bestowed a diagnosis reflecting an imputed underlying pathological process for which proof was rarely sought (e.g., biliary crisis), or a reformulation of the symptoms and signs into a nosological contrivance (e.g., quartan fever). Prognosis trumped diagnosis and formed the basis for a physician's reputation(76). Treatment was probably the least important domain. Surgery was not the exclusive domain of the physician. Other types of healers—bonesetters, lithotomists, midwives, and barbers—served as surgical specialists of a lower professional class. The frequency with which surgery was carried out cannot be accurately estimated. Not all surgery was carried out for medical indications. Ample evidence exists to demonstrate that incisions, piercings, and even craniotomies were performed for ritual and magical purposes.

Principles of Head Injury in the Hippocratic Corpus and the Alexandrian School

The Hippocratic corpus recognized both closed head injury, which received little mention, and open head wounds, which were discussed in detail (243). Trephination was recommended for certain fractures, both open and closed, but not others. For depressed fractures, for example, it was withheld.

It is difficult to understand in modern terms what differentiated injuries that were thought to benefit from trephination from those that were not. Trephination was often carried out prophylactically, perhaps with the intention of reducing "unnatural swelling." Suppuration after surgery was the norm. It seems to have been welcomed, and considered a normal part of the therapeutic continuum, the healing process, or both (243).

Hippocrates (c. 460–377 B.C.E.) advised the surgeon to incise the scalp in a cruciate manner. The next day, the incision was inspected. If the bone was damaged, it was trephined. The inner table was left to be extruded with the suppuration that followed. Hippocrates warned that trephination should be performed early after injury (113). Otherwise, he maintained, sepsis would set in within fourteen days in winter, and seven in summer, often accompanied by delirium, contralateral seizures, and death.

Writings attributed to Celsus or his Alexandrian school of the first century C.E. were more conservative with respect to surgery (36). Like Hippocrates, Celsus continued to distinguish between head injured patients with a good prognosis, who deserved treatment, and those with altered states of consciousness or convulsions, who did not. Celsus recognized that hematomas could develop in the absence of fractures. He remarked upon and recommended surgical exploration for fractures that developed signs of what would now be recognized as infection (35). On this basis, Walker interpreted Celsus to have been an advocate of therapeutic, rather than just prophylactic trephination (243).

The physicians and surgeons of the Roman period were fairly derivative in their practice and teachings. Heliodorus (2nd century, C.E.) believed that the wounds described by Hippocrates could heal by first intention, though less reliably. Suppuration and open drainage was deemed to be safer (196). Even so renowned a figure as Galen (c. 130–201 C.E.) did not substantially advance the treatment of head injury.

Medieval Times

The term "medieval" was invented by the 16th century triumphalists to differentiate themselves and their time from the period between the fall of the Roman Empire and the Renaissance. Although the term may be have been contrived, it is clear that during this period, because of widespread civil unrest, certain classical traditions and teachings had been lost. Scholars preoccupied with preserving knowledge seemed to place little emphasis on innovation. With respect to the practice of medicine, the Hippocratic tradition and Galenic medicine ruled. On the other hand, in many locations, lay healers practiced herbal medicine and surgical procedures were performed by lay practitioners. Ecclesiastical medicine seems to have integrated herbal therapies with rudiments of classical Greek and Hellenistic medicine.

What is known regarding the medieval management of injuries of the head in the West derives almost entirely from later writings. Most concentrated on the management of skull fractures. These injuries were demonstrated by means of ink or black dyes, and variously observed, scraped with a rasp, cut away, or simply dressed. Rhazes (860–932), a Persian physician whose encyclopedic work, the *Continens*, served as a reference for many centuries, introduced the idea that surgery was indicated to relieve compression of the brain. This seems to have been an original idea (243). It did not, however, result in changes in the management of head injury.

Beginning in the eleventh century, a string of medical schools grew up throughout Europe. They were often situated at the junction of Christian and Muslim civilizations, and drew their faculty from both, and also from the Jewish world that bridged the two in many places. The school of Salerno was probably the first. Its teachings on head trauma were represented in the writings of Roger Frugardi and in the textbooks *Rogerina*, the *Surgery of Roland*, and the *Surgery of the Four Masters*. The school of Bologna rose to ascendance in the 12th century. Hugo of Lucca (ca. 1160–1257) was one of the earliest members of the faculty and, by all accounts, a master surgeon. He was probably trained at Salerno, and obtained broad experience in military surgery—including at least one crusade—prior to taking up residence in Bologna (224).

Hugo propounded a somewhat more conservative approach to head injury than that dictated in the Hippocratic and Galenic writings. According to Theodoric (1205–1298), his pupil and, by some accounts, his son, Hugo taught that suppuration was unnecessary. In place of the old method—incising the scalp, debriding or trephining the bone, and packing the wound to achieve healing by secondary intention—he recommended sutures to encourage healing by primary intention. Purging and bleeding, furthermore, were to be replaced by a diet of wine and meat. Hugo's method was detailed in Theodoric's *Surgery* (223, 224) and attributed both to Hugo and to the Arabian physician Avicenna (979–1027), who belonged to a previous generation (224).

In the next generation of surgeons, Henri de Mondeville (1260–1320), a student of Theodoric, followed the conservative method. He, too, disdained suppuration and resisted surgical intervention, except that he resorted to debridement or trephination (the difference was often small) in certain instances of treatment failure or noncompliance. He suggested that dural penetration could be diagnosed by having the patient carry out a Valsalva maneuver. In the case of dural penetration, brain matter would extrude from the wound.

In sum, the issues on which differences depended in this era included: whether scalp injuries should be sutured or packed; whether skull fractures should be left alone, trephined, scraped, or otherwise debrided; the advisability of drains; what dressings should be employed; and whether patients should be bled and purged (243). With minor variations, laceration of the dura and damage to the substance of the brain remained the primary criteria for untreatable wounds. Guy de Chauliac (1300–1368), a Frenchman who exerted a singular influence over surgical teaching for over three centuries, recalled that "as a young man he was quite bewildered by so many schools of different thought and the lack of authoritative guidance" (196). Eventually, he came to favor the healing of wounds by secondary intention, and returned to the idea that suppuration was a favorable, and even necessary event (11).

On the whole, there was more similarity than difference among classical, medieval, and early Renaissance writings, except for the quiet debate regarding the desirability of suppuration. In this matter, the more conservative contingent lost out, at least for a while.

Guy de Chauliac was considered the pre-eminent surgical authority in Francophone Europe until the time of Ambroise Paré (1510–1590). His writings spanned the introduction of gunpowder for the bombardment of cities, but preceded the use of artillery and musketry against troops. There is very little in the way of contemporaneous, early to mid 15th century documentation of early medical experiences with bullet wounds. Nonetheless, works of the second half of the 15th century and later, beginning with Giacomo Berengario da Carpi's (1470–1550) *Tractatus Perutilis et Completus de Fractura Cranei* and *Tractaculus de Fractura Calve sive Cranei* seem to contain the experiences and the thoughts of this early period as well as their own. Firearm injuries were believed to be diabolical because sulfur, saltpeter and charcoal were the materials of hell. It was thought that devils rode the bullets and that bullet wounds were poisoned (11). Magical thinking applied to the treatment of gunshot wounds as well.

Thus, the approach to gunshot wounds, whether of the head or elsewhere, had two components. On the one hand, there were lacerations, fractures, and superficial crush phenomena. With respect to these "ordinary" aspects, the management controversies that preceded the introduction of gunpowder persisted afterwards, with the usual range of variation. On the other hand, the poison had to be drawn.

The military surgeon treated gunshot wounds throughout the body by probing and packing the bullet track with various materials, salves, and solutions. The same technique was initially favored for open head wounds, a legacy of the 11th century that proved invariably fatal when the dura was violated. Death was typically ascribed to the injury rather than the treatment. During the late 15th and early 16th centuries, gunshot wounds were also cauterized to overcome the poison, then packed to stimulate drainage, draw the poison, induce putrefaction, and, eventually, encourage healing by granulation.

The following story is widely known. In 1536, Paré ran out of oil to boil for purposes of cauterization. As an emergency substitute, he compounded a digestive ointment consisting of egg yolk, oil of roses, and turpentine, with the following outcome (11):

> "Those on whom I have used the digestive medication feeling little pain in their wounds, without inflammation and swelling, having rested well through the night. The others on whom I had used the oil I found feverish, with great pain, swelling, and inflammation around their wound."

As a result, he recommended a return to what had been a standard treatment of previous generations, at least in the domain of injuries of the head: linen, silk, hemp or tow packing, sometimes marine sponges, soaked in egg white, rose water, honey (after suppuration had set in) and astringent wines. Dressings were to be changed several times daily according to the season.[3]

Most surgeons continued to trephine for the skull fractures accompanying bullet wounds, for epidural collections of blood and pus, and for other indications. But Arnold of Villanova, an important contemporary of Ambroise Paré, grew skeptical of the trephine. He noted that "the moderns, because of the great dangers which arise from this operation, from which many have died and die daily, have advised other methods. They have invented pigments and powders. . . they give these to the patient and do not perforate his skull, hoping thereby to dissolve his discharges, and many are as a result cured" (235).

Despite his positive experiences with more conservative measures of treating the soft tissue component of bullet wounds, Paré, as well as surgeons belonging to many other schools, continued to insist that trephining was broadly indicated in a number of circumstances including suspected extradural or diplöic hemorrhage, suppuration from a fracture site, and depressed bone fragments (17,183,243). A collateral reason for trephination was the popular belief that undrained blood turned into pus. This contention was later discussed and dismissed by the 18th century English surgeon, Percival Pott (1713–1788) (189). Controversy surrounded the extent of surgery advisable in dural penetration. Paré advocated trephination and aggressive debridement even for penetrating bone spicules (183).

Just as one might expect, these operations were subject to extensive variation, both with respect to indications and with respect to specific techniques. Nonetheless, in principle, all procedures fell into one of these groups. Operations on the *brain*—as opposed to operations on the *scalp* and *calvaria*—were not pursued (except for occasionally probing bullet tracks in the brain). Cranioplasty, while not altogether unknown, rarely met with long-term success. It was deemed a curiosity or a feat of surgical virtuosity rather than a routine operation.

The Debate Over Trephination

The merits of trephination were subject to endless debate centered on three basic issues:

1. should operations be performed on patients with a hopeless prognosis;
2. what, besides reasonable hope for recovery, were proper indications for trephination; and
3. was trephination useful.[4]

This debate simmered for over six hundred years, and did not really end until the modern era. Even though some surgeons could not boast of even a single survivor, proponents of trephination argued that the use of the trephine was not invariably fatal in and of itself, that the operation was harmless, or that it allowed the removal of fragments, blood and pus. These considerations were meant to outweigh the risk. Opponents of trephination suggested both that fractures of the skull were capable of healing without operation, just as other wounds did, and that purging and bleeding accomplished the same goals (reducing inflammation) as trephination (243). A long list of famous surgical figures collected on each side of the argument.

Whether or not their prognostic and pathophysiological significance was appreciated, the phenomena of epidural and subdural hematomata and contre-coup injury were clearly known. Trephination does not appear to have been advocated for these indications specifically, though the case reports documenting the

---

[3]Other seemingly random mixtures utilized as healing salves actually hearkened back to ancient Greek ideas about invoking the forces of nature—earth, air, fire and water—for healing purposes. Ward notes that these practices survived antiquity and entered Christian practice as a middle ground between the extremes of magic and miracle: "he wide area of the use of 'natural' properties was in fact neither magic nor miracle, though in retrospect is was to be confused with both." (246)

[4]The subtext of the last issue alludes to parallel debates, already noted in passing, regarding the merits of suppuration, and the association between retained epidural products of injury and purulence.

TABLE 9.5. *MacLeod's figures on gunshot wounds to the head (159)*

Type	Cases	Deaths
Contusions	630	8
Non-depressed fracture	61	23
Depressed fracture	74	53
Penetrating wounds	67	67
Perforating wounds	19	19
Trephined cases	28	24
Fractures: Alcock's series	28	22
Penetrating injuries:		
Meniere's series	10	10
Cases from India	9	6
Fractures: Lante's series	128	106

finding of epidural blood do assume a triumphant tone.

Pre-modern surgeons knew that hemorrhage could occur in the absence of proven trauma, and certainly in the absence of an obvious fracture, which served primarily to indicate the location for trephination. Rupture of the inner table of the skull without obvious damage to the outer was also recognized. Nonetheless, trephination for control of bleeding and ligation of the middle meningeal artery was not advocated until the nineteenth century.

The Influence of the Napoleonic and Crimean Wars

The 19th century was punctuated by a series of major conflicts. The French military surgeons were highly respected because of their experience in the Napoleonic Wars. During the Crimean War (1853–1856), the British amassed a similar breadth of experience. When the War Between the States (1861–1864) broke out in America, European textbooks of military surgery, written in the wake of these earlier conflicts, served as standard references for both sides.

In 1862, A.N. Talley, president of the medical board of the Confederate Army, arranged with J.W. Randolph in Richmond to reprint an abridged version of George H.B. MacLeod's *Notes on the Surgery of the War in the Crimea, with Remarks on the Treatment of Gunshot Wounds* (the "highest recent authority to which reference could be had.") (159) MacLeod, lec-

turer on Military Surgery at Glasgow, hospital surgeon at Smyrna in Turkey and Sevastopol in Crimea, was an early proponent of scientific approaches to surgery. MacLeod's *Notes* articulate with uncommon clarity the state of the art in the treatment of head injury after the Napoleonic Wars, after Crimea, after the introduction of chloroform, and just before the introduction of Listerian surgery. There would be no further significant change to speak of in the pre-modern era.

MacLeod identified the problem of indriven fragments associated with high energy wounds, the dangers of the ricochet round and the relatively new problem of blast injuries from explosive artillery shells. He understood that not all head injuries were equally severe: he therefore developed a "scale" of severity.[5] He recognized the existence of certain prognostic factors. Younger patients, he wrote, had a higher likelihood of recovery, for example. Finally, he reaffirmed the importance of environmental factors in the avoidance of complications. True to the purpose of providing surgical statistics as well as anecdotes, Table 9.5 offers MacLeod figures regarding gunshot wounds to the head. Of the trephine, he wrote as follows (159):[6]

> . . . .[L]ess difference of opinion, I believe, exists among the experienced army surgeons than among civilians; and I think the decided tendency among them is to endorse the modern "treatment by expectancy," and to avoid operation, except in rare cases. In this, I believe, they judge wisely; for, when we examine the question carefully, we find that there is not one single indication for having recourse to operation, which cannot, by the adduction of pertinent cases, be shown often fallacious; while, if we turn to authorities for advice, we find that not a great name can be ranged on one side,

---

[5]". . .[W]ounds of the side of the head, especially anterior to the ear, are the most dangerous to life; . . . a descending scale will give the following order - the fore-part, the vertex, and the upper part of the occipital region; the last being decidedly the least dangerous." (159)

[6]This section is quoted at length to provide a sense of the reasoning behind MacLeod's assertions, behind the conclusion that trephining should be abandoned, and behind the general attitude towards head injuries amongst experienced surgeons of the time. Another reason for citing at length is that MacLeod's writings, though often referred to, are not readily available.

which cannot be balanced by as illustrious on the other.

Simple contusion, without fracture or depression, caused the old surgeons to ''set on the large crown'' of a trephine, in order to prevent future danger. Fracture, although not accompanied by depression, or any other untoward symptom, called for the trephine in the practice of the Pott school; while many, even now, would operate to cure the local pain which so often remains persistent at the place of injury. Other surgeons, again discarding and condemning all this, say we should trephine only when there is depression; but the amount of depression which demands it, each interprets according to his own fancy. None knows so well as the army surgeon how very considerable a depression may exist, especially at some parts of the head, without any injury to the brain; nor how innumerable are the cases in which great depression has been present, without causing harm at any subsequent period of the patient's life.

A musket ball being the wounding cause, would appear to some a sufficient reason why the trephine should be applied, however slight may be the lesion. ''We should always trephine,'' says Quesney, ''in wounds of the head caused by firearms, although the skull be not fractured.'' ''All the best practitioners,'' says Pott, ''have always agreed in acknowledging the necessity of perforating the skull in the case of a severe stroke made on it by gun-shot, upon the appearance of any threatening symptom, even though the bone should not be broken; and very good practice it is.'' Boyer and Percy are equally urgent when a ball has caused the injury. However, ''the experience of war,'' to which Quesney appeals in confirmation of his opinion, now-a-days completely condemns the practice, whatever it may have done formerly.

Further, ''symptoms of compression'' setting in early or late, are laid down by others as urgently demanding the removal of the bone. ''No injury,'' says John Bell, ''requires operation except compression of the brain, which may arise either from extravasated blood, or from depressed bone, or matter generated within the skull.'' But unfortunately, we can seldom diagnose the existence of compression with any amount of certainty, when it sets in early, and experience teaches us that each and all of those signs which are said to indicate it may, under appropriate treatment, pass away without interference; especially when these symptoms appear early, and often, also, when they set in late. Compression too, when it appears at a late date, if it arise, as it generally

does, from the presence of pus, is well known to be seldom relieved by trephining. Dease first showed it was that the matter was commonly deeply placed or diffused in such cases; and the instances in which it has been found on the surface, or evacuable by such a bold manoeuvre as the well-known thrust of Dupuytren, are exceedingly rare.

Some authors, again, would have us trephine only when the symptoms of compression are severe, go on increasing in severity, and have continued for some time; yet, even under such circumstances, ''recovery not seldom disappoints our fears, and mortifies us by our success.''

But, finally, it is to those surgeons who instruct us to operate when certain pathological conditions exist, which they carefully define, but which experience, unfortunately, tells us do not often manifest themselves by any recognizable signs, that we are chiefly indebted for useful directions to assist us in cases of difficulty. What good can it do to say, you must trephine when the internal table is splintered more extensively than the external, when effusion has taken place on the brain, and so on, when we have often no means of knowing when these conditions exist, or when we are fully aware that they have, each and all, been present and that to a very considerable extent, without any of the appropriate signs being manifest?

...There are three classes to which the trephine is still occasionally applied: 1st, fracture with depression, before symptoms have appeared; 2nd, fracture with depression, attended immediately with signs said to indicate compression; and 3rd, fracture, with or without depression, followed at a late period by symptoms evidencing compression.

...There are, I believe, very few surgeons of experience in the army now-a-days who approve of ''preventive trephining.'' It may be said in our time to be a practice of the past - a practice to be pointed at as a milestone which we have left behind. . . .

The wonderful manner in which the brain accommodates itself to pressure, has been remarked in all times, and the crania in our museums show how extensive the depression may be, and yet the brain escape injury, in which, although the central mass may be pressed upon or hurt, recovery has yet followed. In the cases of fracture with depression which have presented themselves to me during the war, the symptoms and the amount of depression have seldom been in correspondence. . . .

Compression is undoubtedly the evil against

which the trephine is generally employed. But yet, with all that has been said on the subject, in books and lectures, I question whether we are sufficiently acquainted with the nature, seat, or signs of compression, to warrant us in undertaking, at an early period at any rate, an operation of so serious a description, as all recorded experience has shown trephining to be, without more reliable and more clearly-defined evidence of its presence than is commonly thought to denote it. Symptoms which, by the dicta of books, were unquestionably those of compression, have passed off, in the experience of every one, under a treatment of which non-interference was the most important item; while in other cases such large quantities of fluid - blood and pus - have been found, post mortem, on the brain, as all recorded experience tells us *should* have caused a compression which yet never appeared. . . .

It is too much the custom, I think, to deny or overlook the danger which arises from the operation itself. This is no place to inquire what is the source of this danger, whether it be that admission of atmospheric air to the membranes, as supposed by Larrey and Stromeyer, or the renewed irritation and injury of the brain coverings, or, as others say, from pus poisoning; but the fact recurs that the most serious, and at times fatal symptoms, have followed the operation itself, in cases in which, contrary to expectation, the parts below the bone were found sound.

This lengthy section is cited in order to demonstrate how the issues that pre-occupied the practitioner of neurological surgery towards the close of the pre-modern era endured. They would be recognized as legitimate issues even in 1951. While the preponderance of opinion a century earlier favored surgical reticence in closed head injury and in most instances of open head trauma, the controversy was by no means resolved.

The concepts of contre-coup injury, cranial compression, and concussion were recognized fairly early. They had little bearing on therapy, however.

PHASE II: MODERN NEUROSURGERY

Overview

The second phase in the management of head trauma was marked by the introduction of Liste-

rian principles of antisepsis, and of the rudiments of cerebral localization. Listerian precautions made it possible to consider broaching the dura on a regular basis. Not even the introduction of anesthesia had provided so broad a potential: it became feasible to operate on the brain and not just its coverings.

The pre-modern literature is filled with exquisitely detailed case reports specifically relating the location of an injury and the resulting neurological deficit. MacLeod, for example, all but defines the motor strip, and the tongue, hand, and the leg area (159). The key lies in the phrase ''all but.'' Until the modern era, there were many observations regarding diagnosis and technique that *could* have led to operation on the brain, but did not. The explicit recognition that surgery for head trauma had to address compression, penetration, or infection of the *brain*, together with the recognition that the surgery of the brain required specific technique, signaled the beginning of the modern phase of head injury management.

This phase began in the last quarter of the 19th century, and ended after the First World War. During this period, the basic principles of modern wound management, including bacteriological monitoring, were established, and X-ray first came to be used in the field (16). In North America, Harvey Cushing's name is the one most closely associated with the advances in management of head injuries during this period, but there were many other individuals whose names deserve mention. They include Sir Geoffrey Jefferson, Charles A. Elsberg, William Sharpe, Fedor Krause, Ernst von Bergmann, Thierry de Martel de Janville, Gordon Holmes, and Sir Victor Horsley.

The Modern Era

From Sepsis to Neurology

In 1875, Jonathan Hutchinson, Senior Surgeon at the London Hospital, began to publish a series of lectures on injuries to the head (196). Five years earlier, Hughlings Jackson, a close friend, had begun publishing his work on the epilepsies. Under Jackson's influence, Hutchinson suggested that head injuries offered opportunities to observe physiological experiments in nature. In 1867 and again, with further elaboration in 1886, Hutchinson described, for example, the phenomenon of ipsilateral pupillary dilatation associated with middle meningeal hemorrhage, (118, 120). This observation began to address MacLeod's preoccupation with the diagnostic uncertainties in head trauma. In 1878, Hutchinson argued that it would be a mistake to wait until the clinical triad that came to bear his name was fully developed:

> "I am convinced that if we make the diagnosis of compression of the brain only in cases where the pupils are fixed, the countenance bloated, the respiration stertorous and the pulse laboured, we shall fail to recognise it in a majority of cases. This group of symptoms is circulation and a bloodless brain supervene often with met with more frequently after laceration of the brain, whilst in compression often no define symptoms are present until near the patient's death, when those which denote failure of great rapidity." (119)

It seems, however, that Hutchinson hesitated to follow his own advice, and often delayed trephination until the patient was beyond help. His surgical reticence was widely shared, mostly for fear of infection (196).

Like many London surgeons, Hutchinson doubted the efficacy of Lister's antiseptic method. For this reason, he continued to frame the problem of head injury as a problem of sepsis rather than cerebral dysfunction. The discontinuity between pre-modern and modern concepts of head injury turns on this view.

During the pre-modern era, sepsis was deemed to be the cause of death in the majority of those who succumbed, and in many cases, probably was. Neurological damage, while recognized, was not addressed until the very last years of the pre-modern era, when surgeons reporting on successful cases of trephination described relief of localizing signs, and cast the indications for surgery in terms of cerebral compression. Still, surgery in the absence of a fracture was exploratory, and directed, for the most part, at the site of the blow rather than the locus of neurological dysfunction, which, in any event, was not often clearly understood.

In the modern era, the purpose of surgery came to be defined by two problems. The first was the repair of disrupted tissue in order to prevent complications (both septic and non-septic), and to promote neurological recovery. This purpose gradually diminished in importance, and was overtaken by an emphasis on the restoration and preservation of neurological function.[7,8]

Antisepsis and the Prophylaxis of Infection

The introduction of prophylaxis against infection, first through the vehicle of Lister's antiseptic technique, later through aseptic technique, and finally, during the Second World War, through the topical and parenteral application of antibiotics, strongly influenced the management of head trauma. With the adoption of antiseptic and aseptic techniques, surgical outcome improved through a reduction in post-operative infection.

The principles of antisepsis derived from the idea that surgical infection could be prevented by the elimination of airborne, and later skinborne contaminants. Carbolic acid and other antiseptic solutions were aerosolized and sprayed throughout the operating theater during the operation. This technique came to be known as the Listerian method after its developer, Joseph Lord Lister (1827–1912), professor of surgery at Glasgow. Later, the Listerian method was extended to include the use of antiseptic solutions to saturate towels and dressings, to irrigate wounds, and to prep the skin.

The Listerian method came under attack when

---

[7]As a general rule, the surgery of head injury was not as compelling to early surgeons of the modern era as the surgery of epilepsy and brain tumors.

[8]It is often forgotten that the germ theory of disease was still hotly contested in the 1870s. Hutchinson was altogether uncertain, at this juncture, whether microbes had a role in contagion, or whether this role ought to be ascribed to the products of inflammation *per se*. In 1875, he argued *against* the germ theory in a public forum. Oddly enough, this was the same year that the antibiotic effects of the *Penicillium* mold was first noted by John Tyndall, even though nothing further was to be done with this observation for sixty years. It was because the role of germs was not fully comprehended that Lister's antiseptic method was neither quickly adopted, nor immediately recognized as an essential step in the management of head injuries, as well as operations in general.

it was first introduced. Many surgeons did not understand that Lister intended to introduce a new prophylactic principle in surgery, and resented what they presumed to be a self-serving attempt to replace existing methods of treating infected wounds with one bearing his name. Others, notably including William Stewart Halsted of Johns Hopkins, feared that antisepsis would lead to diminished respect for surgical technique. Lister was also criticized for inadequate statistical proof. Nevertheless, most observers who visited Lister and witnessed his results first hand came away firmly convinced of its worth, particularly for saving joints and limbs after open or penetrating injury. William Welch, later of Johns Hopkins, became a convert during his stay in Britain between 1876 and 1877[9] (78).

---

[9]Although some aspects of the history of sterile technique as it applies to neurosurgery are presented elsewhere in this volume, additional elaboration is merited here. Lister left University College, London, to study under Syme in Edinburgh in 1854. The London surgical tradition valued speed above all else (182). Syme, in contrast, emphasized cleanliness, meticulous surgical technique, silver wire suture, drainage, and frequent dressing changes. Nonetheless, Lister's reported mortality rate for amputation, observing these principles, failed to diminish below 45%. Lister was struck by the observation that when a wound healed *per primum*, putrefaction was seldom seen. He studied Pasteur's experiments, contemplated sterilization by means of heat, but concluded that heat could not be applied to wounds. During the 1860s, carbolic acid had been introduced to disinfect sewage. Lister was determined to try this mode of disinfection, and, on August 2, 1865, successfully treated a compound fracture of the tibia utilizing carbolic acid to irrigate and dress the wound. In 1867, he published the results of his "antiseptic surgery." (148) Although Semmelweis was in some respects Lister's forerunner, as Lister himself acknowledged in 1883, Lister deserves the credit for insisting that surgical infection rates could be reduced by the reduction of micro-organisms in a wound.

Other surgeons adopted, modified, and disputed Lister's methods. Some denied that bacteria were pathogenic, but employed soap and scrub brushes for surgical cleanliness with good results. Various antiseptic agents were introduced with varying results. Sterilization with boiling water eventually won out.

Advocates of the aseptic method argued vehemently with the Listerian method for many years. There are some interesting anecdotes attributed to this era. Billroth, early interested in wound infection, remained firmly convinced that one group of bacteria, the so-called (but non-existent) *coccobacteria septica* was the cause of a whole family of diseases. One of Billroth's assistants, Mikulezc, devoted much of his career to neurosurgery and was the first to don gloves for surgery. Charles Ellsberg studied with him. These early gloves, made of cotton, were superseded by the rubber gloves, which Halsted ordered for his nurse because of the skin irritation induced by the mercuric chloride solution he preferred for antiseptic prep (166).

The flaws and shortcomings ascribed to the Listerian method, both real and imagined, led to a search for more satisfactory substitutes. Neurosurgeons figured quite prominently in this process. Sir William Macewen (1848–1924) became a disciple of the antiseptic method as an undergraduate at Glasgow. In 1879, however, Macewen demonstrated microbes growing in pus from wounds packed with carbolized gauze (gauze soaked in carbolic acid), and changed his practice to sterilization of instruments and dressings by boiling (157, 243).

At about the same time, von Bergmann attempted to institute antiseptic technique for the treatment of head injuries on the battlefield. In this, he followed the lead of von Volkmann of Leipzig during the Franco-Prussian War (93, 237, 243). It is often said that von Bergmann abandoned the Listerian method because of its complexity. The real problem, however, turned out to be the topical toxicity of the antiseptic solutions which were utilized to pack wounds open as part of the extended antiseptic method[10] (243). Von Bergmann then turned, like Macewen, to boiling instruments and dressings, and became an advocate of the aseptic method, which required that all material in contact with the wound or the operative site should be prepared in sterile fashion.

On May 25, 1886, Horsley operated on a patient admitted to the service of Ferrier and Jackson at the National Hospital for the Paralysed and Epileptic, at Queen's Square in London. His public demonstration included the use of carbolic spray, and the implementation of the entire antiseptic method propounded by Lister.[11] This

---

[10]Weir, for example, reported packing a brain abscess with the antiseptic iodoform. Respirations ceased but were restored by "artificial respiration, lowering the head, and hypodermic administration of whiskey." (202) Although it is not possible to project in retrospect whether local toxicity was truly the cause of this disturbing event, it was deemed to be so.

[11]Horsley later recounted his method of preparing the scalp as follows: "the day before the operation, the patient's head is shaved and washed with a soft soap and then ether; next the position of the lesion is ascertained by measurement and marked on the scalp. The head is covered with lint, soaked in 1 to 20 solution of carbolic acid, oiled silk and cotton wool, being thus thoroughly carbolised for at least twelve hours before operation" (202).

demonstration did not stay the debate regarding the need for such elaborate precautions, nor did it address the growing tension between the Listerian school of antisepsis and the growing number of advocates for asepsis (181). Horsley's operation did succeed, however, in stimulating surgeons to focus on cerebral localization, neurological diagnosis, and neurosurgical technique. Soon, surgeons throughout Europe began operating on the brain.[12]

Aseptic technique gradually displaced the antiseptic method. The proof of principle required a level of bacteriological sophistication exceeding that available to Lister. The changeover was virtually complete by the early 1900s. Sterilizability figured prominently in the choice of materials for surgical instruments and devices from that point on. Kocher, for example, notes that Cushing had abandoned the use of rubber tourniquets for hemostasis because they did not withstand repeated sterilization[13] (181).

Horsely's public demonstration took place only sixty-five years before the founding of the CNS. This event was directly responsible for making neurosurgery enter the realm of the feasibility.

Compression, Concussion, and Decompression

Unconsciousness without obvious skull injury was described from ancient times, but never understood. Hippocrates' term "cerebral commotion" was often used to describe this phenomenon, but it is unclear how the term was meant. Walker states that Paré also "clearly rec-

ognized [cerebral commotion] as a distinct entity." Again, it is not immediately evident what he recognized. Over the years, "cerebral commotion" was utilized to name, to describe, and ultimately to "explain" unconsciousness (243). After the introduction of the microscope, there were periodic upsurges of interest in this topic. In 1705, for example, Littré discussed a case in which death ensued without evidence of hemorrhage or macroscopic change (149) Additional anecdotes were published over the next sixty years, but no new information was really discovered.

The mechanisms of concussion were subject to increased speculation in the mid of the 19th century. In 1864, Stromeyer, a contemporary of MacLeod's, suggested that a transient compression of the brain from a blow to the head resulted in a local "anemia" that in turn induced unconsciousness (218). Duret argued that the transmission of concussive forces through the aqueduct to the IVth ventricle caused small hemorrhages in the brain stem (65). Others returned to the original meaning of the term "commotion" and determined that the paralysis of vital centers could be ascribed to shaking or movement of the brain during injury. These explanations were largely conjectural. Nonetheless they correctly associated concussion with neurological events. This association was not obvious at the time. It was, however, reinforced through a series of reports at the turn of the twentieth century suggesting that fatal head injuries resulted in degenerative neuronal changes, particularly in the brain stem (204).

The initial wave of European enthusiasm for neurosurgery extended to surgery for head injury as well as space occupying lesions. The renewal of interest in decompressive trephination reflected a sounder scientific basis than in any previous era.

Lumbar puncture was introduced in the late 19th century. This technique made it possible to measure ICP manometrically. Patients with head injury were found to show elevations in pressure. In 1896, Jaboulay suggested trephination for relief of pressure, even when hematomata were not expected (122). In 1908, Cushing advocated subtemporal decompression for elevations

---

[12]This enterprise did not meet with universal success and was soon abandoned by most surgeons. Those that persisted, like Horsley and Cushing, eventually came to the conclusion that this was a special field.

[13]Although it was universally understood that sterile instruments and dressings were more important than antiseptic aerosols in the operating theater, vestiges of antiseptic doctrine remained in force for several generations. From an historical standpoint, the adoption of ultraviolet irradiation of filtered air to reduce the rate of operative infection in the late 1940s and early 1950s at Duke, the Massachusetts General Hospital, and elsewhere, and the virtually universal installation of positive pressure filtered air flow systems in North America, might legitimately be construed as late and technologically advanced vindications of the Listerian method (259).

of ICP. A special retractor was designed for this purpose (49). By 1911, Kocher advocated decompression for all cases of increased ICP:

> It can be confidently asserted that, provided asepsis is guaranteed, there should never be any hesitation about trephining in any case of cerebral pressure. We have regretted many sins of omission in this respect, but very seldom have we had occasion to repeat the performance of an operation (36).

The enthusiasm for decompression did not go unchallenged. Quincke suggested that repeated lumbar taps could do as well as surgery at controlling ICP (191). Fourteen years later, Weed and McKebben demonstrated in animals that dehydration reduced spinal fluid pressure, especially if combined with lumbar puncture (253). Throughout the 1920s, repeated taps, dehydration, and decompression all were utilized. Many surgeons, however, fought the idea of non-operative decompression. Some were uncomfortable with the idea of spinal fluid drainage. Munro fought fluid restriction. Dandy objected to both (243).

The First World War

The First World War broke out in 1914. There was then only one really useful text on war surgery: Sir George Makin's *Surgical Experiences in South Africa, 1899–1900*, based on the Boer War in southern Africa. Other sources of information were more experimental. Rowbotham, for example, writes that the Imperial Royal Prussian War Department had undertaken "extensive researches" on gunshot wounds to the brain "both on the living and on the cadaver," but concludes that these experiments had been carried out twenty years before and were not entirely relevant because of important improvements in firearm technology (196).

For the four years of the war, the trenches became not only killing grounds, but also training grounds for a generation of surgeons (201). One of the best perspectives on medicine on the battlefield can be obtained from William W. Keen's (1837–1932) small book, *The Treatment of War Wounds*. Keen, a Philadelphian, first saw

military service as a surgeon in the Civil War when he was in his mid-twenties.[14] In 1917, at the age of 79, still commissioned as a Major in the Medical Reserve of the U.S. Army, the Emeritus Professor of Surgery at Jefferson Medical College compiled reports from the front at the behest of the Medical Committee of the National Research Council. His charge was to determine the "more important and most recent improvements in the treatment of war wounds" (130).

Keen quotes Cushing verbatim with respect to general principles for dealing with the injured. Cushing came to believe that all penetrating wounds deserved exploration, but that they presented no immediate urgency except in the case of extensive hemorrhage. He recommended evacuating head injured patients to a base hospital staffed by trained specialists with access to fluoroscopy, x-ray, adequate anesthesia, and appropriate surgical instrumentation. "[A] delay of two or three days in forwarding this class of wounded with expedition to a suitable base," he wrote, "is preferable to the delay of two or three days in having them recover from the effects of an incomplete procedure before transportation". (130)

In a statement that determined the course of the military approach to head injury in the English speaking world, Keen concluded:

> Especially do I indorse, on general principles. . . that the only proper hospital to interfere surgically with a cranial wound is one in which facilities and skilled men, both neurologic and surgical, and the best *x*-ray apparatus are to be had. I am told that at present. . . some hospitals much nearer to the trenches than formerly, are thus equipped. An incompletely studied case and an indifferent facility for diagnosis and operation have no place in cranial wounds. The late results of such surgery are lamentable (130).

Keen also endorses the advice of Cushing and others, including Gordon Holmes, Victor Horsley, George Makins, and Geoffrey Jefferson on

---

[14]An early proponent of neurosurgery, he described a point for ventricular puncture, and solicited Cushing's contribution of a section on neurosurgery to his textbook on general surgery (49).

a series of technical suggestions that remain useful:

- the use of Horsley's technique (raw muscle taken from the temporalis flap) for hemostasis;
- the avoidance of dural opening "save to evacuate blood-clots or evidently disorganized brain tissue, to tie bleeding vessels, or for a formal decompression. In these always violently infected wounds this is of especial importance. I cannot subscribe to Burckhardt's statement as to the innocuousness of such incisions. It is best to close the dura and the overlying galea and scalp immediately to avoid a fungus cerebri. Efficient drainage should be provided";
- the utilization of cranial decompression, including contralateral decompression in uninjured tissue;
- the application of pedunculated flaps of pericranium as a dural substitute in contaminated areas without cranioplasty;
- approaching wounds through newly fashioned, clean incisions rather than through the enlargement of existing wound tracks;
- extraction of all foreign bodies in the brain "for in this war practically all such foreign bodies are infected. But the surgeon must use his good judgement and not venture beyond the limits of reasonably legitimate surgery. Sometimes a secondary operation at a much later date will be best. Between the danger of infection and the danger of operation only a large experience and good judgement can decide;"
- radiographic examination of all wounds, insofar as possible;
- physiological monitoring to indicate whether an injured soldier may be moved: "If [the pulse]... be rapid, the patient should not be forwarded at once. A slow pulse favors the presumption of possible recovery. Such patients, as a rule, will bear transportation lasting even for two or three days" (130).

According to Leo M. Davidoff, Cushing issued the following directions to neurosurgical teams while serving as the senior neurosurgical consultant to the American Expeditionary Forces in 1918:

Every scalp wound, no matter how trifling, is a potential penetrating wound of the skull. Many penetrating wounds are met with even among the walking wounded. Only after an x-ray, after shaving the head, and possibly only after exploration, can one be assured that there is or is not a cranial fracture with or without dural penetration.

If a case is operated upon and a penetration found, the operation must be completed, with a primary closure following the special debridement applicable to these injuries. In this respect wounds of the nervous system differ from other wounds which in times of rush should not be subjected to primary wound closure. "All or nothing" is a good rule to apply to craniocerebral injuries - in short, evacuate these cases untreated to the nearest base (except for shaving and the application of a wet antiseptic dressing) rather than do incomplete operations. Patients with craniocerebral injuries stand transportation well before operation; badly during the first few days after operation. This is true of all primary wound closures.

Cranial cases in more or less shock (on arrival at the base) need not undergo a period of resuscitation. The operation should be done under local anesthesia combined with morphine. Consequently the patient can be properly warmed and given fluids during the course of the operation through which he will often sleep. Only in exceptional cases, when patients are irrational or uncooperative, is a general anesthetic necessary. Its administration always adds to the difficulty of the operation, and by increasing intracranial pressure causes extrusion of brain and tends to increase the damage already done.

The chief source of the high mortality in cranial wounds is infection - infection of the meninges; direct infection of the brain leading to encephalitis; infection of the ventricles. Wounds in which the dura has been penetrated are supposed to give a mortality of 50 to 60 per cent, due to infection. It, however, has been shown that experienced neurological surgeons can lower this supposedly inevitable mortality to 25 per cent if the operation can be done with reasonable promptitude in a forward area and the cases retained for a reasonable time after operation. These figures are capable of still further improvement. (57)

In Cushing's hands, the mortality rate for penetrating injuries diminished over three months from "54.4% for the first 44 cases to 28.8% for the 45 cases in the third period - this in spite of the fact that with the advancing line of battle, the interval between the reception of the wounded and the patients' admission averaged at least six hours longer in the last few weeks of the service" (51). The paper in which these results were reported, "A Study of a Series of Wounds Involving the Brain and Its Enveloping Structures," is deemed to be the definitive work on war injuries of this period, and a legitimate reference work still today.

Cushing recommend direct inspection, gentle debridement, and irrigation of the wound track; dural repair; and suture of the galea and the scalp. Both the operative instructions and their accompanying illustrations were widely copied. The operative results established an enduring standard that remains difficult to improve.

The British concurred fairly closely with the American view, which meant Cushing's, for all intents and purposes. G.H. Makins, an English surgeon who made substantial contributions in osteomyelitis and neurosepsis, offered the following observations (130):

> Examination of a considerable number of patients some months after their return to England proved much more satisfactory than had been generally expected. It was found that the proportion of patients who die after transference to England is small; later complications, such as cerebral abscess, are comparatively rare, and serious sequelae, such as insanity and epilepsy, are much less common than had been foretold. In only 15 percent of the patients examined, however, had more than one year elapsed from the date of the injury. It also appeared that many patients with foreign bodies deeply lodged in the brain recover, and are scarcely more liable to serious complications than men in whom the brain has been merely exposed and lacerated. These conclusions are obviously tentative, but as far as they go appear hopeful.

By the war's end, everyone was convinced that for those who did not die at once, the major threats were intradural infection and shock. The first problem was managed by respecting the integrity of the dura mater. The second was managed by retaining the wounded at clearing stations until transportation further down the line

seemed to be safe. Although this approach resulted in a lower *operative* mortality, it later became an issue in determining whether the *case* mortality had been lowered to the extent possible.

There were three publications that closed the first part of the modern phase in the management of head injury. Cushing's series defined the technique of surgery for penetrating head injury. Sir Geoffrey Jefferson published a classic study in Brain in 1919 that delineated the pathology of penetrating head injury. Finally, in 1922, Wagstaffe wrote the official medical history of the war (239). What had been accomplished? The technique of craniotomy had been established. Roentgenological diagnosis, a topic before but one itself which cannot be dealt with here, became standard for penetrating injuries and fractures. A doctrine for the management of penetrating head injuries in wartime was well in place, and easily translated into civilian practice. Outcomes were assayed by means of series, and not just anecdotes. Most importantly, the social value of special expertise in neurosurgery had been demonstrated by means of lowered mortality rates in the field.

As a collateral benefit, the Secretary of War of the United States set up schools to train general surgeons in neurosurgery. These schools were situated in New York, Philadelphia, Chicago and St. Louis. They were, properly speaking, the first formal training programs in neurosurgery. In 1917, a *Manual of Neuro-Surgery* was published under the editorship of Dr. T.H. Weisenburg of Philadelphia. Distribution was "limited to the officers in the Medical Corps of the Army and to libraries receiving Government literature." Extracts were taken from Cushing's chapter on fractures of the skull in Keen's *Surgery* and from his work on the suboccipital approach in *Tumors of the Nervus Acusticus*. They were also taken from Charles H. Frazier's chapter on laminectomy technique in his *Surgery of the Spine and Spinal Cord*, and, particularly in the second and last 1919 revision, from textbooks of neurology, otology, and ophthalmology. There were thirty-one contributors, including essentially all the major figures in American neurosurgery (255).

This manual brought to eight the number of major works published in the modern era with significant coverage of neurosurgery.[15] Only three of the fourteen chapters of the *Manual*, however, dealt specifically with trauma. The others covered the remainder of the standard neurosurgical curriculum. With the exception of technical details, of recommendations regarding the management of infection, and of the treatment of diagnostic technologies, the *Manual* would not be out of place today.

The subject of anesthesia and analgesia has not been mentioned. Both local and general anesthesia was available. Which was utilized became a matter of personal preference. The idea of controlling ventilation to reduce ICP did not become important until much later. The French surgeon de Martel recommended local anesthetic even for posterior fossa operations. The *Manual* of 1919, however, concluded that "ether remains unquestionably the safest [agent], though it admittedly is the most difficult to administer and it possesses the disadvantage of increasing the secretion of the cerebrospinal fluid and thus accentuating tension" (255). Further discussion of anesthetic technique is beyond the scope of this chapter.

PHASE III: CONSOLIDATION

Overview

During the interbellum period between the First and Second World Wars, there were few changes in the management of head trauma. Anesthesia improved. A number of investigators made significant inroads into the pathophysiology of cerebral compression and contusion, and the control of ICP. The roles of dehydration and drainage of spinal fluid for control of ICP were debated. The problem of cerebrospinal fluid fis-

tulae also attracted attention. Finally, the problem of fatalities from road traffic accidents attracted public attention, particularly after Lawrence of Arabia was killed on a motorcycle in Britain at an estimated speed of 80 mph (128).

This period may be called the interbellum, but it was hardly peaceful. The Civil War in Russia raged on for five years. Conflicts on a smaller scale preoccupied Poland and Russia, Finland and Russia, the Far East, and the Middle East. The Spanish Civil War began in 1936, attracted large numbers of volunteers from the United States (the Lincoln Brigade), Nazi Germany (the Condor Legion), Britain, France, and Russia, became a testing ground for Nazi armamentarium, and for the purposeful aërial bombardment of civilian centers, and foreshadowed the worldwide conflict to come.

As a result of these conflicts, several textbooks of war medicine were published around the end of the 1930s. Most reproduced the work of Cushing and the British surgeons of World War I almost *verbatim*, even those emanating from what would become the Axis. The methods published in Russian and French often differed slightly from those advocated in the English speaking world, but the differences tended to be minor, focused on regional preference, and technical, on the whole, rather than conceptual. The most important textbook published in English by Munro was directed broadly at craniocerebral trauma rather than military surgery (175).

In 1927, only 24 years prior to the founding of the CNS, and one generation of neurosurgeons away, an absolutely seminal paper on head injury was published. Vance studied the cause of death in 512 instances of fatal head injury (22), and ranked them as shown in Table 9.6.

Closed head injury or concussion accounted for 27% of all fatalities, subdural hematomas for 26%, and extradural hematomas for 12%. Septic complications accounted for 8% only. In the aggregate, closed head injury was involved in 65% of all fatalities. Here was additional proof that head injury was unequivocally a problem of neurological dysfunction, and not infection, at least in the civilian population.

---

[15]The others were: Archibald's *Surgical Affectations and Wounds of the Head* in Bryant and Buck's *American Practice of Surgery*, 1908; Ballance's *Some Points in the Surgery of the Brain and its Membranes*, 1907; Cushing's chapter in Keen's *Practice*, 1908; Kocher's *Textbook of Operative Surgery*, 1903; Krause's *Surgery of the Brain and Spinal Cord*, 1912; Rawling's *Surgery of the Skull and Brain*, 1912; and von Bergmann's *System of Practical Surgery*, 1904.

TABLE 9.6. *Cause of death in 512 instances of fatal head injury, according to Vance (22)*

Rank	Description	Number
1	Concussion, death within 1–10 hours	139
2	Cerebral compression due to	
	(a) subdural hemorrhage	132
	(b) extradural hemorrhage	61
3	Acute suppurative leptomeningitis	41
4	Injuries to other parts of the body	30
5	Terminal lobar pneumonia	27
6	Unrelated causes	25
7	Extensive laceration of brain	24
8	Exhaustion	14
9	Septic infections including septicemia, extra- and subdural empyema	7

World War II proved the importance of antibiotics, dural closure, and the safety of air evacuation. Improved hemostatic agents were also made available. New methods of cranioplasty were introduced. The value of dedicated neurosurgical units was proven once again. The literature of neurosurgery and of head trauma flourished.

During this same period, basic research into the pathophysiology of concussion received increasing attention. A quantitative, physiologically-based model of head injury gradually displaced the qualitative, histologically-based research paradigm that characterized research prior to the early 1940s. In the civilian sector, the problems associated with high-speed injuries became better understood.

Major Issues

The Causes and Mechanisms of Unconsciousness, Revisited

The causes and mechanisms of unconsciousness after closed head injury were not well understood until the 1940s despite a body of research that had begun half a century before. The earliest investigators pursued a model that depended on histological changes in the brain to elucidate the mechanisms of unconsciousness. In 1878, Duret described petechial hemorrhages in the brain stem after severe head injury (65).

These hemorrhages, which continue to carry his name, proved to be one of the most consistent histological findings, and one of the few whose significance withstood the test of time.

Between 1890 and 1912, the seat of traumatic unconsciousness was generally assumed to lie in the cerebral hemispheres, Duret's hemorrhages notwithstanding. Experimental pathologists focused their search for changes in cortex. The initial series of experiments was both rudimentary and conceptually flawed, however. After 1912, the focus of attention shifted to the brain stem.[16] In 1920, LeCount and Appelbach demonstrated that shearing forces during trauma resulted in axial stretch between the hemispheres and the brain stem (42). In 1924, it became evident that the brain may appear entirely normal after concussion. This fact engendered an acrimonious debate regarding the proper use of the term ''concussion'' (see below). Duret's earlier finding of brain stem hemorrhages was widely reconfirmed at that time, although the relationship of brainstem damage to the preservation of consciousness was not fully comprehended (65). Between 1930 and 1950, several groups of investigators reported reproducible, but seemingly non-specific cellular changes including neuronal vacuolization, chromatin condensation, loss of tigroid material, and neuronal drop-out. The proposition that concussion could be regularly accompanied by minor vascular events, neuronal changes, and alterations in neurofibrillary anatomy was generally accepted. Many researchers also believed that these changes might be reversible.

The questions under investigation during this era are the questions that engaged neurosurgeons and neuroscientists in 1951. They fall into two groups. One group centered around a search for

---

[16]An excellent summary of the research carried out using the models of experimental pathology during this phase is provided by Courville's review in the now generally forgotten text on injuries of the head and spine by the New York neurologist, Samuel Brock. This text, first published in 1940, was considered a standard reference of the time. Together with the first, 1942 edition of Rowbotham's *Acute Injuries of the Head*, Brock delineated the state of the art for the English speaking world during the first part of World War II (22, 196).

the histological changes associated with concussion. The second group centered around an exploration of the phenomena associated with fatal injury. The list of pertinent phenomena was long. It included the focal and generalized changes accompanying hemorrhage into the subarachnoid, subdural, extra-dural and intraparenchymal spaces; lacerations and contusions; post-traumatic encephalitis and abscesses; subdural hygromata; axonal shear injuries; pituitary and hypothalamic damage; and changes in areas remote from the actual site of injury including the brain stem. A significant effort was devoted to establishing a continuum between the two groups. To this end, researchers distinguished between primary and secondary injury, a distinction that was often simplified into early and late or later effects.

Momentary unconsciousness was attributed to early effects. The chain of irrecoverable events that led to death was attributable to later effects. In the neuropathological literature, this distinction was also expressed in terms of primary, and typically focal events such as lacerations and contusions, and secondary, typically more global events such as ischemia and edema (15, 42, 121, 128, 196). The secondary events generally were held responsible for the multifocal changes that characterized severe head injury, especially the changes detected at a distance from the site of trauma (186).

The Pathophysiology of Unconsciousness

The classical methods of histopathology led to an understanding of the secondary, fatal phenomena associated with head trauma, but not so much to the understanding of unconsciousness *per se*. For this reason, investigators addressing the primary events in head injury turned to animal models. Most of these models proposed to demonstrate what happened to the brain when the skull was struck. The range of sophistication embodied in these experiments was quite broad.

Attempts to model head injury began around 1880. Between 1880 and 1920, three key insights were attained. First, a number of studies proved that shock waves were transmitted from the skull to the brain, and that the brain could move freely within the calvaria (66). Second, cortical contusions were correlated in severity and location with the degree to which the brain was accelerated relative to the skull, and with the site at which the brain collided against dural edges and bony irregularities. Third, the characteristically focal injuries produced by small objects striking, penetrating, or perforating the cranium were differentiated from multifocal or generalized damage produced when the moving head struck a solid object. It was established that altered consciousness correlated strongly with multifocal and coup-contrecoup, but not with focal injuries.[17]

In 1941, D. Denny-Brown and W.R. Russell developed a new model of head injury that led to a distinction between concussion associated with dynamic forces such as acceleration, and concussion associated with static forces such as slow compression (58). Dynamic concussion was modeled by a blow to the unrestrained cranium. Static concussion was modeled by a gradual increase in intracranial volume. All other factors held equal, the same degree of concussion required less in the way of dynamic than static forces. Concussion was found to be diminished or eliminated by head restraints (2).

It quickly became obvious that the interplay of forces involved in concussion were extremely complex. Variations and improvements on the Denny-Brown/Russell model were rapidly introduced (196). A.H.S. Holbourn, an Oxford physicist working with gelatin models during the war years, demonstrated that the arrangement of shear-strain damage characteristic of contrecoup injuries followed rotational, rather than linear force patterns. Damage was least where rotation was minimized, and greatest where angular acceleration was maximized. In 1944, Windle, Groat, and Fox utilized the Denny-Brown and Russell concussion model to search for subacute pathological changes in the brain. Previous models had depended almost entirely on acute experiments (219). They demonstrated that some nerve cells underwent chromatolysis be-

---

[17]Children were recognized as exceptions to this rule.

tween 14 and 48 hours after injury, some lost Nissl substance irreversibly over 6–8 days, but others sustained reversible change. These data were proposed as an explanation for the cumulative effects of repeated minor head injury sustained, for example, by pugilists, and as proof of a multifocal mechanism for unconsciousness. A third set of classic experiments revolved around a transparent calvarial prosthesis introduced in 1946 by Pudenz and Shelden. The lucite calvaria allowed direct observation of the brain in monkeys during the application of external forces (190).

Another key figure in the history of head injury research is the American neurosurgeon E.S. Gurdjian. In the early 1940s, Gurdjian pioneered the use of electrophysiological techniques in experimental head trauma. In collaboration with Lissner, Gurdjian demonstrated a relationship between ICP changes and brain damage (100). During the 1950s, Gurdjian collaborated with a number of investigators to develop a quantitative model of skull fracture and concussion. In conjunction with J.E. Webster, he also identified correlations between concussion and certain histopathological changes in the reticular formation[18] (42, 101, 177, 196). This proved to be an important breakthrough, and was reconfirmed in subsequent experiments by Gurdjian, Webster, H.W. McGoun, and others (42).

Although the significance of cerebral edema, increased ICP, cerebral herniation, and disturbances of cerebrovascular autoregulation came to be understood relatively well, advances in the pathophysiology of unconsciousness trailed behind the progress made in anatomy and histopathology (196). This disparity is attributable partially to technological limitations, and partially to other causes. In particular, the possibility that the secondary events in head injury might be related to neurochemical disturbances as well as to neuronal and neurovascular phenomena was not seriously entertained.

This, then, was the conceptual climate that existed when the CNS was founded. It took about two decades longer for other researchers, most notably Adams and Graham in Glasgow, Becker and co-workers in Richmond, and Genarelli and colleagues in Bethesda and Philadelphia, to conclude that the brainstem is ''rarely the main, and never the only site of damage'' (2, 126), and that increased ICP predictably resulted in widespread hypoxic and ischemic injury.[19] The reason these findings had not been described earlier, suggests Bryan Jennett, was because forensic pathologists were required to section the brains of head injury victims while fresh. After neuropathologists in Glasgow arranged to delay brain cutting until fixation was complete, new patterns of damage emerged[20] (126). The detailed description of the pathological sequelae of head trauma is correctly ascribed to the Glasgow group, but the earlier and no less significant contributions of Sir Geoffrey Jefferson, and of Seymour S. Kety and colleagues, all of which were fresh and important in 1951, should not be forgotten (125, 132). The later works of William Caveness, A. Earl Walker, Thomas Langfitt and colleagues, Ayub Ommaya, Adelbert Ames, III and colleagues, as well as many others, depended upon them (31, 34, 140, 141, 179, 180).

Minor Head Injury: Nomenclature and Histopathology

One of the interests of the neurosurgical community in the early 1950s centered upon minor head injury. The origins of the issues in the premodern era have already been outlined. In the 1920s, an important debate about nomenclature developed. The term ''concussion'' came under attack because it did not appear to have a well-defined pathological basis.

Two discriminate factors were proposed: time from injury to recovery, and evidence of struc-

---

[18]The history of studies pertaining to the mechanisms of unconsciousness and the role of the reticular activating system through the early 1960s is painstakingly detailed by Rowbotham (196).

[19]Some of these studies overlap the third and fourth phase of the history of head injury management, but will be discussed here nevertheless for the sake of convenience.

[20]Although this explanation is intriguing, it fails to explain why pathologists in other parts of the world, free from such constraints, had failed to detect these patterns earlier.

tural damage in the CNS. In 1928, Sir Charles Symonds suggested that the term be restricted to an injury from which one recovered within 24 hours, because structural damage would not be expected. George Riddoch agreed. The term "contusion" was designated to refer to neurological deficits of longer duration.

In 1931, Jefferson proposed that the term concussion be abandoned altogether. He argued that unconsciousness invariably involved a true contusion of the brain. Different durations of unconsciousness, and different degrees of severity in closed head injury were correlated simply, in his opinion, with differing extents of petechial hemorrhage.

Several years later, J.G. Greenfield, the British neuropathologist, proposed a compromise in which both terms, concussion and contusion, would be replaced by another that did not embody an implication of histopathological distinction. This compromise never took hold.

In the early 1950s, Greenfield came full circle, and suggested that the term concussion be retained. In 1958 he proposed that it be understood to comprehend the full range of diffuse injury to the brain.[21]

Intracranial Pressure and Cranial Decompression

From an historical perspective, surgery for trauma was justified by many indications. The concept of decompression generally figured prominently among these reasons, and no less so in 1951.

In a work entitled *Observations on the Structure and Function of the Nervous System*, published in 1783, the Scottish physiologist Alexander Monro *secundus* (1733–1817) first suggested that the contents of the skull could be divided into two compartments: blood and brain[22] (174). Because the skull was rigid and neither the brain nor the blood was compressible, Monro concluded that the volume of blood in the brain must be held constant. In 1824, George Kellie published data in support of this hypothesis. In animals, he showed that blood was present in the brain despite exanguination. In man he showed that death by hanging did not increase blood volume (140). The idea that the cranial cavity can be modeled as a rigid box with incompressible contents came to be known as the Monro-Kellie doctrine. Although Valsalva had alluded to a watery fluid in the subarachnoid space of fishes and turtles some seventy-five years earlier, the CSF compartment did not figure in the Monro-Kellie doctrine (231).

It remained for Magendie to demonstrate that fluid filled the ventricular and subarachnoid spaces and passed freely through the foramen that carries his name (82, 160). In 1846, George Burrows repeated some of Kellie's experiments and reinterpreted the results in the light of Magendie's observations. Burrows proposed that the Monro-Kellie doctrine be modified to include three compartments—blood, brain, and CSF—rather than two; that the blood volume of the brain was, in fact, quite capable of change; and that changes in cerebral blood volume would be accompanied by a reciprocal change in the volumes of brain or CSF.[23]

The importance of these ideas was not appreciated initially. Neither in the physiology syllabus at the Harvard Medical School in the 1860s nor in the 1867 edition of Dalton's *Treatise on Human Physiology*—a standard text in the premodern period—was the Monro-Kellie doctrine even mentioned (53).

---

[21]The debate continued beyond the period on which this article is focused. In brief, by the early 1960s, Greenfield focused the term to mean a state of unconsciousness without focal hematoma, contusions, or edema. This restricted definition did not catch on, nor did it become used in this way even after the introduction of sectional imaging techniques in the 1970s. The term reverted to mean "brief loss of consciousness" followed by a variable period of neurological morbidity and a variable degree of disability, the significance of which was widely debated because of its associations with litigation and disability claims. An excellent account of the early debate over the use of this term is given by D.W.C. Northfield (177).

[22]Monro *secundus'* father, Alexander Monro the elder, described the connection between the lateral and the third ventricles.

[23]Additional key work on the subject of CSF was carried out by Luschka, who also confirmed the work of Magendie, in addition to describing the lateral foramina of the fourth ventricle; and by Key and Retzius, who in 1872, published a monograph in Swedish further describing the dynamics of the CSF (82, 133).

Intracranial pressure became clinically interesting when surgeons began operating on space
occupying lesions in the brain Quincke's technique of lumbar puncture, which he had introduced to relieve hydrocephalus in 1891, soon
became adopted as a diagnostic test for measuring ICP, as well as for analyzing CSF. It quickly
became evident, however, that this test was
flawed for two reasons. First, intracranial mass
lesions did not necessarily result in measurably
increased CSF pressures. This observation was
explained by the fact that expanding lesions displaced blood and CSF in a manner that temporarily preserved an equipoise in pressure. Second,
pressure in the lumbar cistern sometimes failed
to reflect ICP.

Theodor Kocher (1841–1917), an early Swiss
neurosurgeon, concluded: "Lumbar puncture
does not give any very certain measure of the
pressure inside the skull, as the pressure may
fall very quickly in the spinal cavity, and remain
high in the cranial cavity"[24] (136). He also
warned that "cases of sudden death have occurred from lumbar puncture, because where
there has been a high intracranial pressure sudden diminution of the pressure in the canal has
caused the cerebellum to be forced down into
the spinal canal, with the result that paralysis of
respiration has occurred from pressure on the
medulla" (136).

Four critical ideas slowly emerged: the idea
of an ICP *dynamic*, subject to change; the idea
that ICP might both reflect and cause clinical
signs; the idea that ICP was subject to *compart-
mentalization*, as demonstrated, for example, by
a differential between the intracranial pressure
and the pressure in the lumbar subarachnoid
space; and the idea of *compensatory mechanisms* that could temporarily buffer increases in
ICP.

Kocher described four stages of cerebral

TABLE 9.7. *Kocher's four stages of cerebral
compression (173, 212)*

Stage	Description
I (Compensated)	No clinical change because of compensatory shifts in blood volume and CSF
II (Incipient Decompensation)	Headache and drowsiness
III (Bulbar Compression)	Depression of consciousness, increase in systemic arterial pressure, bradycardia, irregular respiration
IV (Pre-terminal)	Deep unconsciousness, bilateral fixed and dilated pupils, progressive reduction of systemic arterial pressure

compression: compensated, decompensated,
high, and pre-terminal. The stages are summarized in Table 9.7 (173, 212).

Cushing worked in Kocher's laboratory in
Bern immediately after completing his training
at Johns Hopkins. From 1900 to 1901, he researched the relationship between ICP and systemic blood pressure (7, 44). In 1902, he discussed the experimental aspects of increased
ICP and their clinical implications (45). A similar paper appeared in German (46). In 1903,
Cushing used cases of intracranial hemorrhage
as examples of increased ICP (47). Finally, in
1905, he recommended subtemporal craniectomy or other types of intermuscular calvarial
decompression and the induction of "artificial"
brain herniation through the defect as a strategy
for the management of increased ICP in patients
with inoperable tumors. This sequence of papers
brought to the fore the issues of increased ICP
in neurosurgery.[25]

Prior to the research conducted initially by
Kocher and later continued by Cushing, increased ICP after head injury was regarded as a
local intracranial phenomenon, subject to relief
via trephination. Kocher and Cushing also promoted the idea of elevated ICP as a *global* intra-

---

[24]Professor of Surgery and Director of the Surgical Clinic
at the University of Bern, an early and enthusiastic neurosurgeon who counted Harvey Cushing amongst his students.
Both the German and English editions of his best known
work, the *Textbook of Operative Surgery*, included a comprehensive section on surgery of the nervous system. This
section, based on Kocher's personal experience, went
through several editions and served as one of the earliest
and most widely translated manuals of neurosurgery.

[25]The relationship between Kocher and Cushing was one
of intense mutual respect. Kocher incorporated Cushing's
work on vasomotor aspects of ICP into his own teaching as
early as 1901 (7).

cranial phenomenon. Both Kocher and Cushing, but especially Kocher, believed the relief of elevated ICP to be the chief concern of intracranial surgery (136).[26, 27]

Kocher's classification of intracranial pressure was reproduced with only minor changes in the Army *Manual of Neuro-Surgery* of 1917 and 1919. ICP was by this time well correlated with alterations in temperature, pulse rate, and blood pressure.[28] These physiological changes served to diagnose elevated ICP and cerebral trauma, and to provide indications for treatment (255).[29]

By the 1920s, intracranial tension had come into its own as a pathophysiological mechanism in intracranial disease. It was also recognized as a complication that requiring urgent diagnosis (245).

The association between intracranial pressure and altered CSF dynamics had not escaped notice. Hill, Courtney, and Kocher pioneered research in this area around the turn of the century (41, 112). It was continued by Weed and colleagues soon after the first World War. In a summary paper of 1929, Weed reported that the intravenous administration of hypertonic solutions in experimental animals lowered ICP, and shrank the brain (252). On the basis of this and closely related work, it was generally agreed that the Monro-Kellie doctrine with the Burrows modification provided a reasonable model of ICP dynamics. Langfitt later reflected that, on the basis of these studies, "the craniospinal intradural space was shown to be *nearly* constant in volume and that its contents are *nearly* noncompressible [emphasis original]" (140).

Several alternative approaches to the control of elevated ICP emerged. Some clinicians recommended repeated lumbar puncture for control of increased ICP, in the manner of Quincke. Others favored hypertonic diuresis, after Weed. A third method, that was favored by a significant number of clinicians, was subtemporal decompression as advocated by Cushing.[30]

---

[26]The worst symptoms of disease of the central nervous system are attributable purely to physical and mechanical conditions, as increased tension within the rigid wall of the cranial cavity exerts an injurious and paralysing effect on the central nerve apparatus. Surgery is able, however, to interfere in various ways and reduce this so-called cerebral pressure. It is reprehensible, therefore, not to avail oneself of operative measures immediately the symptoms of pressure make their appearance. Increase of intracranial pressure is readily recognised, and is described in detail in every textbook, both in its chronic and acute form, while every practitioner ought to be familiar with its symptoms. . . .

[27]Cushing introduced a particular method of subtemporal decompression, as well as a retractor with which the exposure was facilitated. Dr. Eben Alexander, Jr. (personal communication) quantitatively investigated the benefits deriving from a typical 5 cm decompression of the type advocated by Cushing, and found that it added approximately 28 cc of volume so long as the dura was opened. Without dural opening, this procedure offered no benefit.

Although subsequent neurosurgeons were wont to refer to cerebral decompression as Cushing's technique, Charles Elsberg (1871–1948), a scholarly contemporary of Cushing's who trained with von Mikulicz in Germany and a founder of the Neurological Institute in New York who eventually served as its chief, noted that the term *decompressive trephining* was first used by the Frenchman Mathieu Jaboulay (1860–1913). Broca and Maubrac, he writes, "were the first to speak of 'cerebral decompression.' " This mode of treatment dates from the observations of Byrom Bramwell (1886), Annandale (1889), and Sahli (1891), and the method has been developed by the researches of Horsley, Keen, Bruns, Saenger, Jaboulay, Cushing, Frazier and Spiller, and many who followed them. Elsberg provides a bibliography of these works (72). Elsberg's biography is sketched in Walker, 1951, pp. 362–363.

[28] Cushing, whose chapter from Keen's textbook was reproduced *verbatim* in the *Manual*, was not mentioned in this context.

[29]. . .An initial rapid pulse may be succeeded by reaction on the part of the patient, manifested by rising temperature, slowing of the pulse, and perhaps a rise in blood pressure with other indications of [intracranial] pressure. It should be remembered that even after minor degrees of brain injury, a slow pulse is common and frequently persistent. While a slow pulse necessitates that close observation be kept, it should not be considered, when no other signs are present,

as a sufficient indication for the surgical relief of pressure. Such a slow pulse is frequently manifest as the only sign indicating a brain injury, and in such a case may not be associated with any rise in blood pressure (255).

[30]Isolation, quiet, sufficient liquids, attention to bowels and avoidance of over filling the bladder, ice packs to the head, are routine.

In those with extreme delirium, restraining sheets may be necessary. Any other method of restraint requires the closest attention to prevent injury. Spinal puncture may be beneficial. The use of bromides and chloral hydrate is seldom of any avail, even in large doses. Morphin [*sic*] is of greater help, but should be given only when rest is essential, and should be combined with atropin [*sic*]. . . .

In the presence of signs of increased intracranial pressure if moderate or increasing, a sub-temporal decompression, as practiced by Cushing, with drainage for 48 hours is advisable.

The operation is upon the side toward which the signs of greater injury point. With general pressure and no other determining factors, the right side is chosen in right-handed people.

Bilateral openings are frequently necessary drain of gutta percha tissue or a strip of rubber dam is placed between the

The remarkable importance attributed to ICP in the management of head trauma can be inferred from surgical texts of the period. In 1921, William Sharpe, an early neurosurgeon in New York, offered the following insights (5, 212):

For many years, the routine treatment of fracture of the skull, whether of the base or of the vault, has been the expectant palliative one; that is, an ice-bag to the head, vigorous catharsis, liquid diet, and absolute rest and quiet, morphia being administered if necessary. Practically all fractures of the base were so treated, it being thought that nothing else could be done for such cases; the mortality was high - more than 50 per cent. Even depressed fractures of the vault, unless there were localized signs of compression, were frequently treated in the same manner.

Naturally, the cases of simple concussion and the mild fractures of the skull. . . have been and are being treated successfully by this method; it is, however, in those cases of fracture of the skull. . . where there are definite signs of an increased intracranial pressure, that this expectant palliative treatment is not sufficient and a more effective method of treatment is essential.

. . .In my opinion, it is not so much a question of ascertaining the presence and the site of the fracture, but rather of finding out whether or not there is an increased intracranial pressure, and if there is, then directing the treatment toward a lowering of this abnormal pressure. For this reason, a careful ophthalmoscopic examination should be made in each case, as the earliest signs of an increased pressure appear in the fundus of the eye, especially about the entrance of the nerve - the so-called optic disc.

These changes in the fundus of the eye are the result of increased intracranial pressure, whether this pressure be due to a slowly growing tumor, to an intracranial hemorrhage, or to a very edematous "swollen" brain resulting from a fracture of the skull. It is this cerebral edema, resulting in varying degrees from any injury of the brain. . . which has been overlooked in the past. . . .

. . .Naturally, I do not advise a decompression in all cases of fracture of the skull, but only in those showing marked signs of increased intracranial pressure.

These ideas were no less authoritative thirty years later, in 1951.

Despite its obvious clinical importance, attempts to develop a cogent approach to the management of head injury based on control of ICP were defeated by three contradictory observations. First, some patients with clinical features of cerebral compression were found to have normal CSF pressures (114). Second, the correlation between lumbar ICP pressure and the changes in systolic arterial pressure predicted by Cushing was imperfect. Finally, the relief of intracranial pressure by the means available did not invariably result in survival or even a satisfactory outcome (23, 173).[31]

As a result of these conceptual difficulties, the problems of ICP and cerebral edema became the object of intensive investigation lasting several decades. During the 1930s, for example, Robert Rand and Cyril Courville attacked the problem of cerebral edema, which they attributed to three mechanisms: transudation of fluid from congested veins; increased secretion from the choroid plexus and ependyma; and intracellular swelling in oligodendroglia (42). In 1938, Jefferson published his classic work on tentorial herniation, in which he posited that neurological deterioration during periods of increased ICP

---

temporal lobe and the base. The drainage of blood-stained cerebrospinal fluid is often most profuse. Such a drain should be removed in 48 hours. A simple decompression without drainage is of little value. In this group of cases the intracranial pressure is due to increased fluid content within the skull. A decompression without drainage merely increases the cranial capacity, and shortly thereafter the original equilibrium is established between the general circulation on the one hand and the cranial fluid content on the other. With drainage of this fluid intracranial tension approaches normal, with consequent readjustment of vasomotor and circulatory control.

This procedure is advisable to relieve acute compression from either free hemorrhage or edema.

. . .Sub-temporal decompression with drainage usually answers all purposes.

. . .[Kocher's] [s]tage four of compression is to be regarded as a terminal condition.

---

[31]A somewhat unrelated frustration had to do with the limitations of diagnosing increased intracranial pressure in timely fashion. The fundoscopic examination did not always demonstrate papilloedema. According to Sharpe, choked discs were never visible before three hours after injury, unless the patient already reached Kocher's stage IV. This made it difficult for relatively inexperienced clinicians to warrant operating upon the group of patients in greatest need of decompression, those with increasing pressure not yet subjected to irreversible medullary compression (212).

might be associated with local shifts of the brain as well as with ischemia (125). In the 1950s, it became evident that the *entire* brain, including the brain stem, was subject to shift (173).[32] Many types of neurological deterioration associated with ICP changes (in retrospect far too many) were ascribed to this mechanism.

Neurological Intensive Care

Relative to 1951, the concept of intensive care, and especially neurological intensive care, is something of an anachronism. The main concern was recovery from surgery and anesthesia, prevention of complications, and first rate patient care whether surgery had been performed or not. The number of neurosurgeons was small relative to the population at large, and more often then not, patients who did not require surgery were treated by neurologists or other medical specialists.

Intensive care as a concept of care evolved out of the recovery room, and came to designate a facility in which intensive nursing care was instituted at a 1:1 or 1:2 patient ratio. In addition, the nurses would be specially trained in physiological monitoring, respirator management (especially following the poliomyelitis epidemics of the 1950s), and resuscitation. The idea of intensive care really took flight in the mid 1960s, when it was shown that survival after myocardial infarction could be improved by continuous monitoring of the EKG and immediate treatment of arrhythmias. But these thoughts had yet to be worked out in the early 1950s. Special units were intended to concentrate neurosurgical patients for the convenience of the surgeon, to provide nurses with experience in the special problems of neurosurgical patients, to segregate neurosurgical patients from other patients (e.g., those undergoing abdominal procedures) who were thought to be more likely to

become infected, and to provide a location in which common and relatively less invasive neurosurgical procedures could be carried out at the bedside with appropriate equipment and assistance.

Some aspects of what is now thought of as intensive care did exist. At the end of the 19th century, Von Bergmann and others had recommended blood-letting to reduce systemic arterial blood pressure after head injury. This practice was abandoned after Cushing argued that hypertension served to protect against cerebral anemia during bouts of increased ICP (212).[33] The relationship of consciousness, blood pressure, pulse and pupillary size and shape to neurological condition resulted in these parameters being measured regularly in neurosurgical patients.

The perceived importance of physiological monitoring did eventually result in a movement to establishment of specialized neurosurgical intensive care units, but not until the late 1960s. In the late 1950s, however, reports appeared of improved outcomes after head injury with spe-

---

[32]This observation led, in turn, to a reformulation of the mechanism for the Cushing reflex as a phenomenon associated with ischemia of the brainstem due to with stretching of the basilar artery and its branches, as well as one associated with compression.

[33]The focus of this chapter dictates that only a very rudimentary discussion of the broader influence of ICP upon the development of neurosurgical technique for non-traumatic indications and spinal cord compression be undertaken. The role of mass lesions in causing hydrocephalus or increased ICP was well understood. Conservative management was identical to that recommended for trauma except that ice packs were not recommended. Ventriculostomy through Kocher's paramedian route, through Keen's point, via Elsberg's transcallosal technique, or through the occipital horns were used for temporary relief of pressure, in the hope of more permanent palliation, and for internal decompression.

Insofar as the diagnostic techniques of the post-World War I period still failed to ensure that masses would be localized with precision or even detected altogether, the need for decompressive craniotomy remained acute. Decompressive craniotomy—trephination or craniectomy with durotomy for control of pressure at a site chosen for reasons other than access to a localized intracranial process—was carried out for palliation under the following conditions: if a tumor could not be found; if a space occupying lesion could not be drained or resected; as an emergency procedure if intracranial pressure reached critical levels before diagnosis could be achieved; or for post-operative control of increased ICP; and for decompression *prior* to surgery if a lesion were localized to an eloquent area of the brain such that intra-operative or post-operative herniation through a dural and calvarial defect might be injurious. A method of decompressive craniotomy was explicitly described in virtually every guide to neurosurgical technique. Concerns about ICP also dictated the choice of anesthesia. See, e.g., Kocher (1911) and Elsberg (1921).

cialized intervention. In 1958, a neurosurgeon, an anesthesiologist, and an otolaryngologist from Newcastle-Upon-Tyne in England reported the advantages of tracheostomy and pharmacological control of spasticity and body temperature after head injury (158). Somewhat later, the advent of simple mechanical ventilators (supplanting the iron lungs that had been utilized during the poliomyelitis epidemics) ushered in the use of controlled hyperventilation and paralysis for control of ICP.

Between 1960 and 1980, the number of intensive care units grew from almost none to 50,000 (127). They were used for postoperative management as well as for acute head injury, and for similar reasons. The number of dedicated neurosurgical intensive care units also grew.

From an historical perspective, the three principle justifications for intensive care units, physiological monitoring, advanced technology, and quick, expert response, were especially germane to the head injured patient. For neurosurgeons, moreover, this idea was rather familiar: both Cushing and Cairn had recommended and implemented specialized expert units for the treatment of head trauma in war time, and believed that their outcomes had improved in consequence. The additional consideration that emerged during the 1960s and 1970s was that the brain was not necessarily benefited by what benefited the body–but this idea had not yet been articulated clearly in the early 1950s (247).

Neurosurgery of Head Trauma

There was comparatively little technical difference between the operations that were carried out at the end of the second phase of the management of head trauma and during the third. The most important changes involved methods of surgical diagnosis; types and timing of surgery; the attitude towards dural closure; the use of antibiotics; and the management of CSF leaks. One might also argue convincingly that changes in instrumentation (e.g., the electrocautery and bipolar coagulator), diagnostic technology (e.g., angiography), implantable materials for hemostasis, dural substitute, and cranioplasty (e.g., gelfoam and methyl methacrylate), in transpor-

tation (e.g., the helicopter), in blood transfusion and the management of shock, in the development of endotracheal and (somewhat later) specifically *neuro*anesthesia, in the funding of neurosurgical research, in the structure of head injury care (e.g., the proliferation of neurosurgeons in the United States and of neurosurgical training programs), and in the dissemination of neurosurgical information (e.g., the founding of the Journal of Neurosurgery, the founding of the CNS, and the publication of *Clinical Neurosurgery*) should be included. A strong case can be made for the importance of each of these factors.

Methods of Surgical Diagnosis, Operations Performed, and the Urgency of Operation

For many years, the preeminent goal of surgical exploration in trauma was to render or to confirm a diagnosis, to prevent infection, and to promote healing. Later, during phases II and III, surgical exploration was also intended to relieve increased ICP without regard to cause, and to decompress specific lesions such as extra-axial hematomas. Surgical options were strongly influenced by diagnostic methods available, and vice versa. Table 9.1 summarizes the changes in diagnostic and surgical focus from phase I to phase IV.

From time immemorial, diagnosis of head injury was based on unconsciousness after injury, with or without skull fracture. These criteria were adequate with regard to injuries of the cranial vault, but not the cranial base. During the last part of the pre-modern period and early phase II, patterns of ecchymosis, bleeding from the nose and ears, CSF rhinorrhea or otorrhea, subconjunctival hemorrhages and related signs became associated with fractures of the base. Later,[34] head injury was reconstrued in terms

---

[34] A process that took some time, *viz.*, the number of *surgical* textbooks that included instructions for executing a neurological examination. The Army *Manual of Neuro-Surgery* of 1917 and 1919 is exemplary in this regard. But even as late as 1947, the editors of the War Supplement Volume of the British Journal of Surgery saw fit to include a section on the ''Neurological State and Post-Operative Course in Penetrating Head Wounds'' by R.P. Jepson and C.W.M. Whitty (pp. 243–250), which begins with a discussion of the value of neurological examination on head wounds, and another on the ''Neurology of Head Wounds'' by R. Ritchie Russell (pp. 250–253).

of neurological impairment.[35] The diagnosis of head injury was also made by lumbar puncture (not deemed generally reliable); glycosuria; and roentgenographic findings. Some surgeons, including Sharpe of New York, continued to rely on inspection of the skull, even to the point of incising the scalp over a suspicious area, years after X-ray devices were widely installed.

During phase I and the early part of phase II, the distinction between open and closed head injury was utilized, both descriptively and prognostically, to articulate the risk of septic complications. The problem of head injury was construed as a function of fracture. Nomenclature followed the orthopedic model (closed versus open fractures of the extremities, closed versus open fractures of the skull) with concessions to differences between penetrating head wounds and simple lacerations of the scalp. The neurological implications embedded in these distinctions did not receive substantial attention before Cushing's work on penetrating head wounds during World War I.

Surgical exploration was for many years the only way to confirm absolutely the nature of a calvarial injury. This tradition seems to be the historical basis for what later became known derisively as "woodpecker surgery." Still, the risks of anesthesia and of other complications, as well as the long history of dismal outcome in head injury, limited enthusiasm for surgery.

There was less hesitation about exploring a compound fracture or a penetrating wound of the skull because the risk of infection was inherent in the injury and was not felt to be significantly increased by intervention. The decision regarding exploration of a closed fracture was described in 1919 as "largely a personal matter. . . [which] depends entirely upon his familiarity with intracranial disturbances which are amenable to operative treatment and his ability to safely cope with them when found" (255). Operation was reserved for patients with progressive signs of medullary compression: bradycardia below 50, systolic systemic blood pressure exceeding 170, and Cheyne-Stokes respirations. Mortality in these pre-terminal cases approximated 90% (212). The thinking in 1951 was not substantially different.

Establishing a Threshold for Surgery

Sharpe believed that the threshold for surgery in closed head injury had been set too high, and his view reflected the majority opinion through the mid- to late 1950s.[36] Sharpe's primary indication for surgery was increased intracranial pressure, followed by focal neurological abnormality in the presence of calvarial depression or deformity. Both elements were required: surgery was not deemed indicated in massive fractures of the vault, for example, on the grounds that a natural decompression had already been afforded by loosened bony fragments.

In the early 1930s, it was generally taught that two types of operation for head injury were to be performed: exploration of the fracture site for diagnosis, debridement, decompression, and dural exploration where indicated; and, in the presence of increased ICP, trephination or craniectomy at the temporal squama for decompression.[37] Surgery was brief—one hour or less—even when both procedures were carried out.

Enthusiasm for subtemporal decompression to diagnose and treat increased intracranial pressure waned in the late 1930s. Max Thorek offered the following aphorisms under the section entitled "Concussion of the Brain" in his classic

---

[35]Significant findings included gaze palsy, hemiparesis, and aphasia; anesthesia; convulsions; reflex asymmetry; and papilloedema.

[36]"For many years," he wrote in 1921, "the routine treatment of fracture of the skull. . . has been the expectant palliative one. . . . Practically all fractures of the base were so treated, it being thought that nothing else could be done for such cases; the mortality was high–more than 50 per cent. Even depressed fractures of the vault, unless there were localized signs of compression, were frequently treated in the same manner. . . ." (212)

[37]The term "surgical decompression" in this context is used to describe an operation for suspected or proven increase in ICP irrespective of, in addition to, or instead of, a direct attack on the cause, and irrespective of whether this condition was recognized *per se*, or was a manifestation of lesions that were unrecognized, unattainable, or undemonstrable by generally available techniques available.

textbook of surgical technique published in 1938 (226)[38]:

> Do not rush the patient to the x-ray room. Get him out of shock first. After shock is combated, get stereo x-rays to ascertain the presence or absence of fracture and its location.
>
> Masterly inactivity - so aptly expressed by Hamilton Bailey - should be the slogan. Good nursing is here superior to medical meddling. . . .
>
> The furor of subtemporal decompression for fractures at the base of the skull (unless definitely indicated) is fortunately passing, except, of course, in definite hemorrhage from the middle meningeal artery. . . .

The operation of subtemporal decompression was still carried out in 1951, however, and the most common debate was not whether subtemporal decompression should be carried out, but whether it afforded sufficient decompression.

Extra-axial Fluid Collections and Intracerebral Hematomas

At the beginning of phase III, there was little comprehension of the role of extra-axial blood or fluid collections or intracerebral hematomas in causing increased ICP. They were categorized simply as ''complications.'' The discussion in the Army *Manual of Neuro-Surgery*, published in 1919, almost identical in flavor to that in Sharpe's textbook in all major aspects, offers a sense of how these ''complications'' were managed (255):

> We are confronted again by the necessity of distinguishing between the management of the fracture itself and the management of its complications. Relatively simple rules can be laid down for the former; for the latter our conduct is largely controlled by physiological laws re-

lating to the circulation of the blood and the cerebrospinal fluid under abnormal conditions. In fractures of the vault, the indication for surgical intervention is usually deformation of fragments, rather than critical cerebral complications. In fractures of the base, it is the reverse, for there intracranial complications are especially serious and deformation is rare.

Exploration for epidural hematoma was indicated by fracture over the middle meningeal region and neurological deterioration. This operation was intended for diagnosis and well as treatment. Neither Thorek nor other writers, however, gave clear advice on how to determine when a subdural hematoma was present. For suspicion of hemorrhage derived from signs of neurological deterioration, with or without fracture, attention was focused upon the middle meningeal artery. When no epidural was found, the dura was opened. If no clot was encountered after lifting the temporal lobe and irrigating, subtemporal decompression was advised (226). Dandy introduced ventriculography in 1918 and encephalography the following year. These were the first means by which the intracranial soft tissues could be in any way visualized. In the first monograph dedicated entirely to this subject, Wakely and Orley's 1938 *Textbook of Neuro-Radiology*, these tests are described as ''the surest way to diagnose and localize a subdural haematoma'' (240). Arteriography, introduced by Moniz in 1927 but not widely available before 1934, was indicated ''only in severe and neurologically obscure cases. . . where there is no proper history of the accident'' (240). In 1951, angiography was still considered a very major procedure, performed via formal exposure of the carotid artery, and still fraught with complications. One important limiting factor was the absence of rapid film changers. The procedure was generally carried out by neurosurgeons, who found exploratory burr holes to be easier, less risky, often faster, and certainly more definitive when a clot was found and could be drained.

Thus, in 1951, the most common method for diagnosing hematomas was via exploratory burr holes. Well prior to the Second World War, exploratory burr holes for hematoma were carried out but with somewhat less urgency than after-

---

[38]Max Thorek was one of the most internationally famous American surgeons of the early twentieth century. He was a true general surgeon who studied with Fedor Krause of Berlin (1857–1937), translating his *Surgery of the Brain and Spinal Cord* into English in 1912. He practiced general and neurosurgery at Cook County Hospital in Chicago, and reflected both European and American thinking in his work. In 1938 he wrote a classic textbook on surgical technique which included neurosurgery. During World War II, the four volumes of this text were reprinted as a special, one volume, war edition that reproduced four pages of the original on one. This text was very widely distributed during the 1940s.

wards (Dr. Eben Alexander, Jr., personal communication). In fact, hematoma was not really perceived to be a salient issue in head trauma at the beginning of the war. In 1940, for example, Cairns wrote that the major problem confronting the neurosurgeon was adequate scalp closure. "The apparently trivial operation of cleaning and suturing a wound of the scalp," he wrote, "is probably the most important neurosurgical operation of the war." Clots were not vigorously pursued in the absence of subacute or delayed deterioration, nor foreign debris other than obviously contaminated material excised, because "every manipulation potentially increases brain damage and diminishes the extent of functional recovery. . . ." (27)

Between 1940 and the end of the Korean War, the importance ascribed to extra-axial collections and intracerebral hematomas increased several fold. This was a gradual process driven by a growing sense that the incidence of such lesions had been severely underestimated. In 1944, Joseph Schorstein calculated the incidence of intracranial hematoma in the North African and Italian campaigns to be 4.2% (83 out of 2000 cases). Three clots were extradural, 11 subdural, 63 intracerebral, and 6 delayed. Cairns' initial assessment appeared justified (209). In 1946, Matson and Wolkin reported 11 hematomas in 305 penetrating wounds (3.6%) (164). They chose to interpret these data quite differently, however:

> It was not until relatively late in the campaign, November 1944, that the significance was appreciated of intracranial hemorrhage on the side opposite from the wound of entrance in retained foreign bodies. Since that time, 11 patients have been operated upon who have had sizable hematomas located either in the opposite subdural space or in the substance of the brain in or adjacent to the tract made by a metallic foreign body at a site distant to the point of penetration. In retrospect, we feel sure that similar lesions were overlooked in earlier cases.

In consequence, Finlayson advocated "early definitive repair" of penetrating head injuries (81). In 1948, Matson called for both an aggressive search for hematomas and for prompt and definitive surgery after penetrating head injury (163). The importance of these paired recommendations rose to the fore in the early 1950s, and was categorically demonstrated during the Korean War.

In 1955, Barnett and Meirowsky published a paper summarizing 316 penetrating wounds treated within 8 hours of injury with the assistance of air evacuation and forward neurosurgical units. They found a hematoma greater than 20 cc in volume in 46.2% of patients overall. The incidence diminished over time to 27% after 12 to 36 hours, and 7% in a group treated 24 to 72 hours after injury (13). Although this paper addressed findings in penetrating head injury only, it demonstrated a clear association between early mortality and the incidence of hematomas. A paradigm of aggressive and early surgery, searching proactively for clots in damaged or deteriorating patients developed.

Prior to the Korean War, the use of exploratory trephination in deteriorating patients was widespread, but by no means universal. Within ten years, exploratory burr holes in search of extra-axial hematomata were the norm in most clinics (196). The method generally recommended involved a series of three burr holes on the side of a fracture or demonstrated external trauma, unless the neurological exam pointed contralaterally. Burr holes were placed frontally, parietally, and temporally. If no lesions were found, or even if they were, the patient then underwent the same exploration on the other side. In some clinics, bilateral posterior fossa burr holes were placed routinely: in others, the additional pair of holes was drilled only if no other lesion sufficient to explain the clinical findings were found. Some schools of thought taught that the dura be opened routinely, and the subdural space explored for hematomas. Others were more reserved. All surgeons were taught to prepare to connect the burr holes into a craniotomy if they had any suspicion of additional damage or if they were dissatisfied with their ability to visualize the cortex and allay any suspicions of hematoma.

Both electroencephalography (EEG) and plain roentgenography were thought initially to hold great promise in diagnosing hematomas. A good deal of research was expended on the first: it was a major investigative paradigm throughout the 1950s. There were several reasons why the EEG was of particular interest. The EEG had first been developed to diagnose organic lesions in psychiatric patients; it was physiological in an era where physiological monitoring of electrical phenomena was high technology and highly admired; it was readily available; and it was generally thought to be highly useful. Unfortunately, it was also highly overread, and highly overrated.

The second method of diagnosis, the plane film, was easily obtained and easily interpreted. It was rarely of significant use, however, except in demonstrating a small repertoire of findings: fractures, pre-existing trauma, pneumocephalus, retained radiodense foreign objects, and chronic, calcified extra-axial collections.

Techniques of Debridement after Penetrating Injury

Many different methods were recommended for debriding head injuries. Cushing advocated debriding the skull *en bloc*. The track was to be gently irrigated and fragments were to be removed with forceps (51). During the British campaign in North Africa, Ashcroft reported that patients treated by partial debridement and packing were inordinately subject to brain abscess, particularly if clusters of bone fragments were left in the wound. His conclusions were skewed by the fact that other foreign material was also often left behind, and patients arrived to the neurosurgical unit only after long delays during which they could not receive optimal wound care. When Kenneth Eden, a New Zealander who died in the war zone of poliomyelitis in 1943, was able to offer definitive operations close to the time of injury, the rate of secondary abscess fell considerably, without aggressive debridement (28).

Nevertheless, the idea that radical debridement was a prerequisite to successful operation was seized upon and championed by a number of neurosurgeons, particularly Meirowsky. This was an important emerging concept in the early 1950s. Meirowsky served with distinction in both the Korean War and World War II. He at-

tained an infection rate of less than 1% by the end of the Korean War. He attributed this success to the deployment of mobile teams close to the battle lines, to very rapid evacuation, and to very early definitive surgery with radical debridement of all missile tracks (147, 169). "Radical" meant, in his parlance, the inclusion of a "narrow surrounding margin of intact cortex" as well as any obviously discolored or devitalized brain. The track was debrided until it was smooth to both palpation and inspection in order to leave a smooth scar (169).[39]

Dural Closure

Prior to the Second World War, little importance was attributed to dural reconstruction. The dura was often left open with the intention of promoting decompression on the one hand, and drainage on the other. The disadvantages of dural opening included spreading infection, wound healing, and cerebral fungus. The dura was closed routinely in complex wounds involving the air sinuses, or in large vertex wounds where the risks of secondary damage from cortical herniation were great. The Nazi surgeons Sorgo and Tönnis advocated closure of the dura with galeo-periosteal flaps and loose closure of the scalp.

During the course of the war, the incidence of deep infection diminished for reasons already suggested. The need for drainage as a means of reducing infection was perceived to have lessened, and experience suggested that adequate decompression could be achieved through debridement. As Cairns put it, "in deeply infected brain wounds if débridement had been done thoroughly a drain was not necessary and that

---

[39]Under the auspices of the Surgeon General of the Army, Meirowsky edited a hugely influential volume entitled *Neurological Surgery of Trauma*. This work came to define the standard treatment of head trauma in Vietnam, as well as in the civilian sector, for almost two decades. Meirowsky advocated repeated operation, if need be, to rid the brain of all radiologically demonstrable bone chips and eliminate delayed infection or abscess (38, 169). This principle was followed *verbatim* at the neurosurgical service of the Walter Reed Army Medical Center for several years under the direction of General W.G. Haynes, despite discouraging neurological deterioration in some instances (Dr. John Slaughter, personal communication).

where débridement was not complete a drain did not suffice. . . . Neurosurgeons learned to recognize the tight brain track as a sign of incomplete debridement. . . .''. (28) As a result, the dura was closed, grafted, or otherwise reconstructed. This tactic represented a change from Cushing's approach of resecting the skull and dural entrance wound *en bloc*. American neurosurgeons in the war zone took the lead in this technique (69, 109, 198). Except in the spine and the posterior fossa, watertight dural closure became the predominant standard of practice after the Second World War. Meirowsky described it as ''established policy'' in Korea, and so it was, for all intents and purposes in 1951 (169).

Antibiotics

The introduction of antibiotics did not change the management of head trauma as much often imagined. It did serve, however, to facilitate bolder surgery and to simplify the management of complications such as wound infection and abscess. In historical terms, antibiotics were long and effectively preceded by antiseptics. Solutions that served antiseptic purposes had been used for centuries in wound dressings, without any real understanding of their mechanisms of action, if any. Listerian technique was introduced in the mid-nineteenth century. Its effects on neurosurgery have already been addressed. The search for improved antiseptics continued through the first part of the twentieth century. The majority, like gentian violet and other supravital stains, were neurotoxic.

Infection during World War I was addressed through surgical debridement, continuous irrigation with Eusol and silver nitrate, and dependence on systemic antisera and antitoxins. These measures were proven again in the Spanish Civil War. They offered but limited value in the brain, even though Dandy and others suggested the use of continuous CSF drainage in meningitis (54).

Infection during the Second World War was, up until the advent of modern antibiotics, managed and treated identically to the First World War.[40] Antibiotic properties of several compounds, including penicillin, were first noted at the end of the nineteenth century, but not understood. First generation antibiotics such as salvarsan and sulfa compounds were brought to market in the early to mid 1930s. The earliest use of antibiotics in neurosurgery was in the treatment of brain abscess (24, 198) In 1938, penicillin was rediscovered by Fleming and co-workers in England. Between 1942 and 1943, penicillin was shown experimentally to control the spread of infection in laboratory models (184). The first large-scale trial of penicillin in neurosurgery was carried out by the British during the Battle of Sicily (July and August, 1943). It effects seemed less impressive in the head than elsewhere (28). Cairns compared a series of cases from May, 1938 and November 1944, with a group after November, 1944, when a mixture of penicillin and sulphamethazine was instilled at the time of surgery. In the first group, there were 51 infections out of 1169 operations (4.8%) and 6 fatalities (11.7%). In the second group, there were 6 infections in 670 cases (0.9%) without fatality. The difference this time was significant. American surgeons, however, reported higher infection rates, even with antibiotics: 23% with sulphonamide alone, and 13% with penicillin. There were no figures to document infection rate without antibiotics altogether (162). Amongst the American forces, penicillin was used routinely after the spring of 1944 (162). Antibiotics were delivered topically, intrathecally, and parenterally (28). Sodium penicillin solution was used for irrigation amongst the Yugoslav partisans, in a method akin to that of Carrel and Dakin during the First War (39).

Despite the reduction of deep infection that followed the introduction of antibiotics in the American theater of operations, and the immeasurable improvements in the treatment of systemic infection, particularly in the multiply wounded, it is interesting to observe the remarkably low incidence of infection in clean or even clean contaminated cases during earlier phases of the war. Antibiotics were broadly, but by no means routinely utilized in 1951.

---

[40]It would be useful to review the history of the treatment of intracranial abscess to fully elucidate the state of the art prior to World War II. This material is summarized in Stern's chapter, ''Surgery of the Craniocerebral Infections,'' in Walker's *History of Neurological Surgery*, pp. 180–212.

CSF Leaks

This section reviews the history of cerebrospinal fluid leaks. The majority of principles for the management of this problem were clarified between 1920 and the mid 1960s. A broader time frame has been selected, however, to provide historical perspective.

In the 17th century, a Dutch surgeon, Bidloo the Elder, first correlated post-traumatic rhinorrhea with the drainage of spinal fluid (146). Cases in which nontraumatic CSF rhinorrhea resulted from increased intracranial pressure were then reported by Miller in 1826, and King in 1834 (52, 172). In view of the limited understanding of CSF dynamics that existed prior to the work of Burrows in 1846, this association was quite remarkable.

The full significance of CSF fistulae was not appreciated, however, until 1884, when Chiari demonstrated a fistulous connection between a pneumatocele in the frontal lobes and the ethmoid sinuses of a patient who died of meningitis following rhinorrhea (37). This finding indicated a mechanism to explain meningitis in this context. Shortly after the introduction of roentgenography, the diagnosis of a fistula was first made in vivo through the recognition of intracranial air as an abnormal intracranial density.[41, 42]

Early repair techniques were not successful. Indeed, the very need for surgical intervention in the management of CSF leaks was questioned as late as the 1930s, when the first lasting repairs

were attained. Combat injuries during World War II rendered the problem of CSF leaks and meningitis more acute. CSF leaks were commonly found in survivors of blast injury, road traffic accidents, and high velocity missile injuries. Meningitis, rather than the leak or the fracture per se, was the issue. By 1944, Dandy advocated surgical repair of any CSF leak within two weeks of onset in order to prevent meningitis (56). This approach was echoed by Walpole Lewin, neurosurgeon to Adenbrooke's Hospital in Cambridge. After a review of the British combat experience and of a large series of basilar skull fractures, Lewin, who is strongly identified with the treatment of head injury in Britain, argued that the spontaneous apparent cessation of a leak did not eliminate the risk of meningitis in the presence of a fistula. He advocated operating on all CSF fistulae that did not close within several days (145, 146). In 1951, this doctrine was widely practiced, but not yet fully articulated.

Nor was there universal agreement about the preferred route for patching a fistula. In 1937, Cairns recommended that leaks be sealed extradurally, by the application of fascia lata to the dural defect. The extradural route was adopted by some neurosurgeons, but most found the intradural approach more familiar (70). The otolaryngologists retained the extradural approach (63). Neurosurgeons did not return to the extradural route routinely until much later (30, 52, 165).

---

[41] "...a middle-aged man was admitted with a head injury. . . . He was x-rayed by Dr. W. H. Stewart, who detected a fracture in the posterior wall of the frontal sinus. The patient was treated conservatively and discharged... but returned some three weeks later having suffered a relapse. On December 14, [1912], a further radiographic examination of the skull was undertaken.... these x-rays showed the ventricles enormously dilated by what was probably air or gas. As a result of these findings Dr. Luckett operated and during the course of the operation tapped one of the ventricles and noticed that air or gas was released. The patient died three days later and at autopsy the fracture in the posterior wall of the frontal sinus was confirmed and part of the bone was found to be depressed about one centimeter." (152)

[42] This observation lead to the development of pneumoencephalography for neurological diagnosis (257). It also contributed conceptually to the development of surgical techniques for the repair of CSF fistulae (55, 95).

CONCLUSION

By 1951, the neurosurgical management of head injury had reached, and, in some respects, recently passed important inflection points. The most important changes included:

1. the shift in thought that moved head injury from a problem of sepsis to one of neurological dysfunction: this shift started well before the Second World War, but was not really completed until the problem of postoperative infection in head trauma was felt to be under good control in the early 1950s;

2. the treatment of head injury by neuro-surgical specialists in dedicated units;

3. technical advances in surgery;

4. improved neuroanesthesia;

5. improved resuscitation and urgent evacuation;

6. antibiotics;

7. outcome studies;

8. the focus on the dissemination of neuro-surgical knowledge, particularly for younger neurosurgeons through the Congress of Neurological Surgeons.

The purpose of this review was to present the state of the management of head trauma in 1951 in its historical context. The history of the management of head trauma reflects the extent to which progress in science and in surgery combines seminal contributions from gifted individuals with ideas that consolidate more slowly and across a broader front. In the first years of the 1950s a fortunate combination of circumstances allowed a number of visionary neurosurgeons access to technical and scientific advances. This combination, together with a dedication to neurosurgery and a passion for teaching successfully advanced the field to the next level of research and practice.

REFERENCES

1. Adams JH. The neuropathology of head injuries, in, Vinken PJ, Bruyn GW (eds): *Handbook of Clinical Neurology: Injuries of the Brain and Skull, Part I,* 1975.

2. Adams H, Graham DI. The pathology of blunt head injuries, in, Critchley M, O'Leary JL, Jennett B (eds): *Scientific Foundations of Neurology.* London: William Heineman Medical Books Ltd., 1972, pp 478–491.

3. Aita J. Modern considerations of the man with brain injury. *J Neurosurg* 4:240–254, 1947.

4. Aitken RR, Drake CG. Continuous spinal drainage in the treatment of postoperative cerebrospinal-fluid fistuale. *J Neurosurg* 21:275–277, 1965.

5. Alexander E. Jr. William Sharpe, MD. Neurosurgeon/Entrepreneur. *Neurosurgery* 22:961–964, 1988.

6. Ambrose J. Computerized transverse axial scanning (tomography). Part II: Clinical application. *Br J Radiol* 46:1023–1047, 1973.

7. American Association of Neurological Surgeons: *A Bibliography of the Writings of Harvey Cushing.* 3rd Edition. Park Ridge, Illinois: American Association of Neurological Surgeons, 1993.

8. Anderson F. Extradural cerebellar hemorrhage: Review of the subject and report of a case. *J Neurosurg* 6:191–196, 1949.

9. Appelbaum E. Meningitis following trauma to the head and face. *JAMA* 173:116–120, 1968.

10. Bacon A. Cerebellar extradural hematoma: Report of a case. *J Neurosurg* 6:8–81, 1949.

11. Bakay, L. *The Treatment of Head Injures in the Thirty Years' War.* Springfield, IL: Charles C. Thomas, 1971.

12. Bakay L, Glasauer FE. *Head Injury.* Boston: Little Brown & Co, 1980.

13. Barnett JC, Meirowsky AM. Intracranial hematomas associated with penetrating wounds of the brain. *J Neurosurg* 12:34–38, 1955.

14. Berry, FB. Foreword, in, *The Surgery of Theodoric, ca A.D. 1267. Translated from the Latin by Eldridge Campbell and James Colton. Volume One (Books I and II).* New York: Appleton-Century-Crofts, Inc, 1955, pp xxxvii–xl.

15. Blackwood W, McMenemey WH, Meyer A, Norman RM, Russell DS. *Greenfield's Neuropathology.* London: Edward Arnold (Publishers) Ltd, 1969.

16. Borden WC. *The Use of the Roentgen Ray by the Medical Department of the United States Army in the War with Spain (1898).* Washington, DC: U.S. Government Printing Office, 1900.

17. Botallus L. *1660 "Opera omnia" medica et chirurgica.* Batavia, Lugdono: D&A a Gaasbeeck. Cited in Walker, 1951, pp 226, 470.

18. Brawley B, Kelly W. Treatment of skull fractures with and without cerebrospinal fluid fistula. *J Neurosurg* 26:57–61, 1967.

19. Breasted JH. *The Edwin Smith Surgical Papyrus (published in facsimile and hieroglyphic transliteration with translation and commentary in two volumes).* Chicago: University of Chicago Press, 1930.

20. Beller A, Peyser E. Extradural cerebellar hematoma. *J Neurosurg* 9:291–298, 1952.

21. Brenner C, Friedman A, Merritt H, Denny-Brown D. Post-traumatic headache. 1:379–391, 1944.

22. Brock, Samuel (ed): *Injuries of the Brain and Spinal Cord.* London: Cassell, 1960.

23. Browder J, Meyers R. Observations on the behavior of the systemic blood pressure, pulse, and spinal fluid pressure following craniocerebral injury. *Am J Surg* 31:403–427, 1936.

24. Bucy PC. Sulfanilamide in the treatment of brain abscess and prevention of meningitis. *JAMA* 11:1639–1641, 1938.

25. Butler E, Puckett W, Harvey E, McMillen J. Experiments on head wounding by high velocity missiles. *J Neurosurg* 2:358–363, 1945.

26. Cairns H. Injuries of the frontal and ethmoidal sinuses with special reference to cerebrospinal fluid rhinorrhea and aeroceles. *J Laryngol Otol* 52:589–623, 1937.

27. Cairns H. Gunshot wounds of the head in 1940. *J R Army Med Corps* 76:12–61, 1941.

28. Cairns H. Neurosurgery in the British Army, 1939–1945. *Br J Surg (War Surg Suppl)* 1:9–26, 1947.

29. Cairns H, Calvert CA, Daniel P, et al. Delayed complications after head wounds with special reference to intracranial infection. *Br J Surg (War Surg Suppl)* 1:1981-243, 1947.

30. Calcatera TC. Extracranial surgical repair of cerebro-spinal rhinorrhea. *Ann Otol* 89:108–116, 1980.

31. Cantu RC, Ames A III, Doxon J, DiGiacinto G. Reversibility of experimental cerebrovascular obstruction induced by complete ischaemia. *J Neurosurg* 31:429–431, 1969.

32. Carmichael F. The reduction of hernia cerebri by tantalum cranioplasty: A preliminary report. *J Neurosurg* 2:379–383, 1945.

33. Carrie A, Jaffe F. Thrombosis of superior sagittal sinus caused by trauma without penetrating injury. *J Neurosurg* 11:173–182, 1954.

34. Caveness WF, Walker AE (eds): *Head Injury*. Philadelphia and Toronto: Lippincott, 1966.

35. Celsus AC. *De Medicina*, translated by WG Spencer. Cambridge: Harvard University Press, 1935.

36. Celsus AC. *De Medicina, Volume 3*, translated by WG Spencer. London: Heinemann, 1938, pp 509–511 (Cited in Rowbotham, 1964, p 7)

37. Chiari, H. Ueber einem Fall von Luftansammlung in den Ventrikeln des menchlichen Gehirns. *Z Heilkd* 5:383–390, 1884.

38. Coates JB Jr, Meirowsky AM (eds): *Neurological Surgery of Trauma*. Washington, DC: Office of the Surgeon General, Department of the Army, 1965.

39. Connoly RC. The management of the untreated brain wound. *Br J Surg (War Surgery Suppl)* 1:168–172, 1947.

40. Cooper A. *Lectures on the Principles and Practice of Surgery*. London: H. Renshaw, 1839.

41. Courtney JW. Traumatic cerebral edema: Its pathology and surgical treatment—A critical study. *Boston Med Surg J* 140:345–347, 1899.

42. Courville CB. General aspects of pathology of craniocerebral injury, in, Brock S (ed): *Injuries of the Brain and Spinal Cord*. London: Cassell, 1960, pp 23–44.

43. Crow W. Aspects of neuroradiology of head injury. *Neurosurg Clin N Am* 2:321–339, 1991.

44. Cushing HM. Concerning a definite regulatory mechanism of the vasomotor center which controls blood pressure during cerebral compression. *Johns Hopkins Hosp Bull* 12:290–292, 1901.

45. Cushing, HM. Some experimental and clinical observations concerning states of increased intracranial tensions. *Am J Med Sci NS* 124:375–400, 1902.

46. Cushing, HM. Physiologische und anatomische Beobachtungen ueber den Einfluss von Hirnkompression auf die intracraniellen Kreislauf und ueber einige hiermit verwandte Erscheinungen. *Mitt Grenzgeb Med Chir* 9:773–808, 1902.

47. Cushing, HM. The blood pressure reaction of acute cerebral compression, illustrated by cases of intracranial hemorrhage. *Am J Med Sci* 125, 1017–1044, 1903.

48. Cushing, HM. The establishment of cerebral hernia as a decompressive measure for inaccessible brain tumors, with the description of intermuscular methods of making the bone defect in temporal and occipital lesions. *Surg Gynecol Obstet* 1:297–314, 1905.

49. Cushing, HM. Subtemporal decompressive operations for the intracranial complications associated with bursting fractures of the skull. *Ann Surg* 47:641–644, 1908.

50. Cushing, HM. Surgery of the Head, in, Keen W (ed): *Surgery-Its Principles and Practice*. Philadelphia and London: W.B. Saunders, 1908, 3:17–276.

51. Cushing, HM. A study of a series of wounds involving the brain and its enveloping structures. *Br J Surg* 5:558–684, 1918.

52. Dagi TF, George ED. The management of cerebrospinal fluid leaks, in, Schmidek HH, Sweet WH (eds): *Operative Neurosurgical Techniques*. Orlando: Grune & Stratton, 1988, pp 57–69.

53. Dalton JC. *A Treatise on Human Physiology Designed for the use of Students and Practioners of Medicine. Fourth Edition*. Philadelphia: Henry C. Lea, 1867.

54. Dandy W. The treatment of staphylococcus and streptococcus meningitis by continuous drainage of the cisterna magna. *Surg Gynecol Obstet* 39:760–744, 1924.

55. Dandy WE. Pneumocephalus (intracranial pneumatocele or aerocele). *Arch Surg* 12:949–982, 1926.

56. Dandy WE. Treatment of rhinorrhea and otorrhea. *Arch Surg* 49:75–85, 1944.

57. Davidoff LM, Feiring EH. Gunshot wounds of the brain and their complications, in, Brock S (ed): *Injuries of the Brain and Spinal Cord*. London: Cassell, 1960, pp 218–254.

58. Denny-Brown D, Russell WR. Experimental cerebral concussion. *Brain* 64:93–164, 1941.

59. Desault PJ. *Oevres Chirugicales*. Maria Xavier Bichat (ed): Paris: Meguigon, 1801–1803.

60. Dickinson E, Pastor B. Two cases of acute subdural hygroma simulating massive intracranial hemorrhage. *J Neurosurg* 5:98–101, 1948.

61. Dionis, P. *Cours d'Operations de Chirurgie*. Paris, 1740. Cited by Rowbotham, 1964, p 9, note 1.

62. Dodge P, Meirowsky A. Tangential wounds of scalp and skull. *J Neurosurg* 9:472–483, 1952.

63. Dohlman, G. Spontaneous cerebrospinal rhinorrhoea: Case operated by rhinologic methods. *Acta Otolaryngol (Stockholm) (Suppl)* 67:20–23, 1948.

64. Dow R, Ulett G, Raaf J. Electroencephalographic studies in head injuries. *J Neurosurg* 2:154–169, 1945.

65. Duret, H. *Etudes experimentales sur les traumatismes cerebraux*. Paris. 1878. Cited by Walker, 1951, p 488, reference 675.

66. Duret, H. *Traumatismes craniocerebraux*. Paris: Librairie Felix Alcan, 1920.

67. Echlim F. Traumatic subdural hematoma—Acute, subacute and chronic: An Analysis of Seventy Operated Cases. *J Neurosurg* 6:294–303, 1949.

68. Ecker A. A bacteriologic study of penetration wounds of the brain, from the surgical point of view. *J Neurosurg* 3:1–6, 1946.

69. Ecker AD. Tight dural closure with pedicled graft in wounds of the brain. *J Neurosurg* 2:384–390, 1945.

70. Eden K. Traumatic cerebrospinal rhinorrhoea: Repair of a fistula by a transfrontal intradural operation. *Br J Surg* 29:299–303, 1941.

71. Einhorn A, Mizrahia EM. Basilar skull fractures in children: Incidence of CNS infection and the use of antibiotics. *Am J Dis Child* 132:1121–1124, 1979.

72. Elsberg CA. Operations on the brain and its membranes, in, Johnson AB (ed): *Operative Therapeusis*. New York and London: D. Appleton and Co, 1921, pp 659–736.

73. Evans J, Scheinker M. Histologic studies of the brain following head trauma; IV. Late changes: Atrophic sclerosis of the white matter. *J Neurosurg* 1:306–320, 1944.

74. Evans J, Scheinker M. Histologic Studies of the brain following head trauma; I. Post-traumatic cerebral swelling and edema. *J Neurosurg* 2:306–314, 1945.

75. Evans J, Scheinker M. Histologic studies of the brain following head trauma; II. Post-traumatic petechial and massive intracerebral hemorrhage. *J Neurosurg* 3:101–113, 1946.

76. Faria Jr, Miguel A. The death of Henry II of France. *J Neurosurg* 77:964–969, 1992.

77. Falconer M, Russell D. Experimental traumatic cerebral cysts in the rabbit. *J Neurosurg* 1:182–189, 1944.

78. Feinstein G, Silver CE. Infection control in head and neck surgery. *J Surg Pract* March/April:13–20, 1979.

79. Fincher E. Microcephalus secondary to birth trauma. *J Neurosurg* 1:265–274, 1944.

80. Findler G, Sahar A, Beller AJ. Continuous lumbar drainage of cerebrospinal fluid in neurosurgical patients. *Surg Neurol* 8:455–457, 1977.

81. Finlayson AI. Penetrating war injuries of the brain. Desirability of early definitive surgery. *Bull US Army Med Dept* 87:61–69, 1945.

82. Fisher RG. Surgery of the congenital anomalies, in, Walker AE (ed): *A History of Neurological Surgery.* Baltimore: Williams and Wilkins, 1951, pp 334–361.

83. Friedman A, Brenner C, Denny-Brown D. Post-traumatic vertigo and dizziness. *J Neurosurg* 2:36–46, 1945.

84. Fuller JFC. *Armament and History.* New York: Charles Scribner & Sons, 1945.

85. Fullerton GD. Basic concepts for nuclear magnetic resonance imaging. *Magn Reson Imaging* 1:39–53, 1982.

86. George ED, Dagi TF. Penetrating missile injuries of the head, in, Schmidek HH, Sweet WH (eds): *Operative Neurosurgical Techniques.* Orlando: Grune & Stratton, 1988, pp 49–55.

87. George ED, Dagi TF. Military penetrating craniocerebral injuries: Applications to civilian triage and management. *Neurosurg Clin NA* 6:753–760, 1995.

88. German W. Neurological surgery: Its past, present and future. *J Neurosurg* 10:526–537, 1953.

89. Giannotta SL, Zee CS. Imaging in acute head injury, in, Pitts LH, Wagner FC (eds): *Craniospinal Trauma.* New York: Thieme Medical Publishers, 1990, pp 25–36.

90. Giordano D. Sulla patria e sulla chirurgia di Frate Teodorico. *Revista di Storia delle Scienze Mediche e Naturali* 21:3–22, 1930.

91. Giordano D. Ancora sulla identita di Teodorico. *Revista di Storia delle Scienze Mediche e Naturali* 21:133–137, 1930.

92. Glaser M, Shafer F. Depressed fractures of the skull: Their surgery, sequelae and disability. *J Neurosurg* 2:140–153, 1945.

93. Goerke, H. Ernst von Bergmann, in, Treue W, Winau R (eds): *Berlinisce Lebensbilder II Mediziner.* Berlin: Colloquium Verlag, 1987, pp 191–202.

94. Gorky P. Case report and technical notes: Extradural hemorrhage of the anterior and posterior fossae. *J Neurosurg* 5:294–298, 1948.

95. Grant FC. Intracranial aerocele following fracture of the skull. Report of a case with review of the literature. *Surg Gynecol Obstet* 36:251–255, 1923.

96. Grantham E. Cranioplasty and the post-traumatic syndrome. *J Neurosurg* 5:19–22, 1948.

97. Greenwood J Jr. Removal of foreign body (bullet) from the third ventricle. *J Neurosurg* 7:169–172, 1950.

98. Groat R, Windle W, Magoun H. Functional and structural changes in the monkey's brain during and after concussion. *J Neurosurg* 2:26–35, 1945.

99. Gross S. Pneumocephalus secondary to a penetrating wound of the brain. *J Neurosurg* 5:405–406, 1948.

100. Gurdjian ES, Lissner HR. Mechanism of head injury as studied by the cathode ray oscilloscope. *J Neurosurg* 1:393–399, 1944.

101. Gurdjian ES, Webster JE. *Head Injuries: Mechanisms, Diagnosis, and Management.* Boston: Little Brown & Co, 1958.

102. Gurdjian E, Webster J, Lissner H. The mechanism of skull fracture. *J Neurosurg* 7:106–114, 1950.

103. Guthkelch A. Extradural haemorrhage as a cause of cortical blindness. *J Neurosurg* 6:180–182, 1949.

104. Hagan RE. Early complications following penetrating wounds of the brain. *J Neurosurg* 34:132–141, 1971.

105. Hamby WB. *Ambroise Paré: Surgeon of the Renaissance.* St. Lous: Warren H. Green, 1967.

106. Hammon WM. Analysis of 2,187 consecutive penetrating wounds of the brain from Vietnam. *J Neurosurg* 34:121–131, 1971a.

107. Hammon WM. Retained intracranial bone fragments: Analysis of 42 patients. *J Neurosurg* 34:142–144, 1971b.

108. Hans JS, et. al. Head trauma evaluated by magnetic resonance and computed tomography: A comparison. *Radiology* 150:71–77, 1984.

109. Haynes WG. Penetrating brain wounds: Analysis of 342 cases. *J Neurosurg* 2:365–378, 1945.

110. Haynes W. Transventricular wounds of the brain. *J Neurosurg* 2:463–468, 1945.

111. Haynes W. Extensive brain wounds: Analysis of 159 cases occurring in a series of 342 penetration war wounds of the brain. *J Neurosurg* 2:469–478, 1945.

112. Hill L. *The Physiology and Pathology of the Cerebral Circulation. An Experimental Research.* London: J & A Churchill, 1896.

113. *Hippocrates On Wounds of the Head.* Translated by Withington. *Loeb Classical Library. Hippocrates, Vol 3.* London: Heinemann, 1927. (Cited in Rowbotham, 1964, p 6, note 2)

114. Hodgson JS. The relationship between increased intracranial pressure and increased intraspinal pressure: Changes in the cerebrospinal fluid in increased intracranial pressure. *Assoc Res Nerv Ment Dis* 8:182–188, 1927.

115. Holbourn A. The mechanics of trauma with special reference to herniation of cerebral tissue. *J Neurosurg* 1:190–200, 1944.

116. Holbourn AHS. The mechanics of brain injuries. *Br Med Bull* 3:147–149, 1945.

117. Hounsfield GN. Computerized transverse axial scanning (tomography). Part I: Description of system. *Br J Radiol* 46:1016–1022, 1973.

118. Hutchinson, J. On compression of the brain. *London Hosp Rep* 4:29, 1867. (Cited by Rowbotham, 1964, p 3, note 4)

119. Hutchinson, J. *Illustrations of Clinical Surgery.* London: Churchill, 1978.

120. Hutchinson, J. On middle meningeal haemorrhage.

Guy's Hosp Rep 43:273, 1886. (Cited by Rowbotham, 1964, p 4, note 1)

121. Irsigler FJ. *The Neurosurgical Approach to Intracranial Infections. A Review of Personal Experiences 1940–1960.* Berlin: Springer-Verlag, 1961.

122. Jaboulay M. La trepanation decompressive. *Lyon Med* 83:73–75, 1896.

123. Jackson I, Speakman T. Chronic extradural hematoma. *J Neurosurg* 7:444–447, 1950.

124. Jefferson, G. Gunshot wounds of the scalp with special reference to the neurological signs presented. *Brain* 42: 93–112, 1919.

125. Jefferson, G. The tentorial pressure cone. *Arch Neurol Psychiatry* 40:857–876, 1938.

126. Jennett B. Historical development of head injury care, in, Pitts LH, Wagner FC (eds): *Craniospinal Trauma.* New York: Thieme Medical Publishers, Inc, 1990, pp 1–10.

127. Jennett B, Teasedale G. *Management of Head Injury.* Philadelphia: FA Davis Company, 1981.

128. Jennett B, Teasdale G, Galbraith S, et. al. Severe head injuries in three countries. *J Neurol Neurosurg Psychiatry* 40:291–298, 1977.

129. Kaplan A. Traumatic pneumocephalus with spontaneous ventriculograms: Report of a case. *J Neurosurg* 1:166–170, 1944.

130. Keen WW. *The Treatment of War Wounds.* Philadelphia and London: Saunders, 1917.

131. Kellie G. An account of the appearances observed in the dissection of two of three individuals presumed to have perished in the storm of the 3d, and whose bodies were discovered in the vicinity of Leith on the morning of the 4th November 1821, with some reflections on the pathology of the brain. *Trans Med-Chir-Soc Edinb* 1:84–169, 1824

132. Kety SS, Shenkin HA, Schmidt CF. The effects of increased intracranial pressure on cerebral circulatory function in man. *J Clin Invest* 27:493–499, 1948.

133. Key A, Retzius G. *Studier I nervsystemets anatomi.* Stockholm. P. A. Norstedt & Soneo, 1872. (Cited by Walker, 1951, note 1237, p 512)

134. Kim PE, Zee CS. The radiologic evaluation of craniocerebral missile injuries. *Neurosurg Clin N Am* 6: 559–687, 1995.

135. Kishore PRS, Hall JA. Radiographic evaluation, in, Cooper P (ed): *Head Injury.* Baltimore: Williams and Wilkins, 1987, pp 51–71.

136. Kocher, T. *Text-book of Operative Surgery. Third English Edition.* Translated from the Fifth German Edition by Harold J. Stiles and C. Balfour Paul. New York: MacMillan, 1911.

137. Kraus JF. Epidemiology of head injury, in, Cooper P (ed): *Head Injury.* Baltimore: Williams and Wilkins, 1987, pp 1–19.

138. Krayenbuhl HA. Questions and answers. *Clin Neurosurg* 14:23–24, 1967.

139. Lanfrank. *Science of Cirurgie. Early English Text Society, Original Series 102.* Berlin: Asher & Co.; New York: C. Scribner & Co.; Philadelphia: J.B. Lippincott & Co., 1894, pp 360. (Cited in Walker, 1951, pp 224, 516)

140. Langfitt TW. Increased intracranial pressure. *Clin Neurosurg* 16:436–471, 1969.

141. Langfitt TW, Tannanbaum HM, Kassell NF. The etiol-

ogy of acute brain swelling following experimental head injury. *J Neurosurg* 24:47–56, 1966.

142. Lanksch W, Gramme TH. *Computed Tomography of Head Injuries.* Berlin: Springer Verlag, 1979.

143. Leech PJ, Patterson R. Conservative and operative management for cerebrospinal leakage after closed head injury. *Lancet* 1:1013–1016, 1973.

144. Lemmen L, Schneider R. Extradural hematomas of the posterior fossa. *J Neurosurg* 9:245–253, 1952.

145. Lewin W. Cerebrospinal fluid rhinorrhea in closed head injuries. *Br J Surg* 42:1–18, 1954.

146. Lewin, W. Cerebrospinal fluid rhinorrhea in non-missile head injuries. *Clin Neurosurg* 12:237–254, 1966.

147. Lewin W, Gibson RM. Missile head wounds in the Korean campaign: Survey of British casualties. *Br J Surg* 43:628–632, 1956.

148. Lister J. On the antiseptic principle in the practice of surgery. *Lancet* 2:353–356, 1867.

149. Littre, A. *Histoire de l'Academie royale des Sciences.* Paris, 1705. (Cited by Walker, 1951, p 519, reference 1399)

150. Livingston C, Lieut U, Davis E. "Delayed recovery" in peripheral nerve lesions caused by high velocity projectile wounding. *J Neurosurg* 2:170–179, 1945.

151. Lockhart W Jr, Van Den Noort G, Kimsey W, Groff R. A comparison of polyethylene and tantalum for cranioplasty. *J Neurosurg* 9:254–257, 1952.

152. Luckett WH. Air in the ventricles of the brain, following a fracture of the skull. Report of a case. *Surg Gynecol Obstet* 17:237–240, 1913.

153. Lundberg N. Continuous recording and control of ventricular fluid pressure in neurosurgical practice. *Acta Psychol Neurol Scand (Suppl)* 36:149, 1960.

154. Lundberg N. Monitoring of the intracranial pressure, in, Critchley M, O'Leary JL, Jennett B (eds): *Scientific Foundations of Neurology.* London: William Heineman Medical Books Ltd., 1972, pp 356–371.

155. MacCallum WG. *William Stewart Halstead.* Baltimore: Johns Hopkins University Press, 1930.

156. MacCarty S, Horning D, Weaver E. Bilateral extradural hematoma: Report of a case. *J Neurosurg* 5: 88–90 1948.

157. Macewen W. Discussion on the aseptic treatment of wounds. *Br Med J* 2:804, 1904.

158. MacIver IN, Frew JC, Matheson JG. The role of respiratory insufficiency in the mortality of severe head injuries. *Lancet* 1:390, 1958. (Cited in Jennett and Teasdale, 1981, p 2, note 27)

159. MacLeod GHB. *Notes on the Surgery of the War in the Crimea, With Remarks on the Treatment of Gunshot Wounds.* Richmond, Va.: J.W. Randolph, 1862.

160. Magendie, F. *Rechereches philosophiques et clinicques sur le liquide cephalorachidien ou cerebrospinal.* Paris: Mequignon-Marvis, 1842.

161. Maltby G. Penetration craniocerebral injuries: Evaluation of the late results in a group of 200 consecutive penetration cranial war wounds. *J Neurosurg* 3: 239–249, 1946.

162. Martin J, Campbell EH Jr. Early complications following penetrating wounds of the skull. *J Neurosurg* 3: 58–73, 1946.

163. Matson DD. *The Treatment of Acute Craniocerebral Injuries due to Missiles.* Springfield, IL: Charles C. Thomas, 1948.

164. Matson DD, Wolin J. Hematomas associated with pen-

etrating wounds of the brain. *J Neurosug* 3:46–53, 1946.

165. McCabe NF. The osteo-mucoperiosteal flap in repair of cerebrospinal fluid rhinorrhea. *Laryngoscope* 86(4): 537–539, 1976.

166. McCallum J, Maroon JC, Janetta PJ. Treatment of postoperative cerebrospinal fluid fistulas by subarachnoid drainage. *J Neurosurg* 42:434–437, 1975.

167. McIntyre, AO. *Medieval Tuscany and Umbria*. San Francisco: Chronicle Books, 1992.

168. Meirowsky A. Wounds of dural sinuses. *J Neurosurg* 10:496–514, 1953.

169. Meirowsky, AM. *Penetrating Craniocerebral Trauma*. Springfield, IL:Charles C. Thomas, 1984.

170. Meredith J. Chronic or subacute subdural hematoma due to indirect head trauma. *J Neurosurg* 8:444–447, 1951.

171. Meyer JS, Welch KMA. Relationship of cerebral blood flow and metabolism to neurological symptoms. *Brain Res* 35:285–348, 1972.

172. Miller C. Case of hydrocephalus chronicus with some unusual symptoms and appearances on dissection. *Trans Med-Chir Soc Edinb* 2:243–248, 1826.

173. Miller D, Adams H. Physiopathology and management of increased intracranial pressure, in, Critchley M, O'Leary JL, Jennett B (eds.): *Scientific Foundations of Neurology*. London: William Heineman Medical Books Ltd., 1972, pp 308–324.

174. Monro, Alexander secundus. *Observations on the Structure and Function of the Nervous System*. Edinburgh: Creech and Johnson, 1783.

175. Munro D. *Cranio-Cerebral Injuries: Their Diagnosis and Treatment*. London, New York, Toronto: Oxford University Press, 1938.

176. Nichols P, Manganiello J. Case reports and technical notes: Traumatic arachnoidal cyst simulating acoustic neurinoma. *J Neurosurg* 10:538–539, 1953.

177. Northfield DWC. *The Surgery of the Central Nervous System*. Oxford: Blackwell Scientific Publications, 1973.

178. Ommaya AK. Spinal fluid fistulae. *Clin Neurosurg* 23: 363–392, 1975.

179. Ommaya AK. Trauma to the nervous system. *Ann R Coll Surg Engl* 39:317–347, 1966.

180. Ommaya AK, Grubb RL, Naumann RA. Coup and contre-coup injury: Observations on the mechanics of visible brain injuries in the rhesus monkey. *J Neurosurg* 38:503–516, 1971.

181. Orr HW. The development of the concept of antisepsis and asepsis from Lister to World War II. *Int Abstracts Surg* 85(3):209–224, 1947.

182. Packard GR. *The Life and Times of Ambroise Paré*. New York: Hoeber, 1926.

183. Paré, A. *La methode curative des playes, et fractures de la test humaine, avec les pourtraits des instruments necessaires pour la curation d'icelles*. Paris: Le Royer, 1561.

184. Pilcher C, Meacham WF. The chemotherapy of intracranial infections. IV. The treatment of pneumococcal meningitis by intrathecal administration of penicillin. *J Neurosurg* I:76–81, 1944.

185. Pitlyk PJ, Tolchin S, Stewart W. The experimental significance of retained intracranial bone fragments. *J Neurosurg* 33:19–24, 1970.

186. Plum F. Organic disturbances in consciousness, in

Critchley M, O'Leary JL, Jennett B (eds): *Scientific Foundations of Neurology*, London: William Heineman Medical Books Ltd., 1972, pp 193–201.

187. Polin RS, Shaffrey MA, Phillips CD, Germanson T, Jane J. Multivariate analysis and prediction of outcome following penetrating head injury. *Neurosurg Clin N Am* 6:689–699, 1995.

188. Pott P. Remarks on that kind of palsy of the lower limbs which is frequently found to accompany a curvature of the spine and is supposed to be caused by it; together with its method of care; etc. London: J. Johnson, 1779.

189. Pott P. *Chirurgical works of Percivall Pott, F.R.S.* Earle J (ed): Philadelphia: J. Webster, 1819. (Cited in Walker, 1951, pp 226, 535 but ascribed in error to Pott, 1779 [q.v.].)

190. Pudenz RH, Shelden CH. The lucite calvarium: A method for direct observation of the brain. II Cranial trauma and brain movement. *J Neurosurg* 3:487–505, 1946.

191. Quincke H. Die Diagnostiche und therapeutische Bedeutung der Lumbarpunktion. Klinischer Vortrag. *Deutsche med Wchnschr* 31:182501828, 1869–1972, 1905.

192. Ramsey R. *Neuroradiology*. Philadelphia: W. B. Saunders, 1987.

193. Raney A, Raney R, Hunter C. Chronic post-traumatic headache and the syndrome of cervical disc lesion following head trauma. *J Neurosurg* 6:458–465, 1949.

194. Ransohoff J. The effects of steroids on brain oedema in man, in, Reulen nad Schurmann (eds): *Steroids and Brain Oedema*. Berlin: Springer Verlag, 1972. (Cited in Jennett and Teasdale, p 242, note 75)

195. Risberg J, Lundberg N, Ingvar DH. Regional cerebral blood volume during acute transient rises of the intracranial pressure (Plateau Waves). *J Neurosurg* 31: 303–310, 1969.

196. Rowbotham GF. *Acute Injuries of the Head: Their Diagnosis, Treatment, Complications and Sequels. 4th Edition*. Edinburgh and London: E & S Livingstone Ltd., 1964.

197. Rowe SN. The use of sulfanilamide in the treatment of brain abscess. Report of two cases. *Ann Surg* 107: 620–626, 1938.

198. Rowe SN, Turner OA. Observations on infection in penetrating wounds of the head. *J Neurosurg* 2: 391–401, 1945.

199. Ruge D. The use of cholinergic blocking agents in the treatment of cranio-cerebral injuries. *J Neurosurg* 11: 77–83, 1954.

200. Salazar AM, Schwab K, Grafman, JH. Penetrating injuries in the Vietnam War: Traumatic unconsciousness, epilepsy, and psychosocial outcome, 1995.

201. Sargent P, Holmes G. The treatment of penetrating wounds of the skull. *Br J Surg* 3:475–489, 1916.

202. Saugous E. *Annual of the Universal Medical Sciences*. Philadelphia: Davis, 1885.

203. Saul TG. Intracranial pressure monitoring and treatment, in, Pitts LH, Wagner FC (ed): *Craniospinal Trauma*. New York: Thieme Medical Publishers, 1990, pp 97–109.

204. Scagliosi G. Ueber die Gehirnschuetterung und die daraus im Gehirn und Rueckenmark hervorgerufnen histologischen Veraenderungen. *Virchows Arch Pathol Anat* 152:487–525, 1898.

205. Scheinker M. Cerebral swelling: Histopathology, clas-

sification and clinical significance of brain edema. *J Neurosurg* 4:255–275, 1947.

206. Schneider R. Fat embolism: A problem in the differential diagnosis of craniocerebral trauma. *J Neurosurg* 9:1–13, 1952.

207. Schneider R, Lemmen L. Traumatic internal carotid artery thrombosis secondary to non-penetrating injuries to the neck. *J Neurosurg* 9:495–507, 1952.

208. Schneider R, Lemmen L, Bagchi B. The syndrome of traumatic intracerebellar hematoma, with contrecoup supratentorial complications. *J Neurosurg* 10:122–137, 1953.

209. Schorstein J. Intracranial hematoma in missile wounds. *Br J Surgery (War Surg Suppl)* 1:96–111, 1947.

210. Schwartz H, Parker J. Early nerve and bone repair in war wounds. *J Neurosurg* 2:510–515, 1945.

211. Sharp S. *A Treatise on the Operations of Surgery with a Description and Representation of the Instruments Used in Performing Them*. London: J and R Tonson and S Draper, 1751.

212. Sharpe W. The treatment of fracture of the skull, in, Johnson AB (ed): *Operative Therapeusis*. New York and London: D Appleton and Co., 1921, pp 581–657.

213. Shoung HM, Sichez JP, Pertuiser B. The early prognosis of craniocerebral gunshot wounds in civilian practice as an aid to the choice of treatment. A review of 49 cases studied by the computerized tomography. *Acta Neurochir (Wien)* 74:27–30, 1985.

214. Smith G, Mosberg W, Pfeil E, Oster R. The electroencephalogram in subdural hematoma; with a review of the literature and the presentation of seven cases. *J Neurosurg* 7:207–218, 1950.

215. Stern WE. Surgery of the craniocerebral infections, in, Walker AE (ed): *A History of Neurological Surgery*. Baltimore: Williams and Wilkins, 1951, pp 180–212.

216. Storey W, Love W. Traumatic bilateral abducent and facial paralysis with good restoration of function: A case report. *J Neurosurg* 6:539–542, 1949.

217. Stortebecker T. Posttramatic oculocardiac syndrome from a neurosurgical point of view. *J Neurosurg* 10:682–685, 1953.

218. Stromeyer L. *Verletzungen und chirirgische Krankheiten des Kopfes*. Freiburg: Herder's Verlag, 1864.

219. Symonds, C. Concussion and contusion of the brain and their sequelae, in, Brock S (ed): *Injuries of the Brain and Spinal Cord*. London: Cassell, 1960, pp 69–116.

220. Taha JM, Saba MI, Brown JA. Missile injuries to the brain treated by simple wound closure: Results of a protocol during the Lebanese conflict. *Neurosurgery* 29:380–383, 1991.

221. Taveras J, Ransohoff J. Leptomeningeal cysts of the brain following trauma with erosion of the skull. *J Neurosurg* 10:233–241, 1953

222. Teasdale G, Jennett B. Assessment of coma and impaired consciousness: A practical scale. *Lancet* 2:81–84, 1974,

223. Theodoric. *Incipit cyrurgia edita et compilata a divino fratre Theodorico episcopo Cerviensi ordinis praedicatorum*. In, Guy de Chauliac, Cyrurgia Guidonis de Cauliaco. Venice, 1499, pp 97–134. (Cited in Walker, 1951, pp 223, 551)

224. Theodoric. *The Surgery of Theodoric, ca A.D. 1267. Translated from the Latin by Eldridge Campbell and James Colton. Volume One (Books I and II)*. New York: Appleton-Century-Crofts, Inc, 1955.

225. Thompson RK, Jacson IJ, Christoferson LA, Strewler GJ, Weaver EN. *Clinical Neurosurgery. Volume I*. Baltimore: Williams and Wilkins, 1955, pp iii.

226. Thorek M. *Modern Surgical Technique*. Philadelphia: JB Lippincott Co, 1938.

227. Troland C, Baxter D, Schatzki R. Observation on encephalographic Findings in cerebral trauma. *J Neurosurg* 3:390–398, 1946.

228. Turnbull F. Extradural cerebellar hematoma: A case report. *J Neurosurg* 1:321–324, 1944.

229. Turner O. Arterio-venous angioma (hamartoma) of the brain with intracerebral hemorrhage: Report of a case with operative removal of the hematoma and recovery. *J Neurosurg* 3:542–548, 1946.

230. Turner O. Tantalum cranioplasty and repeated trauma. *J Neurosurg* 9:100–103, 1952.

231. Valsalva AM. *Joannis Baptistae Morgagni epistolarum anatomicarum duodeviginti ad scripta pertinetium celeberrimi viri Antonii Marie Valsalvae pars altera*. Venice: F Pitterus, 1741. (Cited by Walker, 1951, note 2202, p 553)

232. Verbiest H. Post-traumatic pulsating exophthalmos: Cause by perforation of an eroded orbital roof by a hydrocephalic brain. *J Neurosurg* 10:264–271, 1953.

233. Vidius V. *Chirurgia e Graeco in Latinum conversa*. Paris: Galterius, 1554.

234. Vidius V. *Les Anciencs et Renommes Auctors de la Medicine et chirurgia*. Lyon: Rouille, 1555.

235. Villanova A. *Opera Omnia. Basle*: Perna, 1585. (Cited by Rowbotham, 1967, p 7)

236. Vollmer DG, Dacey RG. Prediction and assessment of outcome following closed head injury, in, Pitts LH, Wagner FC (eds): *Craniospinal Trauma*. New York: Thieme Medical Publishers, 1990, pp 120–140.

237. Von Bergmann E. *Surgical Treatment of Diseases of the Brain: Wood's Medical and Surgical Monographs*. New York: Wm. Wood & Co, 1890.

238. Vourc'h G. Continuous cerebrospinal fluid drainage by indwelling spinal catheter. *Br J Anaesth* 35:118–120, 1963.

239. Wagstaffe WW. *Official History of the War. Medical Services Surgery of the War. Volume 2., Chapter. 1*, 1922. (Cited by Rowbotham, 1964, p 84, note 1)

240. Wakely CPG, Orley A. *A Textbook of Neuro-Radiology*. London: Balliere, Tinadall and Cox, 1938.

241. Walker A, Kollros J, Case T. The Physiological Bases of Concussion. *J Neurosurg* 1:103–116, 144.

242. Walker AE. *Post-Traumatic Epilepsy*. Springfield, Ill. Charles C. Thomas, 1949.

243. Walker, AE. *A History of Neurological Surgery*, Baltimore: Williams & Wilkins Press, 1951.

244. Wannamaker G. Transventricular wounds of the brain. *J Neurosurg* 11:151–160, 1954

245. Ward A Jr. Atropine in the treatment of closed head injury. *J Neurosurg* 7:398–402, 1950.

246. Ward B. *Miracles and the Medieval Mind*. Hampshire: Wildwood House, 1982.

247. Ward JD. Intensive care management of the head-injured patient, in, Pitts LH, Wagner FC (eds): *Craniospinal Trauma*. New York: Thieme Medical Publishers, 1990, pp 88–96.

248. Weaver TA, Fishman AJ. Treatment of craniocerebral wounds. *J Neurosurg* 3:149–156, 1994.

249. Webster J, Dawson R, Gurdjian E. The diagnosis of traumatic intracranial hemorrhage by angiography. *J Neurosurg* 8:368–376, 1951.

250. Webster J, Schneider R, Lofstorm J. Observations on early type of brain abscess following penetrating wounds of the brain. *J Neurosurg* 3:7–14, 1946.

251. Webster J, Schneider R, Lofstorm J. Observations upon the management of orbito-cranial wounds. *J Neurosurg* 3:329–336, 1946.

252. Weed L. Some limitations of the Monro-Kellie hypothesis. *Arch Surg (Chicago)* 18:1049–1068, 1929.

253. Weed LH, McKibben PS. Pressure changes in the cerebrospinal fluid following intravenous injections of solutions of various concentrations. *Am J Physiol* 48: 512–530, 1919.

254. Weed LH, McKibben PS. Experimental alteration of brain bulk. *Am J Physiol* 48:531–555, 1919.

255. Weisenburg TH (ed.): *Manual of Neuro-Surgery*. Washington: Government Printing Office, 1919.

256. White J. Suture of facial nerve after injury at base of skull: Method of gaining exposure and slack by resection of parotid gland. *J Neurosurg* 5:284–287, 1948.

257. Wilkins RH. *Neurosurgical Classics*. New York and London: Johnson Reprint Corporation, 1965, pp 242–256.

258. Windle W, Rambach W, Arellano M, Groat R, Becker R. Water content of the brain after concussion and its noncontributory relation to the histopathology of concussion. *J Neurosurg* 3:157–164, 1946.

259. Woodhall B, Neill RG, Dratz HM. Ultraviolet radiation as an adjunct in the control of post-operative neurosurgical infection. *Ann Surg* 129:4–8, 1949.

260. Zimmerman IM, Veith I. *Great Ideas in the History of Surgery*. Baltimore: Williams and Wilkins, 1961. (Cited as note 1 in Bakay, 1971, p 104)

261. Zimmerman RA, Bialaniuk LT, Genarelli T, Bruce D, Dolinskas C, Uzzell B. Cranial computed tomography and head injury in diagnosis and management of acute head trauma. *Am J Roentgen* 131:27–34, 1978.

10

Pain and the Neurosurgeon

Ronald R. Tasker, MD, MA, FRCS(C)

INTRODUCTION

Pain has always been of primary concern of physicians, and neurosurgery a major agent in its attempted relief. As we review neurosurgical developments from 1950 to 2000, the reader may find it interesting to score the progress in different areas in order to assess how we are doing as we enter the 21st century.

THEORIES OF PAIN

Before reviewing neurosurgical techniques, it is essential to first review how pain is signaled and experienced. Bonica (7) summarized this matter succinctly and noted that in addition to the Aristotelian concept of pain as an affective quality, two conflicting proposals dominated the 19th century. The specificity theory and the intensive or summation theories are illustrated in Figures 10.1 and 10.2. The first is self-explanatory and well illustrated in the famous diagram reproduced in Figure 10.1. The intensive or summation theory proposed that pain resulted from excessive stimulation of the sense of touch, which implied central summation at the dorsal horn. When a critical level of summation was achieved, threshold was exceeded either by excessive stimulation of receptors normally fired by non-noxious stimuli or as the result of patho-

logical processes. As a result, pain was triggered and transmitted centrally. The reader will recognize the essentials of this proposal in contemporary literature. Goldscheider, a major proponent of the summation theory, believed that slowly conducting multisynaptic pathways transmitted the above-described summated effect to the brain, while the dorsal columns carried discriminative information.

Bonica records that in 1943, Livingston (48) devised his own concept of central summation based on ''reverberating activity'' and ''vicious cycles.'' In this author's opinion, Livingston's major contribution was to start the process of recognizing neuropathic pain, already clinically identified by such authors as Weir Mitchell (55) in 1864 and Riddock in 1938 (72) as a distinct entity from nociceptive pain and with a distinct pathophysiology. Livingston's book, entitled *Pain Mechanisms: A Physiologic Interpretation of Causalgia and its Related States,* contains chapters on causalgia and reflex paralysis, minor causalgia, post-traumatic pain syndromes, chronic low back pain disability, facial neuralgias, and phantom limb pain.

At about this time, the fourth theory of pain was postulated. This theory described pain as a dichotomy between a simple neurophysiological process of perception of pain and a complex physiopsychological cognitive reaction to pain.

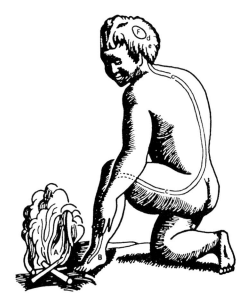

FIGURE 10.1. Descartes' (1664) concept of the pain pathway. He writes, "If for example fire (A) comes near the foot (B), the minute particles of this fire, which as you know move with great velocity, have the power to set in motion the spot of the skin of the foot which they touch, and by this means pulling upon the delicate thread (cc) which is attached to the spot of the skin, they open up at the same instant the pore (de) against which the delicate thread ends, just as by pulling at one end of a rope makes to strike at the same instant a bell which hangs at the other end."

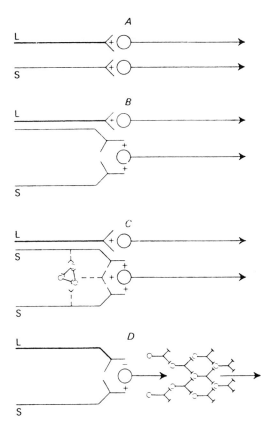

FIGURE 10.2. Diagrammatic representation of historical pain theories.

A. *Specificity Theory*: large fibers (L) transmit the sensation of touch, small (S), pain. (von Frey).

B. *Summation Theory*: large fibers (L) transmit touch, small (S), pain when they converge on dorsal horn (Goldscheider).

C. *Reverberatory Circuits*: pain fibers (S) initiate prolonged activity in a self-exciting chain of neurons that bombard dorsal horn cells which, in turn, transmit abnormally patterned volleys rostrally (Livingston).

D. *Interaction Theory*: large fibers (L) inhibit, small (S) excite central transmission neurons projecting to a multisynaptic system projecting to the brain (Noordenbos).

PAIN NEUROSURGERY UP TO 1950

In 1955, White and Sweet (100)published *Pain: Its Mechanisms and Neurosurgical Control*. This monumental book was based on the authors' experience with 420 pain patients operated upon from 1935 to 1949 in the context of an elaborate discussion and literature review. It established the state of the art as of 1950. Although the authors agreed with Ambroise Paré, who stated in the 16th century "For there is nothing that abateth so much the strength as paine," the book demonstrated how far pain treatment had come since Paré's time. (The latter considered pouring boiling oil into the wound he had made in the arm of Charles IX during bleeding for smallpox, which had inadvertently damaged a sensory nerve and produced neuropathic pain.) The authors quoted Weir Mitchell from the 19th century, who stated "Perhaps few persons who are not physicians can realize the influence which long-continued and unendurable pain may have upon both body and mind."

White and Sweet attribute the first pain textbook that dealt mostly with facial pain and extremity neurectomy to Létiévant. It was published in 1873. They traced the beginning of neurosurgical treatment of pain to Horsley's Gasserian neurectomy for tic douloureux in 1891, leading on to the Frazier procedure in the early years of the 20th century. Meanwhile, in 1911, Abbe drew attention to spinal dorsal rhizotomy and Spiller recognized the spinothalamic tract in the spinal cord in 1905 (which led to the first [open] cordotomy by Martin in 1912). In addition, Foerster mapped spinal dermatomes in 1933 and François-Franck introduced sympathectomy in 1899, which was used by Leriche in 1913 for the treatment of vasoconstrictive disease. The work of Fulton and Jacobsen in 1935 and Moniz in 1936 led to frontal leucotomy, which proved useful in treating certain pain states. Other landmarks recognized by White and Sweet included Mitchell's monographs on pain in 1864 and 1872, and the publications by Foerster in 1927, Lewis in 1942, and Leriche in 1949.

Sir Geoffrey Jefferson's foreword to White and Sweets' book indicates what level the overall philosophy of pain had progressed to at the beginning of the 1950s. He stated ''until it (pain) had been broken down, until its components had been identified in much the same sense as that in which the chemists broke down seemingly homogeneous substances into several different ones in combination, confusion reigned. But once order had been found perhaps we got too simple an idea of what pain really is, neglecting its differences in different sites, 'what it feels like here or there.' '' These words suggest the beginning of a new concept that not all pain syndromes had the same pathophysiology and therefore, would not respond to the same treatment. Jefferson went on to disavow Sir Henry Head's teaching that pain was a ''low or primitive'' type of feeling appropriate to lower animals rather than to men, i.e., ''a debased sort of sensation.''

White and Sweet's book includes a number of topics, such as:

1. percutaneous destructive nerve, spinal root, paravertebral, sympathetic and trigeminal blocks usually made with alcohol
2. open posterior rhizotomy of spinal and cranial nerves including the Frazier procedure

and Dandy's posterior fossa retrogasserian neurectomy
3. open section of trigeminal nerve components
4. medullary section of the descending trigeminal tract
5. greater superficial petrosal neurectomy
6. glossopharyngeal neurectomy
7. open dorsal cordotomy
8. medullary pontine and mesencephalic spinothalamic tractotomy
9. section of Lissauer's tract
10. longitudinal midline myelotomy
11. dorsal cordotomy (of the lateral two-thirds of the ipsilateral dorsal column at C2 for upper limb and at midthoracic level for lower limb, phantom pain)
12. lobotomy
13. cortical resections
14. sympathectomy

Open procedures were generally preferred to percutaneous alcohol injection and strong warnings were given concerning the disabling psychiatric complications of lobotomy.

The third section of the book lists the pain syndromes treated surgically. These include:

1. neuralgias of the peripheral nerves
2. painful neuromata
3. amputation stump and phantom limb pain
4. causalgia and posttraumatic dystrophy
5. painful surgical scars
6. intercostal neuralgia, meralgia paresthetica
7. gangrene of digits
8. degenerative arthritis of the hip
9. facial and cephalic neuralgias
10. cephalic pain whose transmission pathways were uncertain
11. pain of spinal origin
12. pain from involvement of somatic nerves in the neck, thorax, abdomen, pelvis, and extremities
13. pain in diseases of the thoracic and abdominal viscera

The section that deals with the rationale for the various neurosurgical procedures used to relieve pain contains interesting comments that hint at future developments. On page 51, the authors state ''lesions which permanently destroy the original pain pathway may not prevent pain impulses from reaching the sentient areas from some other avenue.'' This was attributed to ''rerouting.'' On pages 91–98, the mechanisms of hyperalgesia and burning pain are discussed and include the concept of two types of pain pathway—a highly differentiated and phylogenetically younger system in the dorsal columns whose activities inhibit those of an ancient pain pathway, as well as a similarly functioning dichotomy of fast and slowly conducting pain fibers. It is suggested that hypersensitivity can be explained as follows: ''The continuous arrival of impulses progressively decreases the threshold of certain neurons.'' White and Sweet conclude, ''There remain extensive gaps in our understanding. We still have no satisfactory method for the interruption of pain in cephalic herpes zoster, the atypical neuralgias of the face and head, and some of the distressing sequelae to amputation and paraplegia.'' As stated on page 3, ''in theory, our present knowledge of anatomy should make it possible for the surgeon to relieve all varieties of intractable pain by specific interruption of afferent pathways, but this is unfortunately far from the case. Frequent failure to benefit herpetic and other neuralgias of the face other than the classical tic douloureux, certain painful phantoms following amputation, and the intensely disagreeable sensations which sometime follow injury of the spinal cord and peripheral nerves remind us that we still have much to learn.'' How much farther have we come at the beginning of the second millennium!

THE 1950s

The status of pain surgery in the 1950s remains clear in my memory, for I was a neurosurgical resident for most of that period and received my FRCSC in 1959. The procedures I was taught by mentors, such as McKenzie, Botterell, Morley, and Lougheed, included alcohol injection into Meckel's cave, peripheral neurectomies, the Frazier procedure and occasionally, posterior fossa rhizotomy for tic douloureux, intercostal neurectomy, dorsal rhizotomy by open laminectomy, open and usually bilateral thoracic cordotomy, open medullary spinothalamic tractotomy, multiple posterior fossa cranial rhi-

zotomy for cancer pain, and infrequently, medullary trigeminal tractotomy.

From that baseline, pain surgery developed remarkably through the 1950s, particularly through technical advances. On the conceptual side, in 1959, Noordenbos (62) elaborated previous suggestions and postulated two pain-conducting systems. One was a slowly conducting, small fiber system summation of whose input at the dorsal horn generates the centripetal patterns that reach the brain and produce the pain, and the other the fast conducting pathway consisting of large diameter fibers which inhibit the small-fiber impulses to prevent summation. He also envisaged a multisynaptic ascending pain-conducting system in the core of the spinal cord (see Figure 10.2).

Paramount amongst technical advances was the introduction of human stereotactic surgery by Spiegel and Wycis in 1948 (85), one of the great advances in pain neurosurgery during the century. Though originally used to treat movement disorders, stereotactic surgery was soon adapted to treat pain. In 1949, Hécaen et al. (30) appeared to be the first to carry out medial thalamotomy in a patient with stroke induced pain. Monnier and Fischer (56) performed both medial and lateral thalamotomies in 1951. The choice of the two targets reflects concepts of pain transmission in two systems—a fast-conducting lateral specific paucisynaptic one through ventrocaudal nucleus of thalamus, and a slowly conducting non-specific multisynaptic one through the medial thalamic nuclei, especially the parafascicular and centromedian nuclei. In 1959, Hassler and Riechert (28,29) showed that pain transmission was associated with a subnucleus of the ventrocaudal nucleus of thalamus, which they named nucleus ventrocaudalis parvocellularis. This led to the performance of basal thalamotomy by which dissociated sensory loss could be achieved at the thalamic level. Whereas in 1948 Spiegel and Wycis (83) reported the first stereotactic mesencephalotomy to relieve pain, the elaboration of stereotactic pain surgery did not take place for another decade.

A seemingly isolated report by Botterell et al. in 1953 (8) anticipated later developments in thinking about central pain. This report showed that in patients with central pain caused by spinal cord lesions, it was the shooting lancinating pain rather than the steady causalgic dysesthetic pain that was relieved by open cordotomy.

Also in the 1950s, it was realized that hypophysectomy could relieve cancer pain, particularly in hormonally-dependent diseases such as breast and prostate cancers (49,80).

THE 1960s

This is a memorable decade since in September 1961, I joined the staff of the Toronto General Hospital. On the conceptual side, 1965 saw the introduction of the Melzack-Wall Gate Theory of pain (52) (Figure 10.3), which combined previous concepts and emphasized the role of modulation (gating) within the nervous system, and predicted that activity in large fibers would inhibit that in small (pain) fibers. Apart from related controversies and modifications of the Gate Theory (Figure 10.4), its importance was to stress the role of modulation in the physiology of pain.

Another 1960s landmark was the publication of the monograph *Central Pain* by Cassinari and Pagni (9). After assimilating the historical clinical facts concerning central pain into a succinct account, they set out to deal with the problem that ''the pathophysiology of central pain has never been thoroughly elucidated.'' In addressing this problem, they showed enormous foresight. ''We have asked ourselves whether the

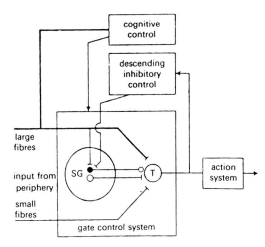

FIGURE 10.4. *The. Modified Gate Control Theory.* Excitatory (white circle) connections have been added to inhibitory (black circle) from substantia gelatinosa (SG) to T cells plus descending inhibitory control from brainstem (Melzack, Wall).

injured sensory systems and the physiopathological mechanisms can be the same in cases with pain in the strict sense, in cases with simple paresthesia, in those with 'spontaneous' symptoms, and in those with 'evoked' phenomena. In the past, few workers asked whether the mechanisms involved might be different for different symptoms; most centered their attention on pain as such.

Because central sensory phenomena may arise as a result of lesions at any level of the central nervous system, from the spinal cord to the cerebral cortex, the question at once arises whether the pathogenetic mechanism is always the same irrespective of the level involved.'' These comments suggest that the authors indeed differentiated between the different mechanisms potentially at work in nociceptive and the different components of neuropathic pain syndromes, while they seriously considered the homogeneity of mechanisms of neuropathic pain whether caused by lesions of the spinal cord or cerebral cortex. The theories proposed to explain central pain at this time were:

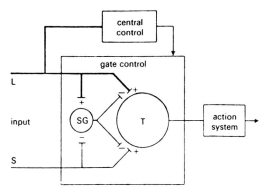

FIGURE 10.3. *The Gate Control Theory:* Large fibers (L) enhance the inhibition of the substantia gelatinosa (SG) and first central transmission cells (T), on afferent fiber terminals while small fibers (S) decrease it (Melzack, Wall).

1. irritation of the sensory pathways or centers
2. alterations of the functional relations between the systems concerned with the elabo-

ration of sensory phenomenon, essentially disinhibition releasing pain

3. loss of a specific thalamic function whose normal activity is to moderate pain
4. irritative impairment of the sympathetic system
5. multifactorial causes.

The reader will at once recognize the persistence of some of these ideas in contemporary thinking, such as denervation neuronal hypersensitivity and the concept of bursting cells, disinhibition based on a number of possible structures, and sympathetically maintained pain.

On the practical side, one of the great developments of the 1960s was that of the radiofrequency (RF) lesion making technique. The percutaneous injection of destructive agents, such as alcohol or percutaneous lesion making using anodal direct current, had been used for a long time (for example, by Kirschner) (41). However, the introduction of the percutaneous RF technique (1,74,87) allowed lesions to be made safely, reproducibly, consistently, and predictably for the first time. RF lesioning of nerves, roots, spinal cord, and deep brain structures flourished and led, particularly in subsequent decades, to a wide variety of neurosurgical pain procedures, most significantly percutaneous cordotomy. In 1963, Mullan et al. (58) first carried out percutaneous cordotomy by the lateral high cervical technique, using a radioactive needle. The conversion to the RF technique made this one of the great procedures in the neurosurgeon's armamentarium. Though Cloward (10) invented an open anterior approach to cordotomy in 1964, this was eclipsed, in the writer's opinion, by the percutaneous technique developed by Lin et al. (47), which consisted of an anterior percutaneous methodology.

In the 1960s, the development of the RF lesioning technique led to a flourishing of stereotactic pain operations, such as RF mecencephalic tractotomy (87) and RF trigeminal tractotomy (11). Mark et al. carried out a detailed study of RF thalamotomy and concluded that medial thalamotomy was superior to lesioning the lemniscal relay nucleus of the thalamus for the relief of pain since it was more effective and caused fewer side effects, such as neuropathic pain (50).

Meanwhile, the Melzack-Wall Gate Theory (52) produced major innovations in the neurosurgical treatment of pain. Since it postulated that activity in large nerve fibers would inhibit activity in the small fibers thought to transmit pain, Wall and Sweet (98) demonstrated pain relief by electrical nerve stimulation. This led Shealey et al. (77) to perform dorsal column stimulation by open laminectomy in 1967.

The publication of *Pain and the Neurosurgeon* by White and Sweet in 1969 (100) fittingly summarizes pain neurosurgery at the end of the 1960s. A follow-up of their earlier work, this book is based on 1287 personal patients. The operations reviewed include cranial neurectomy, posterior rhizotomy, phenol subarachnoid block, sympathectomy, spinothalamic cordotomy, medullary, mesencephalic and pontine tractotomy, commissurotomy, Lissauer tractotomy, dorsal cordotomy, lobotomy, postcentral gyrectomy, stereotactic thalamotomy, and chronic stimulation of peripheral nerves, spinal cord, and brain. Painful diseases treated include injury to peripheral nerves, pain related to amputation, causalgia, posttraumatic arthritis or sympathetic dystrophy, shoulder-hand syndrome, pain in degenerative disease of the hip, pain in ischemia, peripheral neuralgia, tic douloureux, other cephalic neuralgias, pain of spinal origin, pain from malignant disease, and pain from thoracic and abdominal viscera.

This volume also contains comments on procedures that were introduced after the authors' first book was published in 1955. The authors express satisfaction with their modification of Maher's technique of subarachnoid phenol injection, which was introduced in 1957. Maher's technique replaced the traditional alcohol by the substitution of a mixture of glycerin and 5% phenol that was thought to selectively interrupt unmyelinated C fibers. Taarnhøj had introduced a new concept of decompressing the trigeminal nerve in Meckel's cave to relieve tic douloureux in 1952, (88), but it was White and Sweet's experience that vigorous mechanical compression of the nerve was more likely to be successful in relieving trigeminal neuralgia, as advocated by Shelden (78) and Shelden et al. (79). Following the historical work of Dandy (13)(34), which suggested that compression of the trigeminal nerve by a posterior fossa lesion could cause tic, 66 out of 215 of Dandy's lesions being vascular, Gardner (25) supported the same view. However, his work awaited the widespread use of the binocular microscope in Jannetta's hands (38) to popularize microvascular decompression as the best neurosurgical treatment for trigeminal neuralgia at that time. The use of lobotomy to treat some chronic pain syndromes has already been mentioned, as has White and Sweet's warning about the psychological complications of this operation, which was reiterated in their new volume.

A very significant development of the 1960s was the introduction of electrocoagulation of the cingulum by Foltz and White (24) as an alternative to lobotomy for the treatment of pain. This was first performed with the Bovie apparatus, but soon thereafter by RF lesion-making. Cingulotomy appeared to be as effective for pain relief as lobotomy in patients with pain from both cancer and non-malignant disease whenever emotional factors were paramount, yet without the psychological deterioration seen with lobotomy.

THE 1970s

The 1970s were active in the neurosurgical treatment of pain chiefly through the exploitation of three technical advances from the 1960s—RF lesion- making, stereotaxis, and chronic stimulation.

In the 1970s, RF lesions made in Meckel's cave became routine for the treatment of trigeminal neuralgia. Nugent and Berry (63), however, introduced a useful modification. Using a smaller curved electrode, they strove to selectively interrupt the finer pain fibers in the particular area of the patient's tic. Percutaneous RF lesioning of other cranial nerves was introduced.

In 1960, Rees had originally attempted denervation of facet nerves in order to treat chronic back pain using a scalpel (69), but Shealy's introduction of percutaneous RF denervation of facets (76) made the procedure a common and routine event.

Uematsu et al. (96) introduced percutaneous RF posterior rhizotomy that was simpler to perform than the open procedure. However, Smith (82) warned that it might be necessary to per-

form a dorsal ganglionectomy to relieve such pain as intercostal neuralgia in order to interrupt pain afferents to the sympathetic chain, which still required an open approach.

The evolution of the dorsal root entry zone (DREZ) operations began with Hyndman's Lissauer's tract section (36), which was used in an attempt to raise the analgesic level after a cordotomy. Sindou et al. (81) exploited the differential arrangement of pain and other fibers in the dorsal root entry zone of the spinal cord to carry out an open selective posterior rhizotomy of pain fibers using a knife blade. In this author's opinion, essentially the same operation was introduced by Nashold and Ostdahl (60), but the lesions were made in the exposed dorsal cord with RF current rather than Sindou's knife blade. Whereas Sindou's operation was first directed at nociceptive pain, Nashold and Ostdahl's operation was primarily used to treat neuropathic pain. The DREZ operation is one of the few destructive procedures on the central nervous system that will remain an important part of the neurosurgeon's armamentarium. It is particularly useful in treating the pain of brachial plexus avulsion and the shooting, lancinating elements of pain associated with lesions of the conus medullaris and cauda equina.

Midline myelotomy has been mentioned. In 1974, Hitchcock (31) described a stereotactic, percutaneous technique for the operation at the level of C1. The clinical observations led to the conclusion that there was a central pain-conducting pathway in the spinal cord, apart from the spinothalamic tract, that resembled the paleospinothalamic pathway in the brain stem. At the same time, percutaneous RF techniques introduced by Hitchcock et al. and Crue et al. (12,31,32) replaced some open destructive procedures on the trigeminal tracts in the brain stem.

Meanwhile, the growing experience with stereotactic RF mesencephalic tractotomy led to the discovery that the success of the operation depended more upon dividing the more medially-located, non-specific, multisynaptic portion of the mesencephalic pain tract than the spinothalamic tract itself.

Based on known involvement of the hypothalamus in pain conduction as illustrated by Spiegel and Wycis (84), Fairman (23), and Sano (75), these researchers carried out hypothalamotomy for the relief of pain. Sano believed that the hypothalamus was part of an ascending pain pathway involving the medial thalamic nuclei.

Open hypophysectomy for cancer pain has been mentioned, but the impact of this massive procedure on a sick patient was greatly reduced by substituting percutaneous methods that used radioactive seeds and RF current. However, it was the use of percutaneous alcohol injection, first described by Greco et al. (26) but popularized by Moricca in the 1970s (57), that made pituitary destruction a widely used operation to control cancer pain. The procedure was effective whether the cancer was hormone dependent or not, but the mechanism has never been satisfactorily explained.

Another new venture in pain surgery was Leksell's introduction in 1971 of radiosurgery to treat trigeminal neuralgia (45). This has led to the massive growth of radiosurgery extending to such procedures as radiothalamotomy.

However, the most important advance of the 1970s was the elaboration of chronic stimulation techniques for pain relief. Peripheral nerve stimulation, begun in the 1960s, was expanded, though it usually required an open operation for implantation of the electrode. Dorsal column stimulation by open means is still used widely today for the epidural implantation of a paddle type electrode. However, the introduction of the percutaneous technique in 1975 (20,22,33) made dorsal column stimulation the popular operation it is today.

Though "deep brain stimulation" (DBS) had been used in trial studies before, it was not until the 1970s that the marriage of stereotaxis and reliable equipment for chronic stimulation of the nervous system occurred. This made possible concerted studies of DBS on two fronts. Following laboratory work on the rewarding effects from brain stimulation in animals, Richardson and Akil (71) showed that chronic pain could be alleviated by stimulation in the periventricular gray matter (PVG) of man. The advance on the other front was a cephalad extension of dorsal column stimulation to produce paresthesia in the area of the patient's pain by stimulating a stereotactically implanted electrode in the lemniscal relay nucleus of the thalamus. This procedure was introduced by Hosobuchi et al. (34) and Ma-

zars et al. (51). Thus, there were two techniques for DBS for pain relief, one of which, PVG stimulation, seemed more likely to be effective for nociceptive pain, while the other (paresthesia-producing stimulation) seemed more promising in the treatment of neuropathic pain in the same way that dorsal column stimulation is. This dichotomy of effects (PVG DBS for nociceptive pain and paresthesia-producing for neuropathic pain) has not been generally accepted, though the review by Bendok and Levy (2) supports it strongly.

Another major advance of the 1970s was the beginning of what is one of the major techniques in pain surgery, chronic intrathecal spinal opiate infusion (104). This advance, like chronic stimulation, has been very dependent on the development of effective equipment for implantation. However, opiate infusion has had wider implications, and has gradually replaced other neurosurgical interventions, particularly destructive lesioning, for the relief of cancer pain. Furthermore, with the widespread advocacy of the use of oral and parenteral morphine for the treatment of all pain syndromes (not just those related to cancer), opiate infusion has greatly diminished the number of neurosurgical interventions for pain.

THE 1980s

The status of pain neurosurgery in the 1980s has been reviewed by a number of landmark publications. The 1980s comprised the "Decade of the Book." On the fundamental side was Willis' *The Pain System* (102), which updated the neuroanatomical and physiological basis of pain neurosurgery. Another well-known publication from the 1980s is the first edition of the encyclopedic *Textbook of Pain* edited by Melzack and Wall (53). Perhaps not as well-known as it should be is Kandel's *Functional and Stereotactic Neurosurgery* (39). The latter is a scholarly review of the whole field enhanced by Kandel's own experience.

The 1980s also saw two general developments related to pain neurosurgery; both of them are difficult to define. The first was the widespread acceptance of pain clinics and the second was a fuller recognition of neuropathic pain. Bonica, in particular, advanced the acceptance of the role and importance of multidisciplinary pain clinics (6). These clinics have expanded internationally to such a degree as to trigger a thorough reevaluation of their role and cost-effectiveness.

Though the ground work had been laid decades before, it is this author's opinion that it was not until the 1980s that clinicians, including neurosurgeons, became more involved in pain problems. They became generally aware of neuropathic pain as an entity separate from nociceptive pain, with a differing pathophysiology and therefore, requiring separate therapeutic strategies. This was partly the result of the discovery of animal models of neuropathic pain that made it possible to study quantitatively some aspects of the problem, particularly allodynia (4).

The author's interest in this subject began with a review (90) of his experience with percutaneous cordotomy in 1975, further elaborated at the 1989 meeting of the American Association of Neurological Surgeons in Washington (93). This experience, supported by the published work of others, favored a multi-factorial concept of neuropathic pain. The sharp, lancinating elements, especially prevalent in lesions of the conus and cauda equina and after brachial plexus avulsion, responded dramatically to destructive lesions made in the pain pathways, such as cordotomy, cordectomy, and the DREZ procedure. So, too, did the evoked elements of allodynia and hyperpathia. Steady, causalgic, dysesthetic pain, however, did not respond to these destructive procedures, with chronic paresthesia-producing stimulation being the chief method available for its surgical relief. Presumably, the shooting, lancinating pain arises from ectopic impulse generation at the lesion site, with transmission in the spinothalamic tract, thus explaining the response to surgery. Though the concept of disordered processing at the dorsal horn as a mechanism in neuropathic pain was not new, Woolf (103) and others clearly demonstrated this to be the mechanism of allodynia in peripheral neuropathic pain. The disordered processing results in transmission in the spinothalamic tract, and explains the success of cordotomy, cordectomy, and probably the DREZ lesion in relieving this symptom.

Also in the 1980s, Roberts (73) popularized another concept relevant to neuropathic pain—that of sympathetically maintained pain. This field has been minutely scrutinized, both in the laboratory and the operating room, by Jim Campbell and his group (68).

It is difficult to pinpoint the impact of modern brain imaging on pain surgery. Though computerized tomography (CT) became commercially available in the early 1970s, as did modern positron emission tomography (PET) scanning, it was the arrival of magnetic resonance imaging (MRI) in the 1980s that had the greatest impact. Not only did MRI allow more precise anatomical localization based on both the MRI alone and in conjunction with other imaging techniques (through such methodology as image fusion), but it also led to functional MRI, which promises to be of great value in studying the physiological substrate of pain (64).

Another field that is difficult to define is invasive physiological mapping of the brain. Traditionally, stereotactic lesion sites in subcortical structures were confirmed by various means, such as macrostimulation, EEG recording, impedance monitoring, microelectrode recording, and evoked potential recording at the intended target site. Inspired by the brain mapping work of Clinton Woolsey in the laboratory, illustrated with "figurine maps" rather than studying only the target site physiologically, we prepared maps of the thalamus and midbrain (94) in the course of stereotactic operations guided by threshold macrostimulation, stimulating at threshold every 2 mm along every electrode tract used, with the results plotted in computer-generated figurine maps. The technique had the advantage of not only assisting with the operation, but also of studying normal and abnormal brain function. In the 1980s, we replaced macrostimulation brain mapping with microelectrode recording, a technique that had been in use since the 1960s. It used electrodes capable of recording single cells and microstimulation at the same sites. The results were plotted in a similar manner to that used with macrostimulation.

Turning to technical neurosurgical advances, there were several developments in the treatment of trigeminal neuralgia and other forms of facial pain. Based on a serendipitous observation, Håkanson (27) introduced the percutaneous injection of glycerol into the cerebrospinal fluid (CSF) cistern of Meckel's cave—a procedure that has seen wide acceptance for its simplicity and relative safety in treating trigeminal neuralgia. Mullan and Lichtor (59) replaced the previously described open techniques for compression of the trigeminal nerve by a percutaneous one that used an inflated balloon. With increasing interest in the use of chronic stimulation to treat neuropathic pain, in 1980, Meyerson and Håkanson (54) developed a method for chronically stimulating the trigeminal nerve in the middle fossa through an open approach. This was followed by Steude's percutaneous technique (86).

Meanwhile, Nashold et al. extended the concept of the spinal DREZ operation to the trigeminal dorsal root entry zone (60), particularly to treat postherpetic neuralgia.

The 1980s also saw the extension of spinal intrathecal morphine infusion to the ventricles, though the concept was not new (44).

Just at the time the technique of percutaneous cordotomy was suffering from the unavailability of an oil base myelogram dye, CT-guided cordotomy was introduced and popularized by Kanpolat et al. (40), which enormously facilitated the visualization of the target and the execution of the procedure.

THE 1990s

This author finds it difficult to define neurosurgical advances of the 90s. Perhaps the widespread use of opioid therapy has displaced many neurosurgical procedures and diminished the quest for new ones, while the use of DBS has lost support in the United States. In addition, perhaps we stand too close to the 90s to fully assess this decade. Will it prove to have ushered in advances that will only come to fruition in the next millennium? During the 1990s, the production of pain books continued unabated. Notable amongst them was *Textbook of Pain, 4th Edition* by Wall and Melzack (97) and a new edition of Pagni's *Central Pain* still entitled *A Neurosurgical Challenge* (65).

On the conceptual side, awareness of neuropathic pain became universal and pharmacological, and physiological characterization of some

aspects of it advanced thanks to the widespread use of animal models (3). However, it must be kept in mind that models of allodynia in a peripheral neuropathic syndrome have little to do with the most common symptom seen in neuropathic syndromes, the steady causalgic dysesthetic element, and are not necessarily relevant to neuropathic pain caused by more central lesions. For these other aspects of central pain only man, who can describe his sensations, can be a suitable subject upon which to conduct pain research. In this regard, two previously mentioned strategies from the 1980s became truly productive in the 1990s—clinical physiological studies and functional imaging. For example, it has been possible to demonstrate the presence of neurons in the human ventrocaudal nucleus that respond to cold (16,46) and ones in cingulate cortex that respond to pain (35). Somatotopographic reorganization, considered by some to be an important factor in neuropathic pain, has been induced in human ventrocaudal nucleus within minutes using a digital local anesthetic ring block (42). Bursting cells, thought to be markers of denervation neuronal hypersensitivity, also have been thought to play a role in generating neuropathic pain, a notion not supported by studies in man (66).

Turning to functional imaging, using PET or preferably functional MRI, one can track the path of brain activation for a particular function, including pain (37, 89). Such studies implicate the thalamus, areas SI and SII of somatosensory cortex, insula, and anterior cingulate cortex in pain perception, as well as indicating the differing roles of these areas, such as localization of pain affect in cingulate cortex (18). In the 1990s, these imaging studies in particular have focused attention on the cingulate cortex as a major player in the perception of pain. The cingulate cortex is beginning to emerge as a structure consisting of at least two parts that serve as the cortical relay for the medial, nonspecific, spinoreticulothalamic pathway now thought to relay especially in the ventrocaudal portion of the dorsomedian nucleus. The rostral portion of the cingulate cortex (area 24) is seen as involved with pain processing, with the cortex rostral to area 24 concerned with attention-getting and the more caudal cingulate gyrus more involved with affective and evaluative function. This increased awareness of the cingulate cortex has rekindled interest in cingulotomy for the relief of chronic pain (101).

A new technical departure in the neurosurgical treatment of pain was the introduction by Tsubokawa et al. (95) of chronic motor cortex stimulation for the relief of pain. This was based on laboratory demonstration that subthreshold stimulation for motor effects in the area of the patient's pain suppressed denervation neuronal hypersensitivity. The technique has been used to treat the pain of stroke and neuropathic face pain (61). It will be interesting to await accumulating experience that will allows comparison of outcome with that in other procedures.

The 1990s saw rekindled interest in Leksell's radiosurgical technique for treating tic douloureux (43). The use of stereotactic radiosurgery to deliver low dosage radiation to the trigeminal dorsal root entry zone has become a useful treatment dependent on a mechanism that does not involve cellular destruction.

THE FUTURE

What can we expect as we move into the next millennium? Man is not particularly good at predicting the future except as a logical extension of current thinking; conceptual breakthroughs play havoc with such projections. In this author's opinion, neurosurgical advances in the treatment of pain will depend on further unraveling the anatomy, physiology, and pharmacology unique to each of the different pain syndromes (as summarized in the latest edition of the *Textbook of Pain*) (97), and using techniques that further minimize the impact of neurosurgical procedures. Functional imaging and physiological studies in human subjects will prove increasingly productive. This includes microelectrode mapping to elucidate pain processing in general (16,35,46,91) and in specific pain syndromes, in particular (14,15,21,92,98) studies that can be correlated with functional imaging (17,70).

Increased understanding of pain mechanisms and particularly the underlying pharmacology will make possible more sophisticated use of drug infusions or of implanted cell lines, perhaps at specific brain sites. For example, Decosterd et al. (19) reviewed the literature on the antinociceptive effect of infusion of catecholamines into the intrathecal or epidural space and the intrathecal implantation of adrenal chromaffin cells in animals and man. They presented their experience with the use of immunologically shielded xenogeneic adrenal grafts in the lumbar subarachnoid space in a rat model of neuropathic pain.

Finally, evaluation of the results of neurosurgical procedures to relieve pain will have to be evidence based. Groups of patients similarly selected with identical diagnoses will have to receive identical therapy with outcomes evaluated as quantitatively as possible at repeated intervals by disinterested and hopefully blinded observers and the outcomes compared with those in suitable controls.

REFERENCES

1. Aronow S. The use of radiofrequency power in making lesions in the brain. *Neurosurg* 17: 431–438, 1960.
2. Bendok B. Levy RM. Brain stimulation for persistent pain management, in, Gildenberg PL, Tasker RR. (ed): *Textbook of Stereotactic and Functional Neurosurgery*. New York: McGraw Hill, 1998, pp 1539–1556.
3. Bennett GJ. Animal models of neuropathic pain, in, Gebhart GF, Hammond DK, Jensen TS (ed): *Proc 7th World Congress on Pain*. Seattle: IASP Press, 1994, pp 495–510.
4. Bennett GJ, Xie YK. A peripheral mononeuropathy in rat that produces disorders of pain sensation like those seen in man. *Pain* 33:873–107, 1988.
5. Bernard EJ, Nashold BS Jr, Caputi F, et al. Nucleus caudalis DREZ lesions for facial pain. *Brit J Neurosurg* 1:81–92, 1987.
6. Bonica JJ (ed): Evolution of multidisciplinary and interdisciplinary pain programs in pain centers, in, Aronoff GM (ed): *Pain Centers: A Revolution in Health Care*. New York: Raven, 1988, p 55.
7. Bonica JJ. *The Management of Pain, 2nd Edition*. Philadelphia: Lea & Febiger, 1990, pp 6–11.
8. Botterell EH., Callaghan JC, Jousse AT. Pain in paraplegia: Clinical management and surgical treatment. *Proc R Soc Med* 47:17–24, 1953.
9. Cassarini V, Pagni CA. *Central Pain. A Neurological Survey*. Cambridge, Harvard, 1969.
10. Cloward RB. Cervical cordotomy by the anterior approach: Technique and advantages. *J Neurosurg* 21: 19–25, 1964.
11. Crue BL Jr., Todd EM, Carregal, et al. Percutaneous trigeminal tractotomy: Case report utilizing stereotactic radiofrequency lesion. *Bull Los Angeles Neur Soc* 32: 86–92, 1967.

12. Crue BL, Todd EM, Carregal EJA. Percutaneous radio-frequency stereotactic trigeminal tractotomy, in, Crue BL, et al. (ed): *Pain and Suffering.* Springfield: Thomas, 1970, pp 69–80.

13. Dandy WE. Treatment of trigeminal neuralgia by the cerebellar route. *Ann Surg* 96:787–795, 1932.

14. Davis DK, Kiss ZHT, Luo L, et al. Phantom sensations generated by thalamic microstimulation *Nature* 39:385–387, 1998.

15. Davis KD, Kiss ZHT, Tasker RR, et al. Thalamic stimulation-evoked sensations in chronic pain patients and in non-pain (movement disorder) patients. *J Neurophysiol* 75:1026–1037, 1996.

16. Davis KD, Lozano AM, Manduch M, et al. Thalamic relay site for cold perception in humans. *J Neurophysiol* 81:1970–1973, 1999.

17. Davis KD, Taub E, Duffner F, et al. Activation of the anterior cingulate cortex by thalamic stimulation in patients with chronic pain: A positron emission tomography study. *J Neurosurg* 92:64–69, 2000.

18. Davis KD, Wood ML, Crawley AP, et al. MRI of human somatosensory and cingulate cortex during painful electrical nerve stimulation. *NeuroReport* 7:321–325, 1995.

19. Decosterd L, Buchser E, Gilliard N, et al. Intrathecal implants of bovine chromaffin cells alleviate mechanical allodynia in a rat model of neuropathic pain. *Pain* 76:159–166, 1998.

20. Dooley DM. A technique for the epidural percutaneous stimulation of the spinal cord in man. Presented at the Annual Meeting of the AANS, Miami Beach, 1975.

21. Dostrovsky JO, Davis KD, Lee L, et al. *Electrical stimulation: Induced effects in the human thalamus*, in, Devinsky O, Beric A, Dogali M (ed): New York, Raven, 1993, pp 219–229.

22. Erickson DL, Percutaneous trial of stimulation for patient selection for implantable stimulating electrodes. *J Neurosurg* 43:440–444, 1975.

23. Fairman D. Hypothalamotomy as a new perspective for alleviation of intractable pain and regression of metastactic malignant tumours, in, Fusek L, Kunc Z (ed): *Present Limits of Neurosurgery.* Prague: Avicenum, 1972, pp 525–528.

24. Foltz EL, White LE Jr. Pain ''relief'' by frontal cingulumotomy *J Neurosurg.* 19: 89–100, 1962.

25. Gardner WJ. Concerning the mechanisms of trigeminal neuralgia and hemifacial spasm. *J Neurosurg* 19: 947–958, 1962.

26. Greco T, Sbaragli F, Cammilli L. L'alcolizzazione della ipofisi per via transfenoidale nella terapea di particoloari tumor maligni. Settim. *Med* 45:355–356, 1957.

27. Håkanson S. Trigeminal neuralgia treated by the injection of glycerol into the trigeminal cistern. *J Neurosurg* 9:638–646, 1981.

28. Hassler R. The division of pain conduction into systems of pain sensation and pain awareness, in, Janzen R, Keidel WD, Herz A, Steichele C. (ed): *Pain: Basic Principles, Pharmacology, Therapy.* Thieme Stuttgart, 1972, pp 98–112.

29. Hassler R. Riechert. T. Klinische, und anatomische Befunde bei stereotaktischen. Schmerzoperationen im Thalamus. *Arch Psychiat Zges Neurol* 200:93–122, 1959.

30. Hécaen H, Talairach J, David M, et al. Coagulations limitées du thalamus dans les algies du syndrome thalamique. *Rev Neurol Paris* 81:917–931,1949.

31. Hitchcock E. Stereotactic trigeminal tractotomy. *Ann Clin Res* 2:31–135, 1970.

32. Hitchcock ER, Schvarcz JR. Stereotactic trigeminal tractotomy for post-herpetic facial pain. *J Neurosurg* 37:412–417, 1972.

33. Hoppenstein R. Percutaneous implantation of chronic spinal cord electrode for control of intractable pain: Preliminary report. *Surg Neurol* 4:195–198, 1975.

34. Hosobuchi Y, Adams JE, Rutkin B. Chronic thalamic stimulation for the control of facial anesthesia dolorosa. *Arch. Neurol* 29:158–161, 1973.

35. Hutchison WD, Davis KD, Lozano AM, et al. Pain-related neurons in the human cingulate cortex. *Nat Neurosci* 2:403–405, 1999.

36. Hyndman OR. Lissauer's tract section. A contribution to cordotomy for the relief of pain (preliminary report). *J Int Coll Surg* 5:394–400, 1942.

37. Ingvar M, Hsieh JC. The image of pain, in, Wall PD, Melzack R (eds): *Textbook of Pain, 4th Edition.* Edinburgh: Churchill Livingstone, 1999, pp 215–233.

38. Jannetta PJ. Arterial compression of the trigeminal nerve at the pons in patients with trigeminal neuralgia. *J Neurosurg* 26:159–162, 1967.

39. Kandel EL. *Functional and Stereotactic Neurosurgery.* New York: Plenum, 1989.

40. Kanpolat Y, Deda H, Akyar S, et al. CT-guided percutaneous cordotomy. *Acta Neurochir, Suppl* 46:67–68, 1989.

41. Kirschner M. Zur Electrochirurgie. *Arch Klin Chir* 161:761–768, 1931.

42. Kiss ZHT, Davis KD, Tasker RR, et al. Human thalamic neurons develop novel receptive fields within minutes of deafferentation. *Soc Neurosci Abst* 20:119, 1994.

43. Kondziolka D, Lunsford LD, Habeck M, et al. Gamma knife radiosurgery for trigeminal neuralgia. *Neurosurg Clin N Am* 8:79–85, 1997.

44. Leavens ME, Hill CS, Cech DA, et al. Intrathecal and intraventricular morphine for pain in cancer patients: Initial study. *J Neurosurg* 56:241–245, 1982.

45. Leksell L. Stereotactic radiosurgery in trigeminal neuralgia. *Acta Chir Scand* 37:311–314, 1971.

46. Lenz FA, Dougherty PM. Neurons in the human thalamic somatosensory nucleus (ventalis caudalis) respond to innocuous cool and mechanical stimuli. *J Neurophyiol* 79:2227–2230, 1998.

47. Lin PM, Gildenberg PL, Polakoff PP. An anterior approach to percutaneous lower cervical cordotomy. *J Neurosurg* 25:553–560,1966.

48. Livingston WK. *Pain Mechanisms. A Physiological Interpretation of Causalgia and its Related States.* New York: Macmillan, NewYork, 1943.

49. Luft R, Olivecrona H. Experiences with hypophysectomy in man. *J Neurosurg* 301–316, 1953.

50. Mark VH, Ervin FR, Yakovlev PL. Correlation of pain relief, sensory loss, and anatomical lesion sites in pain patients treated by stereotactic thalamotomy. *Trans Am Neurol Assoc* 86:86–90, 1961.

51. Mazars G., Mérienne L, Ciolocca C. Stimulations thalamiques intermittentes antalgiques: Note préliminaire. *Rev Neurol* 128:273–279, 1973.

52. Melzack R, Wall PD. Pain mechanisms: A new theory. *Science* 150:971–978, 1965.

53. Wall PD, Melzack R, (ed): *Textbook of Pain*. Edinburgh: Churchill Livingstone, 1984.

54. Meyerson BA, Håkanson S. Alleviation of atypical trigeminal pain by stimulation of the gasserian ganglion by an implanted electrode. *Acta. Neurochir Suppl* 30: 303–330, 1980.

55. Mitchell SW, Morehouse GE, Keen WW. *Gunshot Wounds and Other Injuries of Nerves*. Philadelphia: Lippincott, 1864.

56. Monnier M, Fischer R. Localisation, stimulation et coagulation du thalmus chez l'homme. *J Physiol Paris*, 43:818, 1951.

57. Moricca G. Chemical hypophysectomy for cancer pain, in, Bonica JJ (ed): *Advances in Neurology, Volume 4*. New York: Raven, 1974, pp 707–714.

58. Mullan S, Harper PV, Hekmatpanah J, et al. Percutaneous interruption of spinal pain tracts by means of a strontium-90 needle. *Neurosurg* 20:931–939, 1963.

59. Mullan S, Lichtor T. Percutaneous microcompression of the trigeminal ganglion for trigeminal neuralgia. *J Neurosurg* 59:1007–1012, 1983.

60. Nashold BS Jr, Ostdahl RH. Dorsal root entry zone lesions for pain relief. *J Neurosurg* 51:59–69, 1979.

61. Nguyen JP, Lefaucheur JP, Decq P, et al. Chronic motor cortex stimulation in the treatment of central and neuropathic pain: Correlations between clinical, electrophysiological and anatomical data. *Pain* 82: 245–251, 1999.

62. Noordenbos W. *Pain*. Amsterdam: Elsevier, 1959.

63. Nugent GR, Berry B. Trigeminal neuralgia treated by differential percutaneous radiofrequency coagulation of the gasserian ganglion. *J Neurosurg* 40:517–523, 1974.

64. Orrison WW Jr, Levine JD, Sanders JA, et al. *Functional Brain Imaging*. St. Louis: Mosby, 1995.

65. Pagni CA. Central Pain: A Neurosurgical Challenge. *Torino Minerva Medica,* 1998.

66. Rahakrishnan V, Tsoukatos J, Davis KD. et al. A comparison of the burst activity of lateral thalamic neurons in chronic pain and non-pain patients. *Pain* 80: 567–575, 1999.

67. Rainville P, Duncan GH, Price DD, et al. Pain affects encoded in human anterior cingulate but not somatosensory cortex. *Science* 277:968–971, 1997.

68. Raja SN, Myer RA, Ringkamp M, et al. Peripheral neural mechanisms of nociception, in, Wall PD, Melzack R (ed): *Textbook of Pain, 4th Edition*. Edinburgh: Churchill Livingstone, 1999, pp 11–57.

69. Rees S. Disconnective neurosurgery, in, Rees S (ed): *The Treatment of Pain as the Major Disability. 2nd Edition*. Australia: Visual Abstracts, 1975.

70. Rezai AR, Lozano AM, Crawley AP, et al. Thalamic stimulation and functional magnetic resonance imaging: Localization of cortical and subcortical activation with implanted electrodes. *J Neurosurg* 90:583–590, 1999.

71. Richardson DE, Akil H. Pain reduction by electrical brain stimulation in man 1. Acute administration in periaqueductal and periventricular sites. *J Neurosurg* 47:178–183, 1977.

72. Riddoch G. Central Pain. *Lancet* 1:1150–1156, 1205–1209, 1938.

73. Roberts WJ. A hypothesis on the physiological basis for causalgia and related pains. *Pain* 24:297–311, 1986.

74. Rosomoff HL, Carroll F, Brown J, et al. Percutaneous radiofrequency cervical cordotomy technique. *J Neurosurg* 23:639–644, 1965.

75. Sano K. Intralaminar thalamotomy (thalamolaminotomy) and posterior hypothalamotomy in the treatment of intractable pain, in, Krayenbühl Maspes PE, Sweet WE (ed): *Progress In Neurological Surgery, Volume 8*. Basel: Karger, 1977, pp 50–103.

76. Shealy CN. Percutaneous radiofrequency denervation of spinal facets: Treatment of chronic back pain and sciatica. *J Neurosurg* 43:448–451, 1975.

77. Shealey CN, Mortimer JT, Reswick JB. Electrical inhibition of pain by stimulation of the dorsal columns: Preliminary clinical report. *Anesth Analg (Cleve)* 46: 489–491, 1967.

78. Shelden CH. Compression procedure for trigeminal neuralgia. *J Neurosurg* 25:374–381, 1966.

79. Shelden CH, Pudenz RH, Freshwater DB, et al. Compression rather than decompression for trigeminal neuralgia. *J Neurosurg* 12:123–126, 1955.

80. Shimken HR, Ortega P, Naffziger HC. Effects of surgical hypophysectomy in a man with malignant melanoma. *J Clin Endocrinol Metab*12:439–453, 1952.

81. Sindou M, Fischer G, Goutelle A, et al. La radiccllotomie postérieure sélective. Premiers résultats dans la chirurgie de la douleur. *Neurochirugie* 20:397–408, 1974.

82. Smith FP. Trans-spinal ganglionectomy for relief of intercostal pain. *J Neurosurg* 32:574–577, 1970.

83. Spiegel EA, Wycis HT. *Mesencephalotomy for relief of pain. Anniversary Volume for O Poetzl*. Vienna, 1948, p 438.

84. Spiegel EA, Wycis HT. *Stereoencephalotomy Part II: Clinical and Physiological Application*. New York: Grune and Stratton, 1962.

85. Spiegel EA, Wycis HT, Marks M, et al. Stereotactic apparatus for operations on the human brain. *Science* 106:349–350, 1946.

86. Steude V. Radiofrequency electrical stimulation of the gasserian ganglion in patients with atypical trigeminal pain. Methods of percutaneous temporary test: Stimulation and permanent inplantation of stimulation devices. *Acta Neurochir Suppl* 33:481–486, 1984.

87. Sweet WH, Mark VH, Hamlin H. Radiofrequency lesions in the central nervous system of man and cat, including case reports of eight bulbar pain-tract interruptions. *Neurosurg* 17:213–225,1960.

88. Taarnhoj P. Decompression of the trigeminal root and the posterior part of the ganglion as a treatment in trigeminal neuralgia: Preliminary communication. *J Neurosurg* 9:288–290, 1952.

89. Talbot JD, Marrett S, Evans AC, et al. Multiple representations of pain in human cerebral cortex. *Science* 251:1355–1358, 1994.

90. Tasker RR. Percutaneous cordotomy. *Compr Ther* 1: 51–56, 1975.

91. Tasker RR. The use of microelectrodes in the human brain, in, Bromm B, Desmedt JE (ed): *Pain and the Brain: From Nociception to Cognition. Advances in Pain Research and Therapy, Volume. 22*, New York: Raven, 1995, pp 143–174.

92. Tasker RR. Can we explain how strokes cause pain? *Pain Forum* 7:18–19, 1998.

93. Tasker RR, de Carvalho GTC, Dolan EJ. Intractable central pain of cord origin: Clinical features and implications for surgery. *J Neurosurg* 77:373–378, 1992.

94. Tasker RR., Organ LW, Hawrylyshyn PA. *The Thalamus and Midbrain of Man. A Physiological Atlas Using Electrical Stimulation.* Springfield: Thomas, 1982.

95. Tsubokawa T, Katayama Y, Yamamoto T, et al. Chronic motor cortex stimulation for the treatment of central pain. *Acta Neurochir Suppl (Wien)* 52: 37–139, 1991.

96. Uematsu S, Udvarhelyi GB, Benson DW, et al. Percutaneous radiofrequency rhizotomy. *Surg Neurol* 2: 319–325, 1974.

97. Wall PD, Melzack R (ed): *Textbook of Pain, 4th Edition.* Edinburgh: Churchill Livingstone, 1999.

98. Wall PD, Sweet WH. Temporary abolition of pain in man. *Science* 155:108–109, 1967.

99. White JC, Sweet WH. *Pain: Its Mechanisms and Neurosurgical Control.* Springfield: Thomas, 1955.

100. White JC, Sweet WH. *Pain and the Neurosurgeon.* Springfield: Thomas, 1969.

101. Wilkinson HA, Davidson KM, Davidson RI. Bilateral anterior cingulotomy for chronic non-cancer pain. *Neurosurgery* 45:1129–1134, 1999.

102. Willis WD. *The Pain System. The Neural Basis of Nociceptive Transmission in the Mammalian Nervous System.* Basel: Karger, 1985.

103. Woolf CJ. Evidence for a central component of post-injury pain hypersensitivity. *Nature* 306:686–688, 1983.

104. Yaksh TL, Rudy TA. Analgesia mediated by a direct spinal action of narcotics. *Science* 192:1357–1358, 1976.

11

Pediatric Neurosurgery

Theodore S. Roberts, MD, Marion L. Walker, MD

The 1970s
The 1980s

The 1990s
The future

Fifty years ago, neurosurgery was a well-established surgical subspecialty with organizations that represented both academic and private practitioners of the specialty. Few neurosurgeons at that time, however, confined their practices to pediatric care only. In reviewing the literature of this era, which includes collected articles from the *Journal of Neurosurgery* (the Congress of Neurological Surgeons' (CNS) publication), *Neurosurgery, and Clinical Neurosurgery* (Proceedings of the CNS), we found that most of these articles are confined to characterization of adult neurosurgical problems. However, intermixed are a number of important pediatric contributions.

By 1950, hydrocephalus was considered to be a treatable disease, though in some clinics, indications for treatment relied on the thickness of the cortical mantle. (Less than 2 cm dimmed the prospects of shunting operations with "successful" outcomes.)

Matson published the results of ventriculo-ureterostomy shunting which required the placement of a polyethylene tube that extended from the cerebral ventricle to the ureter following a nephrectomy (19,20). Chronic problems, such as continued sodium loss, genitourinary infections, and uremic crystallization in and around the catheter/ureter attachment site, became apparent. It is important to note that in the era prior to 1950, desperate measures were often required for control of hydrocephalus. Scarff reported success with endoscopic cauterization of the choroid plexus (30), an operation generally abandoned by the 1950s. Bering, with significant laboratory and clinical observations of the choroid plexus, considered ependyma as another source for cerebrospinal fluid (CSF) production (3). In 1951, Scarff described his treatment of hydrocephalus by puncture of the lamina terminalis and the floor of the third ventricle (29) Figure 11.1. It should be pointed out that in 1922, Dandy described a technique for third ventriculostomy (10). By this time, Torkildson had devised the successful ventricular-cisterna magna shunt (34). The general response from neurosurgeons in the 1950s was that the third ventriculostomy and puncture of the lamina terminalis procedure was "not very successful." Scarff had reported a 40% mortality rate with the technique for obstructive hydrocephalus by the above-mentioned technique. In the 1950s, reports of successful ventriculo-atrial (VA) shunting for hydrocephalus appeared (28).

In 1951, Beller described the syndrome of brain abscess associated with cyanotic congenital heart disease, and presented a case with complete recovery. At that time, this was considered a rare disease entity (2).

In 1967, Ames reported his experience with ventriculo-peritoneal (VP) shunting using a valve to limit the CSF flow (1). By the 1970s, hydrocephalus shunting procedures were moving toward VP shunts in view of the potential chronic complications of a ventriculo-auricular shunt method Figure 11.2. Black drew attention to the phenomenon of a nephrotic syndrome as-

241

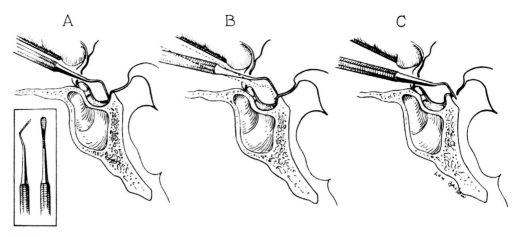

FIGURE 11.1. Technique of puncture of lamina terminalis and floor of third ventricle. (A) The anterior arachnoid walls of the cisterna chiasmatis and the lamina terminalis have been incised, and a dental instrument has been introduced through these incisions into the third ventricle until its tip is brought into contact with the dorsum sellae. (B) The tip of the dental instrument, guided entirely by sense of touch, has been gradually made to "walk up" the inner wall of the dorsum sellae until the tip rests on the lip of the dorsum. (C) The tip of the instrument has been advanced over the lip of the dorsum sellae, tearing a rent in the paper-thin floor of the third ventricle, and thus establishing communication between the ventricle and the interpeduncular cistern. (Scarff JE. Treatment of obstructive hydrocephalus by puncture of the lamina terminalis and floor of the third ventricle. J Neurosurg 8:204–213, 1951.)

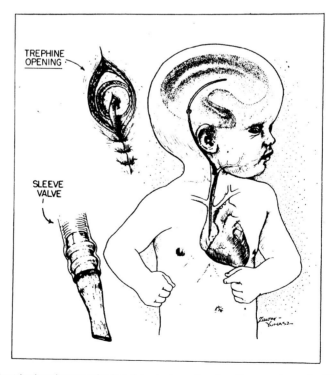

FIGURE 11.2. Ventricular shunt auricular. A technique for shunting cerebrospinal fluid intro the right auricle. (With permission. Pudenz RH, Russell FE, Hurd AH, Sheldon CH. J Neurosurg 14:171–179, 1957.)

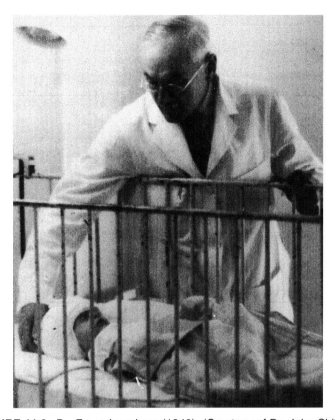

FIGURE 11.3. Dr. Franc Ingraham (1940). (Courtesy of Dr. John Shillito).

sociated with bacteremia following the above-mentioned type of shunt (4). Finney et al. further described this shunt nephritis as a distinct entity readily treatable but often missed because of its occult presentation (11).

In the 1950s, clinicians regarded the diagnosis of posterior fossa medulloblastoma as a disease associated with high morbidity and mortality, despite surgical intervention. In considering the achievements from past decades of neurological surgery, it should be recalled that Cushing (1931) described in detail the clinical presentation of children with cerebellar astrocytomas (9). Around 1929, Dr. Cushing suggested to Dr. Franc Ingraham that he should consider opening a pediatric neurosurgical division at the Children's Hospital in Boston, Massachusetts Figures 11.3, 11.4).

In 1957, Grant and Jones reported their clinical study of 200 posterior fossa gliomas in children (14). They noted a 50% operative mortality rate in the medulloblastoma group with an average survival time of 29 months (14). The recommendation at that time was that medulloblastomas and ependymomas were best treated by biopsy or limited resection alone (establishing a histological diagnosis followed by multiple courses of radiation therapy).

By 1960, Gardner and others had made the association of Arnold Chiari malformation with the presence of syringomyelia (Figure 11.5). He described the craniovertebral decompression, offering significant spinal cord hydromyelia resolution (12).

Management of intractable epilepsy in childhood was advanced by hemispherectomy. Hendrick et al. reported in 1950, that 41 hemispherectomy cases had been reported in the world literature (16). By 1960, it was well appreciated that children subjected to hemispherectomy following a diagnosis of infantile hemiplegia could improve in seizure control and

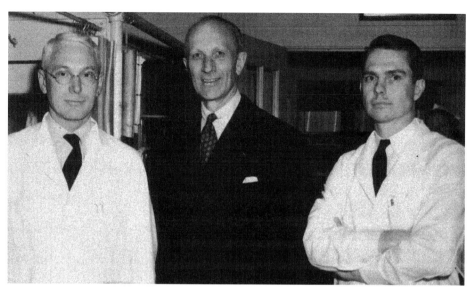

FIGURE 11.4. From left to right, Dr. Franc Ingraham, Dr. Wilder Penfield, and Dr. Donald Matson. (Courtesy of Dr. John Shillito)

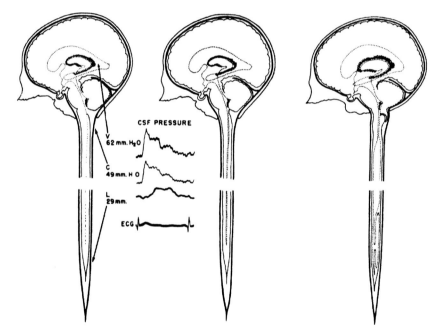

FIGURE 11.5. (Left) Normal adult relationships. The ventricular fluid pulse wave escapes through the 4th ventricle foramina into the subarachnoid space and is progressively damped as it passes down the distensible spinal dural sac. The bypassed central canal is a vestigial structure. (Center) Normal embryonal relationships. The 4th ventricle foramina are closed by semipermeable portions of the rhombic roof and the central canal is an offshoot of the 4th ventricle. (Right) Syringomyelia. The hindbrain hernia interferes with the escape of the ventricular fluid pulse wave through the foramen magnum and directs it into the central canal. A dilation or a diverticulum (syrinx) of the central canal results. (With permission. Gardner JW, Angel J. The mechanism of syringomyelia and its surgical connection. *Clin Neurosurg* 6:131–140, 1959.)

intellectual function. Similarly, surgery for cases with infantile Sturge Weber Syndrome, consisting of hemispherectomy or extensive resection of cortical pial angiomatosis sites, could end the often catastrophic seizures.

Neurosurgery for epilepsy has progressed with greater zeal and increasing emphasis on "invasive" brain monitoring technology and resective procedures.

THE 1970s

In the 1970s, pediatric neurosurgeons continued to focus on the management of hydrocephalus with the general availability of valved shunt systems. The popularity of the ventriculo-atrial (VA) shunt, as previously mentioned, gradually gave way to the VP shunt. Improvements in subcutaneous passage of the distal catheter and peritoneal placement by trocar made the surgical procedure seem less invasive.

The aggressive management of myelomeningoceles began during this decade. With the ability to control hydrocephalus, there was increased interest in achieving the best long-term outcome. It was recognized that most children born with a myelomeningocele would survive even if no treatment was offered at birth. Withholding treatment from these patients resulted in further deterioration of their neurological function (21). To achieve the best outcome, pediatric neurosurgeons began treating patients with early closure of the neural placode, early management of the hydrocephalus, and close observation and follow-up with multispecialty clinics. Long-term outcome studies now confirm the value of this approach (24).

The craniofacial approach to craniosynostosis began in North America during the early 1970s. This surgical concept, developed in France by Tessier, included a team approach to the management of these complex problems (31–33). Pediatric neurosurgeons were well aware of the value of a multispecialty approach to this type of problem, having developed the model in the management of myelomeningocele. The multispecialty approach remains the most common way to manage patients with complex craniosynostosis.

Protocol management of pediatric trauma

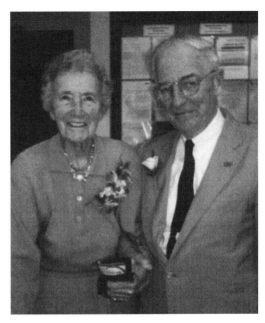

FIGURE 11.6. Mrs. Ingraham and John Shillito. Dedication of the Neurosurgical Suite, Children's Hospital, Boston, 1992. (Courtesy of Dr. John Shillito, Jr.)

began to become prominent and pediatric trauma centers were established (15), The value of air transportation, especially in rural areas was acknowledged and begun (5). Intracranial pressure monitoring became popular. Reports began to show the value of aggressive management of the severely brain injured child in an appropriate Pediatric Intensive Care Unit (7). Fewer patients remained vegetative, with most improving dramatically.

The 1970s also saw an increase in the number of neurosurgeons devoted to pediatric neurosurgery. Centers of excellence had already been established in Toronto, Boston, Philadelphia, Cleveland, Nashville, Columbus, Cincinnati, Chicago, and Los Angeles Figure 11.6. The early developers of this new subspecialty began to expand their specialized knowledge into fields of pediatric neurosurgery that now define it so well. The peculiarities of pediatric brain tumors, developmental anomalies of the brain, the problems of congenital spinal disorders, and the effects of trauma on the developing nervous system are but a few of the areas of interest that they explored. They helped to develop and define pediatric neurosurgery as a subspecialty (35). As these centers trained others, the practice of pediatric neurosurgery began to expand throughout North America. Recognition of the unique diseases and issues of children with neurosurgical problems led to an increasing cadre of young neurosurgeons who devoted their practice to this rapidly expanding subspecialty area of neurosurgery.

As pediatric neurosurgeons began to expand their unique body of knowledge, the desire to form a more recognizable group became an important issue. This led to the formation of the Pediatric Neurosurgery Section of the American Association of Neurological Surgeons (AANS). The Pediatric Section was the first section created within the AANS, and its first meetings were held in conjunction with the annual AANS meeting. It soon became apparent, however, that the time allotted at the AANS meeting was not adequate for scientific meeting coverage and discussion of the evolving issues of pediatric neurosurgery. With this in mind, the Pediatric Section began holding its annual meeting at a separate time so that an adequate scientific forum could be developed for pediatric neurosurgeons. Currently, the scientific program of the annual winter meeting of the Pediatric Section attracts over 200 papers each year. It has served as an ongoing forum for presentation and discussion of the important issues of the subspecialty.

The creation of the Pediatric Section, now a joint AANS/CNS section, which remains open to all AANS and CNS members, pediatric and non-pediatric neurosurgeons alike, posed the problem of identifying and recognizing those neurosurgeons who primarily practiced pediatric neurosurgery. In order to define the criteria more rigidly, the need for an organization to specifically represent pediatric neurosurgery was apparent. This, in turn, led to the birth of the American Society of Pediatric Neurosurgeons (ASPN) in 1978. Although its membership initially appeared exclusive, care was taken to identify all potential members as dedicated pediatric neurosurgeons.

THE 1980s

While recognition of the condition known as ''tethered spinal cord'' began in the 1970s, increased interest and experience made this more an issue for the 1980s. Recognition of the inevitable deterioration of patients with tethering at birth led to an aggressive approach to the problem (23). Others were less aggressive in their initial management but later results began to convince most of those who had taken a more conservative approach of the value of early surgery (8).

The surgical management of medulloblastoma became a model for improved survival in pediatric brain tumors with aggressive management by a team approach. It was discovered that patients who had gross total removal of the tumor had significantly improved long-term survival when surgery was followed by craniospinal radiation and chemotherapy (25). Five-year survival rates went from 35–40% to near 80% for patients with no evidence of CSF spread at the time of first presentation.

Research in developmental neurobiology increased our knowledge of the developing nervous system and led to a greater understanding of the complexities involved in many of the congenital lesions affecting the central nervous system. A unified theory on the development of the Chiari II malformation was developed (22) It linked together the various central nervous system developmental anomalies seen in the child with myelomeningocele. The theory was later validated by research on mice (17). A better understanding of split cord malformations also evolved (26, 27). It was shown that split cord malformations may occur in a single dural sleeve or in separate dural compartments. It was also demonstrated that the split may or may not have bone, cartilage, or fibrous tissue splitting the cord, but that the split cord malformation was always associated with tethering at the level of the split.

As pediatric neurosurgery grew into a subspecialty, an increased awareness of the need to assure optimal training grew. It was realized that post-graduate fellowship training would provide an excellent method to gain additional expertise in pediatric neurosurgery. Attempts to develop a fellowship training program, with the guidance of the Neurosurgical Residency Review Committee (RRC), led to the Accreditation Council for Pediatric Neurosurgical Fellowships (ACPNF). The Accreditation Council's function is somewhat similar to that of the RRC. Fellowship training programs are inspected and approved under the authority of the ACPNF Board of Directors. This board consists of five members—three from the ASPN, one from child neurology, and one from pediatric critical care. The ACPNF also reviews compliance with the pediatric neurosurgical fellowship training guidelines established by the American Board of Pediatric Neurological Surgery.

Another important development toward the advancement of pediatric neurosurgery as a subspecialty was the establishment of a journal devoted to pediatric neurosurgery subjects. This journal is currently titled *Pediatric Neurosurgery*.

THE 1990s

In the early 1990s, endoscopic procedures became increasingly more common in neurosurgery (18). Endoscopic instruments became smaller, images became brighter and clearer, and applications in neurosurgery began to appear. With the long-term complications of shunting becoming ever more apparent, endoscopic third ventriculostomy is now recognized as an alternative for many patients with hydrocephalus. A search for the most appropriate candidates for third ventriculostomy began to define the criteria and improve the chances for success (6). Endoscopic applications for the management of many forms of hydrocephalus and CSF loculations, such as loculated ventricles, slit ventricles, shunt obstruction, unilateral hydrocephalus, and arachnoid cysts, began to appear. Neuroendoscopic procedures are now a part of the normal surgical armamentarium of the pediatric neurosurgeon.

The increasing frustration of pediatric neurosurgeons with shunt problems, especially the concern over chronic over-drainage or the slit ventricle syndrome, led to the development of new designs for shunt systems. The Delta valve (Medtronic PS Medical, Goleta, CA) was felt by

many to be a great step forward in the management of over-drainage. The Orbis Sigma valve (NMT) was another design with limitation of over-drainage in mind. Both shunts have enjoyed long-term success and are very commonly used today. In the later part of the 1990s, the development of programmable valve systems saw the emergence of the Medos valve (Codman, Randolph, MA) into the North American market.

The American Board of Pediatric Neurological Surgery (ABPNS) was formed in September 1991, in order to facilitate the integration of pediatric neurosurgery fellowships and certification with the American Board of Neurological Surgery (ABNS). Counseling began with the American Board of Neurological Surgery, the Neurosurgery RRC, the AANS, ACGME, and pediatric neurosurgeons in order to establish a certificate for fellowship training in pediatric neurosurgery. By 1996, the ABPNS decided to certify pediatric neurosurgeons. Requirements for certification include the following criteria: 1) completion of neurosurgical residency training from an approved training program in the United States or Canada, 2) one year's fellowship training at an approved program, 3) certification in neurosurgery by the ABNS or the Royal College of Surgeons (Canada), 4) passage of a written examination given by the ABPNS, and 5) submission of surgical cases that indicate a practice of at least 75% pediatric cases.

THE FUTURE

As we enter the new millennium, the future development of pediatric neurosurgery appears excellent. We look forward to key developments and improvements in shunt design, more alternatives in the management of hydrocephalus, possible intrauterine surgical treatment of congenital disorders, central nervous system regulation, continued advancements in pediatric neurosurgery, and better strategies for treatment of refractory epilepsy.

The future for the subspecialty of pediatric neurosurgery is exciting and remains an area that is not focused on a single area of interest or surgical technique. Pediatric neurosurgeons treat congenital malformations, hydrocephalus, tumors, intractable epilepsy, infections, trauma, spinal deformities, and vascular problems. They are trained in the use of microscopic technique, frameless stereotaxy, neuroendoscopy, and removal of lesions that affect the skull base.

Opportunities abound for the fellowship trained and ABPNS board eligible pediatric neurosurgeon. Essentially, all academic programs either have or are recruiting such individuals, as are many large private practice groups. The future is bright indeed.

REFERENCES

1. Ames RH. Ventriculo-peritoneal shunt in the management of hydrocephalus. *J Neurosurg* 27:525–529, 1967.
2. Beller AJ. The sydrome of brain abscess with congenital cardiac disease. *J Neurosurg* 8:239, 1951.
3. Bering EA. Problems of the dynamics of the cerebrospinal fluid with particular reference to the formation of cerebrospinal fluid, etc. *Clin Neurosurg* 5:77–99, 1958.
4. Black, JA. Nephrotic syndrome associated with bacteremia after shunt operations for hydrocephalus. *Lancet* 2:9–21, 1965.
5. Black R, Mayer T, Walker M, et al. Special report: Air transport of pediatric emergency cases. *N Engl J Med* 307:1465–1468, 1982.
6. Brockmeyer D, Abtin K, Carey L, Walker M. Endoscopic third ventriculostomy: An outcome analysis. *Pediatr Neurosurg* 28:236–240, 1998.
7. Bruce D, Schut L, Bruno L, Wood J, Sutton L. Outcome following severe head injury in children. *J Neurosurg* 48:679–688, 1978.
8. Byrne R, Hates E, George T, McLone D. Operative resection of 100 spinal lipomas in infants less than 1 year of age. *Pediatr Neurosurg* 23:182–186, 1995.
9. Cushing, H. Experiences with cerebellar astrocytomas: A critical review of 76 cases. *Surg Gynec Obstet* 52:129–204, 1931.
10. Dandy, WE. An operative procedure for hydrocephalus. *Bull Johns Hopkins Hospital* 33:189–190, 1922.
11. Finney HL, Roberts TS. Nephritis secondary to chronic cerebrospinal fluid—vascular shunt infection: Shunt nephritis. *Childs Brain* 6:189–193, 1980.
12. Gardner JW, Angel J. The mechanism of syringomyelia and its surgical connection. *Clin Neurosurg* 6:131–140, 1959.
13. Grantham, EC. Prefrontal lobotomy for relief of pain. *J Neurosurg* 8:405–410, 1951.
14. Grant F, Jones RK. A clinical study of 200 posterior fossa gliomas in children. *Clin Neurosurg (Proceedings Cong. Neurosurg)* 5:1–24, 1957.
15. Haller JJ, Shorter N. Regional pediatric trauma center: Does a system of management improve outcome? *Z Kinderchir* 35:44–45, 1982.
16. Hendrick EB, Hoffman HJ, Hudson AR. Hemispherectomy in children. *Clin Neurosurg* 16:315–327, 1968.
17. Inagaki T, Schoenwolf G, Walker M. Experimental model: Change in the posterior fossa with surgically induced spina bifida aperta in mouse. *Pediatr Neurosurg* 26:185–189, 1997.
18. Jones R, Stenning W, Brydon M. Endoscopic third ventriculostomy. *Neurosurg* 26:86–91, 1990.
19. Matson PD. *Neurosurgery of Infancy and Childhood, 2nd Edition.* Thomas Springfield. 1969, pp 222–258.
20. Matson PD. Ventriculo-ureterostomy. *J Neurosurg* 8:398–404, 1951.
21. McLone D. Treatment of myelomeningocele: Arguments against selection. *J Clin Neurosurg* 33:359–370, 1986.
22. McLone D, Knepper P. The cause of the Chiari II malformation: A unified theory. *Pediatr Neurosci* 15:1–12, 1989.
23. McLone D, La Marca F. The tethered spinal cord: Diagnosis, significance, and management. *Semin Pediatr Neurol* 4:192–208, 1997.
24. Nelson M, Bracchi M, Naidich T, McLone D. The natural history of repaired myelomeningocele. *Radiographics* 8:695–706, 1988.
25. Packer R, Sutton L, Goldwein J, et al. Improved survival with the use of adjuvant chemotherapy in the treatment of medulloblastoma. *J Neurosurg* 747:433–440, 1991.
26. Pang D, Dias M, Ahad-Barmada M. Split cord malformation: Part I: A unified theory of embryogenesis for double spinal cord malformations. *Neurosurgery* 31:451–480, 1992.
27. Pang D. Split cord malformation: Part II: Clinical syndrome. *Neurosurgery* 31:481–500, 1992.
28. Pudenz RH, Russell FE, Hurd AH, Sheldon CH. *J Neurosurg* 14:171–179, 1957.
29. Scarff JE. Treatment of obstructive hydrocephalus by puncture of the lamina terminalis and floor of the third ventricle. *J Neurosurg* 8:204–213, 1951.
30. Scarff JE, Stookey, B. Non-obstructive hydrocephalus: Treatment by endoscopic cauterization of the chorid plexus, long term results. *J Neurosurg* 9:164, 1952.
31. Shillito J Jr, Matson D. Craniosynostosis: A review of 519 surgical cases. *Pediatrics* 41:829–853, 1968.
32. Tessier P. The definitive plastic surgical treatment of the severe facial deformities of craniofacial dysostosis: Crouson's and Apert's diseases. *Plast Reconstr Surg* 48:419–442, 1971.
33. Tessier P, Guiot G, Derome P. Orbital hypertelorism II: Definite treatment of orbital hypertelorism (ORH) by craniofacial or by extracranial osteotomies. *Scan J Plast Reconstr Surg* 7:39–58, 1973.
34. Torkildson A. A new palliative operation in cases of inoperable occulsion of the sylvian aqueduct. *Acta Chir Scand* 82: 117–124, 1939.
35. Walker M. For the Children. *Pediatr Neurosurg* 24:279–284, 1996.

12

History of Peripheral Nerve Surgery

Thomas Kretschmer, MD, David G. Kline, MD

STATUS OF THE SUBSPECIALTY IN 1951

The year 1951 was one of many changes and innovations in peripheral nerve surgery. That year, Max Theiler (1899–1972) was awarded the Nobel prize in Physiology or Medicine for his work related to the diagnosis of and prophylaxis against yellow fever. Other important medical innovations that occurred were the isolation of cephalosporins by Abraham and Burton. The thyreostatic drug carbimazole was synthesized by Lawson et al. For the first time, succinylcholine chloride was used clinically as a muscle relaxant by Bruecke et al. In the surgical field, the first workable prosthetic heart valve was designed and implanted in man by Charles Anton Hufnagel. Charles Dubost et al. successfully resected an abdominal aortic aneurysm and inserted a homologous graft. Nicholas Harold Lloyd Ridley implanted the first intraocular lens.

In addition to these advances in medicine, two important contributors to the medical sciences died in 1951. The first was physiologist Fritz Meyerhof (born 1884), Nobel laureate of 1922, who will always be remembered for the Embden-Meyerhof pathway that described the steps of glycolysis. The second was German surgeon Ferdinand Sauerbruch (born 1875), who influ-enced modern surgery in a diversity of ways. One of his contributions to reconstructive surgery was the Sauerbruch-stump. This was an arm prosthesis that allowed voluntary movement of artificial limbs by insertion of pins attached to pulleys into artificially created muscle channels of the proximal stump.

In 1951, the current knowledge in peripheral nerve surgery was mainly based on the results and experiences treating military casualties of World War II and of prior wars. During World War II, an estimated 25,000 peripheral nerve injuries were treated at 19 neurosurgical US Army centers. General Norman T. Kirk established a peripheral nerve registry to gather data of injuries as well as treatment results (127). By September 1945, 7050 nerve sutures and 67 grafts had been registered. Five centers were established by a Veterans Administration (VA) National Research Council Program and coordinated by a neurosurgeon, Woodhall, of Duke University. The follow-up exams began in 1947 and were published in 1956 as *Peripheral Nerve Regeneration: A Follow-up Study of 3,656 World War II Injuries* (195). The editors were Woodhall (Professor of Neurosurgery, Duke University Medical School, Durham, North Carolina) and Beebe, Ph.D. (Statistician, Follow-up

Agency Division of Medical Sciences, National Research Council, Washington, D.C.). Precise grading scales and statistical analyses were presented. Quite remarkable is that of the 7050 injuries treated by suture, only 67 had grafts. Soldiers on active duty and veterans represented a patient population that was far easier to follow than civilian patients. By regulation, the Army was responsible for treatment and follow-up of injury and illness until maximal medical improvement was reached.

A considerable amount of knowledge used for management of patients with nerve injury was still based on the experiences obtained during World War I and the American Civil War, as times of war always led to a large number of severe nerve injuries not encountered in times of peace. In 1915, Paul H. Hoffman (1884–1962), a physiologist from Freiburg, Germany, and Jules T. Tinel (1879–1952), a neurosurgeon from Paris, published their influential work on recovery of injured nerves and described the sign subsequently named after them. Silas Weir Mitchell was in charge of an army hospital in Turner's Lane, Philadelphia during the American Civil War. Together with his co-workers, he published a little book in 1864 and a more complete work in 1872 that has been considered by some as a foundation of modern knowledge on nerve injuries (114,115). Mitchell made many observations about peripheral nerve injuries and pain syndromes among war victims. In 1864, he coined the term causalgia, although he was not the first to describe the pathology.

A major medical problem during World War I was wound sepsis. The results of infection associated with nerve wounds as experienced by the British forces were published in the British Medical Research Council (BMRC) Special Report series No. 54 in 1920. The authors concluded that the nature of causalgia was still undetermined, that nerve grafting was not justifiable, and that secondary suture produced the best results. At that time, extensive mobilization was used to overcome nerve gaps. The contents of this publication were still regarded as current in the 1940s and thus were reprinted in 1942.

A state-of-the-art publication and reference for many leaders in the field in 1951, from a histopathological point of view, was Lyon's

(then Associate Professor of Anatomy at the University of California Medical School) and Woodhall's *Atlas of Peripheral Nerve Injuries*, published in 1949 (49). As outlined by Spurling in the foreword, this book also was a product of war. It was made possible since the nineteen United States neurosurgical centers established in World War II treated peripheral nerve injuries in high numbers. Another important factor to its publication was the availability of thorough and long-term follow-ups. The pathology reported was seen in patients with war casualties primarily treated at Walter Reed and Halloran General Hospitals from 1943 to 1945. Apart from its clinical value for nerve surgeons for years to come, it accurately reflected the knowledge and current practice at that time.

Severed nerves, lesions in continuity, and sutured and grafted nerves were described pathologically. The sections about lesions in continuity and nerve sutures motivated Kline 12 years later to think about a means to prevent inadvertent resection of injuries that might have potential for spontaneous recovery on the basis of electrophysiological evaluation. This was stimulated by published histological sections of resected lesions in continuity, which appeared to have a fair amount of healthy or regenerating nerve fibers. Other reference works of the 1950s, such as Kahn's *Correlative Neurosurgery,* showed cross sections of resected nerves that retrospectively might have had a potential for regrowth (72). Another neurosurgeon, Mayfield, wrote a book describing his experiences with causalgia (104), while in 1949, Stout published a section on "Tumors of Peripheral Nerves" in the *Atlas of Tumor Pathology* (159).

Challenges and Issues Facing the Subspecialty

The importance of neural fibroblasts for regeneration of nerve was a new issue identified by Denny-Brown in 1946 (36). Interestingly, this subject has gained additional attention in recent years, especially the role of connective tissue factors in functional and non-functional regeneration. Denny-Brown also examined the induction of paralysis of nerve by direct and tourniquet pressure, as well as the effects of transient stretching of peripheral nerve (37,38). These issues had been raised for centuries, not just within the recent decades. Gutmann and Young were interested in the effects of galvanic stimulation on denervated and reinnervated muscle in rabbits and reinnervation of muscle after various periods of atrophy (51,52). Reinnervation, the evaluation of factors influencing this process, and the physiology of nerve regeneration in grafts were of major interest. Hiller (1951) and Hoffman (1950 and 1951) reported their observations and experiments in this field (59,62,63). Guttmann studied various suture materials systematically under experimental conditions (53). Guttmann and Medawar experimented with chemical ways to inhibit fiber regeneration and neuroma formation (54). Lebendenko, in 1943, evaluated the time element for surgery of nerve lesions (85). Livingston and Livingston devoted a fundamental part of their research to pain syndromes of nerves and their mechanisms (87–89). They expanded the hypothesis concerning causalgia and examined the role of neuromas in phantom limb pain. Autonomic function, especially sudomotor changes after peripheral nerve damage, attracted the attention of Kahn, who described changes in sweating with nerve lesions in 1951 (71). Greenfield et al. were interested in another aspect of autonomic function, referable to cold fingertips after nerve injury (49). Other current topics were traction lesions, nerve grafting, damage to nerves by high velocity missiles with and without direct hit, and the pathophysiology of various lesions as well as their reinnervation (1–3, 132,133). Clinical manifestations of congenital neurofibromatosis were described in 1950 by McCarrol, while Mulder discussed the causative mechanism in Morton's metatarsalgia in 1951 (105,117). Sunderland was interested in regenerative rates, the course of recovery after nerve suture, and the pathomorphological changes in severed nerves, and together with Smith, evaluated different suture materials (163,171).

A dominant subject was the usefulness of graft material to restore function. Homografts were compared to other techniques of nerve reunification, such as end-to-end suture, use of tantalum foil, and other tubulation techniques (123). Strange reported an attempt to use a pedi-cled nerve graft, while a two-stage autograft for repair of the sciatic nerve was described by Mac-Carty in 1951 (160,94). Attempts with frozen dried nerve grafts in animals had already been made in 1943 by Weiss (188). He and Taylor had a special interest in repair techniques and were seeking alternative methods of sutureless reunion of severed nerves, such as tubulation and tantalum cuffs (185,186,188). Even then, isotope tracers were used to demonstrate proximo-distal fluid convection in the endoneurial spaces of peripheral nerves. Tantalum and its value in nerve suture and grafting procedures were a major subject of interest (155), especially among the American surgeons (Weiss, White, Spurling). Tantalum was even evaluated by White and Hamlin for its potential to control neuroma formation (189). Later, tantalum was abandoned because it induced scar and could be harmful to nerves. Fibrin glue as a suture substitute had been under investigation during the 1940s and 1950s. Young and Medawar had published a method of fibrin suture in the Lancet as early as 1940 (197). The usefulness of the so-called plasma clot suture for nerve repair had been evaluated and compared to silk sutures histopathologically by Tarlov et al. (172,173). Various types of tissue glues have sparked the interest of surgeons ever since.

Outstanding were the early works of Seddon of Britain (144–152) and Sunderland of Australia (163–171). Their past and subsequent contributions revolutionized peripheral nerve surgery as their systematic anatomic and pathologic studies built the foundation for the principles of nerve injury evaluation and methods of repair which are still valid today.

Seddon made important observations by examining peripheral nerve pathology that included the effect of ischemia and the histology of human ''homograft'' (150). Undoubtedly, the contribution he is remembered for the most is his classification of nerve injury, published in 1943 (145). He coined the terms neuropraxia, axonotmesis, and neurotmesis, which are still in frequent use today as they serve well to distinguish the basic injury types to nerve.

Sunderland provided insights about fascicular anatomy and topography in his early work. He examined the blood supply of different nerves, as well as describing in detail the intraneural topography of the radial, median, and ulnar nerves. He started to examine different lesion mechanisms and the use of autografts to bridge gaps. From the beginning, he attempted to provide an understanding of nerve injury by correlating classical anatomical and pathologic examinations with clinical and surgical experience. This comprehensive and in a sense already multidisciplinary approach was fundamental for his later landmark book of 1968 that influenced nerve surgery in the forthcoming decades (165).

Spurling had an abundant experience with nerve injuries and surgery during and before World War II. His interests lay in tantalum wire and foil for the repair of peripheral nerves, as well as timing of surgery. He reported his results with early nerve surgery in 1944 (156). In his experience, ''whole fresh homogenous nerve grafts'' failed to bring about functionally useful results (157).

As was the case in centuries and decades before (American Civil War, World War I, Russo-Japanese War, Balkan Wars), wartime rekindled an interest in nerve surgery. Thousands of injuries had to be repaired in American, European, and Australian centers. The meticulous collection of data in some centers resulted in a correlation of injuries, type of repair, and time course with results. The great numbers of patients treated led to new conclusions concerning timing, grafting, and level of injuries, as well as site specific differences. In part, this resulted in new strategies of nerve repair. Preliminary data from the American registry were published by Woodhall in 1946 (196). The data, together with detailed statistical analyses, were compiled a few years later in a book. Injuries and their management were then correlated with the follow-up results that had been gathered over several years (195).

Practice Content in the Field by 1951

Resection

It was not until World War I that the practice to resect a neuroma by successive thin slices to a level where the epineurium retracted and nerve fasciculi stood out discretely became accepted.

World War I surgeons were in general agreement that when in doubt, resection of the neuroma followed by nerve suture was preferable to neurolysis (181). The concept of funicular or fascicular matching evolved at about the time of World War I. In 1913, Stoffel reported that a definite intrafunicular anatomy existed in peripheral nerves (158). Early in the history of peripheral nerve surgery, procedures were devised for obtaining end-to-end suture.

Stretching and Positioning

Stretching the nerve and positioning of the limb in a favorable position were earlier techniques that had been extensively used (143, 158). The so-called two-stage bulb suture technique was used extensively by American and British surgeons during World War I in combination with limb positioning to overcome lengthy nerve defects. In principle, the distal (then called gliomatous end) and proximal (then called neuromatous end) bulbous stumps were sutured together without resection to healthy tissue as a first stage to prevent retraction and gain some length via nerve stretching. At the second stage, the definitive suture was placed after neuroma resection.

Nerve Coaptation and Tantalum

Although during World War II many Allied nation surgeons began to favor nerve graft techniques, British surgeons rarely applied the bulb-suture technique (16). In American medical centers, the metallic suture material tantalum (with a thickness of 0.003 inches in diameter) was very popular and regarded as being ideal since it was fine in caliber yet strong and thought to be relatively inert in tissue (Figure 12.1). In addition, the fate of the suture could be followed by x-ray studies. Tantalum was technically more demanding to use. A big problem with all sutures was intraneural fibrosis promoted by the neurorrhaphy itself, as Lyons pointed out from a histologist's viewpoint (93,222). In an effort to prevent this and possibly decrease fibroblastic invasion at the anastomosis site, non-suture methods, such as plasma suture or anastomosis with tantalum and collagen tubes, were tried.

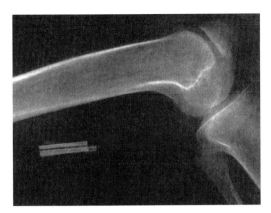

FIGURE 12.1. Radiograph of a tantalum foil around the suture line of a sciatic nerve (from *Atlas of Peripheral Nerve Injuries*, WR Lyons, B Woodhall, W.B. Saunders, 1949).

American surgeons frequently used tantalum foil measuring 0.00025 to 0.00050 inches in thickness to sheath the repair sites (Figure 12.2). The VA Monograph dealing with end-to-end anastomosis performed during World War II by American surgeons reported that 74% of cases were repaired with tantalum wire, and in 98% of cases, the suture site was wrapped in tantalum foil (195).

Despite knowledge of the deleterious effects of stretch injury, bulb-suture techniques were still seen as applicable in cases were a nerve gap

could not be overcome by mobilization, transposition, and/or the use of joint posturing. Grafting was not yet seen as an essential method by the American surgeons during World War II, let alone in 1951. During World War I, results with grafts were so poor that the procedure was mostly utilized as a last resort. Only the encouraging results of Bunnell (1937) and Ballance and Duel (1932) with nerve grafts in facial nerve lesions helped avoid complete abandonment of the method (10,20–22).

Disruptions of suture sites and reactions to sutures and wrapping material as well as suture site neuromas were a frequent source of failure of neurorraphy or grafts. The failure of whole thickness allografts, as well as frozen-dried whole and cabled allografts, was well documented. Nerve autografts were used only with moderate success. Lyons reported a case where fibrin film wrappers (without sutures) were used and failed to keep the graft in good apposition to the nerve stumps (93).

Repair Strategies

In 1949, Lyons summarized the different suture techniques used as follows (93): A ''coaptation suture'' was the temporary apposition of severed nerve ends at the time of debridement to prevent retraction. An ''immediate or emergency suture'' was definitive and performed at

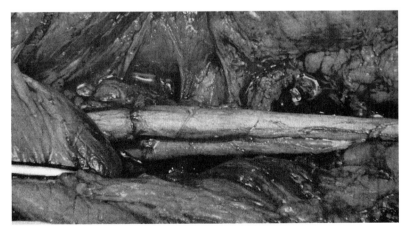

FIGURE 12.2. Completed interrupted epineural suture of peroneal and tibial nerve using a 0.003 inch thick tantalum wire (from *Atlas of Peripheral Nerve Injuries*, WR Lyons, B Woodhall, W.B. Saunders, 1949).

the time of severence or within a few days of that, when further neurosurgical intervention was not intended. For various reasons this variant was not favored very much. As Lyons pointed out, "An important contraindication to the immediate suture of war wounds in peripheral nerves, in addition to the fear of infection and the technical difficulties of suture and nerve segment mobilization, is the inability of the surgeon to evaluate exactly the extent of pathologic changes in the respective nerve ends. The effects of interfascicular hemorrhage and the disorganization of fasciculi are not fully demarcated until the reparative changes associated with fibrosis have time to develop." A series of histologic figures in the same chapter illustrated failures in immediate nerve repair. Even nowadays this is a statement that can be repeated again and again.

"Early suture" was a repair after secondary wound closure. A definitive suture was performed several weeks after injury (average 39 days) following wound debridement, secondary wound closure, and wound healing. Nerve repair after healing of the other soft tissue wounds represented the commonly used method.

The "deferred or delayed suture" was performed several months after injury. Its purpose was to avoid infection due to associated injuries, transport of patients, and the like.

"Secondary suture" described the second, or if necessary, third attempt at nerve repair due to a neuroma formation in the first primary suture, disruption of the first suture line, or failure from other causes. A "bulb-suture" was used if all other attempts to overcome a nerve gap failed and grafting was not considered (Figure 12.3).

In some regards, the Allied surgeons, especially the British, differed in the techniques applied. Seddon felt that in cases were a gap of 10 cm or greater was to be overcome, post-operative methods of stretching, including the bulb-suture technique, invariably resulted in nerve damage to such an extent as to preclude recovery.

Grafting

The British did not feel that grafts were very useful. Summarizing the war results from British centers, Seddon in 1954 concluded: "Heterogenous nerve grafting is useless. Fresh and stored homografts, although promising experimentally, have been tried at two of the British centres and by Spurling, Lyons, Whitcomb and Woodhall in the American army, and have been found wanting" (147, p 389). Seddon explained that the success of autografts in experimental settings was no longer in doubt and that it was evident that if certain conditions were met, the results with human autografts might equal those of well-executed sutures. It appeared to him that the likelihood of success or failure would be mainly determined by technique. In his section on technical considerations in the BMRC report, he described that the donor nerve should have a cross-sectional area that would at least be equal

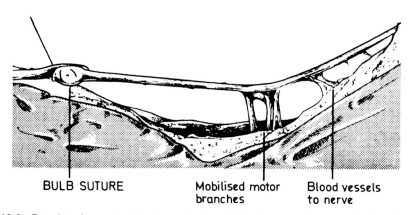

BULB SUTURE   Mobilised motor   Blood vessels
                     branches   to nerve

FIGURE 12.3. Drawing demonstrating the principle of a bulb suture to gradually lengthen a nerve (from *Surgical Disorders of the Peripheral Nerves,* HJ Seddon, Williams & Wilkins, 1972).

to that of the distal stump of the damaged nerve. In the BMRC patient population, autologous nerve grafting was performed on 70 patients and nerve pedicle operations on 4 patients in the period from 1941–1947 (147). Recovery was good in 42% in optimally repaired relatively simple cases. Overall, results were between 33–50%. If cases with partial recovery were included, the grafting procedure yielded useful return in 68% of cases.

Predegenerated Grafts

Another issue at that time was the use of pre-degenerated grafts. Abercombie and Johnson in 1942 noted that if the degenerated axons and myelin had been phagocytized, there might then be "open" channels waiting to receive the new outgrowing axons (1,2). The activity of the Schwann cells was found to be greatly increased (3). The Schwann cells' important role in nerve sprouting was already well appreciated. Despite these observations, predegenerated grafts never found widespread use. Instead, more importance was attached to a clean bed for the graft to ensure that proper vascularization was not hindered by a badly scarred bed.

Plasma Clot Suture

Plasma clot suture was found to be useful for some cutaneous nerve grafts because of their loose structure and the mobility of their sheath. The concept was introduced by Young and Medawar. Fibrinogen was mixed with thrombin and dripped with a fine pipette onto the wound site. A sutureless technique for securing union between divided nerve ends was described by Ballance and Duel as early as 1932 (10). They discovered that when a nerve graft was placed within the facial canal, it was soon fixed firmly in place by the clotting of plasma. Thus, they advocated the procedure for the repair of infratemporal facial nerve injuries. In 1940, Young and Medawar described fibrin suture of nerves in rabbits using cockerel plasma fortified with fibrinogen (197). Two years later, Seddon and Medawar gave this method a clinical trial. The original preparation of Young and Medawar consisted of cockerel plasma fortified by dissolving fibrinogen so that its normal concentration was increased up to ten-fold. This was superseded by human material, which in Britain was obtained from the Lister Institute, Elstree, Hertfordshire. It was found to be of no value when the suture site was under tension or when a pool of plasma could not be obtained about the nerve ends. Tarlov described modifications in the technique in an attempt to overcome these obstacles (Figure 12.4) (172).

Tantalum's Fate

Autologous plasma compared favorably with silk, whereas tantalum nerve sutures, introduced by Spurling, were thought to incite no more of a response then was consistent with sutural trauma alone (93). Tantalum sutures were also praised for their additional advantage of allowing the diagnosis of suture line separation to be made by roentgenography. The early promises of tantalum, however, have not been sustained by the test of time. Tantalum sutures were found to be no better than silk and furthermore, a severe late reaction could be observed. Initial claims that the material was inert in tissues appeared to be based on inadequate experimental studies, according to Sunderland in 1968. When the nerve was wrapped with tantalum, failure was thought to be related to folding and fragmentation of the foil as well as to a reaction induced by the foil itself (165, p 659). For the sake of historical interest, it should be mentioned that Sargent and Greenfield in 1919, as well as Guttmann in 1943, systematically investigated different suture materials with regard to their adaptability for nerve (53,142). The latter demonstrated in an experimental setting that catgut sutures resulted in a marked fibroblastic reaction that could impede regeneration. Interestingly, among the materials studied, women's hair, plain linen thread, and silk caused the least irritation, whereas gut, dyed silk, and impregnated sutures caused a more severe reaction.

Conduits

Attempts to use various types of conduits to guide nerve fibers across a gap had already been made prior to and throughout the 19th century. (181). Tubulation, although inventive, was not

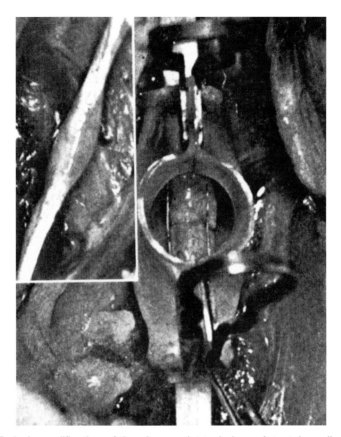

FIGURE 12.4. Tarlov's modification of the plasma clot technique. A tantalum sling suture relieved tension at the nerve ends. The removable mold device was used to facilitate the encasing of the apposed nerves with plasma (from *A History of Neurological Surgery,* EA Walker, Williams & Wilkins).

very successful or persuasive. Von Büngner successfully bridged a nerve gap with a segment of human brachial artery and reported this in 1891 (23,181). During the Russo-Japanese War, formalin-hardened arteries were used (58), while fascial tubes were tried during the Balkan Wars (35). In World War I, German surgeons tried agar tubes (42). During World War II, American medical officers used tantalum sleeves extensively for a period of time. Until 1951, no method of tubulization proved to be very useful. Another interesting approach to overcome a nerve gap was the interposition of formalin-fixed spinal cords of animals, which was tried during World War II with discouraging results by a Scandinavian surgeon (13).

Clinical Electrophysiology

The technical means to evaluate peripheral nerve function were only available at a very modest level in current practice in 1951 (33). However, with the development of electroencephalography and the need for better methods to study peripheral nerve injuries in World War II, interest in electromyography experienced a revival (70). The initial impetus to use clinical electromyography was given by Piper in 1912, although the electrical phenomena associated with muscular contraction were known earlier (130).

In 1947, Nulsen and Lewey described intraneural bipolar stimulation as a new intraoperative aid in the assessment of nerve injuries (124). Intraoperative stimulation was accepted so slowly that Seddon, in his 1972 edition of *Surgical Disorders of the Peripheral Nerves,* felt an urge to express his astonishment that ". . .in an age of technical idolatry, exploration of nerves is still being performed without the aid of a nerve stimulator, although already. . .our surgical grandparents used a faradic coil. . ." (149,249). Moreover, he described that any instrument would be suitable as long as it delivered a stimulus of a duration not exceeding a thousandth of a second of controllable intensity, and preferably with an interval of half a second between the pulses. He underlined that bipolar stimulation should always be used.

Leaders in the Field in 1951

The leaders in the field, in 1951, have already been mentioned, as most were involved in the war effort or in research post-World War II. Sir Sydney Sunderland provided his five grade classification of peripheral nerve injuries during 1951 (164). His work has been cited repeatedly throughout the following decades. Born in 1910 in Brisbane, Australia he received his M.B., D.Sc., M.D., and LL.D. (honorary) degrees from the University of Melbourne. It was at the University of Melbourne that he began his career as Lecturer in Anatomy and Neurology in 1937. He was appointed to the Chair of Anatomy at the age of 27 and became Professor of Anatomy and then of Experimental Neurology at the same institution, publishing a remarkably large volume of original experimental work concerning the anatomy and regeneration of the peripheral nervous system. He was a visiting Specialist in Peripheral Nerve Injuries at the 115th Australian General Military Hospital and the Commonwealth Repatriation Department in Melbourne from 1941 to 1945, where servicemen in the Australian Forces who sustained peripheral nerve injuries in the Middle East were treated. He worked with Hugh Trumble, a neurosurgeon. Later, he served as Dean of the University of Melbourne from 1953 to 1971, worked as a member and eventually became Chairman of the Royal Australian College of Surgeons Certification Committee between 1945 and 1969, and

served on many governmental and academic councils in Australia and New Zealand. In addition to being knighted by the Queen of England in 1971, he spent time as a demonstrator in Anatomy at Oxford, as a Visiting Professor in Anatomy at Johns Hopkins Hospital/University, and as a Fogarty Scholar at the National Institute of Health (NIH). He is best known for his work with fascicular anatomy and the changing topography of these intraneural structures. Sir Sydney also made singular contributions to the understanding of oculomotor involvement by uncal herniation as well as the mechanisms involved in nerve root or spinal nerve stretch and avulsion.

Sir Herbert Seddon, his British counterpart, began his career slightly earlier than Sunderland, and was highly recognized as a surgeon and scientist. Many aspects of his professional life bear a striking similarity to Sunderland's contributions and professional interests. He proposed a very simple classification of injuries, wrote about nerve anatomy as well as lesion mechanisms, and played a major role in the development of the field. Sir James Learmonth, Sir Harry Platt, and J.Z. Young served together in 1953 on the Nerve Injury Committee of the BMRC, with Seddon as chairman. By that time, they were famous orthopedists with a special interest in peripheral nerves. Submuscular transposition of the ulnar nerve was originally described by Learmonth. Young, in the early 1940s, produced an extensive number of important papers that covered peripheral nerve topics from basic science (anatomy and regeneration) to technical aspects (functional repair and suture alternatives). Platt had experimented with autogenous fascial tubulization and autogenous nerve grafts as far back as 1920. He published a book in 1921 about peripheral nerve injuries based on experiences in World War I, and in the 1930s and early 1940s, went on to expand his knowledge about nerve injuries and traction lesions.

Meanwhile, in the United States, by 1951, G. E. Spurling had years of expertise in the field. However, the sign that bears his name is related to cervical pathology. A positive Spurling's maneuver is indicative of nerve root compression in the neural foramen. In the 1930s, he advocated dorsal sympathetic ganglionectomy to treat upper extremity causalgia, which helped to make the possibility of sympathectomies more generally known. Spurling made other important contributions related to spinal surgery.

Sterling B. Bunnell (1882–1957) of San Francisco already had surpassed the zenith of his clinical work. He will be remembered as a surgeon with a special interest in hand surgery and peripheral nerves. He pioneered nerve grafting techniques and reported his first promising results in 1927. Most famous, however, are Bunnell's tendon suture, Bunnell's suture with a pullout wire, and Bunnell's no man's land (the palm area being not ideal for tendon suture). In 1944, his text *Surgery of the Hand* was published and was one of the early works with limited references to peripheral nerves (followed by *Hand Surgery in WWII* in 1955). His French counterpart was Marc Iselin (born in 1898), whose book *Surgery of the Hand*, published in 1942, likewise presented outlines of peripheral nerve management.

Neurosurgeon Frank Nulsen had a special interest in peripheral nerve surgery because of his profound experience with nerve injuries sustained in Korea and cared for in the United States at the Valley Forge Hospital. Nulsen made important observations concerning lesions in continuity that were included subsequently in the VA Monograph of 1956.

Barnes Woodhall (1905–1985) initially worked on a range of neurosurgical topics at Duke University as an assistant professor. In 1942, he enlisted in the Army Medical Corps (after a short period at Ashford General Hospital), and served as Chief of Neurosurgery at the Walter Reed General Hospital in Washington, D.C. until 1946. During that time, he accumulated his experience with peripheral nerve injuries. Woodhall (Figure 12.5) returned to Duke University in 1946 as Professor and Chairman of the Division of Neurosurgery. His important contributions to peripheral nerve surgery were published between 1946 and 1956. In his later career, he was deeply involved in various other clinical and administrative areas (193).

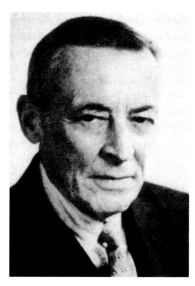

FIGURE 12.5. Portrait of Barnes Woodhall (from *History of the Congress of Neurological Surgeons,* JM Thompson, Williams & Wilkins).

PROGRESS, INNOVATIONS, AND ACCOMPLISHMENTS BY DECADE

1950s

Seddon expanded the understanding of traumatic nerve lesions with his publications from 1943 to 1954. He reported results with cable grafts, described the steps of regeneration, presented methods to evaluate and monitor the latter, and introduced a simple system of injury types. The BMRC Special Report series was published in 1954. Woodhall and Beebe reported in the VA Monograph of 1956 on their results with tantalum foil in 984 of 3656 World War II cases. In 1954, Bunnell authored *Hand Surgery in World War II*, a book with limited references to peripheral nerve.

BMRC Series

The BMRC Special Report Series from 1954 was one of the early multicenter studies in the field (147). Different centers in Britain devoted their work to systematically study different medical topics with standardized investigations, uniform data collection, and precise statistical analysis (at all centers). Special areas addressed included results of nerve suture, vasomotor phenomena, autonomic function, and effects of galvanism on denervated muscle. The latter was investigated in detail using animal models at the Oxford center. The whole idea and concept of this multicenter study was not new, but based on the former BMRC committee work and their report from 1920. The so-called special report series No. 54 had reported results of World War I surgery. At that time, the dominant issues included the nature of causalgia (which remained undetermined), coaptation of nerve stumps and timing thereof, and means to overcome nerve gaps and infection. Because of poor results, nerve grafting was found to be unjustifiable, and secondary suture was felt to be more reliable. Extensive mobilization of nerve stumps was the most commonly used method to overcome nerve gaps. The overwhelming problem, however, was sepsis, which probably was a major cause for poor results. The successor of this volume was the 1954 report, which again was a result of war. Perhaps most influential to workers in the field for decades to come was the chapter on histopathology. A substantial part was based on Seddon's publication of 1943, where he described his three categories of nerve injury, namely, neuropraxia, axonotmesis, and neurotmesis (143). Finally, the BMRC system to grade muscle power was introduced, which is still the one most widely used today.

BMRC Results

The principles of neurolysis for lesions in continuity were discussed by the BMRC and, most notably, did not support the practice of neurolysis. "The use of internal neurolysis by longitudinal incision of the sheath of the nerve or by intraneural injection of saline has little to support it either in theory or in practice" (147, p 81). The results were tabulated in precise tables and a clear-cut conclusion on the results of nerve suture was provided. In divided nerves, the prospect of functional return varied from nerve to nerve, and was altered by level of injury, delay, and gap. Favorable results with radial repair were mentioned. Surprisingly, ulnar nerves did

as well. Recovery of sciatic function had been considered so poor that in cases of transection, amputation of the leg was sometimes advocated. The tibial nerve showed far better recovery as compared to the peroneal nerve. Only 20% of high sutures of the peroneal nerve proved to be worthwhile. A definite point was made that final outcome could not be evaluated until three years had elapsed. Delay, high level of injury, and extensive resection had been associated with an unfavorable result (147, pp 377–378). Their results indicated that primary suture could no longer be regarded as ideal, even in aseptic wounds, although it must be remembered that most of these data were based on gunshot injuries. With the development of new drugs and antibiotics, sepsis was better controlled than during World War I.

A hypothesis on the cause of causalgia was formulated that stressed the role of a dysfunctional sympathetic nervous system, as sympathectomy was found to be helpful in its treatment.

Sympathectomy

After Spurling had proposed sympathectomy via a posterior approach for the treatment of causalgia in 1930 (154,181), patients who underwent sympathectomy usually had their stellate ganglion and the T2 to T3 thoracic ganglions removed, which usually left them with a permanent Horner's syndrome. In 1955, Palumbo first described and performed a method to prevent a Horner's syndrome by removal of only the lower third of the stellate ganglion (128).

Sensibility and Sweating

Around 1958, Moberg introduced new methods for evaluating sensibility testing (Figure 12.6) (116). He demonstrated the importance of two-point discrimination and the ninhydrin test in evaluating the return of sensory function. Kahn reported a fairly easy method to evaluate sudomotor paralysis qualitatively by direct observation of beads of sweat through the plus 20 lens of an ophthalmoscope (71).

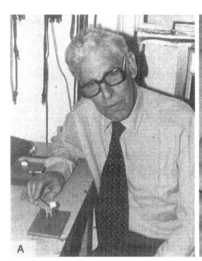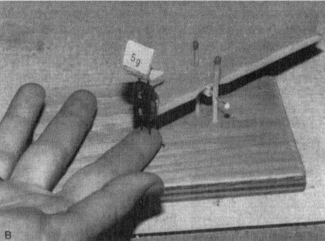

FIGURE 12.6. Eric Moberg and one of his devices for sensibility testing (from *Management of Nerve Problems,*" GE Omer Jr, M Spinner, AL Van Beek, W. B. Saunders).

VA Study

In 1956, the American counterpart to the BMRC was the VA Medical Monograph *Peripheral Nerve Regeneration: A Follow-up Study of 3,656 World War II Injuries.* Other VA Monographs reported on prisoners of war, tuberculosis in the army, and war neuroses. Included in the 1956 volume on nerves were some important results of Nulsens' experiences with Korean casualties at the Valley Forge Army Hospital from 1951 to 1953. Portions of one chapter were devoted to the problem of lesions in continuity. "The problem of the neuroma in continuity whose status cannot be determined by visualization is a frequent one and it is therefore necessary to go to some pains to define certain evidence for unsatisfactory regeneration when this cannot be settled by the gross appearance of the lesion"(195, p 586). The chapter on neurosurgical implications addressed one major drawback of the usual intraoperative nerve evaluation of those days prior to direct intraoperative nerve action potential recording. "Unfortunately, the extent of injury to a peripheral nerve cannot be determined by gross inspection unless it be divided; nor can one reliably infer the extent of injury from the functional deficit."

Equipment

One section of the VA Monograph outlines a checklist of the essential and desirable equipment of that time. Essential items included peripheral diagnosis and operating room charts, atraumatic .003 tantalum wire and atraumatic ophthalmologic silk suture, a spring algesiometer, von Frey's hairs (a set of hairs and brushes of scaled thickness used in the evaluation of touch sensation and discrimination), spring scales for recording muscle strength, and an operating room nerve stimulator. An electromyographic unit consisting of an oscillograph, preamplifier and a precision stimulator, a Richter dermometer, a skin temperature recorder, and a chronaximeter were seen as desirable equipment.

VA Results

VA data showed that the emergency suture of war wounds of peripheral nerves was followed by a failure to regenerate in over 50% of cases. These results were reported by the best surgeons, as experience and training background of surgeons had been considered and evaluated as well. Therefore, immediate or emergency peripheral nerve surgery was seen as contraindicated. One exception was the rare case of an expanding hematoma, the precursor of a false aneurysm, with progressive peripheral nerve dysfunction caused by pressure. In their conclusion, the authors indicated that no statistically significant positive effect of the type of suture material (silk versus tantalum, tantalum foil reinforcement, plasma clot suture) on outcome could be detected. Suture line disruptions reportedly were a frequent reason for failure of regeneration. This was especially so in the lower extremity related to excessive suture line tension. Combined nerve and arterial injuries in the upper extremities were proven to have an unfavorable outcome, as were nerves that were affected at a very proximal level. Concerning timing of surgery, it was recognized that favorable results could still be obtained within eight to nine months after injury, whereas repairs after a year post-injury showed significantly worse outcomes.

Other neurosurgical books with extensive chapters on peripheral nerve surgery include Volume Two of *Surgery in World War II* published by the Medical Department of the United States Army and edited by Spurling and Woodhall in 1959, and *Correlative Neurosurgery* published in 1955.

1960s

Sunderland's Classification

Sunderland's work suggested that the morphological and pathophysiological knowledge of peripheral nerves was not yet complete. His anatomical studies on the internal constitution of nerves and nerve trunks led to a totally new understanding of nerve injuries and the importance of injury level. Of significant importance was his classification of nerve injuries (Sunderland Grades I to V, first published in 1951) that was provided in the first edition of *Nerves and Nerve Injuries*, published in 1968 (164,165). This monumental book was a comprehensive guide to the subject and also included the practical important aspects of diagnosis and treatment.

As Sunderland stated in the preface, it was an account of the thoughts, experience, and investigations of one individual and represented 25 years of personal endeavor in the field. Descriptions of operative procedures were omitted on purpose, with the intent of concentrating on establishing the scientific criteria for the techniques employed to repair damaged nerve. Although published in 1968, the book was a result of activities in the laboratory and the clinic from 1940 to 1957.

Another individual who contributed to the understanding of internal neuroanatomy was Kaplan. Substantial studies on the subject at the beginning of this century were performed by the German anatomist, Ranschburg (1917), and the clinician, Stoffel (1913) (135,158).

Roos devoted his efforts to detection and management of the thoracic outlet syndrome and described a transaxillary approach for first rib resection in 1966 that gave rise to controversy that still persists today (136–138).

A milestone which is discussed in more detail in the pain section of this volume was White and Sweet's forty year résumé in 1969 of their work on pain (191).

Microsurgery

Most importantly, the 1960s saw the onset, development, and the increasing application of microsurgery. The introduction and application of microsurgical techniques certainly marked a turning point in this century's history of peripheral nerve surgery. While the term microsurgery was used as early as 1892, it referred to the study of neurologic pathways in amphibia. In these studies, the neural crest was removed after closure of the neural tube (40). Jacobson (a vascular surgeon from Vermont) and Suarez are thought to be the first to use the term with today's meaning and implications. In 1960, they used the term ''microsurgery'' in the title of a paper that described small vessel repair in laboratory animals (68). Earlier, however, Michon et al. applied microsurgical techniques in 1964 to peripheral nerve surgery (109,153).

Microsurgery has two mainstays apart from

the surgical skill—proper magnification and instrumentation. The use of the operating microscope, again, had its definite roots in laboratory work on animals. This fact makes it quite difficult to exactly trace its introduction, as many scientists were experimenting with microscope-like devices on animal dissections. In the mid-1950s, Lougheed and Morely of Toronto began to work with a microscope in order to study the effects of subarachnoid blood on vessels of the circle of Willis. They reported this method in 1961 (90). Also in the mid-1950s, another celebrity in the neurosurgical field, Malis, used microscopic magnification for his experiments on the cerebral cortex of cats. Along the way he discovered that the bipolar coagulator, invented by Greenwood in 1940, was quite a helpful tool to improve hemostasis (40, 50). After a few technical alterations, it turned out to be one of the most important microsurgical tools (Figure 12.7).

The Surgical Microscope

At the turn of the century, Maier and Lion had already used microscopes to study animals (99). The first to apply the surgical microscope clinically were otologists (134). They employed them in the treatment of middle ear diseases since magnifying loupes were not completely satisfactory. In 1921, Nylen used a monocular dissecting microscope on two patients, one suffering from chronic otitis and the other from labyrinthine fistulas (125). Apparently at Nylen's suggestion, Holmgreen performed fenestration under a microscope and described his experiences with the microscope for use in otosclerosis (64,134). The binocular operating microscope as a clinical tool was used by Nylen in 1954 for otological surgery (125), whereas a monocular device had been applied as early as 1923 by Holmgreen for otosclerosis surgery (64). Kurze (Figure 12.8) (of the University of California)

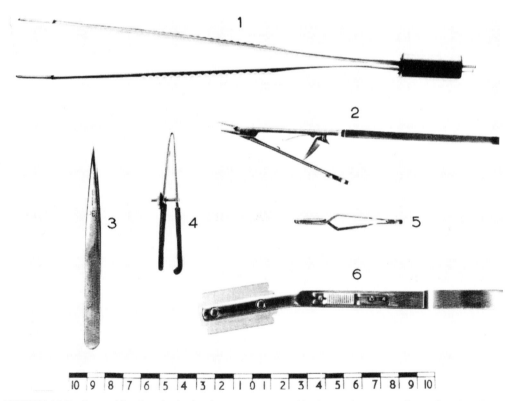

FIGURE 12.7. Assembly of typical microinstruments used in the early 1970s. (from *Surgical Disorders of the Peripheral Nerves,* HJ Seddon, Williams & Wilkins, 1972).

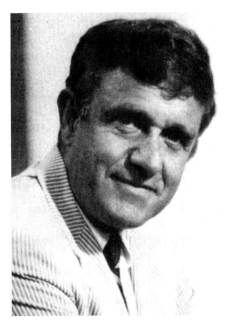

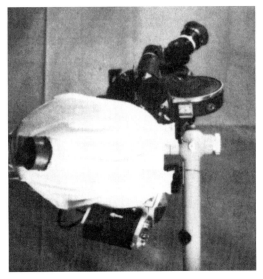

FIGURE 12.9. Operating microscope in 1960 (from *Neurosurgery,* RH Wilkins and SS Rengachary, McGraw-Hill).

FIGURE 12.8. Portrait of Theodor Kurze, who probably performed the first craniotomy in 1957 using the operating microscope (from *Neurosurgery,* RH Wilkins and SS Rengachary, McGraw-Hill).

and House, his collaborator from the ear-nose-throat (ENT) faculty, became interested in developing an improved route for surgery on acoustic neurinomas. It is reported that Kurze performed a craniotomy under the microscope on a human being as early as 1957 (40). In 1961, House, and in 1962, Kurze and Doyle, reported on subtemporal middle fossa approaches to the internal auditory canal for removal of acoustic tumors by using microdissection techniques (40, 84). Prior to the advent of practically usable binocular operating microscopes in the late 1950s, nerve repairs were technically very ungratifying. Smith had used the surgical microscope (Figure 12.9) in peripheral nerve reconstruction since 1962, and Kurze detailed his early experience in 1964. Millesi, a plastic surgeon, is recognized for contributing much to the popularity and refinement of microscopic techniques for nerves. He and his co-workers continuously developed and advanced microsurgical methods (111–113). Higher magnification and the advantage of focused and high power illumination were factors to help the manual process of repair. In addition, evaluation of the pathology could be improved many fold.

1970s

Needle and Suture Refinement

Probably the most important next step into the microsurgical era was the introduction of other fine instrumentation. Acland, in 1972, and Buncke, in 1971, developed small needles and fine metallic sutures for use in experimental replantation and transplantation (4,19). For some observers, this marks the actual breakthrough in miscrosurgery, for now, bulky sutures could be discarded. Thus, the suture lines became smooth and accurate, and satisfied the very critical eye. With the new suture, material trauma was minimized and coaptation could be achieved without inducing scar tissue on an interfascicular level. Employing the new equipment, Buncke managed to place arterial grafts of less than one mm (19).

Phalen

Phalen had been diagnosing and treating patients with carpal tunnel syndrome since 1947 and will be remembered by the sign that bears his name and which is provoked by a maneuver that is used for evaluation of median nerve compression. In 1970, he was able to reflect on a 21-year experience with the compression neuropathy and the test that is associated with his name (129). He frequently had reported about his experiences with carpal tunnel syndrome since 1951. In 1950, he presented a report entitled ''Spontaneous Compression of the Median Nerve at the Wrist'' at the 99th Annual Meeting of the American Medical Association before the section on Orthopedic Surgery. His report was based on his experience with his first 11 patients. During the discussion, he felt that he presented a clinical syndrome ''unknown to almost all of the physicians attending that meeting,'' as noted in his 1970 paper. This is an interesting comment, considering that today carpal tunnel syndrome is probably the most frequently treated peripheral nerve syndrome.

Seddon and Sunderland

Seddon published *Surgical Disorders of the Peripheral Nerves* in 1972, another landmark work that embraced the field of peripheral nerve surgery from structure to treatment (149). His knowledge, which was founded on a clinical basis, added further to the understanding of traumatic lesions. Very important for the advancement and direction of the field were his studies on the results of cable grafts to bridge gaps, the rate of neural regeneration, and his standardized way and method to evaluate lesions and lesion levels.

Over a three-decade period, Sunderland supplied detailed information about the internal neuroanatomy of peripheral nerves. In 1978, a second extensively revised and updated edition of his *Nerves and Nerve Injuries* was published. Microsurgery progressed in big steps as an increasing number of surgeons applied the new techniques and were seeking more and more precise coaptation techniques.

Microsurgical Research Centers

Specialized replantation and microsurgical research centers were built around the world mostly under the guidance of orthopedic and hand surgeons, such as Kleinert and Kutz in Louisville, Kentucky, O'Brien in Melbourne, Australia, and Tamai in Tokyo, Japan. Buncke at the University of California in San Francisco, Strauch at the Albert Einstein College of Medicine, Urbaniak at Duke University, and E. Meyer at the University of Zürich in Switzerland, created microscopic teaching laboratories (127).

In the 1960s, Millesi, at the University of Vienna, had already begun to refine microsurgical grafting methods with his co-workers Meissl and Berger. He propagated a new interfunicular grafting technique that offered a means to restore neural continuity and function where recovery was impossible in the past. He was a strong advocate of the operating microscope and cable grafting, and reported his results therewith (112,113). Concerning the classification of peripheral nerve injuries, he later added further subgrouping to Sunderland's five grade classification that took the extent and localization of the fibrotic reaction (intrafascicular, interfascicular, or epifascicular fibrosis) into consideration (43). The intent was to supplement the Sunderland classification from a surgical viewpoint to help operative decision-making (epineuriotomy versus epineurectomy versus neurolysis versus resection and grafting). Millesi et al. also introduced and advocated the principle of no-tension-repair (98).

Lack of Neurosurgeons in the Field

During the 1960s and 1970s, neurosurgeons played a significant role in the further development of peripheral nerve microsurgery. Donaghy speculated that after the poor success rates of nerve grafting in World War I, many neurosurgeons paid scant attention to these techniques; hence, a big part of the development and research in the field was accomplished by orthopedic and plastic surgeons, especially in the 1970s and 1980s (40). An exception to the rule was facial nerve repair. Neurosurgeons demonstrated new methods of repair and developed decompression techniques of cranial nerves (69). One of the exceptional neurosurgeons was Samii, who operated on a number of nerve patients in Germany. By applying microsurgical techniques in a very meticulous way to suture small nerves under the microscope, he was able to obtain high recovery rates in the 1970s (140,141). Kline in America and Hudson in Canada devoted their clinical and research interest to peripheral nerves and advocated grafting techniques as well as intraoperative recordings (47,61,74–82).

Nerve Action Potential

A key to Kline's operative approach to peripheral nerves was a new way of intraoperative evaluation of nerve damage by applying the electrophysiological method of nerve action potential (NAP) measurement. He had been encouraged to find a means against inadvertent resection of nerves that still had potential for recovery. He was inspired by histopathological demonstrations of supposedly irreversibly damaged and thus resected nerves with a fair amount of at least morphologically intact-looking axons. Despite the great progress that had been made with the new microsurgical concepts, a major problem remained unsolved. What were the objective signs that indicated that a nerve segment was damaged irreversibly, hence needing resection and graft repair? How could one sort out those nerve segments that appeared normal from the outside and yet were nonfunctional? On the other hand, how could one prevent resection of nerves that had a potential for spontaneous recovery? Mere electrical stimulation, as previously mentioned, was not sufficient. A solely axonotmetic nerve with an excellent potential for spontaneous recovery could demonstrate a nerve conduction block marked enough to prevent a muscle contraction, which, however, did not mean that all axons were dysfunctional. There were just not enough distal functional ones to elicit a visible muscle contraction. It takes many months for enough axons to grow down the distal stump, reach muscle, and reconstruct motor end plates well enough for stimulation to provide muscle contraction.

After experimental work on macaque rhesus monkeys, Kline and Dejonge found a solution in evoked compound nerve action potentials. The amplitude and pattern of potentials were related to axon counts and distribution as to the size at the recording sites. A method to directly stimulate and record from the nerve intraoperatively to guide the decision-making process was described (74). The proposed method provided information about regeneration across a lesion in continuity that was otherwise not available. The first paper describing this new method was published in 1968 yet it was not until 1998 that Spinner wrote the following in the second edition of *Management of Peripheral Nerve Problems* (16 years after the first edition). ''Interfascicular nerve grafting and intraoperative electrical evaluation of neural lesions in continuity . . . are now established techniques.''

Spinner presented important anatomical variations in the forearm in 1972 and published the first edition of the monograph *Injuries to the Major Branches of Peripheral Nerves of the Forearm,* followed by the second edition in 1978.

Vascularized Nerve Grafts

Inspired by the breathtaking new possibilities that the new microsurgical techniques offered, vascularized nerve grafts (VNG) were clinically applied, with the idea of supplying better chances for the sprouting of new axons along the natural guiding tracks by preventing ischemia of the graft. Taylor and Ham reported the new technique of VNG in 1976 (175). In 1981, Fachinelli et al. reported the use of VNG (44), while in 1984, Bonney et al. (peripheral nerve specialists from Great Britain) reported promising results (14), as did Merle et al. in 1985 (108) and Doi et al. in 1984 (39). In principle, a nerve graft was moved with its blood supply. The theory behind the technique was to prevent a lengthy period of ischemia in the recipient nerve bed that might damage Schwann cells. Schwann cells had been recognized as being essential for a successful graft repair. A vascularized graft was thought to improve and better maintain the Schwann cell population and along with increased vascularity, a faster and more complete axonal regeneration was expected (127).

Conduits

Lundborg, from the Department of Hand Surgery, Malmö Hospital, Sweden, resumed the ancient attempt of finding an optimal tube for sprouting axons to overcome gaps and find the distal stump (91,92). He first experimented with mesothelial tubes in rats. As is known today, the results of nerve grafting in a rat model differ crucially from humans. One of the biggest drawbacks of rat models is the far better result that will always be obtained when compared to any human model, as sprouting axons almost miraculously will find ways to distal stumps. As a consequence, the initial positive results in rats might have been overrated. Terzis further refined and proved the importance of the new microsurgical grafting methods and their superiority over the older concept of suture under tension.

1980s

In his Surgical Neurology editorial *Where Has Peripheral Nerve Surgery Gone?*, White complained that surgical treatment and experimentation dealing with nerve trauma seemed to be no longer part of neurosurgical practice. "With the exception of the stimulating studies of Kline and Ducker, one has the strong impression that the neurosurgical interest in the surgical techniques appropriate to the repair of damaged nerves and the investigation of nerve regeneration is now at an all-time low. As a matter of fact, the most active and innovative clinical and research activity in this important field is now being undertaken by plastic and orthopedic surgeons" (192).

Sunderland Society

On an organizational level, the need for a nerve study group was seen and a group of surgeons interested in peripheral nerve pathology met at Duke University in 1978, hosted by Goldner. A biannual program was discussed and a preliminary society formed, with Curtis, Goldner, Kline, Omer, and Spinner as the founding senior members (127). In 1979, The Peripheral Nerve Study Group was founded. Its purpose was to "study in depth difficult problems and advances in peripheral nerve anatomy, physiology, and surgery." The first formal program was held July 1980, in Glen Cove, New York, with Spinner as president. Sunderland was the invited guest speaker. Kline was elected to be the next president and Omer was elected as the succeeding president. Membership quickly expanded and a multinational society was formed, with members from Australia, Austria, Canada, France, Italy, Sweden, Switzerland, and West Germany. In September 1980, Kline proposed a name change, since the group's name was similar to The Neurological Nerve Study Group, which already had met for a number of years. At the second formal meeting in New Orleans in November 1981, the group changed its name to The Sunderland Society, as suggested by Spinner and his executive committee, in appreciation of Sunderland's professional contributions. Today, the group meets every two years and has become a forum for exchange of clinical and scientific novelties, ideas, and results in the field.

After three years of work, Omer and Spinner edited a multi-authored book entitled *Management of Peripheral Nerve Problems,* with the intention of presenting the state-of-the-art for those physicians actively involved in the management of peripheral nerve problems. One of its aims was to combine results of research and clinical activities in a single volume for surgically orientated readers, and outline methods of care for all the major nerves of the body.

Fascicular NAPs and Intraoperative Histochemistry

Hudson and Kline applied their intraoperative method of evaluating nerve damage by evoked compound NAPs routinely in every single case since the 1970s and frequently reported on the advantages of the method and their results. Another driving force in the development of microsurgical techniques and an early advocate of tension free repair was Terzis. In her 1987 monograph, she described a single fascicular recording setup for compound action potentials as another intraoperative tool aiding in the evaluation of peripheral nerves (176). Another topic that was meticulously pursued involved histochemical means to differentiate intraoperatively between motor and sensory fibers in order to obtain superior fascicular matches. The histochemical methods available still lacked practicability in an operative setting and still do at the present time. (One of the fastest methods to date, the ACE histochemical method, still has results only available within 2 hours.) (178).

Nerve Coaptation Alternatives

After it was realized that even the finest microsurgical sutures placed in the epineurium or perineurium could lead to fibroblastic proliferation and possibly cause compression, scarring, and misdirection of axonal tissue, attempts at sutureless coaptation were investigated. Even though microsuture coaptation was the most commonly used technique, various research centers were busily working on alternative methods

for nerve coaptation. Laser nerve welding was at the top of the list. Laser neurorrhaphy, however, seemed to lack tensile strength, which diminished the possible advantage of avoiding placement of foreign material into the repair site and inducing less scar tissue (45,60,89,101,122). Experiments with fibrin glue saw another revival as well.

Fibrin Glue

In his 1988 report, Narakas summarized the reasons preventing the broader application of fibrin glue. At the same time, he explained its proper use and indications (Figure 12.10a, Figure 12.10b) (118). Due to problems with the Food and Drug Administration (FDA) approval in the United States, fibrin glue was used on a regular basis much longer in Europe, (e.g., for dural repairs). Therefore, a fundamental number of experiments with fibrin glue as adjunct in nerve surgery were being performed in Europe (11,43,101,118,120).

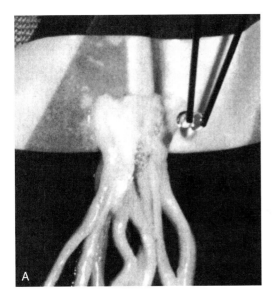 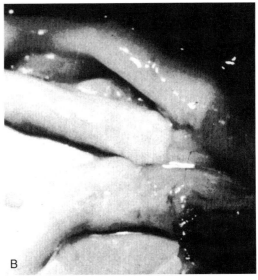

FIGURE 12.10A and B. Examples of Fibrin glue technique as used by A. Narakas. (A) Grafts are assembled to form a multistrand cable and glued together over a distance of 0.5–1.0 cm. Droplets of the compound glue can be seen. (B) Fascicular group grafting using glue without stay stitches. The "naked" fasciculi can be seen at the end of the cables (from A Narakas, The use of fibrin glue in repair of peripheral nerves, *Orthop Clin North Am* 19(1),187–199, 1988, W.B. Saunders).

Fascicular Versus Epineurial Repair

At the very beginning of the 1980s, fascicular nerve versus epineurial nerve repair was a very popular topic among microsurgeons. Results and the different indications are mirrored in several publications, including works by Millesi and Terzis in 1984 (111), Hudson et al. in 1979 (61), Sunderland in 1979 (167), and an experimental study by Kline et al. in 1981 (81). Results indicated that epineurial repair should be employed when differentiation of the motor and sensory branches was not clear cut, which seemed to apply especially to upper arm injuries. In injuries where motor and sensory branches were clearly distinguishable, for example with some wrist level injuries, a grouped fascicular technique seemed to yield better results "with or without epineurial stint" (167). Documentation indicated that better alignment yielded better results, but surprisingly in many of the reports, the final conclusion of epineurial versus perineurial repairs (and as such fascicular repairs) in predominantly motor or sensory nerves showed little differences in final results. As was known for many years, one of the most important factors in determining the long-term results was the patient's age (61,81,179).

Neurotrophic and Neurotropic Factors

From the 1950s through the 1970s, the approach to peripheral nerve repair was changing from a pure mechanistic one to a more biological approach, while in the 1980s, the importance of various factors at a molecular biological level was strongly stressed (139). Current research was more and more focused on different neurotrophic and neurotropic factors that could possibly aid in nerve repair by supporting, inducing, or maintaining axon sprouting, guided by grafts and different types of conduits. Since the 19th century it was known that a peripheral nerve could sometimes regenerate across small gaps when some sort of tubulization guidance was provided. Lundborg et al. (92), Chiu et al. (26), Strauch et al. (161), and Mackinnon and Dellon (95–97) showed a special interest in different sorts of tubulization techniques. Preformed pseudosynovial tubes, autogenous vein grafts, and bioabsorbable polyglycolic acid tubes served as sheath material. First successes were obtained with conduits that covered nerve defects of 3 cm or less and in sensory digital nerve injuries where only small gaps had to be overcome. The next step in this development was to equip the conduits with different neurotropic and trophic factors in an attempt to attract the sprouting axons faster and in greater number and thus, improve the functional result. Mackinnon, Hudson, and Midha also revived research on human allografts, after new methods of immunosuppression became available, which helped to overcome some of the old obstacles of general transplant surgery (96,98). The new developments concerning immunological aspects involved either manipulation of the host's immune system or modification of the donor graft by pretreating it with lyophilization or high-dose irradiation to decrease antigenicity (55,98). Unfortunately, suppression of the host's immune system is still necessary if allografts are used. A diversity of conduit types have been advocated, a trend that is still present at the turn of the 20th century. So once again, a main challenge was to find means to overcome a nerve gap other than by sacrificing an intact autologous nerve. Mackinnon and Dellon published a very popular book in 1988 that covered all aspects of clinical nerve surgery as well as current research topics, with an extensive section devoted to their new approaches towards allograft and tubulization techniques (96).

The knowledge of intraneural anatomy still was far from complete due to the complexity and frequency of fascicular changes and the unknown degree of axonal mixing within fascicles, for example, in the upper extremity nerves. Often, the plexiform pattern of the fascicles within proximal nerves limits the prospect of surgical success. Therefore, also in the 1980s, anatomic dissections and cross-sectional studies of intraneural topography were performed to yield information that would possibly help in surgery. Chow et al., in 1985, showed that the motor branch of the ulnar nerve at wrist level in 98% of cadavers was lying either dorsal or ulnar and dorsal (28). Watchmaker et al. found that the median nerve at the distal forearm and wrist level contained three separate groups of fascicles with the motor branch traveling along the third group on the radial or volar radial aspect of the nerve (183). Further insight into fascicular patterns led to a better understanding of lesion mechanisms and their repair, especially when split repair was needed.

Molecular Biology

Research began to focus on the molecular biological approach towards nerve injuries and regeneration, as reflected by a growing number of publications devoted to these topics (95,178, 182). The concepts of neurotropism and neurotrophism were not exactly new, but now they began to influence the management of nerve injuries and inspired experimental settings that tried to support nerve repair on a molecular biological level (for extensive review see (46)). In a very broad sense, ''neurotropism implies an ability to influence the direction of nerve regeneration, while neurotrophism refers to an ability to influence the development and maturation of the nerve'' (178,220). Over 100 years ago, Forssman, in 1898, described an early appreciation of neurotropism. It concerned the nerve's attraction to its distal stump or an appropriate end organ (178). In 1982, Politis extended this concept when he discovered that when using Y chambers as conduits for sprouting axons, they would selectively grow down the channel that contained the distal nerve stump (131). Brushart, in 1987, noticed that proximal motor stumps selectively reinnervated distal motor nerve stumps rather than sensory ones (18).

The concept of neurotrophism had been formulated in 1951 by Levi-Montalcini and Hamburger (86). They discovered that mouse sarcoma had selective stimulating effects on the sensory and sympathetic nervous system of the chick embryo. After additional experiments, they found several tissues that were able to stimulate nerve growth and proliferation in culture. In 1959, together with Cohen, they isolated and purified a substance, and named it nerve growth factor (NGF) (29). Soon, it became obvious that not only a transected nerve itself excreted factors to attract (tropins) and nourish (trophins) nerve sprouts, but also the surrounding fibroblasts. This line of research indicated that the apparent role of the surrounding fibrous tissue in nerve repair might have been underestimated. In 1989, Cordeiro found evidence that acidic fibroblast growth factor enhanced peripheral nerve regeneration in vivo (31). In the 1990s, NGF-related research launched an overwhelming interest in factors that were able to influence nerve growth and repair.

Over the decades, mere mechanical principles were replaced by biological and physiological-based concepts that were now supplemented to a growing extent by approaches on a molecular biological level.

Nerve Tumors

Significant changes also came about in clinical work, as peripheral nerve tumors and brachial plexus injuries were operated on in increasing frequency. After the introduction and broad availability of magnetic resonance imaging (MRI), peripheral nerve tumors could be diagnosed at earlier stages. Furthermore, it became possible to appreciate their relation to surrounding structures preoperatively significantly more precisely, which in turn permitted one to choose a more focused surgical approach (e.g., posterior versus anterior approach to the brachial plexus). MRI of the soft tissue and particularly nerves turned out to be extremely useful in determining the location and involvement of neoplasias, especially in primary nerve tumors (30). Formerly rare pathologies, such as desmoid tumors, were diagnosed with higher frequency. Subsequently, incidence rates for several types of nerve tumor are changing. In spite of the research on nonsurgical therapies, surgical removal has remained the cornerstone for treatment. Neurofibromas, which formerly were felt to be unresectable without major deficit, now often can be resected with little or minimal deficit thanks to changes in methods of dissection and use of intraoperative electrophysiological techniques (41).

Brachial Plexus Injuries

Profound changes in attitude and management of brachial plexus injury took place after Seddon's 1963 address to the Royal College of Surgeons, in which he stated that repair of traction injuries of the brachial plexus was sufficiently disappointing (except for the upper trunk) as to essentially preclude it (148). In the late 1970s, more plexus repairs were performed, and throughout the 1980s, systematic approaches to repair were established in most peripheral nerve repair centers. One of the early researchers who greatly influenced this very specialized field was Narakas (1927–1993). He was born in Lithuania and later adopted Swiss citizenship and spent his professional life in Lausanne. His admirers described him as a multigifted and multilingual individual who paired great surgical dexterity with artistic capability and compassion, testified to by hundreds of drawings made by him to document his cases. He was greatly recognized and

highly appreciated for his devoted and very unique way of teaching. In order to share his knowledge, he organized symposia. The first of these took place in Lausanne in 1976. This plexus symposium was attended by Sunderland (Figure 12.11). It is said that part of Narakas' surgical dexterity was related to his wide experience in different surgical fields. Apart from complete training in general surgery, his postgraduate training included two years of neurosurgery, two years of orthopedic surgery, one year of ear-nose-throat and plastic surgery, and then four years of hand and peripheral nerve surgery. He was introduced to peripheral nerve repair, grafting, and brachial plexus explorations by his former chief, Verdan, in the early1960s.

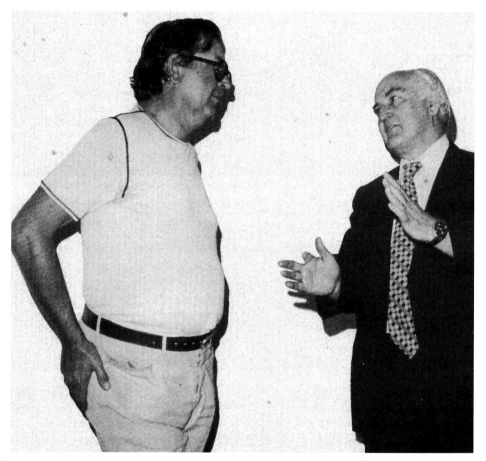

FIGURE 12.11. Sir Sydney Sunderland and Dr. Narakas during the first plexus Symposium in Lausanne, Switzerland, 1976 (from *Brachial Plexus Lesions,* C Bonnard and ACJ Sloof, Springer).

Very early on he was interested in microsurgery for which he was initially trained by Yasargil in Zürich. His work showed that remarkable results could be achieved with brachial plexus injuries when expertise in the microsurgical principles of graft repair and neurotization (nerve transfer) techniques were applied at the right time for the right reason.

Birth Palsies

After some delay, the attitude towards birth palsies changed as well, and different plexus repair procedures and nerve transfers began to be applied. A landmark reference to compare operative results against spontaneous recovery was the series by Tassin from 1983, who followed 44 children with birth palsy who did not receive a brachial plexus operation (174). Management of birth palsies is still one of the most controversial topics in nerve surgery, especially in terms of appropriate timing for surgery. Gilbert and Tassin are certainly among those who are to be credited with the renewed surgical efforts in this field because of their work which suggested the efficacy of early operative intervention and repair by grafts (48).

1990s

Endoscopic Carpal Tunnel Release

While endoscopic carpal tunnel release (CTR) became a very popular technique during the 1990s, potential risks of the procedure are still controversial and often discussed. In 1983, Paine described a retinaculotome placed through a small incision on the volar wrist crease to divide the transverse carpal ligament (127). The drawbacks of such a technique became apparent with incomplete division, palmar hematoma, or in some instances, direct nerve damage. As a result, several surgeons independently developed and described a modified Paine procedure, the endoscopic technique. The first reported endoscopic technique applied was the Okutsu Universal Subcutaneous method, described in 1987 as a single port technique with incision of the ligament in a distal-to-proximal direction (126).

Chow, in 1989, described a two portal method (27), while in 1992, Agee, and in 1993, Menon, described other single port techniques (5,107).

Peripheral Nerve Stimulation

Peripheral nerve stimulation for focused pain after peripheral nerve injury certainly was not invented in the 1990s, but has been used by various pain centers. In the 1960s, the first trials with peripheral nerve stimulation that used placement of cuffs proximal to the injury sites were performed. Today, stimulation leads are placed beneath the involved nerve proximal to the nerve damage, with the nerve separated from the lead by fascia or intermuscular septum. Peripheral nerve stimulation may nowadays be considered when surgery on the nerve and/or conservative therapy fails in cases where pain is highly focused in one particular nerve, or involves not more than one or two nerve roots in its distribution. In 1990, Gybels et al. reported remarkable success rates (81%) in their very carefully selected patient pool (56,127).

Laser Coaptation

Further work with laser coaptation indicated that the method was not yet a valid alternative to suture. Dehiscence rates as high as 12–20% were seen in CO_2 laser-spot welding of the epineurium. Compared to suture repair, the surgical time could be decreased by one-third. However, bonding strength was measured to be approximately 10% that of a suture repair initially. After 8 days, bonding strength was found to equal that of suture repair (60,106).

Allografts

In allograft research, a new generation of immunosuppressants such as cyclosporin A and FK-506, promised to reduce rejection rates with increased potency and less toxicity. Recent data from Midha, Mackinnon, and others suggest that host axon regeneration across peripheral nerve allografts continues after cessation of immunosuppression with FK-506 (178, p 220).

Nerve Transfers

Although sporadically used much earlier with fairly good success in cases of irreparable nerve damage of brachial plexus segments due to root avulsions, "neurotizations," or nerve transfers began to be favored and performed routinely at a growing number of centers in the 1990s. The differing potentials of transferred and recipient nerve combinations, such as spinal accessory to suprascapular nerve and intercostals to musculocutaneous nerve, or more recently, medial pectoral to musculocutaneous nerve, are current operations. The question remains as to which functioning nerve should be transected, rerouted, or transferred to which distal recipient nerve in an attempt to innnervate a non-functioning muscle. Only recently, results of longer follow-up periods and greater case numbers were available. Once again, Narakas was the neurosurgeon who greatly influenced the development of this repair variant, applicable in brachial plexus nerve root avulsions (119,120,121). He not only reported very good results, but also documented his operative approaches beautifully with his own drawings. A selection of 60 of his cases, along with his drawings, was posthumously published in 1999 as edited by B. Sloof and C. Bonnard. They are not only beautiful to look at but nicely illustrate the pathology, and give interesting insights to the different repair steps. In combination with the case histories, his drawings allow one to see how he deduced the most efficient way of performing a repair. Narakas died in November 1993. During his academic career, he authored a total of 216 papers relating to the field of nerve transfers and repairs.

In 1991, Sunderland made his last extensive contribution to the field in the form of a monographic critical appraisal of nerve injuries and repair (168). This book was based on his lifetime study of nerves and reflected on selected and sometimes controversial topics of the field. Sunderland died in Melbourne, Australia on August 27, 1993, at the age of 82.

In 1995, the first edition of Kline and Hudson's book *Nerve Injuries–Operative Results for Major Nerve Injuries, Entrapments, and Tumors* was published (76). It reviewed the results of treatment over a 30-year period, and took over 9 years to write. Clinical data from more than 3000 surgical cases were evaluated after extensive follow-up periods and presented together with current knowledge, as well as personal experience with management of the different pathologies. The book's style was one of dual authorship and differed from the currently available multi-authored reference monographs in the field. The authors felt "that a comprehensive and yet readable analysis of results in this field appeared indicated and had not been done since publication of the VA Medical Monograph: Peripheral Nerve Regeneration of 1956."

In 1998, a second edition of Omer and Spinner's *Management of Peripheral Nerve Problems* was published. It contained major revisions of past chapters and the addition of new ones. Birch, Bonney, and Wynn-Parry put together their outstanding experience in the field in their 1998 *Surgical Disorders of the Peripheral Nerves*, which presented extensive chapters on pain and iatrogenic peripheral nerve injuries (12).

End-to-side Anastomosis

Clinically oriented techniques still being researched include nerve lengthening, allografts, tubulization techniques, and end-to-side anastomosis. Initial cases of end-to-side anastomosis in humans were presented at the July 1999 meeting of the Sunderland Society in London. Earlier animal models showed that a distal nonfunctional nerve stump can be connected end-to-side with a functioning nerve and induce nerve sprouting from the proximal functioning nerve down to the distal stump without sacrificing existing function. Missing proximal nerve stumps are seen as another good indication. First repairs using this promising new technique were performed in humans in 1997 and 1998 in Vienna by Frey. In order to induce sprouting, a small epineurectomy was performed on the donor nerve to expose the fascicles. Interestingly, the best results were obtained when additional trauma at the epineurectomy site occurred. This could be provoked by a slight pinch with the forceps. Such injury might incite neurotropic factors.

Nerve Expanders

Van Beek, plastic surgeon and former president of the American Society of Reconstructive Microsurgery, advocates nerve lengthening procedures to overcome nerve gaps by use of expanders. He supports using nerve lengthening rather than nerve grafting in severe fibrosis of the recipient bed, which would preclude adequate outcomes with autologous grafting, as well as in cases of inadequate donor nerve supply (127). Freeze dried muscle grafts with retained basal laminae have also been tried as scaffolding for sprouting axons.

Neurobiology

Summarizing the important scientific novelties in the field during the 1990s is equivalent to a molecular biological excursion. This in itself says a lot about the gradually changing foci of interest in the nerve field. As can be observed in all medical fields, research has made ample use of available methods in genetics and molecular biology. Envisioned research goals are now quite often aimed at actually altering and actively influencing defects and deficiencies at cellular and genomic levels. Thus, an overview of this burgeoning area of science is difficult. Neurotropic factors, receptors, second messengers, and arrays of trophic factors from multiple sources, including neurotrophins, neuropoietic cytokines, insulin-like growth factors, and glial cell line-derived neurotrophic factors, have all been discovered. Some of these factors appear to significantly influence functional recovery of neurons (46,178). It remains to be seen which factors actually turn out to be of clinical relevance.

In 1995, Demirkan et al. discovered that serum of a transected distal nerve stump exerted an influence on sprouting axons (34). When they reinjected axoplasmic fluid from the site of nerve transection beneath the epineurium distal and proximal to the stump, they could enhance regeneration of conventionally repaired nerves. In 1994, Kim et al. tried to use labeled Schwann cell transplants in nerve repair, as it was found that nerve regeneration is not directed or limited by axonal growth but to a major extent by Schwann cells and some of their cell products (73). Several factors, such as insulin-like growth factor (IGF), have been found to enhance regeneration.

Finally, we now recognize that nerve injuries alter genetics. The newest term used is "immediate early genes", or IEGs. Following a nerve injury, different types of IEGs are locally upregulated, and result in increased levels of proteins that could be indicative of ongoing repair mechanisms, such as c-fos, c-jun, jun-b. For example, c-fos protein increased in spinal cord cells after root avulsions at corresponding levels, which implies locally upregulated transcription of genetic messages as compared to controls (198). Interestingly, NGFs seemed to prevent upregulation of IEGs. Whenever IEGs were upregulated, intracellular calcium and CAMP levels increased as well (102). Furthermore, other multifunctional proteins related to neurodegeneration could be isolated, such as hsp 70 in 1988 and SGP-2 in 1992 (103,180).

CHALLENGES AND ISSUES AT THE TURN OF THE CENTURY

Genetics

One of the overall goals of molecular biology will be to weave the patches of applicable knowledge into a sound fabric in order to generate a chemically therapeutic and maybe even a gene therapeutic model for peripheral nerve regeneration. Growth promoting substances that can influence genes might eventually be isolated. In gene therapy, replication-deficient retroviruses already are used as carriers for transferring a desired specific gene. Therefore, if the genes that are important for nerve regeneration are detected and isolated, they could be delivered locally to the target cells. Clinical models already exist for gene therapy of Parkinson's disease and amyotrophic lateral sclerosis. Other growth promoting substances and markers for the potential of regrowth and recovery are being sought. However, these are not the only aspects of nerve repair that have been and will be followed. The exciting and sometimes frightening world of genetic techniques also comprise genetic engineering. This involves the controlled production of designed substances via manipulated host cells. A good example of the successes and benefits to be gained is the production of genetically engineered human insulin. One of the implications of this line of reasoning would be to clone nerve fibers to use them as autologous grafts. A very closely related area is tissue engineering, which has already been developed and followed by plastic surgeons and dermatologists to produce appropriate skin grafts for burn victims. Remarkable results have been achieved by culturing autologous keratinocytes in burn victims (65). Of course, nerves are different than tissue and keratinocytes are probably among the easiest cells to culture.

Neurobionics

Another promising and emerging area is neurobionics, where electronically or mechanically operated body parts are steered by volitional control via an interface between brain and machine. In 1992, Kovacs et al. was the first to begin work in this area (83). They grew a nerve through holes in a silicon wafer that was hooked to an electrical microcircuit. This allowed subsequent stimulation and recording of the traversing axons. Such technology, if further advanced, could perhaps support faster regeneration, as well as motor and sensory reeducation. In 1994, Akin et al. used a similar device that was implanted between the cut ends of the glossopharyngeal nerve to examine nerve regeneration (6). They implanted a silicone sieve with more than 700 etched holes and managed to actually demonstrate functional regeneration of the nerve across the device. It should be noted that the different fields might merge together and become truly multidisciplinary, as more and more integration of these areas occurs.

Although this historical outline covers a period from 1951 to 2000, the reader should be aware that most of the problems discussed are not new and have been discussed for centuries. Somehow, they continually appeared on the research agenda. However, the approaches to solve these problems have changed. The future definitely will bring clinically applicable microbiological and perhaps biotechnical answers to

support and improve the existing armamentarium of peripheral nerve microsurgery.

Aspects to be Addressed

As exciting as these perspectives may sound, there are still enough mundane aspects of peripheral nerve surgery that need to be addressed. For example, research on connective tissue needs to be fortified, especially as it concerns the role of endoneurial and perineurial fibroblasts, as these are the cells that produce scarring. Even nerve grafts need further refinement. A task that all too easily can be disregarded in times of very sophisticated basic science endeavors is continued research on outcomes of surgical disorders of nerves, since results should guide our management. A huge field waiting to be explored is pain of nerve origin, since a need for more effective pain management exists. Intraoperative neurophysiologic studies should be improved and extended. Somatosensory-evoked potentials and evoked cortical responses are being refined to evaluate spinal nerve and root integrity, but no simple procedure exists that can reliably certify or exclude avulsions or differentiate, for that matter, at a peripheral level only regenerative motor from sensory fibers. This could greatly facilitate the decision for a particular repair type. The potential role of magnetic stimulation over cortex with recordings from roots or very proximal muscles should be explored.

A fascinating approach by Carlstedt et al. that recently received attention has been the implantation of avulsed nerve roots or spinal nerves into spinal cord (24). At some stage, MRI techniques might even advance to document not only very early degeneration (which is already possible) but also early and hopefully significant degrees of regeneration.

Surgical resection has remained the mainstay of therapy for peripheral nerve tumors in spite of all efforts for biochemical or radiotherapeutic solutions. Removal of benign nerve sheath tumors can be quite a rewarding task. Some changes in management involve neurofibroma, which can now sometimes be resected with little or minimal deficit due to altered dissection principles and electrophysiologic evaluation. In this regard, in spite of all envisioned advances, we believe that management of nerve tumors and most nerve injuries will remain a surgical task for a long time to come.

As this chapter is intended to be a historic review, and medical history as such should in part serve for future attempts, we want to close with some thoughts from Sunderland. In a sense, his words almost perfectly describe today's dilemma of clinical science in a world of information explosion. "As specialisation increases and the advantage of knowledge further outstrips the capacity of the mind to keep pace with it, the threads of science gradually become tangled and disconnected, perspective becomes blurred, and inquiries come to lack design and purpose. This results in knowledge taking on a patchwork form rather than a continuous and meaningful design woven into the fabric of medicine. If new information is to be fully effective it will be necessary to preserve the closest possible integration of knowledge against those forces that are tending to destroy it." (165)

REFERENCES

1. Abercombie M, Johnson ML. The outwandering of cells in tissue cultures of nerves undergoing Wallerian degeneration. *J Exp Biol* 19:266, 1942.
2. Abercombie M, Johnson ML. The effect of reinnervation on collagen formation in degenerating sciatic nerves of rabbits. *J Neurol Neurosurg Psychiatry* 10:89, 1947.
3. Abercombie M, Johnson ML, Thomas GA. The influence of nerve fibers on Schwann cell migration investigated in tissue culture. *Proc R Soc Ser B* 136:448, 1949.
4. Acland R. New instruments for microvascular surgery. *Br J Surg* 59:181–184, 1972.
5. Agee JM, McCaroll HR, Tortosa RD, et al. Endoscopic release of the carpal tunnel: A randomized prospective multicenter study. *J Hand Surg* 17A:987–995, 1992.
6. Akin T, Najafi K, Smoke RH, et al. A micromachined silicon sieve electrode for nerve regeneration applications. IEEE Transactions on Biomedical Engineering 41:305–313, 1994.
7. Allbrook DB, Aitken JT. Reinnervation of striated muscle after acute ischemia. *J Anat* 85:376, 1951.
8. Almquist EE. Nerve repair by laser. *Orthop Clin North Am* 19(1)201–208, 1988.
9. Almquist EE. Adjuncts to suture repair of peripheral nerves: Laser, glue, and other techniques, in, Omer GE Jr, Spinner M, Van Beek AL (eds): *Management of Peripheral Nerve Problems, 2nd Edition.* Philadelphia: W.B. Saunders Company, 1998, pp 311–318.
10. Ballance CA, Duel AB. The operative treatment of facial palsy. *Arch Otolaryngol* 15:1–70, 1932.
11. Bertelli JA, Mira JC. Nerve repair using freezing and fibrin glue: Immediate histologic improvement of axonal coaptation? *Microsurgery* 14:135, 1993.
12. Birch R, Bonney G, Wynn-Parry C. *Surgical Disorders of the Peripheral Nerves.* Edinburgh: Churchill Livingston, 1999.
13. Björkesten G. Suture of war injuries to peripheral nerves: Clinical studies of results. *Acta Chir Scandinav Suppl* 95(119):188, 1947.
14. Bonney G, Birch R, Jamieson AM, et al. Experiences with vascularized nerve grafts. *Clin Plast Surg* 11:137–142, 1984.
15. Bratton BR, Coleman W, Hudson A, Kline DG. Experimental interfascicular nerve grafting. *J Neurosurg* 15:323–332, 1979.
16. Bristow WR. Injuries of peripheral nerves in two world wars. *Br J Surg* 34:333–348, 1947.
17. Brunelli GA, Vigasio A, Brunelli GR. Different conduits in peripheral nerve surgery. *Microsurgery* 15:176–178, 1994.
18. Brushart TM. Selective reinnervation of distal motor stumps by peripheral motor axons. *Exp Neurol* 97:289, 1987.
19. Buncke HJ, Murray DE. Autogenous arterial interposition graft of less than 1 mm in external diameter. *Trans Int Congr Plast Reconstr Surg* Melbourne, 1971.
20. Bunnell S. Surgery of nerves of the hand. *Surg Gynecol Obstet* 44: 45, 1927.
21. Bunnell S. Surgical repair of the facial nerve. *Arch Otolaryngol* 25:235–259, 1937.
22. Bunnell S, Boyes JH Nerve grafts. *Am J Surg* 44:64, 1939.
23. von Büngner O. Über die Degenerations- und Regenerationsvorgänge am Nerven nach Verletzungen. *Beitr Pathol Anat* 10:321–393, 1891.
24. Carlstedt T, Grane P, Hallin RG, et al. Return of function after spinal cord implantation of avulsed spinal nerve roots. *Lancet* 346:1323–1325, 1995.
25. Chiu DTW, Strauch B. A prospective clinical evaluation of autogenous vein grafts used as a nerve conduit for distal sensory nerve defects of 3 cm or less. *Plast Reconstr Surg* 86:928, 1990.
26. Chiu DTW, Janecka I, Krizek TI, et al. Autogenous vein graft as a conduit for nerve regeneration. *Surgery* 91:226, 1982.
27. Chow JC. Endoscopic release of the carpal ligament: A new technique for carpal tunnel syndrome. *Arthroscopy* 5:19–24, 1989.
28. Chow JC, Van Beek AL, Meyer DL, et al. Surgical significance of the motor fascicular group of the ulnar nerve in the forearm. *J Hand Surg Am* 10:867–872, 1985.
29. Cohen S. Purification and metabolic effects of a nerve growth-promoting protein from snake venom. *J Biol Chem* 234:129, 1959.
30. Collins JD, Shaver ML, Disher AC, Miller TQ. Bilateral magnetic resonance imaging of the brachial plexus and peripheral nerve imaging: Technique and three-dimensional color, in, Omer GE Jr, Spinner M, Van Beek AL (ed): *Management of Peripheral Nerve Problems, 2nd Edition.* Philadelphia: W. B. Saunders, Philadelphia, 1998, pp 82–93.
31. Cordeiro PG, Seckel PR, Lipton SA, et al. Acidic fibroblast growth factor enhances peripheral nerve regener-

ation in vivo. *Plast Reconstr Surg* 83:1013–1021, 1989.

32. Davis L, Perret G. Methods of nerve repair. *S Clin N America* 27:117, 1947.

33. Dawson GD, Scott JW. The recording of nerve action potentials through skin in man. *J Neurol Neurosurg Psychiatry* 12:259, 1949.

34. Demirkan F, Snyder CC, Latifoglu O, et al. A method of enhancing regeneration of conventionally repaired peripheral nerves. *Ann Plast Surg* 34:67–72, 1995.

35. Denk W. Über Schussverletzungen der Nerven. Beitr. *Z Klin Chir* 91:217–221, 1914.

36. Denny-Brown D. The importance of neural fibroblasts in the regeneration of nerve. *Arch Neurol Psychiatry* 55:171, 1946.

37. Denny-Brown D, Brenner C. Paralysis of nerve induced by direct pressure and by tourniquet. *Arch Neurol Psychiatry* 53:88, 1945.

38. Denny-Brown D, Doherty MM. Effects of transient stretching of peripheral nerve. *Arch Neurol Psychiatry* 54:116, 1945.

39. Doi K, Kuwata N, Kawakami F, et al. The free vascularized sural nerve graft. *Microsurgery* 5:175, 1984.

40. Donaghy RMP. History of microneurosurgery, in, Wilkins RH, Rengachary, SS (ed): *Neurosurgery*, New York: McGraw-Hill, 1996, pp 37–42.

41. Donner TR, Voorhies RM, Kline DG. Neural sheath tumors of major nerves. *J Neurosurg* 81:362–373, 1994.

42. Edinger L. Über die Vereinigung getrennter Nerven. Grundsätzliches und Mitteilung eines neuen Verfahrens. *Münchner med Wchnschr* 63:225–228, 1916.

43. Egloff DV, Narakas A. Nerve anastomoses with human fibrin: Preliminary clinical report (56 cases). *Ann Chir Main Memb Super* 2:101, 1983.

44. Fachinelli A, Masquelet A, Restrepo J, Gilbert A. The vascularized sural nerve. *Int J Microsurg* 3:57, 1981.

45. Fischer DW, Beggs JL, Kenshalo DL, Shetter AG. Comparative study of microepineurial anastomosis with the use of CO2 laser and suture technique in rat sciatic nerves: Part I. *Neurosurgery* 17:300, 1985.

46. Fu SY, Gordon T. The cellular and molecular basis of peripheral nerve regeneration. *Mol Neurobiol* 14(1–2):67–116, 1997.

47. Gentilli F, Hudson A, Kline D, et al. Peripheral nerve injection injury. An experimental study. *Neurosurgery* 4:244–253, 1979.

48. Gilbert A, Razabonic R, Amar-Khodja S. Indications and results of brachial plexus surgery in obstetrical palsy. *Orthop Clin North Am* 19:91–105, 1988.

49. Greenfield AD, Shepherd JT, Whelan RF. The part played by the nervous system in the response to cold of the circulation through the finger-tip. *Clin Sci* 10:347, 1951.

50. Greenwood J Jr. Two-point coagulation: A new principle and instrument for applying coagulation current in neurosurgery. *Am J Surg* 50:267–270, 1940.

51. Gutmann E, Guttmann L. Effect of galvanic exercise in denervated and re-innervated muscle in rabbits. *J Neurol Neurosurg Psychiatry* 7:7, 1944.

52. Gutmann E, Young JZ. The re-innervation of muscle after various periods of atrophy. *J Anat* 78:15, 1944.

53. Guttmann L. Experimental study of nerve suture with various suture materials. *Br J Surg* 30:370–375, 1943.

54. Guttmann L, Medawar PB. The chemical inhibition of fiber regeneration and neuroma formation in peripheral nerves. *J Neurol Neurosurg Psychiatry* 5:130, 1942.

55. Guttmann RD. Developing ways of reducing allograft immunogenicity. *Can Med Assoc J* 124:143, 1981.

56. Gybels J, Van Calenbergh F. The treatment of pain due to peripheral nerve injury by electrical stimulation of the nerve. *Adv Pain Res Ther* 13:217–222, 1990.

57. Happel LT, Kline DG. Nerve Lesions in Continuity, in, Gelberman, R. (ed): *Operative Nerve Repair and Reconstruction*. Philadelphia: J.B. Lippincott, 1991, pp 601–616.

58. Hashimoto T, Tokuoka H. Über die Schussverletzungen peripherer Nerven und ihre Behandlung (Tubulisation). *Arch F Klin Chir* 84:354–402, 1907.

59. Hiller F. Nerve regeneration in grafts. *J Neuropathol Clin Neurol* 1:5, 1951.

60. Huang TC, Blanks RH, Berns MW, Crumley RL. Laser vs. suture nerve anastomosis. *Otolaryngol Head Neck Surg* 107:14, 1992.

61. Hudson AR, Hunter D, Kline DG, Bratton BR. Histological studies of experimental interfascicular graft repairs. *J Neurosurg* 51(3):333–340, 1979.

62. Hoffman H. Local re-innervation in partially denervated muscle: A histophysiological study. *Aust J Exp Biol Med Sci* 28:383, 1950.

63. Hoffman H. A study of the factors influencing innervation of muscles by implanted nerves. *Aust J Exp Biol Med Sci* 29:289, 1951.

64. Holmgreen G. Some experiences in surgery of otosclerosis. *Acta Otolaryngol* 5:460–466, 1923.

65. Horch RE, Bannasch H, Kopp J, et al. Single-cell suspensions of cultured human keratinocytes in fibrin-glue reconstitute the epidermis. *Cell Transplant* 7(3):309–317, 1998.

66. House WF. Surgical exposure of the internal auditory canal and its contents through the middle cranial fossa. *Laryngoscope* 71:1363–1385, 1961.

67. Ishii DN, Glazner GW, Pu SF. Role of insulin-like growth factors in peripheral nerve regeneration [Review]. *Pharmacol Ther* 62:125–144, 1994.

68. Jacobson JH II, Suarez EL. Microsurgery in anastomosis of small vessels. *Surg Forum* 11:243–245, 1960.

69. Jannetta PJ, Rand RW. Vascular compression of the trigeminal nerve at the pons in patients with trigeminal neuralgia, in, Donaghy, RMP, Yasargil MG (ed): *Micro-Vascular Surgery*, Stuttgart, Georg Thieme Verlag, 1967, p 150.

70. Jasper H, Ballem G. Unipolar electromyogram of normal and denervated human muscle. *J Neurophysiol* 12:231–244, 1949.

71. Kahn EA. Direct observation of sweating in peripheral nerve lesions. *Surg Gynecol Obstet* 92:22, 1951.

72. Kahn EA, Bassett RC, Schneider RC, et al. (ed): *Correlative Neurosurgery*, Springfield, Illinois, Charles C. Thomas, 1955.

73. Kim DH, Connolly SE, Kline DG, et al. Labeled Schwann cell transplants versus sural nerve grafts in nerve repair. *J Neurosurg* 80:254–260, 1994.

74. Kline DG, Dejonge BR. Evoked potentials to evaluate peripheral nerve injuries. *Surg Gynecol Obstet* 127:1239–1248, 1968.

75. Kline DG, Happel LT. A quarter century's experience with intraoperative nerve action potential recording. *Can J Neurol Sci* 20:3–10, 1992.

76. Kline DG, Hudson AR. *Nerve Injuries. Operative Re-*

sults for Major Nerve Injuries, Entrapments, and Tumors, Philadelphia: W. B. Saunders, 1995.

77. Kline DG, Judic DJ. Operative management of selected brachial plexus lesions. *J Neurosurg* 58:631–649, 1983.

78. Kline DG, Nulsen FE. The neuroma in continuity: Its preoperative and operative management. *Surg Clin North Am* 52:1189–1209, 1972.

79. Kline DG, Hackett ER, Davis GD, Myers MB. Effect of mobilization on the blood supply and regeneration of injured nerves. *J Surg Res* 12:254–266, 1972.

80. Kline DG, Hackett ER, Happel LH. Surgery for lesions of the brachial plexus. *Arch Neurol* 43:170–81, 1986.

81. Kline DG, Hudson AR, Bratton BR. Experimental study of fascicular nerve repair with and without epineurial closure. *J Neurosurg* 54:513–520, 1981.

82. Kline DG, Hackett ER, Sumner AJ. Management of the neuroma in continuity, in, Wilkins RH, Rengachary SS (ed): *Neurosurgery, 2nd Edition.* New York: McGraw-Hill, 1996, pp 3169–3177.

83. Kovacs GT, Storment CW, Rosen JM. Regeneration microelectrode array for peripheral nerve recording and stimulation. *IEEE Trans Biomed Eng* 39:893–902, 1992.

84. Kurze T, Doyle B Jr. Extradural intracranial (middle fossa) approach to the internal auditory canal. *J Neurosurg* 19:1033–1037, 1962.

85. Lebendenko VV. Time element in restorative surgery of peripheral nerve lesions. *Am Rev Sov Med* 1:23, 1943.

86. Levi-Montalcini R, Hamburger V. Selective growth stimulation of mouse sarcoma on sensory and sympathetic nervous system of the chick embryo. *J Exp Zool* 116:321, 1951.

87. Livingston KE. The phantom limb syndrome: A discussion of the role of major peripheral nerve neuromas. *J Neurosurg* 2:251, 1945.

88. Livingston WK. *Pain Mechanisms. A Physiologic Interpretation of Causalgia and its Related States.* New York: Macmillan, 1943.

89. Livingston WK, Davis EW, Livingston KE. Delayed recovery in peripheral nerve lesions caused by high velocity projectile wounding. *J Neurosurg* 2:170, 1945.

90. Lougheed WM, Morely T. A method of introducing blood into the subarachnoid space in the circle of Willis in dogs. *Can J Surg* 4:329–337, 1961.

91. Lundborg G, Hansson HA. Regeneration of peripheral nerve through a preformed tissue space: Preliminary observation on the reorganization of regenerating nerve fibers and perineurium. *Brain Res* 178:573, 1979.

92. Lundborg G, Hansson HA. Nerve regeneration through preformed pseudosynovial tubes. *J Hand Surg* 5:35, 1980.

93. Lyons WR, Woodhall B. *Atlas of Peripheral Nerve Injuries.* Philadelphia: W. B. Saunders, 1949.

94. MacCarty CS. Two-stage autograft for repair of extensive damage to sciatic nerve. *J Neurosurg* 8:319, 1951.

95. Mackinnon SE. New directions in peripheral nerve surgery. *Ann Plast Surg* 22(3):257–273, 1989.

96. Mackinnon SE, Dellon A.L. *Surgery of the Peripheral Nerve.* New York: Thieme, 1988.

97. Mackinnon SE, Dellon AL. Clinical nerve reconstruc-

tion with bioabsorbable polyglycolic acid tube. *Plast Reconstr Surg* 85:419, 1990.

98. Mackinnon SE, Hudson AR, Falk RE, et al. Peripheral nerve allograft: An immunological assessment of pretreatment methods. *Neurosurgery* 14:167, 1984.

99. Maier M, Lion H. Experimenteller Nachweis der Endolymfbewegung. *Arch f d ges Physiol Berl* 187:47–74, 1921.

100. Maragh H, Hawn RS, Gould JD, Terzis JK. Is laser nerve repair comparable tomicrosuture coaptation? *J Reconstr Microsurg* 4:189, 1988.

101. Maragh H, Meyer BS, Davenport D, et al. Morphofunctional evaluation of fibrin glue versus microsuture nerve repairs. *J Reconstr Microsurg* 6:331, 1990.

102. Mattson MP, Cheng B. Growth factors protect neurons against excitotoxic/ischemic damage by stabilizing calcium homeostasis. *Stroke* 24(Suppl 12):1136, 1993.

103. May, PC, Finch CE. Sulfated glycoprotein 2: New relationships of this multifunctional protein to neurodegeneration. *Trends Neurosci* 15:391, 1992.

104. Mayfield FH. *Causalgia.* Springfield, Illinois: Charles C. Thomas, 1951.

105. McCarrol HR. Clinical manifestations of congenital neurofibromatosis. *J Bone Joint Surg* 32A:601, 1950.

106. Mcgillicuddy J. Techniques of nerve repair, in, Wilkins RH, Rengachary SS (ed): *Neurosurgery, 2nd Edition.* New York:McGraw Hill, 1996, pp 3179–3197.

107. Menon J. Endoscopic carpal tunnel release: A single portal technique. *Contemp Orthopaed* 26:109–116, 1993.

108. Merle M, Lebreton E, Foucher G, et al. Vascularized nerve grafts: Preliminiary results. Presented to the American Society for Reconstructive Microsurgery, Las Vegas, 1985, in, Omer GE Jr, Spinner M, Van Beek AL, (ed): *Management of Peripheral Nerve Problems, 2nd Edition.* Philadelphia: W.B. Saunders, 1998, pp 295–304.

109. Michon J, Masse P. Le moment optimum de la suture nerveuse dans les plaies du membre superior. *Rev Chir Orthop* 50:205–212, 1964.

110. Millesi H. *Chirurgie der peripheren Nerven,* München: Urban und Schwarzenberg Verlag, 1992.

111. Millesi H, Terzis JK. Nomenclature in peripheral nerve surgery. *Clin Plast Surg* 11:3, 1984.

112. Millesi H, Meissl G, Berger A. The interfascicular nerve grafting of the median and ulnar nerves. *J Bone Joint Surg* 54A:727–750, 1972.

113. Millesi H, Meissl G, and Berger A. Further experience with interfascicular grafting of the median, ulnar, and radial nerves. *J Bone Joint Surg* 58A:209–218, 1976.

114. Mitchell SW. *Injuries of Nerves.* Philadelphia, Lippincott, 1872.

115. Mitchell SW, Morehouse GR, Keen WW. *Gunshot Wounds and other Injuries of Nerves.* Philadelphia: Lippincott, 1864.

116. Moberg E. Objective methods for determining the functional value of sensibility in the hand. *J Bone Joint Surg* 40B:454–476, 1958.

117. Mulder JD. The causative mechanism in Morton's metatarsalgia. *J Bone Joint Surg* 33B:94, 1951.

118. Narakas A. Brachial plexus surgery. *Orthop Clin North Am* 12:303–323, 1984.

119. Narakas A. The use of fibrin glue in repair of peripheral nerves. *Orthop Clin North Am* 19(1):187–199, 1988.

120. Narakas, A Les lesions dans les elongations du plexus

brachial: Differentes posibilities et associations lesio-
nelles. *Rev Chir Orthop* 63:44–54, 1977.

121. Narakas A, Hentz VR. Neurotization in brachial plexus
injuries: Indication and results. *Clin Orthop* 237:
43–56, 1988.

122. Neblett CR, Morris JR, Thomsen S. Laser assisted microsurgical anastomosis. *Neurosurgery.* 19:914, 1986.

123. Norcross NC, Bakody JT. Observations on the use of
tantalum foil in peripheral nerve surgery. *J Neurosurg*
4:69, 1947.

124. Nulsen FE, Lewey FH. Intraneural bipolar stimulation:
A new aid in the assessment of nerve injuries. *Science*
106:301, 1947.

125. Nylen CO. The microscope in aural surgery, its first
use and later development. *Acta Otolaryngol* 116:
226–240, 1954.

126. Okutsu I, Ninomiya S, Takatori Y, et. al. Subcutaneous
operation under the universal subcutaneous endoscope.
Arthroscopy 12:77–81, 1987.

127. Omer GE Jr, Spinner M, Van Beek AL (ed): *Management of Peripheral Nerve Problems, 2nd Edition.* Philadelphia: W.B. Saunders, 1998.

128. Palumbo LT. Upper dorsal sympathectomy without
Horner's syndrome. *Arch Surg* 71:743–751, 1955.

129. Phalen GS. Reflections on 21 years experience with the
carpal-tunnel syndrome. *JAMA* 212:1365–1367, 1970.

130. Piper HE. *Elektrophysiologie menschlicher Muskeln.*
Berlin: J. Springer, Berlin, 1912, p 163.

131. Politis MJ, Ederle K, Spencer PS. Tropism in nerve
regneration in vivo: Attraction of regenerating axons
by diffusable factors derived from cells in distal nerve
stumps of transected peripheral nerves. *Brain Res* 253:
1–12, 1982.

132. Platt H. Traction lesions of the external popliteal nerve.
Lancet 2:612, 1940.

133. Puckett WO, Grundfest H, Mcelroy WD, et al. Damage
to peripheral nerves by high velocity missiles without
direct hit. *J Neurosurg* 3:294, 1946.

134. Rand RW. (ed): *Microneurosurgery.* Saint Louis: C.V.
Mosby Company, 1969.

135. Ranschburg P. Über die Anastomosen der Nerven der
oberen Extremität des Menschen mit Rücksicht auf
ihre Neurologische und Nerven Chirurgische Bedeutung. *Neurol Centralbl* 36:521–534, 1917.

136. Roos DB. Transaxillary approach for first rib resection
to relieve thoracic outlet syndrome. *Ann Surg* 163:
354–358, 1966.

137. Roos DB. Experience with first rib resection for thoracic outlet syndrome. *Ann Surg* 173:429–442, 1971.

138. Roos DB, Owens JC. Thoracic outlet syndrome. *Arch
Surg* 93:71–74, 1966.

139. Sames M. Development of peripheral nerve surgery.
[article in Czech]. *Rohzl Chir* 77(3):110–116, 1998.

140. Samii M. Die operative Wiederherstellung verletzter
Nerven. *Langenbecks Arch Chir* 27:87–110, 1972.

141. Samii M. Use of microtechniques in peripheral nerve
surgery: Experience with over 300 cases, in, Handa H
(ed): *Microneurosurgery.* Tokoyo: Igaku-Shoin, 1973,
pp 85–93.

142. Sargent P, Greenfield JG. An experimental investigation of certain materials used for nerve suture. *Br Med
J* 2:407–410, 1919.

143. Schüller A. Die Verwendung der Nervendehnung zur
operativen Heilung von Substanzverlusten am Nerven.
Wien med. *Presse Nr 5 Jahrg* 29:146–150, 1888.

144. Seddon HJ. Classification of nerve injuries. *Br Med J*
2:237, 1942.

145. Seddon HJ. Three types of nerve injury. *Brain* 66:237,
1943.

146. Seddon HJ. The early management of peripheral nerve
injuries. *Practitioner* 152:101, 1944.

147. Seddon HJ. (ed): *Peripheral Nerve Injuries. Medical
Research Council Special Report Series No. 282.* London: Her Majesty's Stationary Office, 1954.

148. Seddon HJ. Nerve grafting: Fourth Watson-Jones Lecture of the Royal College of Surgeons of England 1963.
J Bone Joint Surg 45 B:447–461, 1963.

149. Seddon HJ. *Surgical Disorders of the Peripheral
Nerves.* Baltimore: Williams&Wilkins, 1972.

150. Seddon HJ, Holmes W. The late condition of nerve
homografts in man. *Surg Gynecol Obstet* 79(4):
342–351, 1944.

151. Seddon HJ, Medawar PB. Fibrin suture of human
nerves. *Lancet* 2:87, 1942.

152. Seddon HJ, Medawar PB, Smith H. Rate of regeneration of peripheral nerves in man. *J Physiol* 102:191,
1943.

153. Smith JW. Microsurgery of peripheral nerves. *Plast
Reconstr Surg* 33:317–329, 1964.

154. Spurling RG. Causalgia of the upper extremity: Treatment by dorsal sympathetic ganglionectomy. *Arch
Neurol Psychiatry* 23:784–788, 1930.

155. Spurling RG. The use of tantalum wire and foil in the
repair of peripheral nerves. *S Clin N Am* 23:
1491–1504, 1943.

156. Spurling RG. Peripheral nerve surgery-technical considerations. *J Neurosurg* 1:133, 1944.

157. Spurling RG, Lyons WR, Whitcomb BB, et al. The
failure of whole fresh homogenous nerve grafts in man.
J Neurosurg 2:79, 1945.

158. Stoffel A. Beiträge zu einer rationellen Nervenchirur-
gie. *Münch med Wchnschr* 60:175–179, 1913.

159. Stout A P. Tumors of the peripheral nervous system, in,
National Research Council Committee on Pathology,
(Ed): *Atlas of Tumor Pathology, Section 2, Fascicle 6,*
Washington, D.C.: Armed Forces Institute of Pathol-
ogy, Washington DC, 1949.

160. Strange FG, Strange C. Case report on pedicled nerve
graft. *Br J Surg* 37:331, 1950.

161. Strauch B, Ferder M, Lovelle -Allen S, et al. Determining the maximal length of a vein conduit used as an
interposition graft for nerve regeneration. *J Reconstr
Microsurg* 12:521, 1996.

162. Suematsu N. Tubulation for peripheral nerve gap: Its
history and possibility. *Microsurgery* 10(1):71–74,
1989.

163. Sunderland S. Observations on the course of recovery
and late end results in series of cases of peripheral
nerve suture. *Aust NZ J Surg* 18:4, 1949.

164. Sunderland S A classification of peripheral nerve injuries producing loss of function. *Brain* 74:491, 1951.

165. Sunderland S. *Nerves and Nerve Injuries.* Baltimore:
Williams & Wilkins, 1968.

166. Sunderland S. Mechanisms of cervical root avulsion
in injuries of the neck and shoulder. *J Neurosurg* 41:
705–714, 1974.

167. Sunderland S. The pros and cons of funicular nerve
repair. Founder's Lecture, The American Society for
Surgery of the Hand. *J Hand Surg* 4:201, 1979.

168. Sunderland S. *Nerve Injuries and Their Repair: A Crit-*

ical Appraisal. Edinburgh:Churchill Livingstone, 1991.

169. Sunderland S, Bradley KC. The cross sectional area of peripheral nerve trunks devoted to nerve fibers. *Brain* 72:428, 1949.

170. Sunderland S, Bradley KC. Endoneurial tube shrinkage in the distal segment of a severed nerve. *J Comp Neurol* 93:411, 1950.

171. Sunderland S, and Smith GK. The relative merits of various suture materials for the repair of severed nerves. *Aust NZ J Surg* 20:85, 1950.

172. Tarlov IM. Plasma clot suture of nerves, illustrated technique. *Surgery* 15:257–269, 1944.

173. Tarlov IM, Benjamin B, Goldfort AI. Autologous and heterologous plasma clot and silk sutures of nerves: An experimental study of comparative tissue reactions. *J Neuropathol Exp Neurol* 1:449, 1942.

174. Tassin JL. *Paralysies obstetrical du plexus brachial: Evolution spontaneé, resultats des interventions reparatrices précoces.* Thesis, Université Paris VII, 1983.

175. Taylor IG, Ham FJ. The free vascularized nerve graft. *Plast Reconstr Surg* 57:143, 1976.

176. Terzis JK. *Microreconstruction of nerve injuries.* Philadelphia: W. B. Saunders, 1987.

177. Terzis JK, Faibisoff BA, Williams HB. The nerve gap: Suture under tension vs. graft. *Plast Reconstr Surg* 56: 166, 1975.

178. Terzis JK, Sun O, Thomas P. Historical and basic science review: Past, present, and future of nerve repair. *Reconstr Microsurg* 13:215–225, 1997.

179. Tupper JW, Crick JC, Matteck LR. Fascicular nerve repairs. A comparative study of epineurial and fascicular perineurial techniques. *Orthop Clin North Am* 19(1):57–69, 1988.

180. Vass K, Welch W, Nowak T. Localization of 70 kDa stress protein induction in gerbil brain after ischemia. *Acta Neuropathol* 77:128, 1988.

181. Walker E A (ed): *A History of Neurological Surgery, Facs. of 1951 Edition.* New York: Hafner Publishing Company, 1967.

182. Watchmaker GP, Mackinnon SE. Advances in Peripheral Nerve Repair. *Clin Plast Surg* 24(1):63–73, 1997.

183. Watchmaker GP, Gumucio CA, Crandall RE, et al. Fascicular topography of the median nerve: A computer-based study to identify branching patterns. *J Hand Surg Am* 16:53–59, 1991.

184. Weinzweig N, Grindel S, Ganzales M. et al. Successful regeneration across nerve allografts in rats receiving transient and long-term immunosuppression with FK-506. Presented at the 40th Annual Meeting, Plastic Surgery Research council, NY, May, 1995, in, Terzis JK, Danny DS, Thanos PK. Historical and Basic Science Review: Past, Present, and Future of Nerve Repair. *J Reconstr Microsurg* 13:215–225, 1997.

185. Weiss P. Sutureless reunion of severed nerves with elastic cuffs of tantalum. *J Neurosurg* 1:219, 1944.

186. Weiss P. The technology of nerve regeneration: A review. Sutureless tubulation and related methods of nerve repair. *J Neurosurg* 1:400, 1944.

187. Weiss P. Functional nerve regeneration through frozen-dried nerve grafts in cats and monkeys. *Proc Soc Exp Biol Med* 54:277, 1945.

188. Weiss P, Taylor AC. Repair of peripheral nerves by grafts of frozen-dried nerves. *Proc Soc Exp Biol Med* 52:326, 1943.

189. Weiss P, Taylor AC. Guides for nerve regeneration across gaps. *J Neurosurg* 3:375, 1946.

190. White JC, Hamlin H. New uses of tantalum in nerve suture: Control of neuroma formation. *J Neurosurg* 2: 402, 1945.

191. White JC, Sweet WH. *Pain and the neurosurgeon: A Forty Year Experience.* Springfield: Charles C. Thomas, 1969.

192. White RJ. Where has peripheral nerve surgery gone? *Surg Neurol* 13(5):373, 1980.

193. Wilkins RH, Woodhall B, in, Thompson JM (ed): *History of the Congress of Neurological Surgeons 1951–1991.* Baltimore: Williams and Wilkins, 1992, pp 84–87.

194. Williams HB, Terzis JK. Single fascicular recordings: An intraoperative diagnostic tool for the management of peripheral nerve lesions. *Plast Reconstr Surg* 57: 562–569, 1976.

195. Woodhall B, Beebe GW. (eds): *Peripheral Nerve Regeneration. A Follow-Up Study of 3,656 World War II Injuries. VA Medical Monograph.* Washington, D.C.: US Government Printing Office, 1956.

196. Woodhall B, Lyons WR. Peripheral nerve injuries. I. The results of ''early'' nerve suture. *Surgery* 19:757, 1946.

197. Young JZ. Structure, degeneration and repair of nerve fibers. *Nature* 156:132, 1945.

198. Young JZ, Medawar PB. Fibrin suture of peripheral nerves. *Lancet* 2:126–128, 1940.

199. Zhao S, Pang Y, Beuerman RW, Thompson HW, Kline DG. Expression of c-Fos protein in the spinal cord after brachial plexus injury: Comparison of root avulsion and distal nerve transection. *Neurosurgery* 42(6)1357–1362, 1998.

13

Spinal Surgery from the Eisenhower Years to the Third Millennium

Nicholas Theodore, MD, Volker K. H. Sonntag, MD

". . . the existence of the operating specialist, as contrasted with the general surgeon, is justified only if the former takes advantage of his opportunities to contribute to the knowledge of the disorders he specially treats. When progress ceases to be made, through the intensive studies which the smaller field of work permits, there is every reason why the vagrant specialty should be called back under the wing of its parent, general surgery, from whom under no circumstances should it ever be permitted to wander too far." (37)

It is doubtful that even our visionary neurosurgical forefathers, such as Horsley, Cushing, and Dandy, could have imagined the dramatic changes that have occurred in the field of spinal surgery in the last 50 years. Cushing's early views of the field of neurosurgery were conservative. As the above quote indicates, he felt that when and if the mysteries of the nervous system were completely defined, neurosurgery would be relegated to the place of its birthright—general surgery. Thankfully, the total knowledge in the field of neurosurgery in general and in spinal surgery in particular has continued to grow exponentially. Spinal surgery today bears little resemblance to that practiced in 1950 and will continue to be refined throughout the third millennium.

In 1950, the field of neurosurgery was blossoming, with considerably more interest and attention being directed toward cranial surgery than spinal disorders. The appeal of being a "brain surgeon" seemed to be greater than handling the mundane issues of the spine. Martin (122) probably spoke for most neurosurgeons when he stated in his article entitled "Recent Trends in Neurosurgery" that "the spinal cord continues to arouse much less interest, both as to pathology and physiology, than do the intracranial contents, and much of the literature concerning the cord has to do with case histories." The field of spinal surgery, however, has become a distinct region under the umbrella of neurosurgery. In fact, issues of subspecialization loom on the horizon and could one day divide the field of neurosurgery into several distinct entities.

1950s

As the 1950s began, it briefly seemed as if spinal surgery was generating equal interest with the cranial aspects of neurosurgery. For example, five of the nine articles in the first issue of the *Journal of Neurosurgery*, published in 1950, involved the spine. At that time, spinal surgery was essentially confined to the posterior approaches. Plain radiography, myelography, and lumbar puncture were the diagnostic modalities of choice. Although the use of myelography increased during this decade, it was by no means embraced by all neurosurgeons. In an editorial essay published in 1958, Semmes proffered his view that even though myelography was routinely used by some neurosurgeons, "the clinical picture is far more reliable and every patient who has had both myelography and surgery insists that the myelography is more painful and trying" (169).

Several major clinical entities were described during the 1950s; one of the most significant was neurogenic claudication (188). In a seminal contribution, Verbiest first detailed the symptoms associated with congenital stenosis of the lumbar region and later expounded on the condition in greater detail (189).

Another clinical landmark occurred when Schneider et al. (163) described the "syndrome of acute central cervical cord injury" in 1954. They detailed nine cases of central cord syndrome of their own along with six other cases from the literature, and concluded that the "degree of recovery is directly proportional to the amount of edema as compared to hematoma, ranging from complete recovery to total destruction with ascending hematomyelia and death." They observed that central cord syndrome was often associated with facial injuries. Schneider et al. proposed hyperextension injuries as the cause of central cord syndrome by applying the earlier work of Taylor (182), and they dispelled the belief that all cases are associated with hematomyelia. Ultimately, Schneider et al. concluded that cervical myelography may be contraindicated because of the hyperextension necessary to avoid the upward passage of contrast agent through the foramen magnum. They left neurosurgeons of the day with the haunting dictum that "decompressive laminectomy is futile" for the treatment of central cord syndrome and that once the diagnosis has been made, "surgical intervention is contraindicated."

During the 1950s, advances were also made in the field of spondylolisthesis. Meyerding described his original method of measurement in 1932 (129). In 1954, Taillard (180) then introduced his classic measurement system as it applied to his experience in treating 50 children and adolescents with spondylolisthesis.

Although posterior approaches to spinal pathologies were the most common during the 1950s, several significant advances were also made. For example, in 1954, Capener (22) described the "lateral rhachotomy," which was essentially a posterolateral approach to the spine. Soon thereafter followed Hodgson and Stock's (96) description of a transthoracic retroperitoneal approach for spinal fusion in the treatment of Pott's disease, an entity that helped define an entire era of spinal surgery.

Other advances in lumbar surgery included descriptions by Woolsey (195) and by Gill et al. (71) of an operative treatment for spondylolisthesis that involved no fusion but only the resection of the loose neural arch and fibrocartilaginous mass. Although these techniques were not necessarily innovative, the issue of deciding which patients with spondylolisthesis would benefit from fusion gained attention. Woolsey (195) believed that younger patients with a significant degree of spondylolisthesis would benefit from fusion but on a case-by-case basis. He thought that "the orthopedic surgeon and the neurosurgeon should determine the necessity for lumbosacral fusion" because "fusion is not necessarily indicated in all patients."

During the 1950s, advances in cervical spine surgery were nothing short of revolutionary. The description of anterior cervical disk removal and subsequent interbody fusion with autograft bone by Robinson and Smith (155) and the ingenious circular grafting technique devised by Cloward (29) represented milestones in spinal neurosurgery. The discussion that follows Cloward's original description of his technique is invigorating to say the least. Dr. John Raaf stated that he had "been trying to decide whether anterior cervical fusion is in the same category as Russian tonsillectomy. . . because the Russian citizen is not allowed to open his mouth" (29). Besides this skepticism, several thoughtful criticisms were made. For example, Dr. William B. Scoville (29) asked the following: "May not fusion of a cervical interspace cause this same stress on adjacent interspaces?" His comment is most likely the first reference to the now commonplace term, *adjacent level instability* with respect to the changes that follow anterior cervical surgery with fusion.

Even though atlantoaxial instability had been discussed in the literature since Mixter and Osgood's description in 1910 (130), its treatment was controversial. In 1958, Alexander et al. (5) described 25 patients with odontoid fractures, 15 of whom underwent posterior fusion. Only one patient died—secondary to pulmonary embolism. Their in-depth analysis detailed the technique of C1–3 fusion, which they advocated be performed early after an odontoid fracture to avoid potential late neurological sequelae associated with the injury.

With respect to the treatment of traumatic spinal disorders, Tarlov's monograph entitled *Spinal Cord Compression. Mechanism of Paralysis and Treatment* was considered a classic (181). Another major contribution included Wannamaker's landmark review of the treatment of 300 consecutive spinal cord injuries sustained during the Korean conflict (190). He recommended performing "laminectomies on all patients with penetrating wounds of the spine, [and] early laminectomies in all cases of closed injuries with fracture dislocation" (190). Wannamaker reported 279 laminectomies with an overall mortality rate of 1% and no deaths immediately attributable to surgery.

The treatment of acute spinal disorders also received a boost with the introduction of the halo vest by Perry and Nickel in 1959 (147). Although halo vests now bear little resemblance to their prototype, this device represented a significant innovation that allowed mobilization of patients previously confined to bed rest while their fractures healed.

Other topics of interest during the 1950s included the danger of intrathecal methylene blue (19), curtailing a common practice for diagnosing cerebrospinal fluid (CSF) fistulae. The treatment of spastic paraplegia by selective spinal cordectomy or other ablative measures also became an area of intense interest (30,117–119, 162,170).

Although not as pervasive as today, economic issues still confronted neurosurgeons in the 1950s. Turnbull (186) realized the importance of medical economics when he referred to "the responsibility of the neurosurgeon to the medical profession as a whole, having in mind the problems of medical economics." He believed that because neurosurgeons had contact with many referring physicians and enjoyed a "relative absence of competition," they should actively participate in the politics of medicine. Ultimately, Turnbull was correct in predicting the encroachments that would later affect physicians in North America. As he said, it is "surprising to sense the unwitting faith in our organization that is implied by our demand for continuance of a large measure of self-government" (186). These words began to ring true as the field of spinal neurosurgery evolved.

1960s

The 1960s ushered in an era of technical developments that began to change the practice of spinal surgery forever. Although diagnostic modalities were similar to those employed in the 1950s, advances in radiologic technology introduced by Oldendorf (139) and Cormack (31) laid the framework for the development of computerized tomography (CT). Another advance in diagnosis was the description of a measurement system for spondylolisthesis, as developed by Laurent and Einola (110), which helped to maintain interest in this field. The method most commonly used today, however, continues to be Taillard's (180).

Advances in basic science during this decade included the description of bone morphogenetic proteins (BMPs) by Urist (187). Although the importance of this discovery was not recognized at the time, BMPs now represent the forefront of strategies for spinal fusion.

Technical advances in visualization with the aid of the operating microscope also entered the arena of spinal surgery with Yaşargil's (197) and Caspar's (24) independent descriptions of the use of the microscope for the treatment of herniated lumbar disks. Both reports were published in 1977, but Yaşargil actually began using the operating microscope for lumbar disk surgery in 1967.

Surgical advances in this decade included refinements of anterior lumbar surgery supplemented with fusion using a compression plate attached to the vertebral bodies with screws (99). This technique did not become popular at the time, but similar techniques involving variations on the fusion technique became standard practice in the 1990s.

Another surgical variation was Hirsch's description of anterior cervical diskectomy without fusion in 1960 (94). This report ushered in a period of conservatism and offered an option for those interested in adopting anterior cervical methods without adding fusion to the procedure. In general, the procedure consisted of incising the anterior annulus and removing the disk while leaving the posterior annulus and ligament intact. The increased popularity of the anterior approaches for cervical disk surgery prompted Mayfield to compare the two methodologies in 1965 (125); he continued to advocate the posterior approach.

Other landmark advances included the development of the first widely available spinal instrumentation-fixation system by Harrington (86,87). Although relatively simplistic by contemporary standards, Harrington's system revolutionized the field of spinal surgery and opened the door for the development of countless variations.

For many years, the transoral approach had been used to drain retropharyngeal abscesses. Neurosurgery, however, did not embrace this approach to gain anterior exposure of the atlantoaxial region because of early reports of infection, CSF leakage, and limited exposure. That situation changed in 1962 with Fang and Ong's (56) description of a direct transoral approach to the upper cervical region. They advocated using this new technique to treat atlantoaxial instability by fusion and to remove tuberculous lesions.

Also of note was the development of the transthoracic approach for thoracic disk herniations below T4 positioned central or centrolateral to the spinal cord. Independently described by Perot and Munro (146) and Ransohoff et al. (149), this technique has become commonplace for thoracic pathologies that require ventral decompression. Other surgical advances in the 1960s included the description of occipitocervical fusion by Newman and Sweetnam (136) and the introduction of an anterior approach for the treatment of scoliosis (47).

Biological advances in the 1960s included the discovery by Smith et al. of an enzyme with the capability of dissolving the nucleus pulposus in a rabbit (174). Soon thereafter, the technique of chemonucleolysis was applied to the first human patient (173). The technique is still practiced but remains controversial.

In the 1960s, the treatment of spinal cord injury was still conservative and no major advances, per se, were made. One area explored was the role of hypothermia in the treatment of spinal cord injury (1,2,134). The results were promising in animal models, but hypothermia was never tested in a rigorous clinical trial of human spinal cord injury.

1970s

Of the past 50 years, the 1970s stand out as the decade associated with the most significant advances in the field of neurological imaging. In 1972, Hounsfield (98) developed CT and built the first scanner. The first CT scanner in the United States was purchased and installed at the Massachusetts General Hospital in 1972. For the first time, the spine could be imaged with a modality other than plain radiography or myelography. Ultimately, CT gave spinal surgeons the ability to detect small fractures and other abnormalities almost certainly overlooked in earlier times.

Soon after the introduction of CT, magnetic resonance imaging (MRI) was developed. The first MR scanner was built at Nottingham University in England in 1976 (93). However, several years elapsed before refinements in this technology made it widely available. MRI offers unprecedented anatomic definition of structures as elusive as the transverse ligament (42,93) and as small as a 1 mm hemangioblastoma of the spinal cord.

The use of the operating microscope increased in the 1970s. In 1973, Robertson (154) described his microsurgical technique of anterior cervical diskectomy without fusion for the treatment of cervical disk disease. Soon thereafter followed the description by Hankinson and Wilson (84), which similarly took advantage of the operating microscope.

Whether to fuse patients after an anterior cervical diskectomy was not answered during the 1970s. The debate, which began during the period of Smith and Robinson (172) and Cloward (29), continued with both sides offering commentaries and opinions (46,123).

An important surgical advance of the 1970s was the advent of minimally invasive procedures. Williams popularized microdiskectomy in 1978 with his article ''Microlumbar Diskectomy: A Conservative Approach to the Virgin Herniated Lumbar Disk'' (194). Another minimally invasive technique introduced in the 1970s was the percutaneous removal of a lumbar disk herniation, a procedure first described by Hijikata (92). Numerous variations on instrumentation and technique followed, all designed to spare patients a large incision and extensive dissection of soft tissue.

The treatment of atlantoaxial instability also improved compared with older methods. Brooks and Jenkins introduced wedge-compression bone grafting (20). Of their 15 patients, 13 developed solid fusions after surgery and postoperative treatment with an external orthosis. Both patients who failed treatment had rheumatoid arthritis. The authors concluded that their technique should not be used in such patients.

Fusion techniques were also refined during the 1970s. Innovations included techniques such as the transposition of a vascularized rib for the stabilization of progressive kyphosis (156). Numerous descriptions of metallic implants for the internal fixation of the spine ultimately served as the foundation for today's sophisticated instrumentation systems (58,86,97,140,185,193).

The treatment of thoracic disk herniations witnessed an innovation with Patterson and Arbit's description of a transpedicular approach to these problematic lesions (144). This technique offered a viable option for the treatment of lateral disk herniations and avoided the hazards associated with a simple laminectomy.

The treatment of spondylolisthesis witnessed yet another twist when Freebody et al. introduced the anterior transperitoneal approach for the direct repair and fusion of this condition (62). Numerous methods were advocated for the treatment of this disorder, but no consensus was reached.

Other surgical innovations included Hattori's description of cervical laminoplasty in 1973 (88). This technique was a great advance since it offered the ability to treat spinal stenosis and theoretically to prevent the development of kyphosis afterward. This contention, however, has never been firmly established. Other solutions for the treatment of spinal stenosis were proffered by surgeons such as Southwick et al. (176) and Callahan et al. (21). They advocated lateral facet fusion after laminectomy using corticocancellous bone struts attached to the facets by various wiring techniques. Roy-Camille et al. (158) took these techniques one step further with their introduction of lateral mass screw-plate fixation for posterior fusion of the cervical spine after trauma.

Spinal cord injury was governed by the conservative therapies espoused by Guttmann and others that had prevailed since World War II. Spinal cord injury was considered irreversible and as a result, research was minimal (78,79). Finally, in the 1970s, spinal cord injury research got the breath of life that it had so desperately needed. Individuals such as Osterholm and Mathews (141,142) reported a series of experiments that outlined the potential role of catecholamines in the pathophysiology of spinal cord injury. These experiments suggested that after injury, norepinephrine was released from injured neurons in the central gray matter of the spinal cord. Although these experiments could not be replicated in other laboratories, the study signaled the advent of investigations into the use of pharmacotherapy for acute spinal cord injury. Early decompressive surgery also was advocated (158).

Perhaps the rapid growth of knowledge in the field of spinal neurosurgery inspired the American Association of Neurological Surgeons and the Congress of Neurological Surgeons to establish the Joint Section on Disorders of the Spine and Peripheral Nerves in 1979. This organization serves as a unified body between the two organizations to promote the advancement of spinal surgery. Not surprisingly, it is one of the most heavily attended specialty sections in all of organized neurosurgery in the United States.

1980s

The explosive growth in the field of spinal surgery in the 1970s was far exceeded by that of the next decade. During the 1980s, little time was spent reflecting on the innovations of the previous decade since technological innovations were being made at a tremendous pace. One innovation was the idea of frameless stereotaxy, as proposed by Gildenberg et al. in 1982 (69,70). Although easily overlooked by practitioners of spinal surgery at the time, these concepts laid the foundation for the development of first cranial and then spinal applications for image-guided surgery.

Diagnostic concepts established in the 1980s included Denis' description of the three-column model for the classification of acute thoracolumbar injuries (38). Besides establishing a cogent treatment philosophy for fractures in this region, Denis' model accounted for the inherent biomechanical properties of the spine and served as a springboard for the laboratory studies that would follow.

Surgical advances in the 1980s were overwhelming. For the treatment of the lumbar spine, individuals such as Luque described methods for segmental instrumentation of the spine that are still practiced (115,116). Other surgical advances, such as pedicle screw fixation and stabilization, were introduced by innovators such as Magerl (120), Roy-Camille et al. (159), Louis (113,114), Dick (40), Steffee et al. (177,178), and Cotrel et al. (32). Even though the above mentioned methods were developed by orthopedic surgeons, spinal neurosurgeons soon embraced and expanded upon them.

During this decade, anterior approaches to the thoracolumbar spine were also refined, and a number of stabilization methods were introduced (45,107,109). These advances are now taken for granted. At that time, however, they filled the void for a method to fixate the spine after a ventral decompression.

In terms of spondylolisthesis, Morscher et al. (133) were the first to propose direct repair of the defect. Their technique consisted of bone grafting and a hook-screw construct that stabilized the spondylolytic defect directly. Soon thereafter, Bradford and Iza (17) described seg-mental wire fixation and bone grafting to repair this condition.

Minimally invasive techniques also expanded, and earlier methods of percutaneous lumbar diskectomy were refined. Coincident with innovations in optics and illumination, several variations on this technique were described, including a lateral approach (105), the introduction of diskoscopy (166), and automated diskectomy (121).

Tremendous strides were made in the treatment of the cervical spine, including the introduction of an elegant method to repair a fractured odontoid directly via an anterior approach (14). Odontoid screw fixation, as this method is now known, has become a valuable addition to the spinal surgeon's armamentarium and is one of the few procedures that permits a spinal fracture to be repaired without sacrificing motion. Magerl then introduced his brilliant technique of transarticular screw fixation of C1–2, which also has become a valuable tool for the treatment of complex atlantoaxial conditions (73,74,103).

Bone fusion research increased with analyses of various allograft fixation techniques and investigations into the usage of demineralized bone matrix (34,91). The use of direct current to stimulate bone growth for spinal fusion was also introduced (106).The field of spinal cord injury research was also gaining momentum in the 1980s. In addition to the pattern of catecholamine release (4), the role of endorphins and opiate antagonists also garnered considerable interest (50–52,55,60,80–82,85,102,199). Other treatment strategies under investigation in this decade included calcium-channel blockers, thyrotropin-releasing hormone, dexamethasone, and hyperbaric oxygen (53,54,64,179).

Another advance that would later become popular was the introduction of vertebroplasty in 1988 (8). Although not fully established until recently, this modality offered a nonsurgical approach for the treatment of insufficiency fractures for which options were severely lacking.

1990s AND THE THIRD MILLENNIUM

Today, spinal surgery bears little resemblance to that practiced during the Eisenhower years. Innovations are now made almost daily. The fields of biotechnology, engineering, and medicine have coalesced into a unified front for the treatment of spinal disorders. In the field of imaging, frameless stereotaxy for use during spinal surgery has been a real advantage. Especially in the treatment of complex atlantoaxial conditions, it can be used to define a safe route for transarticular screw placement, to help position thoracic and lumbar pedicle screws, and to resect various spinal tumors (23,104,128,192). The ability to use CT and MRI (or a combination of the two) in real-time to define anatomic locations with pinpoint accuracy will take the field of spinal surgery to new heights in the 21st century. The morbidity associated with some procedures should decrease concomitantly. The addition of fluoroscopic registration to image-guided surgery further improves current technologies and possibly decreases the exposure to radiation inherent in the prolonged use of fluoroscopy during spinal instrumentation surgery.

Other advances include the introduction of intraoperative imaging. Although currently undergoing clinical trials, this technology is still cumbersome (9,75,83,124,167,168). However, anatomical landmarks can be updated continuously, thereby providing accurate information on an ongoing basis. Future imaging technologies will most likely marry the concept of global positioning satellites with intraoperative imaging strategies to provide real-time anatomic localization and continuously updated views of the region of interest.

The treatment of intervertebral disk disease also will likely change in this new millennium. A number of artificial disks have been described and have undergone clinical testing. The solution to degenerated disks, however, is probably biological rather than biomechanical (7,28, 36,48,72,111). Nishimura and Mochida (137) recently described the percutaneous insertion of autologous nucleus pulposus into a degenerated disk model. The degeneration of remaining structures was delayed. More recently, Annunen et al. (6) identified a possible genetic defect in patients with intervertebral disk disease. Notochordal cell transplantation and genetic procedures for the diagnosis and treatment of disk disorders will most likely become commonplace in the third millennium.

Innovations in minimally invasive surgical techniques include the development of thoracoscopic and laparoscopic surgery (157). These video-assisted techniques combine high-intensity illumination with state-of-the-art cameras to provide unparalleled three-dimensional views of spinal anatomy. Thoracoscopic surgery is becoming common for the treatment of thoracic disk herniations, sympathectomies, biopsies, deformity corrections, and tumor resections (10, 35,41,43,143,145). Laparoscopic surgery is being used to treat disk herniations as well as to implant interbody fusion devices (126,151–153, 171,200).

Other percutaneous innovations include the increasing usage of vertebroplasty (13,27, 33,39,65) and the transpedicular injection of ethanol for the treatment of vertebral hemangiomas (90). Future percutaneous approaches may involve the direct injection of osteoinductive agents in an osteoconductive matrix directly into an osteoporotic vertebra to enhance healing or to prepare adjacent levels for surgery. Stem cells and other biological enhancements may also be used. Spinal surgery of the 21st century will evolve toward less open procedures as the reliance on minimal access techniques increases.

The enhancement of bone fusion will also change as BMPs become commercially available for clinical use. Many studies have proven the efficacy of BMPs in animal models (11, 89,100), but human trials have only recently begun appearing in the literature (12). Another potential use includes the development of instrumentation that is "coated" with a mixture of osteoinductive and conductive agents to ensure a rapid, solid fusion. As the technology is refined, one could envision percutaneous fusion strategies for the treatment of certain disorders (3).

As the treatment of spinal disorders progresses, the biomechanical aspects of the spine become increasingly important. In the past several years, advances in computer technology have encouraged the development of finite-element modeling of the spine, which can be used to predict stresses on the spine during various normal and pathological maneuvers (66,108, 160). Realizing the patterns of injury caused by repetitive stresses and blunt trauma can help in the design of strategies to prevent these problems and to ensure their effective treatment.

Of all the strategies investigated for the treatment of spinal cord injury in the 1980s, only methylprednisolone was shown to be effective (15,16,135). The advances of the past decade and those most promising in the 21st century center around the field of neurobiology. A major advance includes the discovery that the central nervous system (CNS) contains a population of stem cells that can be purified, expanded, and transplanted, and under certain conditions, can form viable synaptic connections (61,63,127, 148,175,191). This discovery shattered the long-held belief that the CNS cannot regenerate and opens the door for a myriad of potential therapies to replace cells after spinal cord injury.

Another advance includes the inhibitory role that CNS myelin plays after spinal cord injury. Recent efforts have concentrated on using antibodies against these myelin-associated growth inhibitors, both to overcome the inhibition and to enhance repair after spinal cord injury (18, 164,165,183).

Understanding the role of trophic factors, scarring, and inflammation after spinal cord injury may also lead to effective treatments. A recent strategy involves the role of activated macrophages and has shown significant promise (95,150). Other strategies involve neural transplantation and regeneration based on the recent work of Cheng et al. (25,26), Guest et al. (76,77), and others (101,112,196). Perhaps one day, these strategies may allow a damaged region of spinal cord to be "bypassed" or directly repaired using a combination of transplanted tissue and other biological repair-enhancing techniques. There is little doubt that the treatment of acute spinal cord injury should improve significantly during the third millennium. Ultimately, a combination of techniques will likely overcome the inhibitory effects of myelin and enhance the proper growth and recovery of injured axons.

The final frontiers in spinal surgery will affirm that current and future techniques are safe, efficacious, and improve outcomes as compared with conservative therapy. Managed care and the insinuation of third-party payers into the medical decision-making process make it imperative to establish the benefit of spinal procedures unequivocally.

Internal medicine has rallied to the cause of evidence-based medicine, but the field of spinal surgery has been slow to follow. Recently, a large randomized, placebo-controlled, multicenter study of postmenopausal women with osteoporosis demonstrated the efficacy of raloxifene hydrochloride, a selective estrogen-receptor modulator, in preventing vertebral fractures (49). Indeed, to date, the most widely studied procedure in neurosurgery has been carotid endarterectomy, which clearly prevents stroke in certain patients (57,68,131,132,138,198). Similar studies in spinal surgery have been scarce.

Two recent studies examined the efficacy and outcomes in patients undergoing lumbar spinal fusion with and without instrumentation (59,184). One study used pedicle screws to augment single-level fusions. The procedure increased the rate of fusion but did not improve clinical outcomes with respect to pain (59). The other study demonstrated improved functional outcomes after posterolateral lumbar fusion with or without instrumentation (184). Both studies concluded that the routine use of pedicle screw fixation may be unnecessary. Similar controversy surrounds cervical diskectomy as compared to diskectomy and fusion (44,161).

The goal of organized spinal surgery in the third millennium will be to establish large multicenter, randomized, controlled trials to define which procedures are beneficial to patients. By incorporating these studies into practice, the "art" of spinal surgery assumes a more scientifically acceptable mantle. The result will be improvement in the well being of patients.

Whereas before the 1990s economic issues in spinal surgery took a back seat to scientific and technical advances, this era ultimately ended. The insidious control exerted by the practices of managed care will take its toll on the treatment of spinal disorders. A rude awakening for all spinal surgeons occurred with the class-action pedicle screw litigation of the 1990s, which injected the device classification system of the Food and Drug Administration into a malpractice-type lawsuit (67). After a hard-fought battle that pitted both organized neurosurgery and orthopedic surgery against the plaintiff's attorneys, this issue was resolved in favor of the neurosurgeon, but only after extensive time and money were invested. Organized spinal surgery has learned some important lessons from this environment and has become more cautious before embracing new techniques. One would hope that as we enter the 21st century, the medical economic climate could be directed toward providing the highest level of care for patients with spinal disorders while ensuring fair compensation for spinal surgeons.

CONCLUSION

The colorful characters that defined spinal surgery in the 1950s are gone. It is doubtful that we will ever again liken the draping of a patient as being as ''ritualistic and time-consuming as a Mormon wedding!'' as did Semmes (169), or describe an increase usage of blood transfusions as ''killing more patients than appendicitis'' (169). Semmes attributed his conservative approach to Dr. Wilhelm Kohlmer, who stated, ''as less you do, better ist'' (169). The passing of these philosophies defined the end of an era. Since the 1960s, the unprecedented growth in technology and knowledge has allowed treatment options to be developed that would have been considered science fiction in 1950. Only by studying the past and the historical evolution of spinal surgery can one effectively predict the future and focus efforts and limited resources on improving the outcome of all patients with spinal disorders.

REFERENCES

1. Albin MS, White RJ, Acosta-Rua G, et al. Study of functional recovery produced by delayed localized cooling after spinal cord injury in primates. *J Neurosurg* 29:113–120, 1968.
2. Albin MS, White RJ, Yashon D, et al. Effects of localized cooling on spinal cord trauma. *J Trauma* 9: 1000–1008, 1969.
3. Alden TD, Pittman DD, Beres EJ, et al. Percutaneous spinal fusion using bone morphogenetic protein-2 gene therapy. *J Neurosurg (Spine 1)* 90:109–114, 1999.
4. Alderman JL, Osterholm JL, D'Amore BR, et al. Catecholamine alterations attending spinal cord injury: A reanalysis. *Neurosurgery* 6:412–417, 1980.
5. Alexander E, Jr, Forsyth HF, Davis CH, Jr, et al. Dislocation of the atlas on the axis: The value of early fusion of C1, C2, and C3. *J Neurosurg* 15:353–371, 1958.
6. Annunen S, Paassilta P, Lohiniva J, et al. An allele of COL9A2 associated with intervertebral disc disease. *Science* 285:409–412, 1999.
7. Bao QB, McCullen GM, Higham PA, et al. The artificial disc: Theory, design and materials. *Biomaterials* 17:1157–1167, 1996.
8. Bascoulergue Y. Percutaneous injection of methyl methacrylate in the vertebral body for the treatment of various diseases. *74th Annual Meeting of the Radiological Society of North America.* Chicago, November, 1988.
9. Black PM, Alexander E 3rd, et al. Craniotomy for tumor treatment in an intraoperative magnetic resonance imaging unit. *Neurosurgery* 45:423–433, 1999.
10. Blackman RG, Luque E. Endoscopic anterior correction of idiopathic scoliosis. in, Dickman CA, Rosenthal DJ, Perin NI (eds): *Thoracoscopic Spine Surgery.* New York: Thieme, 1999.
11. Boden SD, Martin GJ Jr, Morone MA, et al. Posterolateral lumbar intertransverse process spine arthrodesis with recombinant human bone morphogenetic protein 2/hydroxyapatite-tricalcium phosphate after laminectomy in the nonhuman primate. *Spine* 24:1179–1185, 1999.
12. Boden SD, Zdeblick TA, Sandhu HS, et al. The use of rhBMP-2 in interbody fusion cages. Definitive evidence of osteoinduction in humans: A preliminary report. *Spine* 25:376–381, 2000.
13. Bostrom MPG, Lane JM. Future directions: Augmentation of osteoporotic vertebral bodies. *Spine* 22: 38S–42S, 1997.
14. Böhler J. Anterior stabilization for acute fractures and non-unions of the dens. *J Bone Joint Surg* 64A:18–27, 1982.
15. Bracken MB, Shepard MJ, Collins WF, et al. A randomized, controlled trial of methylprednisolone or naloxone in the treatment of acute spinal-cord injury. Results of the Second National Acute Spinal Cord Injury Study. *N Engl J Med* 322:1405–1411, 1990.
16. Bracken MB, Shepard MJ, Holford TR, et al. Administration of methylprednisolone for 24 or 48 hours or tirilazad mesylate for 48 hours in the treatment of acute spinal cord injury. Results of the Third National Acute Spinal Cord Injury Randomized Controlled Trial. National Acute Spinal Cord Injury Study. *JAMA* 277: 1597–1604, 1997.
17. Bradford DS, Iza J. Repair of the defect in spondylolysis of minimal degrees of spondylolisthesis by segmental wire fixation and bone grafting. *Spine* 10: 673–679, 1985.
18. Bregman BS, Kunkel-Bagden E, Schnell L, et al. Recovery from spinal cord injury mediated by antibodies in neurite growth inhibitors. *Nature* 378:498–501, 1995.
19. Brihaye J, Lorthioir J Jr. Observation clinique d'un syndrome de la queue de cheval après injection de bleu

de méthylène dans le cul-de-sac arachnoidien lombo-
sacré. *Acta Chir Belg* 56:312–316, 1957.

20. Brooks AL, Jenkins EB. Atlanto-axial arthrodesis by
the wedge compression method. *J Bone Joint Surg*
60A:279–284, 1978.

21. Callahan RA, Johnson RM, Margolis RN, et al. Cervical facet fusion for control of instability following laminectomy. *J Bone Joint Surg* 59A:991–1002, 1977.

22. Capener N. The evolution of lateral rhachotomy. *J
Bone Joint Surg Br* 36:173–179, 1954.

23. Carl AL, Khanuja HS, Sachs BL, et al. In vitro simula-
tion: Early results of stereotaxy for pedicle screw
placement. *Spine* 22:1160–1164, 1997.

24. Caspar W. A new surgical procedure for lumbar disc
herniation causing less tissue damage through a microsurgical approach. *Adv Neurosur* 4:74–80, 1977.

25. Cheng H, Cao Y, Olson L. Spinal cord repair in adult
paraplegic rats: Partial restoration of hind limb function. *Science* 273:510–513, 1996.

26. Cheng H, Hoffer B, Stromberg I, et al. The effect of
glial cell line-derived neurotrophic factor in fibrin glue
on developing dopamine neurons. *Exp Brain Res* 104:
199–206, 1995.

27. Chiras J, Depriester C, Weill A, et al. Percutaneous
vertebral surgery: Technic and indications [French]. *J
Neuroradiol* 24:45–59, 1997.

28. Cinotti G, David T, Postacchini F. Results of disc prosthesis after a minimum follow-up period of 2 years.
Spine 21:995–1000, 1996.

29. Cloward RB. The anterior approach for removal of
ruptured cervical disks. *J Neurosurg* 15:602–617,
1958.

30. Cooper IS, MacCarty CS, Rynearson EH, et al. Metabolic consequences of spinal cordectomy. *Proc Mayo
Clin* 24:620–627, 1949.

31. Cormack AM. Representation of a function by its line
integrals, with some radiological applications. *J Appl
Phys* 34:2722–2727, 1963.

32. Cotrel Y, Dubousset J, Guillaumat M. New universal
instrumentation in spinal surgery. *Clin Orthop* 227:
10–23, 1988.

33. Cotten A, Boutry N, Cortet B, et al. Percutaneous vertebroplasty: State of the art. *Radiographics* 18:311–323,
1998.

34. Covey DC, Albright JA. Clinical induction of bone
repair with demineralized bone matrix or a bone morphogenetic protein. *Orthop Rev* 18:857–863, 1989.

35. Crawford AH. Anterior release of spinal deformities,
in, Dickman CA, Rosenthal DJ, Perin NI (eds): *Thoracoscopic Spine Surgery.* New York: Thieme, 1999.

36. Cummings BH, Robertson JT, Gill SS. Surgical experience with an implanted artificial cervical joint. *J Neurosurg* 88:943–948, 1998.

37. Cushing H. *Consecratio Medici and Other Papers.*
Boston: Little, Brown, and Company, 1928.

38. Denis F. The three column injury and its significance
in the classification of acute thoracolumbar spinal injuries. *Spine* 8:817–831, 1983.

39. Deramond H, Depriester C, Galibert P, et al. Percutane-
ous vertebroplasty with polymethylmethacrylate:
Technique, indications, and results. *Radiol Clin North
Am* 36:533–546, 1998.

40. Dick W. The ''fixateur interne'' as a versatile implant
for spine surgery. *Spine* 12:882–900, 1987.

41. Dickman CA, Apfelbaum RI. Thoracoscopic resection

of intrathoracic neurogenic tumors, in, Dickman CA,
Rosenthal DJ, Perin NI (eds): *Thoracoscopic Spine
Surgery.* New York: Thieme, 1999.

42. Dickman CA, Mamourian A, Sonntag VKH, et al.
Magnetic resonance imaging of the transverse atlantal
ligament for the evaluation of atlantoaxial instability.
J Neurosurg 75:221–227, 1991.

43. Dickman CA, Rosenthal DJ, Perin NI. Thoracoscopic
microsurgical discectomy, in, Dickman CA, Rosenthal
DJ, Perin NI (eds): *Thoracoscopic Spine Surgery.* New
York: Thieme, 1999.

44. Dowd GC, Wirth FP. Anterior cervical discectomy: Is
fusion necessary? *J Neurosurg* 90:8–12, 1999.

45. Dunn, HK. Anterior stabilization of thoracolumbar injuries. *Clin Orthop* 189:116–124, 1984.

46. Dunsker SB. Anterior cervical discectomy with and
without fusion. *Clin Neurosurg* 24:516–521, 1977.

47. Dwyer AF, Newton NC, Sherwood AA. An anterior
approach to scoliosis: A preliminary report. *Clin Orthop* 62:192–202, 1969.

48. Enker P, Steffee A, Mcmillin C, et al. Artificial disc
replacement: Preliminary report with a 3-year minimum follow-up. *Spine* 18:1061–1070, 1993.

49. Ettinger B, Black DM, Mitlak BH, et al. Reduction of
vertebral fracture risk in postmenopausal women with
osteoporosis treated with raloxifene: Results from a
3-year randomized clinical trial. *JAMA* 282:637–645,
1999.

50. Faden AI. Pharmacotherapy in spinal cord injury: A
critical review of recent developments. *Clin Neuro-
pharmacol* 10:193–204, 1987.

51. Faden AI, Jacobs TP, Holaday JW. Opiate antagonist
improves neurologic recovery after spinal injury. *Science* 211:493–494, 1981.

52. Faden AI, Jacobs TP, Mougey E, et al. Endorphins in
experimental spinal injury: Therapeutic effect of naloxone. *Ann Neurol* 10:326–332, 1981.

53. Faden AI, Jacobs TP, Smith MT. Evaluation of the
calcium channel antagonist nimodipine in experimental spinal cord ischemia. *J Neurosurg* 60:796–799,
1984.

54. Faden AI, Jacobs TP, Smith MT, et al. Comparison of
thyrotropin-releasing hormone (TRH), naloxone, and
dexamethasone treatments in experimental spinal injury. *Neurology* 33:673–678, 1983.

55. Faden AI, Jacobs TP, Smith MT, et al. Naloxone in
experimental spinal cord ischemia: Dose-response
studies. *Eur J Pharmacol* 103:115–120, 1984.

56. Fang HSY, Ong GB. Direct anterior approach to the
upper cervical spine. *J Bone Joint Surg* 44A:
1588–1604, 1962.

57. Ferguson GG, Eliasziw M, Barr HW, et al. The North
American Symptomatic Carotid Endarterectomy Trial:
Surgical results in 1415 patients. *Stroke* 30:
1751–1758, 1999.

58. Fielding JW, Pyle RN Jr, Fietti VG Jr. Anterior cervical
vertebral body resection and bone-grafting for benign
and malignant tumors: A survey under the auspices of
the Cervical Spine Research Society. *J Bone Joint Surg
Am* 61:251–253, 1979.

59. Fischgrund JS, Mackay M, Herkowitz HN, et al. 1997
Volvo Award winner in clinical studies. Degenerative
lumbar spondylolisthesis with spinal stenosis: A prospective, randomized study comparing decompressive

laminectomy and arthrodesis with and without spinal instrumentation. *Spine* 22:2807–2812, 1997.

60. Flamm ES, Young W, Demopoulos HB, et al. Experimental spinal cord injury: Treatment with naloxone. *Neurosurgery* 10:227–231, 1982.

61. Flax JD, Aurora S, Yang C, et al. Engraftable human neural stem cells respond to developmental cues, replace neurons, and express foreign genes. *Nat Biotechnol* 16:1033–1039, 1998.

62. Freebody D, Bendall R, Taylor RD. Anterior transperitoneal lumbar fusion. *J Bone Joint Surg Br* 53:617–627, 1971.

63. Fricker RA, Carpenter MK, Winkler C, et al. Site-specific migration and neuronal differentiation of human neural progenitor cells after transplantation in the adult rat brain. *J Neurosci* 19:5990–6005, 1999.

64. Gamache FW Jr, Myers RAM, Ducker TB, et al. The clinical application of hyperbaric oxygen therapy in spinal cord injury: A preliminary report. *Surg Neurol* 15:85–87, 1981.

65. Gangi A, Kastler BA, Dietemann J-L. Percutaneous vertebroplasty guided by a combination of CT and fluoroscopy. *AJNR* 15:83–86, 1994.

66. Gardner WJ. The principle of spring-loaded points for cervical traction. *J Neurosurg* 39:543–544, 1973.

67. Garfin SR, Yuan HA. Food and Drug Administration regulation of spinal implant fixation devices. *Clin Orthop* 335:32–38, 1997.

68. Gasecki AP, Eliasziw M, Ferguson GG, et al. Long-term prognosis and effect of endarterectomy in patients with symptomatic severe carotid stenosis and contralateral carotid stenosis or occlusion: Results from NASCET. North American Symptomatic Carotid Endarterectomy Trial (NASCET) Group. *J Neurosurg* 83:778–782, 1995.

69. Gildenberg PL, Kaufman HH. Direct calculation of stereotactic coordinates from CT scans. *Appl Neurophysiol* 45:347–351, 1982.

70. Gildenberg PL, Kaufman HH, Murthy KS. Calculation of stereotactic coordinates from the computed tomographic scan. *Neurosurgery* 10:580–586, 1982.

71. Gill GG, Manning JG, White HL. Surgical treatment of spondylolisthesis without spine fusion: Excision of loose lamina with decompression of the nerve roots. *J Bone Joint Surg Am* 37:493–520, 1955.

72. Griffith SL, Shelokov AP, Buttner-Janz K, et al. A multicenter retrospective study of the clinical results of the LINK SB Charite intervertebral prosthesis: The initial European experience. *Spine* 19:1842–1849, 1994.

73. Grob D, Magerl F. Dorsal spondylodesis of the cervical spine using a hooked plate [German]. *Orthopade* 16:55–61, 1987a.

74. Grob D, Magerl F. Surgical stabilization of C1 and C2 fractures [German]. *Orthopade* 16:46–54, 1987b.

75. Grunert P, Muller-Forell W, Darabi K, et al. Basic principles and clinical applications of neuronavigation and intraoperative computed tomography. *Comput Aided Surg* 3:166–173, 1998.

76. Guest JD, Hesse D, Schnell L, et al. Influence of IN-1 antibody and acidic FGF-fibrin glue on the response of injured corticospinal tract axons to human Schwann cell grafts. *J Neurosci Res* 50:888–905, 1997.

77. Guest JD, Rao A, Olson L, et al. The ability of human Schwann cell grafts to promote regeneration in the transected nude rat spinal cord. *Exp Neurol* 148:502–522, 1997.

78. Guttmann L. *Spinal Cord Injuries—Comprehensive Management and Research.* Oxford, England: Blackwell Scientific, 1973.

79. Guttmann L. The conservative management of closed injuries of the vertebral column resulting in damage to the spinal cord and spinal roots. In, Vinkin PJ, Bruyn GW, Braakman R (eds): *Handbook of Clinical Neurology: Vol. 26. Injuries of the Spine and Spinal Cord—Part II.* Amsterdam: North-Holland, 1976.

80. Hall ED, Braughler JM. Effects of intravenous methylprednisolone on spinal cord lipid peroxidation and $(Na^+ + K^+)$-ATPase activity: Dose-response analysis during 1st hour after contusion injury in the cat. *J Neurosurg* 57:247–253, 1982.

81. Hall ED, and Braughler JM. Glucocorticoid mechanisms in acute spinal cord injury: A review and therapeutic rationale. *Surg Neurol* 18:320–327, 1988.

82. Hall ED, Braughler JM, McCall JM. New pharmacological treatment of acute spinal cord trauma. *J Neurotrauma* 5:81–89, 1988.

83. Hall WA, Martin AJ, Liu H, et al. Brain biopsy using high-field strength interventional magnetic resonance imaging. *Neurosurgery* 44:807–814, 1999.

84. Hankinson HL, Wilson CB. Use of the operating microscope in anterior cervical discectomy without fusion. *J Neurosurg* 43:452–456, 1975.

85. Hansebout RR. A comprehensive review of methods of improving cord recovery after acute spinal cord injury, in, Tator CH (ed): *Early Management of Acute Spinal Cord Injury.* New York: Raven, 1982.

86. Harrington PR. The history and development of Harrington instrumentation. *Clin Orthop* 93:110–112, 1973.

87. Harrington PR, Dickson JH. Spinal instrumentation in the treatment of severe progressive spondylolisthesis. *Clin Orthop* 117:157–163, 1976.

88. Hattori S. A new method of cervical laminectomy. *Central Jpn J Orthop Traumatic Surg* 16:792–794, 1973.

89. Hecht BP, Fischgrund JS, Herkowitz HN, et al. The use of recombinant human bone morphogenetic protein 2 (rhBMP-2) to promote spinal fusion in a non-human primate anterior interbody fusion model. *Spine* 24:629–636, 1999.

90. Heiss JD, Doppman JL, Oldfield EH. Brief report: Relief of spinal cord compression from vertebral hemangioma by intralesional injection of absolute ethanol. *N Engl J Med* 331:508–511, 1994.

91. Herron LD, Newman MH. The failure of ethylene oxide gas-sterilized freeze-dried bone graft for thoracic and lumbar spinal fusion. *Spine* 14:496–500, 1989.

92. Hijikata S. Percutaneous nucleotomy: A new concept technique and 12 years' experience. *Clin Orthop* 238:9–23, 1989.

93. Hinshaw WS, Bottomley PA, Holland GN. Radiographic thin-section of the human wrist by nuclear magnetic resonance. *Nature* 270:722–723, 1977.

94. Hirsch C. Cervical disk rupture: Diagnosis and therapy. *Acta Orthop Scand* 30:172–186, 1960.

95. Hirschberg DL, Yoles E, Belkin M, et al. Inflammation after axonal injury has conflicting consequences for recovery of function: Rescue of spared axons is im-

paired but regeneration is supported. *J Neuroimmunol* 50:9–16, 1994.

96. Hodgson AR, Stock FE. Anterior spinal fusion: A preliminary communication on the radical treatment of Pott's disease and Pott's paraplegia. *Br J Surg* 44: 266–275, 1956.

97. Holdsworth F. Fractures, dislocations, and fracture-dislocations of the spine. *J Bone Joint Surg Am* 52: 1534–1550, 1970.

98. Hounsfield GN. Computerized transverse axial scanning (tomography). 1. Description of system. *Br J Radiol* 46:1016–1022, 1973.

99. Humphries AW, Hawk WA, Berndt AL. Anterior interbody fusion of lumbar vertebrae: A surgical technique. *Surg Clin North Am* 41:1685–1700, 1961.

100. Itoh H, Ebara S, Kamimura M, et al. Experimental spinal fusion with use of recombinant human bone morphogenetic protein 2. *Spine* 24:1402–1405, 1999.

101. Iwashita Y, Kawaguchi S, Murata M. Restoration of function by replacement of spinal cord segments in the rat. *Nature* 367:167–170, 1994.

102. Janssen L, Hansebout RR. Pathogenesis of spinal cord injury and newer treatments: A review. *Spine* 14: 23–32, 1989.

103. Jeanneret B, Magerl F. Primary posterior fusion C1/2 in odontoid fractures: Indications, technique, and results of transarticular screw fixation. *J Spinal Disord* 5:464–475, 1992.

104. Kalfas IH, Kormos DW, Murphy MA, et al. Application of frameless stereotaxy to pedicle screw fixation of the spine. *J Neurosurg* 83:641–647, 1995.

105. Kambin P, Gellman H. Percutaneous lateral discectomy of the lumbar spine. *Clin Orthop* 174:127–132, 1983.

106. Kane WJ. Direct current electrical bone growth stimulation for spinal fusion. *Spine* 13:363–365, 1988.

107. Kaneda K, Abumi K, Fujiya M. Burst fractures with neurologic deficits of the thoracolumbar-lumbar spine: Results of anterior decompression and stabilization with anterior instrumentation. *Spine* 9:788–795, 1984.

108. Kong WZ, Goel VK, Gilbertson LG. Prediction of biomechanical parameters in the lumbar spine during static sagittal plane lifting. *J Biomech Eng* 120: 273–280, 1998.

109. Kostuik JP. Anterior spinal cord decompression for lesions of the thoracic and lumbar spine, techniques, new methods of internal fixation results. *Spine* 8: 512–531, 1983.

110. Laurent LE, Einola S. Spondylolisthesis in children and adolescents. *Acta Orthop Scand* 31:45–64, 1961.

111. LeMaire JP, Skalli W, Lavaste F, et al. Intervertebral disc prosthesis: Results and prospects for the year 2000. *Clin Orthop* 337:64–76, 1997.

112. Li Y, Field PM, Raisman G. Regeneration of adult rat corticospinal axons induced by transplanted olfactory ensheathing cells. *J Neurosci* 18:10514–10524, 1998.

113. Louis R. Fusion of the lumbar and sacral spine by internal fixation with screw plates. *Clin Orthop* 203:18–33, 1986.

114. Louis R. Pars interarticularis reconstruction of spondylolysis using plates and screws with grafting without arthrodesis. Apropos of 78 cases [French]. *Rev Chir Orthop Reparatrice Appar Mot* 74:549–557, 1988.

115. Luque ER. The anatomic basis and development of segmental spinal instrumentation. *Spine* 7:256–259, 1982.

116. Luque ER. Interpeduncular segmental fixation. *Clin Orthop* 203:54–57, 1986.

117. MacCarty CS. The treatment of spastic paraplegia by selective spinal cordectomy. *J Neurosurg* 11: 5539–5545, 1954.

118. MacCarty CS, Kiefer EJ. Thoracic, lumbar and sacral spinal cordectomy: Preliminary report. *Proc Mayo Clin* 24:108–115, 1949.

119. MacCarty CS, Roth GM, Thompson GJ. Physiologic observations after thoracic, lumbar and sacral cordectomy. *Proc Mayo Clin* 26:113–120, 1951.

120. Magerl F. External skeletal fixation of the lower thoracic and lumbar spine. In, Uhthoff HK, Stahl E (eds): *Current Concepts of External Fixation of Fractures.* Berlin: Springer-Verlag, 1982.

121. Maroon JC, Onik G. Percutaneous automated discectomy: A new method for lumbar disc removal. Technical note. *J Neurosurg* 66:143–146, 1987.

122. Martin J. Recent trends in neurosurgery. *J Neurosurg* 15:674–687, 1958.

123. Martins AN. Anterior cervical discectomy with and without interbody bone graft. *J Neurosurg* 44: 290–295, 1976.

124. Matula C, Rossler K, Reddy M, et al. Intraoperative computed tomography guided neuronavigation: Concepts, efficiency, and work flow. *Comput Aided Surg* 3:174–182, 1998.

125. Mayfield FH. Cervical spondylosis: A comparison of the anterior and posterior approaches. *Clin Neurosurg* 13:181–188, 1965.

126. McAfee PC, Regan JJ, Geis WP, et al. Minimally invasive anterior retroperitoneal approach to the lumbar spine: Emphasis on the lateral BAK. *Spine* 23: 1476–1484, 1998.

127. McKay RD. Brain stem cells change their identity. *Nat Med* 5:261–262, 1999.

128. Merloz P, Tonetti J, Pittet L, et al. Pedicle screw placement using image guided techniques. *Clin Orthop* 354: 39–48, 1998.

129. Meyerding HW. Spondylolisthesis. *Surg Gynecol* 54: 371–377, 1932.

130. Mixter SJ, Osgood RB. Traumatic lesions of the atlas and axis. *Ann Surg* 51:193–207, 1910.

131. Moore WS, Young B, Baker WH, et al. Surgical results: A justification of the surgeon selection process for the ACAS trial. The ACAS Investigators. *J Vasc Surg* 23:323–328, 1996.

132. Morgenstern LB, Fox AJ, Sharpe BL, et al. The risks and benefits of carotid endarterectomy in patients with near occlusion of the carotid artery. North American Symptomatic Carotid Endarterectomy Trial (NASCET) Group. *Neurology* 48:911–915, 1997.

133. Morscher E, Gerber B, Fasel J. Surgical treatment of spondylolisthesis by bone grafting and direct stabilization of spondylolysis by means of a hook screw. *Arch Orthop Trauma Surg* 103:175–178, 1984.

134. Negrin J Jr. Extravascular perfusion for selective regional hypothermia of the central nervous system (brain or spinal cord). *Acta Neurochir (Wien)* 12: 88–95, 1964.

135. Nesathurai S. Steroids and spinal cord injury: Revisiting the NASCIS 2 and NASCIS 3 trials. *J Trauma* 45:1088–1093, 1998.

136. Newman P, Sweetnam R. Occipito-cervical fusion: An operative technique and its indications. *J Bone Joint Surg Br* 51:423–431, 1969.

137. Nishimura K, Mochida J. Percutaneous reinsertion of the nucleus pulposus: An experimental study. *Spine* 23:1531–1539, 1998.

138. North American Symptomatic Carotid Endarterectomy Trial (NASCET) Investigators Clinical alert: Benefit of carotid endarterectomy for patients with high-grade stenosis of the internal carotid artery. National Institute of Neurological Disorders and Stroke and Trauma Division. *Stroke* 22:816–817, 1991.

139. Oldendorf WH. Isolated flying spot detection of radiodensity discontinuities—displaying the internal structural pattern of a complex object. *Trans Bio Med Elect* 8:68–72, 1961.

140. Orozco R, and Llovet J. Osteosinterior en las fracturas del raquir cervical. *Rev Ortop Traumatol* 14:285–288, 1970.

141. Osterholm JL, Mathews GJ. Altered norepinephrine metabolism following experimental spinal cord injury. 1. Relationship to hemorrhagic necrosis and post-wounding neurological deficits. *J Neurosurg* 36:386–394, 1972.

142. Osterholm JL, Mathews GJ. Altered norepinephrine metabolism, following experimental spinal cord injury. 2. Protection against traumatic spinal cord hemorrhagic necrosis by norepinephrine synthesis blockade with alpha methyl tyrosine. *J Neurosurg* 36:395–401, 1972.

143. Papadopoulos SM, Dickman CA. Thoracoscopic sympathectomy, in, Dickman CA, Rosenthal DJ, Perin NI (eds): *Thoracoscopic Spine Surgery.* New York: Thieme, 1999.

144. Patterson RH, Arbit E. A surgical approach through the pedicle to protruded thoracic discs. *J Neurosurg* 48:768–772, 1978.

145. Perin NI. Biopsy of vertebral lesions. In, Dickman CA, Rosenthal DJ, Perin NI. (eds): *Thoracoscopic Spine Surgery.* New York: Thieme, 1999.

146. Perot PL, Munro DD. Transthoracic removal of midline thoracic disc protrusions causing spinal cord compression. *J Neurosurg* 31:452–458, 1969.

147. Perry J, Nickel VL. Total cervical-spine fusion for neck paralysis. *J Bone Joint Surg Am* 41:37–60, 1959.

148. Rakic P. Young neurons for old brains? *Nat Neurosci* 1:645–647, 1998.

149. Ransohoff J, Spencer F, Siew F. Transthoracic removal of thoracic disc: Report of three cases. *J Neurosurg* 31:459–461, 1969.

150. Rapalino O, Lazarov-Spiegler O, Agranov E, et al. Implantation of stimulated homologous macrophages results in partial recovery of paraplegic rats. *Nat Med* 4:814–821, 1998.

151. Regan JJ, Guyer RD. Endoscopic techniques in spinal surgery. *Clin Orthop* 335:122–139, 1997.

152. Regan JJ, McAfee PC, Guyer RD, et al. Laparoscopic fusion of the lumbar spine in a multicenter series of the first 34 consecutive patients. *Surg Laparosc Endosc* 6:459–468, 1996.

153. Regan JJ, Yuan H, McAfee PC. Laparoscopic fusion of the lumbar spine: Minimally invasive spine surgery. A prospective multicenter study evaluating open and laparoscopic lumbar fusion. *Spine* 24:402–411, 1999.

154. Robertson JT. Anterior removal of cervical disc without fusion. *Clin Neurosurg* 20:259–261, 1973.

155. Robinson RA, Smith GW. Anterolateral cervical disc removal and interbody fusion for cervical disc syndrome. *Bull Johns Hopkins Hosp* 96:223,1955.

156. Rose GK, Owen R, Sanderson JM. Transposition of rib with blood supply for the stabilisation of spinal kyphosis (Abstract). *J Bone Joint Surg Br* 57:112,1975.

157. Rosenthal DJ, Dickman CA. The history of thoraco-scopic spine surgery, in, Dickman CA, Rosenthal DJ, Perin NI (eds): *Thoracoscopic Spine Surgery.* New York: Thieme, 1999.

158. Roy-Camille R, Saillant G, Bertaux D, et al. Early management of spinal injuries, in, McKibbin B (ed): *Recent Advances in Orthopaedics.* Edinburgh: Churchill Livingstone, 1979.

159 Roy-Camille R, Saillant G, Mazel C. Internal fixation of the lumbar spine with pedicle screw plating. *Clin Orthop* 203:7–17, 1986.

160. Sanan A, Rengachary SS. The history of spinal biomechanics. *Neurosurgery* 39:657–669, 1996.

161. Savolainen S, Rinne J, Hernesniemi J. A prospective randomized study of anterior single-level cervical disc operations with long-term follow-up: Surgical fusion is unnecessary. *Neurosurgery* 43:51–55, 1998.

162. Scarff JE, Pool JL. Factors causing massive spasm following transection of the cord in man. *J Neurosurg* 3:285–293, 1946.

163. Schneider RC, Cherry G, Pantek H. The syndrome of acute central cervical spinal cord injury: With special reference to the mechanisms involved in hyperextension injuries of cervical spine. *J Neurosurg* 11:546–577, 1954.

164. Schnell L, Schwab ME. Axonal regeneration in the rat spinal cord produced by an antibody against myelin-associated neurite growth inhibitors. *Nature* 343:269–272, 1990.

165. Schnell L, Schneider R, Kolbeck R, et al. Neurotrophin-3 enhances sprouting of corticospinal tract during development and after adult spinal cord lesion. *Nature* 367:170–173, 1994

166. Schreiber A, Suezawa Y, Leu H. Does percutaneous nucleotomy with discoscopy replace conventional discectomy? Eight years of experience and results in treatment of herniated lumbar disc. *Clin Orthop* 238:35–42, 1989.

167. Schwartz RB, Hsu L, Wong TZ, et al. Intraoperative MR imaging guidance for intracranial neurosurgery: Experience with the first 200 cases. *Radiology* 211:477–488, 1999.

168. Seifert V, Zimmermann M, Trantakis C, et al. Open MRI-guided neurosurgery. *Acta Neurochir (Wien)* 141:455–464, 1999.

169. Semmes RE. In favor of simplicity: Applied to medicine in general and neurosurgery in particular. *J Neurosurg* 15:1–3, 1958.

170. Shelden CH, Bors E. Subarachnoid alcohol block in paraplegia. Its beneficial effect on mass reflexes and bladder dysfunction. *J Neurosurg* 5:385–391, 1948.

171. Silcox DH, 3rd. Laparoscopic bone dowel fusions of the lumbar spine. *Orthop Clin North Am* 29:655–663, 1998.

172. Smith GW, Robinson RA. The treatment of certain cervical-spine disorders by anterior removal of the intervertebral disc and interbody fusion. *J Bone Joint Surg Am* 40:607–624, 1958

173. Smith L. Chemonucleolysis. *Clin Orthop* 67:72–80, 1969.
174. Smith L, Garvin PJ, Jennings RB, et al. Enzyme dissolution of the nucleus pulposus. *Nature* 198:1311–1312, 1963.
175. Snyder EY, Yoon C, Flax JD, et al. Multipotent neural precursors can differentiate toward replacement of neurons undergoing targeted apoptotic degeneration in adult mouse neocortex. *Proc Natl Acad Sci USA* 94:11663–11668, 1997.
176. Southwick WO, Johnson RM, Callahan RA, et al. Cervical laminectomy and facet fusion: Fifteen years' experience (Abstract). *J Bone Joint Surg Br* 59:121,1977.
177. Steffee AD, Sitkowski DJ. Reduction and stabilization of grade IV spondylolisthesis. *Clin Orthop* 227:82–89, 1988.
178. Steffee AD, Biscup RS, Sitkowski DJ. Segmental spine plates with pedicle screw fixation: A new internal fixation device for disorders of the lumbar and thoracolumbar spine. *Clin Orthop* 203:45–53, 1986.
179. Sukoff MH. Review and update of cerebral edema and spinal cord injuries. *Hyperbaric Oxygen Rev* 1:189–195, 1980.
180. Taillard W. Le spondylolisthesis chez l'enfant et l'adolescent (etude de 50 cas). *Acta Orthop Scand* 24:115–144, 1954.
181. Tarlov IM. *Spinal Cord Compression. Mechanism of Paralysis and Treatment.* Springfield, Illinois: Charles C Thomas, 1957.
182. Taylor AR. The mechanism of injury to the spinal cord in the neck without damage to the vertebral column. *J Bone Joint Surg Br* 33:543–547, 1951.
183. Thallmair M, Metz GA, Z'Graggen WJ, et al. Neurite growth inhibitors restrict plasticity and functional recovery following corticospinal tract lesions. *Nat Neurosci* 1:124–131, 1998.
184. Thomsen K, Christensen FB, Eiskjaer SP, et al. 1997 Volvo Award winner in clinical studies. The effect of pedicle screw instrumentation on functional outcome and fusion rates in posterolateral lumbar spinal fusion: A prospective, randomized clinical study. *Spine* 22:2813–2822, 1997.
185. Tucker HH. Technical report: Method of fixation of

subluxed or dislocated cervical spine below C1–C2. *Can J Neurol Sci* 2:381–382, 1975.
186. Turnbull F. Neurosurgery is what you make it: At the beginning. *J Neurosurg* 7:289–293, 1950.
187. Urist MR. The first three decades of bone morphogenetic protein research. *Osteologie* 4:207–223, 1995.
188. Verbiest H. A radicular syndrome from developmental narrowing of the lumbar vertebral canal. *J Bone Joint Surg Br* 36:230–237, 1954.
189. Verbiest H. *Neurogenic Intermittent Claudication.* Amsterdam: North Holland, 1976.
190. Wannamaker GT. Spinal cord injuries: A review of the early treatment in 300 consecutive cases during the Korean Conflict. *J Neurosurg* 11:517–524, 1954.
191. Weiss S, Dunne C, Hewson J, et al. Multipotent CNS stem cells are present in the adult mammalian spinal cord and ventricular neuroaxis. *J Neurosci* 16:7599–7609, 1996.
192. Welch WC, Subach BR, Pollack IF, et al. Frameless stereotactic guidance for surgery of the upper cervical spine. *Neurosurgery* 40:958–964, 1997.
193. Werlinich M. Anterior interbody fusion and stabilization with metal fixation. *Int Surg* 59:269–273, 1974.
194. Williams RW. Microlumbar discectomy: A conservative surgical approach to the virgin herniated lumbar disc. *Spine* 3:175–182, 1978.
195. Woolsey RD. The mechanism of neurological symptoms and signs in spondylolisthesis at the fifth lumbar, first sacral level. *J Neurosurg* 11:67–76, 1954.
196. Xu XM, Zhang SX, Li H, et al. Regrowth of axons into the distal spinal cord through a Schwann-cell-seeded mini-channel implanted into hemisected adult rat spinal cord. *Eur J Neurosci* 11:1723–1240, 1999.
197. Yasargil MG. Microsurgical operation of herniated lumbar disc. *Adv Neurosurg* 4:81,1977.
198. Young B, Moore WS, Robertson JT, et al. An analysis of perioperative surgical mortality and morbidity in the asymptomatic carotid atherosclerosis study. ACAS Investigators. Asymptomatic Carotid Artheriosclerosis Study. *Stroke* 27:2216–2224, 1996.
199. Young W, Flamm ES, Demopoulos HB, et al. Effect of naloxone on posttraumatic ischemia in experimental spinal contusion. *J Neurosurg* 55:209–219, 1981.
200. Zdeblick TA. Laparoscopic spinal fusion. *Orthop Clin North Am* 29:635–645, 1998.

14

Fifty Years of Stereotactic and Functional Neurosurgery

Philip L. Gildenberg, MD, PhD

INTRODUCTION

Human stereotactic surgery was born 53 years ago. Since then, it has developed from a unique clinical experiment to a science that permeates every aspect of neurosurgery (Table 14.1). The rapid and exciting growth of this field has taken advantage of scientific advances in several disciplines and has incorporated them into useful and practical techniques.

THE WAY IT WAS

Although the object of this book is to give a history of human stereotactic surgery of the past 50 years, I have taken the liberty of beginning the story in 1947, for that is when this field began. In order to set the stage, it is necessary to review functional neurosurgery at that time, which is defined as that aspect of neurosurgery intended to change the function (usually abnormal) of the nervous system.

In 1947, the primary indication for functional neurosurgery was pain control. At that time, little distinction was given between cancer pain and chronic pain of noncancer origin. The rather naive consideration was that interruption of the spinothalamic tract (the primary pain pathway) anywhere along its course would control pain.

The most common procedure for pain was a laminectomy, with anterolateral cordotomy at either the cervical or thoracic level. Interruption of the spinothalamic tract in the brain for head or facial pain required a craniotomy, with estimation of the position of the spinothalamic tract just below the surface in the peduncle (212) or in the medulla (187).

The second most common functional neurosurgical procedure, after cordotomy, was prefrontal lobotomy. In the days before ataractics or tranquilizers, prefrontal lobotomy was performed for a variety of indications, most commonly for violent or agitated schizophrenics, since physical restraint and/or incarceration were the only other options. Patients with damaging obsessive-compulsive disorder also were treated with prefrontal lobotomy, with profoundly depressed patients less so since they were less visible. "Violent behavior" was con-

TABLE 14.1. *Stereotactic and functional neurosurgery time line*

Date	Technology	Movement disorders	Pain	Psychosurgery	Image guided surgery	Radiosurgery
1950	First stereotactic frames, Pneumoencephalography	Pallidotomy, Parkinson's disease	Cordotomy, mesencephalotomy, lemniscal lesions	Prefrontal lobotomy, Dorsomedial thalamotomy		Leksell's orthovoltage apparatus
1955	Radiofrequency lesions	Thalamotomy				Charged particle radiation
1960	Positive contrast ventriculography, Cryoprobe	Widespread use of thalamotomy	Extralemniscal mesencephalotomy and thalamotomy	Cingulotomy		
1965	Microelectrodes	L-dopa introduced				First Gamma Knife
1970		Little stereotactic activity	Spinal cord stimulation	Campaign against psychosurgery		
1975		L-dopa plus surgery	Deep brain stimulation		CT/MRI-stereotaxis began	Second Gamma Knife
1980	Computer analysis of physiologic data		Implantable spinal pumps	Little psychosurgery activity	N-shape fiducial system, Biopsy	Early linac system development
1985	Long-term epilepsy monitoring	Adrenal transplantation	Multidisciplinary pain programs		Volumetric target	Commercial Gamma Knife
1990		Fetal tissue transplantation, Rebirth of pallidotomy			Frameless articulated arm	Gamma Knife proliferation
1995		Brain stimulators for movement disorders			Frameless-armless systems, Intraoperative MR	Linac system proliferation, Fractionated stereotactic radiotherapy

sidered an appropriate indication for this procedure. These prefrontal lobotomies were often done by long blades (''ice picks'') inserted through the thin roof of the orbit and moved from side to side, sometimes on many patients lined up on a single day (66). Needless to say, the operation was often followed by severe intellectual deficit, even in those patients who otherwise might have had a reasonable psychiatric clinical result.

Prefrontal lobotomy appalled Spiegel. It was the desire to refine psychosurgery by making a minimally invasive lesion in the dorsomedial nucleus of the thalamus to interrupt the thalamofrontal projection without destroying the function of the frontal lobes that was the motivation for developing human stereotactic surgery (194). Even so, the first patients treated with stereotactic surgery primarily had movement disorders; stereotactic psychosurgery came later.

In 1886, a young Victor Horsley performed the first epilepsy surgery with extirpation of injured brain tissue (60). Electroencephalography, which became widely used only in the 1940s, often made it possible to determine the region of the epileptogenic focus. In 1928, this led to the introduction of temporal lobectomy by Penfield (59). The electroencephalographic recording, and intraoperative stimulation techniques developed for temporal lobectomy awaited application in stereotactic surgery.

Surgery for movement disorders developed slowly and carried a great risk. Following the influenza epidemic of 1918–1920, large numbers of patients survived encephalitis only to develop Parkinson's disease two decades later. Medications were primarily anticholinergic and not very effective, especially in the later stages, since the concept of basal ganglion dopamine depletion-causing parkinsonism had not been developed.

Movement disorder surgery initially concerned ablation of the sensorimotor cortex, as demonstrated first by Horsley as early as 1909 (106). Patients might experience great reduction in tremor with only moderate impairment of voluntary function. Bucy (34) reintroduced that operation in 1939 (and ever after, when extrapyramidal surgery had been proven, insisted that it was necessary to include the corticospinal pathways in any lesion used to treat Parkinson's disease).

By the 1920s, the concept of the role of the extrapyramidal system in regulating movement was developed (218). However, many physicians were reluctant to attempt interruption of those pathways for movement disorders. Even an icon such as Dandy (50) stated that interruption of basal ganglion pathways would be fatal. It took an adventurous soul, Russell Meyers (157,159), to prove Dandy wrong in 1939 by successfully treating movement disorders by basal ganglia surgery. In 1942, he developed operations to extirpate the head of the caudate nucleus, interrupt the extrapyramidal bundles in the peduncle, or interrupt the ansa lenticularis as it emerged from the globus pallidus by an interhemispheric approach (159). He reported a mortality rate of 15.7%, and even he advocated abandoning such surgery (159). Ansotomy was later refined by Fenelon (61), who introduced an electrode into the area of the ansa lenticularis through a less adventurous subfrontal route.

In 1947, Walker (213) refined his pedunculotomy for pain to interrupt the extrapyramidal fibers for hemiballismus and later for other movement disorders (214). His procedure was used even after the introduction of stereotactic surgery (which impacts on a later development in functional neurosurgery). The corticospinal projection passes through the middle third of the mesencephalic peduncle as it descends through the brain stem. At that point, it lies just below the surface and is vulnerable to surgical attack.

It was in 1948 that Browder (30) resected part of the head of the caudate nucleus and divided the anterior limb of the internal capsule to treat Parkinson's disease. Although it had a beneficial effect on tremor, persistent paresis or apraxia often resulted.

Technology

Certain technological advances converged in 1947 to make stereotactic surgery feasible. One of the most valuable instruments used in the neurophysiology laboratory was the Horsley-Clarke stereotaxic apparatus, which was invented in 1906 (107). It was based on a Cartesian coordinate system, that is, the definition of a point in space by noting its relationship to three planes mutually at right angles intersecting at a single point. In other words, a point in space could be defined by three numbers—an anterior-posterior (AP), lateral, and vertical coordinate. The Horsley-Clarke apparatus secured the head of an experimental animal to the frame by earplugs and tabs that rested on the inferior orbital rims. The AP coordinate lay a measured distance in front of or behind the plane of the ear plugs, the vertical coordinate above or below the plane defined by the earplugs and the orbital tabs, and the lateral measurement from the midline, which defined the three stereotactic coordinates. An electrode holder could be adjusted so that the electrode could be advanced accurately by a microdrive to the target point. An atlas of the animal's brain that consisted of sections taken in reference to these three planes allowed the investigator to define the coordinates that lay within the target structure.

Neurophysiology had progressed to offer a number of potential targets for clinical use, and much of that information had been obtained using animal stereotaxic[1] techniques. The primary and immediate extralemniscal pain pathways were well demonstrated, including the periaqueductal and periventricular gray and intralaminar thalamus; however, the endorphin transmitters had not been isolated. The extrapyramidal feedback loops had been defined anatomically, but animal models of most extrapyramidal motor dysfunctions were still unknown. Papez' circuit expressed emotional characteristics, along with the reverberating circuits between the medial thalamus and the frontal lobes.

Neurophysiologic techniques at that time included stimulation with recording of evoked potentials, so hardware for both intraoperative stimulation and recording was well developed. Wiring in buildings was not yet generally insulated or shielded, so it was necessary to record

from within a grounded cage. Lesions were made for neurophysiologic investigations by injecting alcohol or similar substances or by application of direct current to produce electrolytic lesions, a technique described 40 years before (107).

Chief among the technological advances converging at this time was the possibility of intraoperative x-ray. Film processing had become more rapid, and most operating rooms were equipped with portable x-ray machines. In order to use internal cerebral landmarks for targeting, it was necessary to visualize them roentgenographically. Pneumoencephalography had been introduced by Dandy in 1918 (49), and by the 1940s, it was commonly used to visualize the anatomy of the foramen of Monro as it entered the third ventricle, as well as the pineal gland (the landmarks originally used for stereotactic localization), along with fiducials on the stereotactic frame that permitted accurate orthogonal alignment.

Computers were in their infancy and would not impact on stereotactic surgery for another two decades. The most advanced computer of the day was the Eniac, a top-secret military project that took up an entire floor of College Hall at the University of Pennsylvania. It was not until the later development of the transistor that computers could be brought into the laboratory and eventually into the operating room.

THE BIRTH OF HUMAN STEREOTACTIC SURGERY

The two major players in the development of human stereotactic surgery were Spiegel and Wycis. Dr. Ernst Spiegel was a neurologist who had fled Vienna when the Nazis took over. Even though he had been the youngest docent, a stellar investigator, and an outstanding faculty member of the University of Vienna, he lost his laboratory and was at risk of losing his students in 1936. Dr. William Parkinson, then the Dean of Temple Medical School in Philadelphia, learned of his plight, and invited Dr. Spiegel to develop a Laboratory of Experimental Neurology. His wife, Dr. Mona Spiegel-Adolph received a position in the adjacent Laboratory of Colloid Chemistry. In Philadelphia, Dr. Spiegel's physiologic

---

[1]Horsley and Clarke used the spelling "stereotaxic," which is still used in the experimental laboratory. Spiegel and Wycis originally used the term "stereoencephalotomy," which was changed to "stereotactic" when the American and World Societies for Stereotactic and Functional Neurosurgery were founded in 1973. It was felt that "tactus," from the Latin to touch, was a more accurate description of the science than the Greek "taxic," meaning an arrangement (78).

studies mainly involved the extrapyramidal system, and he had a limited clinical practice. In 1938, he was invited by a friend and a fellow Jewish refugee in Switzerland, publisher Samuel Karger, to edit a journal devoted to information that linked neurology to other related experimental and clinical fields. The journal was called **Confinia neurologica,** or borderlands of neurology (which was later changed to **Applied Neurophysiology** when I became Editor in 1975 and **Stereotactic and Functional Neurosurgery** in 1988). The journal was a major implement to disseminate information about stereotactic surgery to a cadre of interested neurosurgeons.

Dr. Henry Wycis grew up in a small town in Pennsylvania. He worked his way through college as a semi-professional baseball player and, some say, a poker player. While a student at Temple Medical School, from which he graduated with two records (the most classes missed and the highest graduating average), he began to work in Spiegel's laboratory (hence the missed classes). He continued that collaboration during his neurosurgical residency, as a faculty member at the same institution, and throughout his life.

The first human stereotactic apparatus designed by Spiegel and Wycis was essentially a Horsley-Clarke apparatus suspended from a plaster cap, which held a ring about the patient's head. The original Model I Spiegel-Wycis stereoencephalatome is presently housed at the Smithsonian Institute. It included fiducial marks that could be superimposed on AP and lateral x-rays to assure an orthogonal arrangement and to provide reference lines from which the location of visualized and calculated structures could be measured. The position of the electrode could be adjusted by sliding the electrode holder along AP or lateral bars. The electrode holder allowed only a vertical insertion of the electrode, and a microdrive was used to advance an electrode to the desired vertical coordinate.

Spiegel and Wycis simultaneously developed the first human stereotactic atlas, which was later published in 1952 (195). It allowed an estimation of the target point. Variability among individual brains could be estimated from variability tables published in the atlas' appendix as well as in a series of published articles.

Although the motivation for the development of human stereotactic surgery was to improve psychosurgery, the initial patients were treated for movement disorders. The first patient had severe chorea as part of Huntington's disease. Lesions were made by injection of alcohol in hopes of sparing *fibres de passage.* Two targets were selected. An injection was made into the globus pallidus in order to interrupt the extrapyramidal pathway. A second injection was made into the dorsomedian nucleus of the thalamus, since it had been recognized that the involuntary movement increased when the patient became upset and eased when he was more tranquil. The patient had good but only temporary improvement as the disease progressed. Nevertheless, it was demonstrated that it was possible to interrupt the extrapyramidal pathway with improvement in motor function, rather than deterioration of control as had been feared, with the same minimally invasive techniques that had been successful in the laboratory.

THE FIRST "DECADE," 1947–1959

As our story begins, stereotactic surgery had just been introduced at a single institution. By the end of the first decade, it was practiced at perhaps 40 institutions throughout the world. Most of the indications for stereotactic surgery (and several for image-guided surgery) had been sampled, international communication had been established among practitioners of this infant field, and a journal had become established as the repository of information in the field. Yet, stereotactic surgery was almost completely ignored by the neurosurgical community as a whole.

From the beginning, the philosophy was to use every insertion of an electrode into a human brain as an opportunity to study human neurophysiology. Many observations made in the laboratory were documented in humans. The pathophysiology of every disease under treatment was studied, as well. The information obtained in the operating room was valuable to help localize the electrode position, and the information obtained about the pathophysiology was used to develop new indications and targets for stereotactic surgery. Thus, many of the neurologists and neurosurgeons involved in stereotactic surgery were also involved in basic and clinical research.

In 1948, the year after Spiegel and Wycis introduced stereotactic surgery, they were visited by Lars Leksell (144). He designed the first arc quadrant stereotactic apparatus after returning to Sweden. The following year, Talairach (102) in Paris developed a stereotactic apparatus with a fixed grid system. In 1951, Riechert and Wolff (179) in Germany described an apparatus with a phantom base to determine the settings mechanically. That same year, Bailey and Stein (10) demonstrated their burr hole mounted system at a meeting in the United States. At the same time, a remarkable story was developing in Japan. Narabayashi, who was isolated from the Western medical literature after the Second World War, independently developed a human stereotactic apparatus in 1951 (167,211). During the 1950s, there were at least 40 different stereotactic apparatuses designed in various centers throughout the world. There were no commercial systems available, and each neurosurgeon had to have a custom apparatus built.

In 1956, I was a freshman student at Temple Medical School looking for a summer research project. There was no neurophysiologist in residence, so the head of the Department of Physiology directed me to the laboratory of his old teacher, Ernst Spiegel. I spent 13 of the next 16 years with Dr. Spiegel and Dr. Wycis, which was an amazingly exciting period in the development of stereotactic surgery (84).

Technology

The Spiegel-Wycis apparatus was redesigned several times during the first few years, until their Model V, which was used until they retired, allowed accurate reapplication. It was secured to four screwed-in posts that projected through the scalp, and could be adjusted by altering the length of the legs and diagonal brackets. The reapplicability was important, since during the first decade it was necessary to visualize internal landmarks by pneumoencephalography. Their program called for a pneumoencephalogram on Tuesday, and then allowed the patient to recover until the surgery itself was done on Thursday. During the latter part of the 1950s, positive contrast ventriculography was introduced, which made it possible to perform the operation in a single day. Polaroid x-ray film was developed, so rapid processing could be done in the operating room.

A major concern during the first stereotactic decade was how to make a lesion in the brain. Although the first procedures involved the injection of alcohol (202) or other substances, such as procaine-oil or wax (41,168), these agents diffused along pathways in unpredictable patterns (73). Some authors (195) continued to use direct current electrolytic lesions, as reported 50 years earlier by Horsley and Clarke (107).

Hassler and Riechert (95) used ideas from a device reported by a colleague in 1945 (221) and used a high frequency current to heat the tissue around the tip of the electrode. Although early electrodes had the risk of lesions along the shaft from current leakage (74), such technical problems were being solved and radiofrequency generators were available by the end of the decade (47). In 1958, an elaborate system of making lesions with focused ultrasound was reported by Meyers (160), who was a pioneer in extrapyramidal surgery prior to the introduction of stereotaxis.

The original Spiegel-Wycis atlas was published in 1952 as *Stereoencephalotomy, Volume I* (195).

Stereotactic Radiosurgery

As early as 1951, Leksell described and invented stereotactic radiosurgery (145). He attached an orthovoltage x-ray device to an enlarged version of his arc quadrant apparatus to bombard the target from many angles, thereby minimizing radiation to surrounding areas. Although the original intention was to produce lesions for functional neurosurgery, the device was probably not accurate enough; therefore, the first use was to treat a craniopharyngioma (7). Soon after, he treated trigeminal neuralgia by irradiating the gasserian ganglion (150).

In 1954, Lawrence, at Berkeley, used focused charged particle irradiation for pituitary suppression, (150) and in 1958, Leksell's collaborator, Larsson in Sweden together with Leksell, used a proton beam as a stereotactic radiosurgical tool (141). Both used stereotactic techniques to localize the beam of ionizing radiation.

Clinical Progress

Most of the diseases that responded to stereotactic intervention were sampled during the 1950s. During a period of unrivaled empirical human experimentation, stereotactic surgery was used for movement disorders, pain, psychiatric problems, and even for tumors.

Movement Disorders

Although the first movement disorder treated was Huntington's chorea, Parkinson's disease rapidly became the primary indication for functional stereotactic surgery, and remains so today. Spiegel and Wycis initially were reluctant to make a lesion in the globus pallidus for Parkinson's disease for fear of increasing the bradykinesia or akinesia that accompanies that disease. However, in 1951, Hassler and Riechert (95) successfully treated Parkinson's disease with lesions in the ventrolateral thalamus. With the safety of extrapyramidal lesions being established in parkinsonism, Spiegel and Wycis (198) treated that disease the following year by lesioning the ansa lenticularis fibers as they emerged from the globus pallidus, a procedure they called pallidoansotomy. That same year, Narabayashi and Okuma (168) reported the use of pallidotomy in Parkinson's disease. In fact, as early as 1952 Spiegel and Wycis (196) wrote a paper that compared mesencephalotomy, thalamotomy, and ansotomy for Parkinson's disease.

In 1952, Irving Cooper experienced a "surgical accident" (39). He was performing a nonstereotactic mesencephalic pedunculotomy, as had been described as a treatment for Parkinson's disease in 1949 by Walker (213), when he accidentally disrupted the anterior choroidal artery. He stopped the procedure without making the intended incision in the peduncle. The patient awoke from anesthesia much improved without neurological deficit. This chance observation led Cooper (40) to advocate ligation of the anterior choroidal artery for treatment of Parkinson's disease. Despite initial optimistic reports, the operation proved to be unreliable, with a significant risk of hemiplegia. Cooper considered what structures had been infarcted on ligation of that

vessel to provide clinical improvement, and theorized that the globus pallidus was the most likely target, especially since other reports of pallidotomy were just appearing. In 1955, he advocated the injection of alcohol into the globus pallidus, a procedure he called chemopallidectomy (41). He did not use stereotactic techniques, however, and his approach to the pallidum to insert a needle or balloon cannula (42) upward through the temporal lobe, a trajectory that coincidentally pointed also to the ventrolateral thalamus. Another surgical accident occurred around this time. It is not certain whether the misplacement of the injection was discovered on checking the calculations of an assistant (119) or on examining a patient's brain at autopsy after an unrelated death (83), but Cooper discovered that one of his best results occurred after a lesion that was intended for the pallidum ended up in the thalamus. In 1958, he moved his intended target to the ventrolateral thalamus (46), essentially the same target advocated by Hassler and Riechert (95) in 1954. Cooper's major contribution was his vast experience (1000 cases by 1960) (44) and the dissemination of information to the public about functional neurosurgery (51).

By 1954, Hassler and Riechert (95) had defined their thalamic target more precisely, with the ventralis oralis posterior (Vop) recommended for tremor and the ventralis oralis anterior (Voa) for spasticity. Studies on brains of patients who had undergone stereotactic surgery (96) contributed significantly to Hassler's redefining the subnuclei of the thalamus. By the end of the 1950s, most neurosurgeons had followed Hassler and Riechert's lead, and the thalamus became the target of choice for Parkinson's disease. For bradykinesia and ataxia, however, Leksell advocated lesions in the pallidum somewhat more posterior and ventral than other neurosurgeons, as reported later by Svennilson et al. (209) in 1960.

During the first decade of stereotactic surgery, other movement disorders were also treated with stereotactic techniques. Intention tremor was treated with lesions in the ventrolateral thalamus, essentially the same target as for Parkinson tremor (43). Choreoathetosis was treated with lesions in the pallidum (200).

Pain

One of the earliest indications for stereotactic surgery was the treatment of intractable pain. Interruption of the lemniscal pain pathway in the mesencephalon was a logical choice, since the tract was comprised of a tight bundle of fibers at that point and the location of the pathway could be measured. Lemniscal mesencephalotomy was described as early as 1953 (197), although the original procedure was modified by subsequent observations in the following decade.

It was during the 1950s that it became apparent that the extralemniscal pathways play a role in perception of pain (82). In 1949, Hécaen et al. (102) suggested that a thalamotomy lesion for treatment of pain might be more effective if it included the centrum medianum in addition to the ventrobasal complex.

Psychosurgery

Dorsomedian thalamotomy was already used for psychosurgery at the beginning of the 1950s, as well as hypothalamotomy for agitated behavior and psychosis (203).

Epilepsy

For the purposes of this review, only those procedures used in the management of epilepsy that involved stereotactic techniques will be considered. During the period before and during the 1950s, epilepsy surgery was born and developed significantly along scientific principles. Many of the techniques used in epilepsy surgery were adopted into stereotaxis, much of the scientific apparatus was the same, and many of the same surgeons were involved.

Brain Tumors

A prescient report in 1956 concerned stereotactic insertion of a needle to aspirate a craniopharyngioma cyst (165). Since that partially calcified tumor could be visualized directly and outlined by air on x-ray, it was possible to calculate the stereotactic coordinates. It was not until the advent of computed tomographic (CT) imaging that such procedures became widespread.

THE DECADE 1960–1969

Stereotactic surgery in the 1960s began on an upswing. Surgery for Parkinson's disease was becoming increasingly popular and well-known to the general public. Technology was progressing rapidly, which allowed stereotactic procedures to become routine. By the end of the decade, however, the field almost died with the introduction of l-dopa in 1968.

The 1960s began with the first international symposium of stereotactic surgery in Philadelphia in 1961 (199). Surgeons were invited to bring their stereotactic apparatuses, many of which were lined up on the benches in the chemistry laboratory of Temple Medical School as the scientific exhibit. There was a feeling of comradeship and openness. Most of the neurosurgeons performing stereotactic surgery throughout the world were present in one room. On the first day of the symposium, Cooper introduced a patient who demonstrated how well he could write after surgery. The following morning, Wycis, not to be outdone, introduced his patient who played the piano. Most of the papers presented were in English, but those that were not were translated line-for-line by Spiegel (who also spoke German, French, Spanish, Italian, Latin, and Greek).

Technology

By the beginning of the 1960s, radiofrequency had become the standard means of lesion production. However, in 1961, a new technique brought together two stereotactic personalities. Cooper wanted to develop a means of freezing tissue at the end of a probe, with the idea that a reversible test lesion could first be made by moderate cooling. He recruited Arnold St. J. Lee as a consulting engineer to design the cryoprobe (45). Lee had been Spiegel's laboratory assistant in 1947, and was the fourth author of the original paper on the introduction of human stereotactic surgery (202).

During this decade stereotactic devices became generally available. In the United States, the Todd-Wells apparatus was the most popular, and in Europe, the Leksell and the Riechert-Mundinger systems were used.

Perhaps the greatest technologic feat of the decade was the introduction of microelectrode recording into the operating room by Abel-Fessard et al. (1) in 1961. At first, this permitted mapping of field potentials and then, mapping of single units to determine the boundaries of the anatomical structures and to identify the location of those cells firing synchronously with tremor. Recording technology was so difficult to use, however, that microelectrode recordings were performed in very few medical centers throughout the 1960s, mainly as a research tool, and were not generally used.

Stereotactic Radiosurgery

The Gamma Knife was developed in 1967 (146). Leksell's experiments with an orthovoltage radiotherapy device did not result in a technique that was accurate enough to be adopted for general clinical use. He needed a system that was mechanically stable. Consequently, he arranged cobalt sources around a portion of a large steel hemisphere, each collimated to focus the energy at a single point, with a stereotactic head holder that could be adjusted to bring the target within the brain coincident with that point. Although the original intention was to produce lesions for functional neurosurgery, it was used little for that purpose; however, many other indications gradually appeared.

Clinical Progress

Movement Disorders

Although Parkinson's disease remained the primary indication for stereotactic surgery, other movement disorders were treated during the 1960s. For instance, myoclonia was treated by making a lesion in Forel's field (220). Hyperkinesia and hemiballismus were treated with lesions in the thalamus and/or globus pallidus (5,164), although hemiballismus was also reported as a complication of thalamotomy (28). The internal capsule was used as a target for dystonia and athetosis of cerebral palsy (56), as was the dentate nucleus (101).

The major emphasis of stereotactic surgery was Parkinson's disease. No effective medications to treat the disease were available and the postencephalitic parkinsonian patients were still of surgical age. More and more neurosurgeons were deciding to perform a basic thalamotomy, although sometimes with questionable control or experience. It was estimated that more than 25,000 procedures had been performed and the numbers were increasing rapidly. The mortality rate had dropped from the prestereotactic level of more than 15% (158), to 2% in 1958 (201), and less than 1% in 1960 (178), where it remains today.

At the academic centers, the search for the best target continued. Most neurosurgeons by that time had followed Hassler and Riechert to the thalamus, with pallidotomy being performed in a few places (138,209). Spiegel and Wycis, not satisfied that the most optimal results were being obtained (and not wishing to follow others), examined the effect of lesions in the head of the caudate nucleus (206) (the target of tissue transplantation many years later). They finally settled, however, or Forel's field, where the axons emerging from the globus pallidus in the ansa lenticularis and the lenticular fasciculus come together into a compact bundle, so that the smallest lesion would interrupt the most pallidofugal fibers (204).

Those neurosurgeons concentrating on the thalamus sought a more critically defined target, based on microelectrode recording. In 1966, Bertrand and Jasper suggested the ventralis intermedialis nucleus (Vim) for both Parkinson's disease (20) (which still remains the optimal target for tremor) and dyskinesia (114).

The ax fell in 1968, when L-dopa became generally available to treat Parkinson's disease (48). Neurologists originally thought that this medication and its later refinements would indefinitely control parkinsonian symptoms with minimal side effects. They were so reluctant to consider otherwise that it was almost a decade before patients were again referred for neurosurgical management. By then, a combination of medication and surgery was thought to be optimal (120). By the end of the 1960s, almost no surgery was being performed for Parkinson's disease, with the result that stereotactic surgery died at all but a few medical centers.

Pain

The concept of pain perception changed significantly during the 1960s (82). In 1965, Melzack and Wall (156) presented their gate theory of pain perception. This theory postulated that there were more influences than the primary pain pathway in the spinothalamic tract, and emphasized both the importance of the extralemniscal system and the ability to modify pain perception by increasing nonpainful input, as well as providing a physiological basis for psychological influences in pain management.

The theory prompted several important modifications of stereotactic pain surgery. Nashold studied the pathways in patients undergoing mesencephalotomy (169) and advocated moving the lesion more medially so it would encroach significantly on the multisynaptic pathway in the central gray. The same target was advocated for pain of the thalamic syndrome (166). The interruption of extralemniscal pathways in (186) or at the base of the thalamus (205) often provided good pain relief, even if the primary pain pathway was not interrupted. The limbic system became a target for the treatment of pain, as Ballantine (112) observed relief of cancer pain by interruption of the cingululate gyrus, the same target he had used for psychosurgery.

The Melzack-Wall concept that a nonpainful stimulation might inhibit pain perception (if you rub it, it feels better) led to the use of implanted stimulators for pain management. In 1967, Wall and Sweet (215) observed that electrical stimulation of their own infraorbital nerves provided local analgesia. The following year, Sweet and Wepsic (210) described alleviation of pain in the distribution of a peripheral nerve by chronic stimulation of that nerve. About that same time, Shealy et al. (188) reported that stimulation of the tactile and proprioceptive nerves in the dorsal columns of the spinal cord provided relief of pain, and introduced spinal cord stimulation as a treatment for pain. Although these procedures are not stereotactic per se, they led to the commercial development of implantable neural stimulators. Also, in 1960, Heath and Mickle (98) and Gol (93) in 1967 reported that patients might obtain relief of pain by chronic stimulation in the septal area, the same area where experimental animals would seek stimulation, as reported by

Olds and Milner (173) in 1954. The stage was set for the introduction of deep brain stimulation for pain management in the 1970s.

Psychosurgery

The 1960s was the last decade in which psychosurgery was used freely. Psychotropic drugs were just beginning to appear. The belief that surgery was needed where drugs failed encouraged clinical trials, especially in aggressive patients where the only other options might be incarceration or restraints. Medial thalamotomy was used for hyperactive and aggressive behavior by Andy (6) and other surgeons (13). Both thalamotomy and hypothalamotomy were used for frank psychosis (54,203). Even anorexia nervosa was sometimes treated successfully with hypothalamotomy (53).

Epilepsy

Stereotactic lesions were used for treatment of various convulsive disorders. Some success was reported with lesions in Forel's field (115) or other parts of the basal ganglia (11). Thalamotomy was used for myoclonic epilepsy (135). In addition, stereotactic techniques were introduced to insert electrodes for evaluation of epileptic foci (163), which remains one of the major uses of stereotactic surgery in epilepsy management.

THE DECADE 1970–1979

At the beginning of the 1970s, stereotactic surgery was in an almost dormant state. The few remaining cases were concentrated in several academic centers. Both the general neurosurgical and neurological communities had lost interest in this procedure. A further blow was to be given to psychosurgery.

By the end of the decade, a series of developments led to the rebirth of stereotaxis, with its potential to be even greater. Progress in computer science made CT and magnetic resonance imaging (MRI) scanning available, and both were rapidly incorporated into stereotactic technology. As a result, the field of stereotactic surgery expanded into every corner of the realm of neurosurgery. Toward the end of this decade, it became increasingly apparent that L-dopa was not the panacea for Parkinson's disease as had been thought, and attention began to return to surgical management.

Technology

Image Guided Surgery

The scientific advance that initiated the rebirth of stereotactic surgery was the development of small, relatively inexpensive computers that could be used practically and economically in medicine. In the late 1970s this led to the introduction of computerized scanning, which became generally available in the early 1980s. The marriage between CT scanning and stereotactic surgery was only natural (76). Both depended on spatial identification of structures within the brain. The structures that were used as stereotactic landmarks were visualized on CT scans. The data for both were organized in a Cartesian orientation. The structures within the head did not move significantly between the time of scanning and surgery. It was possible to attach the stereotactic frame securely to the skull so the orientation between the stereotactic coordinates and the anatomy visualized on the scan could be maintained throughout the procedure. In addition, for the first time it was possible to visualize the pathology directly, especially masses or tumors, which opened a host of new indications for stereotactic techniques. When MRI was introduced in the middle of the 1980s, stereotactic surgery adapted to it as soon as it became assured that the MR images were not too distorted, so that targeting might be accurate.

The first attempts during the 1970s to orient the stereotactic frame with a CT scan involved attaching the frame to the scanner, using a variety of variable length fiducial rods, or orienting the vertical coordinate to the individual slice of a brain CT scan (88). The way was prepared to open the next decade with techniques that would provide stereotactic localization directly from the CT scan. As a result, a new field was born—image-guided neurosurgery.

Microelectrode Recording

As recording technology improved, microelectrode recording became more practical for clinical use (70). Although it was possible to delineate such targets as Vim with more confidence, the level of activity in surgery for movement disorders began to increase only toward the end of the 1970s.

Stereotactic Radiosurgery

Although little progress in functional stereotactic surgery was made during this decade, significant advances were made in stereotactic radiosurgery. The technology of the Leksell Gamma Knife had been developed, but indications for its use were lacking. In 1970, Steiner began to use this device for treatment of cerebral arteriovenous malformations (207). A second generation Gamma Knife was developed (150), which produced a more spherical field that was used to treat various mass lesions, such as tumors; however, these were the only two in operation.

Clinical Progress

Despite technological advances during the 1970s, clinical progress in the management of movement disorders was minimal. Somewhat more progress was made in pain management and the gradual development of new techniques in epilepsy surgery, while a disastrous political upheaval that damaged psychosurgery occurred.

Movement Disorders

Major interest in movement disorders concerned the investigation of the underlying mechanisms of Parkinson's disease, using techniques developed in the laboratory to study dopamine pharmacology (172,180). Throughout the early 1970s, few surgeries were performed for parkinsonism, but by the end of the decade, a combination of medical and surgical management was deemed best for many patients (120,189).

Pain

Several important concepts in pain management emerged during the 1970s. The concept of the difference between chronic pain of nonmalignant origin and persistent pain of cancer was formulated, and was used by Bonica and Fordyce (63) in their multidisciplinary program for management of chronic pain. Less emphasis was placed on interruption of the primary pain pathway (82). It was believed that stimulation of pain suppression areas might be more advantageous than interruption of neurons for management of chronic pain.

In the early 1970s, implantable spinal cord stimulators became available. Electrodes that required laminectomy for insertion were for the most part supplanted by electrodes that could be inserted percutaneously (110), and the use of spinal cord stimulators became more common.

Chronic stimulation of the somatosensory thalamus for management of denervation pain was introduced by Hosobuchi and Adams (109) in 1973. Soon thereafter, stimulation of the periventricular or periaqueductal area for treatment of other types of persistent pain was applied by implanted deep brain stimulators (108). The series reported in 1977 by Richardson and Akil (177) indicated a 70% success rate.

Management of cancer pain was advanced by introduction of implantable pumps that could deliver a low dose of narcotic to the spinal cord (216).

Psychosurgery

The beginning of the 1970s saw considerable activity in the area of psychosurgery. Indications by this time were primarily for depression and obsessive-compulsive disorder, since sedative ataractic medication had meanwhile been developed to help in the management of the most aggressive or schizophrenic patients (103). Various targets were advocated (111), such as the genu of the corpus callosum (136), the cingulate gyrus (112), and the hypothalamus (22). The use of psychosurgery for drug addiction (14), for patients with aggressive or violent behavior (154,185), and for those with sexual dysfunction was advocated by some (55,182).

In 1972, a campaign against psychosurgery was begun (27). It equated psychosurgery to the type of lobotomy that had essentially been discontinued over a decade before. It also alleged that psychosurgery was being used primarily to subdue aggressive persons, especial minorities, always resulted in severe mental incapacity, and was of no psychological benefit. A commission was established to study these allegations by retrospectively interviewing a number of patients who had undergone cingulotomy. They found that the procedure was generally of great benefit and that patients functioned much better after surgery than they had before (170). Although the commission recommended that psychosurgery warranted increased research funding since it held much promise, the political upheaval that had been generated caused most neurosurgeons throughout the world to abandon the field. As a result, psychosurgery never fully recovered or gained back its popularity.

THE DECADE 1980–1989

The 1980s saw the solidification of stereotactic and functional neurosurgery as a vital and growing field. In an editorial published in 1987 in Neurosurgery, I asked, "Whatever happened to stereotactic surgery"? (77) The answer was, "It is coming back and will be larger than ever!"

Technology

Image Guided Surgery

The breakthrough in orienting the stereotactic frame to a CT image came in 1980. A medical student at the University of Utah Medical School designed a fiducial system that contained nine rods in three sets of three, each set oriented like the letter "N," so that all the information for three-dimensional targeting was contained on an individual two-dimensional image (31). This system was subsequently adapted to most other stereotactic apparatus. By the end of the decade, similar systems were used for localization in almost all the major stereotactic frames. The system was soon adapted to MRI, which showed exquisite detail of both normal and pathological anatomy. The age of image guided stereotactic surgery was off to a vigorous start.

Imaging systems became more elaborate, with CT scanners being installed in the operating rooms of some busy services (149), or being designed around stereotactic applications (133).

As technology became available to target any point that could be identified on a CT or MR scan, computers became more accessible for surgical planning. The use of volume-in-space, as opposed to point-in-space, opened new prospects in brain tumor surgery. Between 1980 and 1983, this led Kelly (121,123) to provide the most significant contribution of the 1980s, the use of an entire tumor volume in space as the stereotactic target. His technique involved the computer reconstruction of a virtual tumor volume by outlining the tumor margin on each slice, stacking the slices, and interpolating the margin to render a smooth outline. Since the scan had been taken with the stereotactic frame in place, the stereotactic localization of the tumor was known. The surgeon could be guided to the tumor, and the outline of the margin displayed through the microscope to direct the resection. Other techniques used computer workstations to facilitate tumor resection in various ways (92,224). Thus, irregular, indistinct, or deep-seated tumors could be resected with minimal damage to the surrounding brain.

Other techniques omitted the need for the stereotactic frame. In 1986, Roberts (181) used sonic triangulation to align the operating microscope to the surgical field, at which point frameless stereotactic surgery was born. Similar techniques employed the optical localization of light-emitting diodes or other fiducials secured to the patient's head, operating instruments, or microscope, which avoided some of the instability of the sonic system.

Stereotactic Radiosurgery

The 1980s witnessed a revolution in stereotactic radiosurgery. At the beginning of the decade, new techniques were developed in rapid succession. Fabrikant et al. (58) used the helium ion beam clinically, at first for vascular malformations. A second cyclotron unit opened in Boston (127). The Leksell Gamma Knife was produced commercially, and by the end of the decade, a proliferation of Gamma Knife centers were established.

The event that made stereotactic radiosurgery generally available in the 1990s occurred around 1982 in several locations, when the linear accelerator was adapted to the stereotactic frame. The

first report was that of Colombo (38) in Italy. That was followed soon after by Betti (21) in Paris and Buenos Aires, and Barcia-Solario (16) in Spain. Several years later, Winston and Lutz (219) and, by the end of the decade, Friedman and Bova (67), introduced techniques in the United States that made it possible to adapt existing linear accelerators to stereotactic frames. At the end of the decade, these linac techniques were not yet commercially available.

Clinical Progress

The 1980s saw an impressive surge in clinical activity in stereotactic surgery. The field was reborn and expanded, and surpassed even the level of activity in the mid-1960s. The indications for stereotactic techniques exceeded the functional procedures of the earlier stereotactic era and began to extend into almost all aspects of neurosurgery.

Image-Guided Neurosurgery

The initial use of image-guided stereotaxis was for biopsy (125), its most frequent indication even today. During the 1980s, stereotactic biopsy became an important procedure in the diagnosis of patients with acquired immuno-deficiency syndrome (AIDS), many of whom also had lesions or masses in the brain (87,89,147).

Stereotactic aspiration of cysts or brain abscesses has become the treatment of choice (29). Aspiration of intracerebral hematomas (4,8), sometimes followed by urokinase administration (171) provides a relatively atraumatic technique for treatment of that condition.

The use of stereotactic guidance for tumor resection has provided a significant advance. Many neurosurgeons use a conventional frame with the inserted cannula guiding them to the target tumor or for identification of the tumor boundary (94,152).

It has been long recognized that the boundary of low or middle grade gliomas is more distinct when it is defined by MRI (than can been seen by eye in the operating room). The problem has been to present this information to the surgeon in the most efficient manner possible. This border can now be incorporated into the surgeon's vision as he or she looks at the operative field, so that the resection can be guided by the greater information content presented by imaging. Kelly's use of volumetric stereotactic-guided tumor resection provided the opportunity for more complete resection with greater sparing of surrounding tissue than had previously been possible (124). It also provided the opportunity to confirm that tumor cells infiltrate beyond the apparent boundary of gliomas (52).

Movement Disorders

Surgery for movement disorders progressively increased during the 1980s, as more and more Parkinson's patients began to break through the benefit of L-dopa or succumbed to its side effects. The main procedure remained thalamotomy, although the exact target varied greatly (137).

Near the beginning of 1980, however, a different tack was taken to treat Parkinson's disease. An attempt was made to insert cells that would produce the deficient dopamine into the basal ganglia. In 1985, Backlund et al. in Sweden (9) reported two patients in whom they had transplanted adrenal medullary tissue, rich in catecholamines, into the head of the caudate nucleus. They indicated that results were encouraging, but not good enough to consider this procedure as a treatment, and advised further study. In 1987, Madrazo et al. in Mexico (153) reported more encouraging results, which prompted many similar series (3,104,175). Although there were significant complications reported with open surgery to implant the adrenal tissue (64,113), the use of stereotactic injection of adrenal tissue avoided those problems (91). Even so, the surgery to remove the adrenal gland was stressful to this fragile group of patients, and the adrenal gland was often found to be atrophic (35). Therefore, the procedure was abandoned after several years.

A more complex but seemingly more promising approach was the transplantation of fetal nigral cells to the basal ganglia in hopes they might reestablish dopaminergic connections. The concept for transplantation of fetal cells had been explored at a conference in 1984 (155), and laboratory investigations had documented its potential (12,32,65). Again, the first patients were operated in Sweden by Brundin et al. (33). Although the results were encouraging, the procedure for obtaining fetal cells and coordinating their transplantation into the caudate of a Parkinson's disease patient were daunting, so that by the end of the decade few centers engaged in this investigational treatment (37,105).

In the 1980s, the seeds were planted for a procedure that was introduced in the next decade and today shows promise of becoming the predominant stereotactic surgical management option for tremor and Parkinson's disease. In 1982, but not reported until 1987, Siegfried (190) noted that a patient with a deep brain stimulator implanted for pain management had suppression of dyskinetic movements. In 1987 as well, Benabid (19) reported a decrease in Parkinson tremor in a pain patient similarly implanted with a thalamic stimulator. It was not until the following decade that these observations took root and the use of implanted stimulators specifically for management of movement disorders began.

Pain

During the 1980s, a considerable consolidation of physiologic information about pain perception and a gradual shift of attitudes toward comprehensive multidisciplinary management occurred, much of which did not involve surgery (85). The chronic pain syndrome became identified with depression, addiction, psychological and physical regression, and intolerance to stress. The differences between acute pain, cancer pain, and chronic pain of noncancer origin became more greatly appreciated (79).

The most important development in pain management was the increased use of intrathecal narcotics for management of cancer pain, and the availability of implantable pumps to deliver intrathecal morphine in a slow, controlled fashion (176).

Several new techniques for treatment of trigeminal neuralgia emerged. Håkanson (97) introduced retrogasserian glycerol injection, which was at first thought to provide relief with no sensory loss. Mullan (162) developed a percutaneous technique to insert a compression balloon into Meckel's cave to produce hypesthesia in the trigeminal distribution.

It was during the 1980s that the use of implanted deep brain stimulators for pain management dwindled. This occurred for several reasons. As with all pain management techniques, patient selection was a problem. It was difficult to identify pain patients who might benefit due to the many physical and psychological confounding factors that were not well defined (84). Criteria for success were universally accepted. Conservative, comprehensive management of chronic pain was a time consuming and sometimes expensive endeavor, which even today is not generally appreciated by insurance payers. And, finally, at least in the United States, deep brain stimulators for pain management was disapproved by the Food and Drug Administration (FDA), since proof of efficacy was not forthcoming.

Psychosurgery

There was amazingly little activity in this field throughout the 1980s. In fact, the International Conference of Psychosurgery was not held due to the lack of new information. The political upheaval in this field that began in the United States appeared to have taken its toll in the rest of the world.

Epilepsy

The advances in technology were quickly incorporated into management of epilepsy. Long-term video/EEG monitoring with computerized data management was implemented, so that patient selection became more refined. Advances in imaging, particularly functional imaging, were introduced and studies began to assess their use in localization of seizure activity.

Stereotactic Radiosurgery

The 1980s saw the development of the technology that would make stereotactic radiosurgery generally available in the 1990s. Several new Gamma Knife centers were established throughout the world, including the first one in the United States. Lunsford (151) navigated the daunting maze of regulatory agencies and import requirements to install the first unit at the University of Pittsburgh. He established the precedent that allowed additional installations in many other centers during the following decade. As more centers meant more patients for follow-up, the indications, complications, and long-term implications rapidly expanded (208).

THE DECADE 1990–1999

The 1990s witnessed the most rapid advance in stereotactic technology and the most rapid dissemination of stereotactic techniques ever seen throughout the neurosurgical community, as well as the popularization of stereotactic radiosurgery and the rebirth of functional neurosurgery for movement disorders. At the beginning of the decade, stereotactic surgery was the realm of a relatively small group of subspecialists. By the end of the decade, more stereotactic surgery was being practiced by more neurosurgeons than ever before, and stereotactic techniques made inroads to become needed skills for every practicing neurosurgeon. At the end of the decade, the rate of progress continued to accelerate, and promised even greater gains during the next decades.

Technology

Just as technology blossomed everywhere during the 1990s, new technology was being integrated into stereotactic surgery. To be part of this revolution has been both exciting and frustrating. As new technology appears at an ever more rapid rate, changes in health care financing make it more and more difficult to bring this technology to the patient.

Although stereotactic frames are still required to access small targets or for most functional neurosurgery, the 1990s marked the transition from frame-based to frameless navigation systems for targeting during craniotomy. With that, stereotactic surgery made the transition of becoming a necessary technique for general neurosurgery. In addition, a renaissance in functional neurosurgery occurred. The decade began with the resurrection of stereotactic pallidotomy and ending with the rapid growth of the use of implanted stimulators for movement disorders.

Image Guided Surgery

Originally, CT or MR images were incorporated into stereotactic space with various stereotactic frames. The development of graphic intensive computer workstations made it possible to employ new techniques to relate the position of the actual head to a target within the virtual head. As the cost of computers has dropped, such devices became not only practical but desirable. Software has been developed to merge CT with MR and other images (132). It displays the images to the surgeon in the operating room, manipulates the images for optimal use of the information, and relates those images to stereotactic space (118,124). Generally, the relationship is obtained by securing several fiducials to the scalp, so that they can be visualized both on the scalp and at surgery. As the surgeon applies the pointer to each fiducial in turn, the computer registers the real and virtual position to each other, superimposing the virtual and real head in space (71).

The first commercially available systems to relate the virtual image to the real image involved an articulated arm. As the pointer at the end of the arm was positioned in space, the sensors at each joint were used to calculate the precise position and trajectory of the pointer (71). These systems were used in surgery (57) with considerable accuracy (192).

As a reflection of how fast technology has been advancing, they were quickly supplanted by frameless-armless systems that allow freer use of the pointer in space with equivalent accuracy (17). Localization of a pointer is accomplished by identification of several fiducials on the pointer or surgical instrument by two or three video cameras (100) or other detectors (193) that calculate the position of each fiducial by triangulation (71). Similar techniques are used to localize a microscope in space, so it accurately focuses on the target point within the brain (126).

Toward the end of the decade, further refinements were being introduced to allow registration without the use of fiducials (69). As computers rapidly become more powerful, intraoperative technology will advance at an ever increasing rate.

These techniques allow the surgeon to indicate a point-in-space as the target. However, the efficiency of tumor resection is improved significantly by using a volume-in-space as the target. This concept was pioneered by Kelly (122) in the 1980s. The system uses a dedicated microscope with a heads-up display that demonstrates the outline at any given depth (122,183). Another system that employs a volume as the target is the Exoscope developed by Gildenberg (90), which integrates a video image of the surgical field with a three-dimensional computer-generated image of the tumor.

Such technology allows a smaller, critically planned craniotomy opening, optimal exposure of the tumor with minimal manipulation of surrounding tissue, and a shorter operating time (2).

The most complete approach to guided craniotomy involves combining intraoperative MRI with frameless guidance (23). To bring the MRI into the operating room, all instrumentation had to be redesigned to compensate for the hostile magnetic environment. The ability to scan periodically throughout the surgery allows the surgeon to compensate for brain shift, monitor the progress of resection, or detect potential complications.

Stereotactic Radiosurgery

Until the 1990s, radiosurgery was performed either with the Leksell Gamma Knife or in a specialized institution that incorporated a high energy radiation source. In the 1990s, stereotactic radiosurgery expanded rapidly and became available to most patients throughout the world. Two developments from the 1980s made this possible. First, the Leksell Gamma Knife became widely commercially available. Second, progress in computer science made it possible to program linear accelerators (present in almost every major hospital) to be used for stereotactic radiosurgery.

The developmental activity of the prior decade paid off. In 1992, the first commercially available, dedicated radiosurgery linear accelerator was built after the design developed by Kooy et al. (131) at the Joint Center in Boston. The key to its development was the user-friendly computer interface that allowed sophisticated, three-dimensional planning to provide maximal radiation to the target while sparing nearby radiosensitive structures. Soon thereafter, the system developed by Friedman and Bova (67,68) at the University of Florida also became available. This program used a mechanical device for accurate alignment of the collimator, assuring its accuracy and facilitating the incorporation of stereotactic radiosurgery into a linear accelerator. This procedure is also used for conventional radiation therapy.

The 1990s have seen a rapid proliferation of linear accelerator-based stereotactic radiosurgery programs, since they are affordable at most hospitals with a radiation oncology department. At the same time, Leksell Gamma Knife units were being installed throughout the world. In 1990, there were five Gamma Knife installations in the United States and four elsewhere in the world, for a total of nine. By the end of the decade, there were 55 in the US and an additional 77 throughout the rest of the world, for a total of 132 installations. In 1990, there were perhaps a dozen centers dedicated to the development of linear accelerator radiosurgical technology, but none commercially available. It is estimated that there were 500 linac programs at the turn of the millennium. In general, each Gamma Knife center, where the instrument was not used for any other application, did more procedures than each linac center, where the equipment was almost always shared with other radiation oncological procedures.

One of the great technological differences between the Gamma Knife and linac-based programs is the ability to provide fractionated treatments with the linac systems, which has been termed stereotactic radiotherapy. It is a well accepted radiobiological phenomenon that fractionating a radiation treatment, that is, giving the treatment in divided doses over several days provides greater safety to normal tissues, which

can then tolerate a higher dose of radiation without adverse effects. At the same time, fractionation increases the therapeutic effectiveness against some neoplasms, which are irradiated throughout more vulnerable parts of the cell cycle. Since the Gamma Knife requires firm fixation of the stereotactic frame to hold the head in position, it can be used only with single dose stereotactic radiosurgery. Several noninvasive techniques have been developed for linac systems that reposition the patient's head accurately each day for a treatment session. This makes it possible to provide stereotactic-directed, fractionated radiation (81,130), which opens the door to more effective, less risky treatment for many conditions.

A direct offshoot of the computer dosimetry developed for these programs has been stereotactic conformal radiotherapy. This bridges the gap between stereotactic radiotherapy and conventional radiotherapy in that it provides radiation to large areas of the brain or the entire brain, but shapes the field to provide different doses to different structures within the head (36). As a result, it is possible to provide a larger than usual dose to a glioma, while delivering a modest dose to the brain stem and a minimal dose to the eyes and optic nerves.

Functional Neurosurgery

The 1990s produced a particularly significant technological advance in the treatment of movement disorders. It had long been recognized that during surgery, tremor could be modified by stimulation of various parts of the extrapyramidal loop, which had been used for physiologic mapping of the target since the inception of stereotactic techniques. In particular, high frequency stimulation had the same effect as producing a lesion. This observation led to the use of implanted spinal cord stimulators in the 1970s for treatment of spasmodic torticollis (75). During the 1980s, it was used in several patients with both movement disorders and pain, and both were improved when a deep brain stimulator was implanted for pain management (24,190). During the 1990s, the implantation of stimulators specifically for management of movement disorders was instituted. By the end of the decade, deep brain stimulators were becoming the preferred surgical treatment for tremor or Parkinson's disease.

Clinical Progress

The 1990s saw an explosion of activity in stereotactic surgery for movement disorders, stereotactic radiosurgery, and image-guided neurosurgery. More and more neurosurgeons are becoming interested in stereotactic techniques, bringing diverse ideas into the field and introducing stereotaxis into every aspect of neurosurgery.

Image-Guided Neurosurgery

The 1990s saw the consolidation and dissemination of the use of stereotactic localizing techniques as part of the standard armamentarium of neurosurgery to approach masses or anatomical targets visualized on imaging studies. During the first part of the decade, guidance was used with frame-based systems for single target points, such as for biopsy, as well as aspiration of abscesses, cysts, or hematomas. Cannulae were inserted to a target point for ventriculostomy, or urokinase irrigation of hematomas following aspiration. Electrodes were inserted for long-term monitoring for epilepsy (222). A deep volume, such as a metastatic tumor, could be approached stereotactically and then resected along a natural plane.

As image-guided neurosurgery began to mature, the frame was replaced by frameless systems, initially with an articulated arm and then with a pointer or instrument that could be positioned in space by visualization of attached fiducials. The ever more sophisticated work stations allowed visualization of the actual or reconstructed planes of the CT or MR scans taken preoperatively. The reconstructed volume of a tumor was first used as a volumetric target with frame-based guidance during the 1980s (117) and extended to other stereotactic frames during the 1990s (90,224). Subsequently, frameless systems began to incorporate three-dimensional visualization for intraoperative guidance, as well

(116). Since contrast-enhanced imaging often allows better definition of tumor margins than the eye of the surgeon, computer guidance frequently allows more complete tumor resection, while minimizing the operative exposure and trauma to surrounding tissues.

Movement Disorders

The early part of the 1990s produced several papers that were instrumental in the rebirth of functional stereotactic surgery. Laitinen (139,140) resurrected an old paper in which Svennilson (209) reviewed Leksell's (138) target for pallidotomy for treatment of Parkinson's disease, which was somewhat more posterior and ventral than the usual target. Good results were reported in managing bradykinesia, medication-induced dyskinesia, and rigidity, which are the most disabling complaints of patients who have exhausted management with L-dopa. The gradual development of widespread use of that target reawakened interest in surgical management of Parkinson's disease.

With the use of implanted stimulators rather than lesions, surgery for Parkinson's disease or essential tremor became less hazardous, with the same clinical result. Tremor is treated with chronic-stimulating electrodes in the same Vim thalamic target that has been used for tremor of various etiologies (25). Siegfried (191) implanted stimulating electrodes into the pallidum and observed the same benefit as with pallidotomy—improvement in the motor disorder, but with no modification in medication requirement. Benabid (18) thereafter used the subthalamic nucleus as the target (a target which had not been used for lesion production because of fear of hemiballismus) (134), with both improvement in motor function and a decreased need for medication (72).

Near the end of the decade, some neurosurgeons had used the Gamma Knife to produce lesions for treatment of movement disorders (223). This technique, however, has not generally been accepted, since it precludes the opportunity for physiologic mapping of the target, where mapping is a necessary part of the procedure. It may prove to be useful, however, in those procedures where the target is based on anatomical criteria alone or for ablation of epileptic foci (148).

Pain

The 1990s have seen little progress in pain management. The general philosophy advocates again unrestricted use of narcotics, de-emphasis on a multidisciplinary, psychologically-oriented approach, and the naive use of indiscriminate blocks for all sorts of chronic pain (86).

The Gamma Knife has been used for treatment of trigeminal neuralgia with often good but delayed response (128).

Psychosurgery

Only a few articles concerning the benefits of psychosurgery for obsessive compulsive disorder have been published (161,184), but better psychiatric medication and loss of interest in this field have produced a relative quiescence.

Epilepsy

Radiosurgery has been used for functional procedures where the target can be visualized by imaging. Perhaps the best example of this is callosotomy for management of seizures (174). Some believe that stereotactic radiosurgery may make it possible to stop epileptogenic activity without tissue destruction (15,99,217).

Stereotactic Radiosurgery

The proliferation of stereotactic radiosurgery during the 1990s has produced a huge clinical experience, inasmuch as both indications and results are better defined. Radiosurgery for arteriovenous malformations continues to be an important treatment. The use of radiosurgery for the treatment of tumors is now the most common indication. Metastatic tumors of various types respond to radiosurgery and are the most commonly treated (26). Although it has long been recognized that meningiomas respond to radiation, the use of single dose radiosurgery (129) or fractionated stereotactic or conformal radio-

therapy allows efficient treatment with minimal radiation of surrounding structures. Other benign tumors, such as pituitary adenomas or acoustic schwannomas may be treated successfully with minimal risk (62). The use of hypofractionation (very few treatment sessions, usually two to five) allows almost complete control of acoustic tumors with almost no cranial nerve VII or VIII complications in early analysis (143). Pituitary adenomas that infiltrate into the cavernous sinus may respond well to radiosurgery or conformal stereotactic radiotherapy (142).

The opportunities to treat residual tumors with stereotactic radiosurgery after partial resection make it possible to be more conservative in surgery to avoid sacrificing neurological function. Every neurosurgeon should be aware of the capability of stereotactic radiosurgery to allow him or her to make the wisest decision during surgery.

THE DAWN OF THE NEW MILLENNIUM

Looking forward to stereotactic and functional neurosurgery in the new millennium, one can only anticipate a continued rapid growth. It will soon be the norm to use guidance techniques in essentially every neurosurgical procedure. As molecular and genetic treatments become available for brain diseases, many procedures will require stereotactic techniques for definitive diagnosis in order to obtain tissue to customize the treatment, or to deliver the treatment directly to the site of pathology. The ever more rapid advances in computer technology will find their way into the neurosurgical operating room through stereotactic surgery, which will play an ever increasing role in neurosurgical developments.

REFERENCES

1. Abel-Fessard D, Arfel G, Guiot G, et al. Identification et délimitation précise de certaines structures souscorticales de l'homme par l'electro-physiologie. *CR Acad Sci (Paris)* 243:2412–2414, 1961.
2. Alberti O, Dorward NL, Kitchen ND, et al. Neuronavigation: Impact on operating time. *Stereotact Funct Neurosurg* 68:44–48, 1997.

3. Allen GS, Burns RS, Tulipan NB, et al. Adrenal medullary transplantation to the caudate nucleus in Parkinson's disease: Initial clinical results in 18 patients. *Arch Neurol* 46:487–491, 1989.

4. Amano K, Kawamura H, Tanikawa T, et al. Surgical treatment of hypertensive intracerebral haematoma by CT-guided stereotactic surgery. *Acta Neurochir Suppl (Wien)* 39:41–44, 1987.

5. Andy OJ. Diencephalic coagulation in the treatment of hemiballism. *Conf Neurol* 22:346–350, 1962.

6. Andy OJ. Thalamotomy in hyperactive and aggressive behavior. *Conf Neurol* 32:322–325, 1970.

7. Backlund EO. The history and development of radiosurgery, in, Lunsford LD (ed): *Stereotactic Radiosurgery Update*. New York: Elsevier, 1992, pp 3–9.

8. Backlund EO, von Holst H. Controlled subtotal evacuation of intracerebral hematomas by stereotactic technique. *Surg Neurol* 9:99–101, 1978.

9. Backlund EO, Granberg PO, Hamberger B, et al. Transplantation of adrenal medullary tissue to striatum in parkinsonism: First clinical trials. *J Neurosurg* 62:169–173, 1985.

10. Bailey P, Stein SN. A stereotaxic apparatus for use on the human brain: AMA Scientific Exhibit, Atlantic City, 1951.

11. Baird HWI, Wycis HT, Spiegel EA. Convulsions in tuberous sclerosis controlled by elimination of impulses in the basal ganglia. *J Pediatr* 49:165–172, 1956.

12. Bakay RA. Central nervous system grafting: Animal and clinical results. *Stereotact Funct Neurosurg* 58:67–78, 1992.

13. Balasubramaniam V, Kanaka TS, Ramanujam PV, et al. Sedative neurosurgery: A contribution to the behavioural sciences. *J Indian Med Assoc* 53:377–381, 1969.

14. Balasubramaniam V, Kanaka TS, Rumanujam PB. Stereotaxic cingulumotomy for drug addiction. *Neurology (Madras)* 21:63–66, 1973.

15. Barcia Salorio JL, Barcia JA, Roldan P, et al. Radiosurgery of epilepsy. *Acta Neurochir Suppl (Wien)* 58:195–197, 1993.

16. Barcia-Salorio JL, Soler F, Hernandez G, et al. Radiosurgical treatment of low flow carotid-cavernous fistulae. *Acta Neurochir Suppl (Wien)* 52:93–95, 1991.

17. Barnett GH, Kormos DW, Steiner CP, et al. Intraoperative localization using an armless, frameless stereotactic wand. Technical note. *J Neurosurg* 78:510–514, 1993.

18. Benabid AL, Pollak P, Gross C, et al. Acute and long-term effects of subthalamic nucleus stimulation in Parkinson's disease. *Stereotact Funct Neurosurg* 62:76–84, 1994.

19. Benabid AL, Pollak P, Hommel M, et al. Treatment of Parkinson tremor by chronic stimulation of the ventral intermediate nucleus of the thalamus. *Rev Neurol (Paris)* 145:320–323, 1989.

20. Bertrand G, Jasper H. Microelectrode recording of unit activity in the human thalamus. *Confin Neurol* 26:205–208, 1965.

21. Betti O, Derechinsky V. Hyperselective encephalic irradiation with a linear accelerator. *Acta Neurochir Suppl* 33:385–390, 1984.

22. Black P, Uematsu S, Walker AE. Stereotaxic hypothalamotomy for control of violent, aggressive behavior. *Conf Neurol* 37:187–188, 1975.

23. Black PM, Moriarty T, Alexander E, et al. Development and implementation of intraoperative magnetic resonance imaging and its neurosurgical applications. *Neurosurgery* 41:831–842, 1997.

24. Blond S, Siegfried J: Thalamic stimulation for the treatment of tremor and other movement disorders. *Acta Neurochir Suppl (Wien)* 52:109–111, 1991.

25. Blond S, Caparros-Lefebvre D, Parker F, et al. Control of tremor and involuntary movement disorders by chronic stimulation of the ventral intermediate thalamic nucleus. *J Neurosurg* 77:62–68, 1992.

26. Boyd TS, Mehta MP. Radiosurgery for brain metastases. *Neurosurg Clin N Am* 10:337–350, 1999.

27. Breggin PR. The return of lobotomy and psychosurgery. *Congressional Record* 118:26–24, 1972.

28. Brion S, Guiot G, Derome P, et al. Postoperative hemiballism during stereotaxic surgery: Apropos of 12 cases, two of them anatomo-clinical, in a series of 850 operations. *Rev Neurol (Paris)* 112:410–443, 1965.

29. Broggi G, Franzini A, Peluchetti D, et al. Treatment of deep brain abscesses by stereotactic implantation of an intracavitary device for evacuation and local application of antibiotics. *Acta Neurochir (Wien)* 76:94–98, 1985.

30. Browder J. Section of the fibers of the anterior limb of the internal capsule in Parkinsonism. *Am J Surg* 75:264–268, 1948.

31. Brown RA, Roberts TS, Osborn AG. Stereotaxic frame and computer software for CT-directed neurosurgical localization. *Invest Radiol* 15:308–312, 1980.

32. Brundin P, Barbin G, Isacson O, et al. Survival of intracerebrally grafted rat dopamine neurons previously cultured in vitro. *Neurosci Lett* 61:79–84, 1985.

33. Brundin P, Bjorklund A, Lindvall O. Practical aspects of the use of human fetal brain tissue for intracerebral grafting. *Prog Brain Res* 82:707–714, 1990.

34. Bucy PC, Case TJ. Tremor: Physiologic mechanism and abolition by surgical means. *Arch Neurol Psychiatry* 41:721–746, 1939.

35. Carmichael SW, Wilson RJ, Brimijoin WS, et al. Decreased catecholamines in the adrenal medulla of patients with parkinsonism. *N Engl J Med* 318:254, 1988.

36. Carol M, Grant WH, III, Pavord D, et al. Initial clinical experience with the Peacock intensity modulation of a 3-D conformal radiation therapy system. *Stereotact Funct Neurosurg* 66:30–34, 1996.

37. Clarkson ED, Freed CR. Development of fetal neural transplantation as a treatment for Parkinson's disease. *Life Sci* 65:2427–2437, 1999.

38. Colombo F, Benedetti A, Pozza F, et al. Stereotactic radiosurgery utilizing a linear accelerator. *Appl Neurophysiol* 48:133–145, 1985.

39. Cooper IS. Ligation of the anterior choroidal artery for involuntary movements of parkinsonism. *Psychiatr Q* 27:317–319, 1953.

40. Cooper IS. Surgical alleviation of parkinsonism: Effects of occlusion of the anterior choroidal artery. *J Am Geriatr Soc* 11:691–717, 1954.

41. Cooper IS. Chemopallidectomy. *Science* 121:217, 1955.

42. Cooper IS. Clinical results and follow-up studies in a personal series of 300 operations for parkinsonism. *J Am Geriatr Soc* 4:1171–1181, 1956.

43. Cooper IS. Neurosurgical alleviation of intention

tremor of multiple sclerosis and cerebellar disease. *N Engl J Med* 263:441–444, 1960.

44. Cooper IS. Results of 1000 consecutive basal ganglia operations for parkinsonism. *Ann Intern Med* 52:483–499, 1960.

45. Cooper IS, Lee AStJ. Cryostatic congelation. *J Nerv Ment Dis* 133:259–263, 1961.

46. Cooper IS, Bravo G, Riklan M, et al. Chemopallidectomy and chemothalamectomy for parkinsonism. *Geriatrics* 13:127–147, 1958.

47. Cosman E. Radiofrequency lesions, in, Gildenberg P, Tasker RR (ed): *Textbook of Stereotactic and Functional Neurosurgery.* New York: McGraw-Hill, 1998, pp 973–985.

48. Cotzias GC, VanWoert MH, Schiffer LM. Aromatic amino acids and modification of parkinsonism. *N Engl J Med* 276:374–379, 1967.

49. Dandy WE. Ventriculography following the injection of air into the cerebral ventricles. *Ann Surg* 68:5–11, 1918.

50. Dandy WE. Changes in our conceptions of localization of certain functions in the brain. *Am J Physiol* 93:643–647, 1930.

51. Das K, Benzil DL, Rovit RL, et al. Irving S. Cooper (1922–1985): A pioneer in functional neurosurgery. *J Neurosurg* 89:865–873, 1998.

52. Daumas Duport C, Scheithauer BW, Kelly PJ. A histologic and cytologic method for the spatial definition of gliomas. *Mayo Clin Proc* 62:435–449, 1987.

53. Demoulin C. Anorexia nervosa. A general review of recent works *Ann Med Psychol (Paris)* 1:375–393, 1969.

54. Diaz Perez G, Chiorino R, Donoso P, et al. Posterior hypothalamotomy using the stereotaxic method in the treatment of erethism and aggressiveness. *Neurocirugia* 26:12–18, 1968.

55. Dieckmann G, Hassler R. Unilateral hypothalamotomy in sexual delinquents: Report on six cases. *Confin Neurol* 37:177–186, 1975.

56. Dierssen G. Treatment of dystonic and athetoid symptoms by lesions in the sensory portion of the internal capsule. *Confin Neurol* 26:404–406, 1965.

57. Doshi PK, Lemmieux L, Fish DR, et al. Frameless stereotaxy and interactive neurosurgery with the ISG viewing wand. *Acta Neurochir Suppl (Wien)* 64:49–53, 1995.

58. Fabrikant JI, Lyman JT, Frankel KA. Heavy charged-particle Bragg peak radiosurgery for intracranial vascular disorders. *Radiat Res Suppl* 8:S244–S258, 1985.

59. Feindel W: Toward a surgical cure for epilepsy: The work of Wilder Penfield and his school at the Montreal Neurological Institute, in, Engel J, Jr. (ed): *Surgical Treatment of the Epilepsies, 2nd Edition.* New York: Raven Press, 1993, pp 1–9.

60. Feindel W, Leblanc R, Villemure J-G. History of the surgical treatment of epilepsy, in, Greenblatt SH, Dagi TF, Epstein MH (ed): *A History of Neurosurgery.* Park Ridge, Illinois: American Association of Neurological Surgeons, 1997, pp 465–488.

61. Fenelon F. Essais de traitement ceurochirurgical du syndrome parkinsonien par intervention directe sur les voies extrapyramidales immédiatement sous striopallidales (anse lenticulaire): Communication suivie de projection du film d'un opérés pris avant at après l'intervention. *Rev Neurol (Paris)* 83:437–440, 1950.

62. Foote KD, Friedman WA, Buatti JM, et al. Linear accelerator radiosurgery in brain tumor management. *Neurosurg Clin N Am* 10:203–242, 1999.

63. Fordyce WE, Roberts AH, Sternbach RA. The behavioral management of chronic pain: A response to critics. *Pain* 22:113–125, 1985.

64. Forno LS, Langston JW. Unfavorable outcome of adrenal medullary transplant for Parkinson's disease. *Acta Neuropathol (Berl)* 81:691–694, 1991.

65. Freed WJ, Cannon-Spoor HE, Wyatt RJ. Embryonic brain grafts in an animal model of Parkinson's disease: Criteria for human application. *Appl Neurophysiol* 47:16–22, 1984.

66. Freeman W, Watts JW. *Psychosurgery: Intelligence, Emotional and Social Behavior Following Prefrontal Lobotomy for Mental Disorders.* Springfield: Thomas, 1942.

67. Friedman WA, Bova F. The University of Florida radiosurgery system. *Surg Neurol* 32:334–342, 1989.

68. Friedman WA, Bova FJ, Spiegelmann R. Linear accelerator radiosurgery at the University of Florida. *Neurosurg Clin N Am* 3:141–166, 1992.

69. Friets EM, Strohbehn JW, Roberts DW. Curvature-based nonfiducial registration for the Frameless Stereotactic Operating Microscope. *IEEE Trans Biomed Eng* 42:867–878, 1995.

70. Fukamachi A, Ohye C, Narabayashi H. Delineation of the thalamic nuclei with a microelectrode in stereotaxic surgery for parkinsonism and cerebral palsy. *J Neurosurg* 39:214–225, 1973.

71. Galloway RL. Orientation and registration of three-dimensional images, in, Gildenberg PL, Tasker RR (ed): *Textbook of Stereotactic and Functional Neurosurgery.* New York: McGraw-Hill, 1998, pp 331–337.

72. Gentil M, Garcia-Ruiz P, Pollak P, et al. Effect of stimulation of the subthalamic nucleus on oral control of patients with parkinsonism. *J Neurol Neurosurg Psychiatry* 67:329–333, 1999.

73. Gildenberg PL. Studies in stereoencephalotomy VIII: Comparison of the variability of subcortical lesions produced by various procedures. *Confin Neurol* 17:299–301, 1957.

74. Gildenberg PL. Variability of subcortical lesions produced by a heating electrode and Cooper's balloon cannula. *Confin Neurol* 20:53–65, 1960.

75. Gildenberg PL. Treatment of spasmodic torticollis by dorsal column stimulation. *Appl Neurophysiol* 41:113–121, 1978.

76. Gildenberg PL. Computerized tomography and stereotactic surgery, in, Spiegel EA (ed): *Guided Brain Operations.* Basel Karger, 1982, pp 24–34.

77. Gildenberg PL. Whatever happened to stereotactic surgery? *Neurosurgery* 20:983–987, 1987.

78. Gildenberg PL. "Stereotaxic" versus "stereotactic." *Neurosurgery* 32:965–966, 1993.

79. Gildenberg PL. General and psychological assessment of the pain patient, in, Tindall GT, Cooper PR, Barrow DL (ed): *The Practice of Neurosurgery.* Baltimore: Williams and Wilkins, 1996, pp 2987–2996.

80. Gildenberg PL. Gildenberg-Laitinen Adapter Device (GLAD): A non-invasive reapplication system for stereotactic head rings, in, Gildenberg PL, Tasker RR

(ed): *Textbook of Stereotactic and Functional Neurosurgery.* New York: McGraw-Hill, 1997, pp 211–215.

81. Gildenberg PL. History of pain management, in, Greenblatt SH, Dagi TF (ed): *A History of Neurosurgery.* Park Ridge, Illinois: American Association of Neurological Surgeons, 1997, pp 465–488.

82. Gildenberg PL. General principles and selection of techniques in the management of pain of benign origin, in, Gildenberg PL, Tasker RR (ed): *Textbook of Stereotactic and Functional Neurosurgery.* New York: McGraw-Hill, 1998, pp 1321–1336.

83. Gildenberg PL. The history of surgery for movement disorders. *Neurosurg Clin N Am* 9:283–294, 1998.

84. Gildenberg PL. History of movement disorder surgery, in, Lozano A (ed): *Movement Disorder Surgry: Progress and Challenges.* Basel: S Karger, 2000, pp. 1–20.

85. Gildenberg PL, De Vaul RA. *The Chronic Pain Patient: Evaluation and Management. Basel:* Karger, 1985.

86. Gildenberg PL, DeVaul RA. Medical management of chronic pain, in, Youmans JR (ed): *Neurological Surgery, 4th Edition.* Philadelphia: Saunders, 1995, pp 5073–5089.

87. Gildenberg PL, Gathe JC, Jr., Kim JH. Stereotacic biopsy in AIDS patients. *Clin Infectious Dis* 30: 491–499, 2000.

88. Gildenberg PL, Kaufman HH, Murthy KS. Calculation of stereotactic coordinates from the computed tomographic scan. *Neurosurgery* 10:580–586, 1982.

89. Gildenberg PL, Langford L, Kim JH, et al. Stereotactic biopsy in cerebral lesions of AIDS. *Acta Neurochir Suppl (Wien)* 58:68–70, 1993.

90. Gildenberg PL, Ledoux R, Cosman E, et al. The Exoscope—a frame-based video/graphics system for intraoperative guidance of surgical resection. *Stereotact Funct Neurosurg* 63:23–25, 1994.

91. Gildenberg PL, Pettigrew LC, Merrell R, et al. Transplantation of adrenal medullary tissue to caudate nucleus using stereotactic techniques. *Stereotact Funct Neurosurg* 54–55:268–271, 1990.

92. Giorgi C, Broggi G, Garibotto G, et al. Three-dimensional neuroanatomic images in CT-guided stereotaxic neurosurgery. *AJNR* 4:719–721, 1983.

93. Gol A. Relief of pain by electrical stimulation of the septal area. *J Neurol Sci* 5:115–120, 1967.

94. Hariz MI, Fodstad H. Stereotactic localization of small subcortical brain tumors for open surgery. *Surg Neurol* 28:345–350, 1987.

95. Hassler R, Riechert T. Indikationen und Lokalisationsmethode der gezielten Hirnoperationen. *Nervenarzt* 25: 441–447, 1954.

96. Hassler R, Riechert T, Mundinger F. The precision in anatomical localization of stereotactic Parkinson operations checked with data from autopsies. *Arch Psychiatr Nervenkr* 212:97–116, 1969.

97. Håkanson S. Trigeminal neuralgia treated by the injection of glycerol into the trigeminal cistern. *Neurosurgery* 9:638–646, 1981.

98. Heath RG, Mickle WA. Evaluation of seven years experience with depth electrode studies in human patients, in, Ramey, O'Doherty (ed): *Electrical Studies on the Unanesthetized Brain.* New York: Hoeber, 1960, pp 214–228.

99. Heikkinen ER, Heikkinen MI, Sotaniemi K. Stereotactic radiotherapy instead of conventional epilepsy surgery: A case report. *Acta Neurochir (Wien)* 119: 159–160, 1992.

100. Heilbrun MP, Koehler S, MacDonald P, et al. Preliminary experience using an optimized three-point transformation algorithm for spatial registration of coordinate systems: A method of noninvasive localization using frame-based stereotactic guidance systems. *J. Neurosurg* 81:676–682, 1994.

101. Heimburger RF, Whitlock CC. Steretotaxic destruction of the human dentate nucleus. *Confin Neurol* 26: 346–358, 1965.

102. Hécaen H, Talairach T, David M, et al. Mémoires originaux: Coagulations limitées du thalamus dans les algies du syndrome thalamique. *Rev Neurol* 81:917–931, 1949.

103. Hitchcock E. Psychosurgery today. *Ann Clin Res* 3: 187–198, 1971.

104. Hitchcock ER, Clough CG, Hughes RC, et al. Transplantation in Parkinson's disease: Stereotactic implantation of adrenal medulla and foetal mesencephalon. *Acta Neurochir Suppl (Wien)* 46:48–50, 1989.

105. Hitchcock ER, Kenny BG, Clough CG, et al. Stereotactic implantation of fetal mesencephalon. *Stereotact Funct Neurosurg* 54–55:282–289, 1990.

106. Horsley V. The Linacre Lecture on the function of the so-called motor area of the brain. *Br Med J* ii:125–132, 1909.

107. Horsley V, Clarke RH. The structure and functions of the cerebellum examined by a new method. *Brain* 31: 45–124, 1908.

108. Hosobuchi Y, Adams JE, Linchitz R. Pain relief by electrical stimulation of the central gray matter in humans and its reversal by naloxone. *Science* 197: 183–186, 1977.

109. Hosobuchi Y, Adams JE, Rutkins B. Chronic thalamic stimulation for the control of facial anesthesia dolorosas. *Arch Neurol* 29:158–161, 1973.

110. Hosobuchi Y, Adams JE, Weinstein PR. Preliminary percutaneous dorsal column stimulation prior to permanent implantation: Technical note. *J Neurosug* 37: 242–245, 1972.

111. Hunter SE. Stereotactic hypothalamotomy, in, Gildenberg PL, Tasker RR (ed): *Textbook of Stereotactic and Functional Neurosurgery.* New York: McGraw-Hill, 1998, pp 1507–1517.

112. Hurt RW, Ballentine HT, Jr. Stereotactic anterior cingulate lesions for persistent pain: A report of 68 cases. *Clin Neurosurg* 21:334–351, 1974.

113. Jankovic J, Grossman R, Goodman C, et al. Clinical, biochemical, and neuropathologic findings following transplantation of adrenal medulla to the caudate nucleus for treatment of Parkinson's disease. *Neurology* 39:1227–1234, 1989.

114. Jasper H, Bertrand G. Stereotaxic microelectrode studies of single thalamic cells and fibres in patients with dyskinesia. *Trans Am Neurol Assoc* 89:79–82, 1964.

115. Jinnai D, Nishimoto A. Stereotaxic destruction of Forel H for treatment of epilepsy. *Neurochirurgia (Stuttgart)* 6:164–176, 1963.

116. Kall BA, Goerss SJ, Kelly PJ, et al. Three-dimensional display in the evaluation and performance of neurosurgery without a stereotactic frame: More than a pretty picture? *Stereotact Funct Neurosurg* 63:69–75, 1994.

117. Kall BA, Kelly PJ, Goerss SJ. Interactive stereotactic surgical system for the removal of intracranial tumors utilizing the CO_2 laser and CT-derived database. *IEEE Trans Biomed Eng* 32:112–116, 1985.

118. Kelly PJ. *Tumor Stereotaxis.* Philadelphia: Saunders, 1991.

119. Kelly PJ. Stereotactic surgery: What is past is prologue. *Neurosurgery* 46:16–27, 2000.

120. Kelly PJ, Gillingham FJ. The long-term results of stereotaxic surgery and L-dopa therapy in patients with Parkinson's disease: A 10-year follow-up study. *J Neurosurg* 53:332–337, 1980.

121. Kelly PJ, Alker GJ Jr, Kall BA, et al. Method of computed tomography-based stereotactic biopsy with arteriographic control. *Neurosurgery* 14:172–177, 1984.

122. Kelly PJ, Earnest F, Kall BA, et al. Surgical options for patients with deep-seated brain tumors: Computer-assisted stereotactic biopsy. *Mayo Clin Proc* 60:223–229, 1985.

123. Kelly PJ, Kall B, Goerss S, et al. Precision resection of intra-axial CNS lesions by CT-based stereotactic craniotomy and computer monitored CO_2 laser. *Acta Neurochir (Wien)* 68:1–9, 1983.

124. Kelly PJ, Kall BA, Goerss S, et al. Results of computer-assisted stereotactic laser resection of deep-seated intracranial lesions. *Mayo Clin Proc* 61:20–27, 1986.

125. Kim JH, Gildenberg PL. Stereotactic biopsy, in, Gildenberg PL, Tasker RR (ed): *Textbook of Stereotactic and Functional Neurosurgery.* New York: McGraw-Hill, 1998, pp 387–396.

126. Kiya N, Dureza C, Fukushima T, et al. Computer navigational microscope for minimally invasive neurosurgery. *Minim Invasive Neurosurg* 40:110–115, 1997.

127. Kjellberg RN, Hanamura T, Davis KR, et al. Bragg-peak proton-beam therapy for arteriovenous malformations of the brain. *N Engl J Med* 309:269–274, 1983.

128. Kondziolka D, Lunsford LD, Flickinger JC, et al. Stereotactic radiosurgery for trigeminal neuralgia: A multi-institutional study using the gamma unit. *J Neurosurg* 84:940–945, 1996.

129. Kondziolka D, Niranjan A, Lunsford LD, et al. Stereotactic radiosurgery for meningiomas. *Neurosurg Clin N Am* 10:317–325, 1999.

130. Kooy HM, Dunbar SF, Tarbell NJ, et al. Adaptation and verification of the relocatable Gill-Thomas-Cosman frame in stereotactic radiotherapy. *Int J Radiat Oncol Biol Phys* 30:685–691, 1994.

131. Kooy HM, Nedzi LA, Loeffler JS, et al. Treatment planning for stereotactic radiosurgery of intracranial lesions. *Int J Radiat Oncol Biol Phys* 21:683–693, 1991.

132. Kooy HM, van Herk M, Barnes PD, et al. Image fusion for stereotactic radiotherapy and radiosurgery treatment planning. *Int J Radiat Oncol Biol Phys* 28:1229–1234, 1994.

133. Koslow M, Abele MG. A fully interfaced computerized tomographic-stereotactic surgical system. *Appl Neurophysiol* 43:174–175, 1980.

134. LaFia DJ. Hemiballismus as a complication of thalamotomy: Report of two cases. *Confin Neurol* 31:42–47, 1969.

135. Laitinen LV. Thalamotomy in progressive myoclonus epilepsy. *Acta Neurol Scand* 43:31–47, 1967.

136. Laitinen LV. Stereotactic lesions in the knee of the corpus callosum in the treatment of emotional disorders. *Lancet* 1:472–475, 1972.

137. Laitinen LV. Brain targets in surgery for Parkinson's disease: Results of a survey of neurosurgeons. *J Neurosurg* 62:349–351, 1985.

138. Laitinen LV. Leksell's unpublished pallidotomies of 1958–62. *Stereotac Funct Neurosurg* In press, 2000.

139. Laitinen LV, Bergenheim AT, Hariz MI. Leksell's posteroventral pallidotomy in the treatment of Parkinson's disease. *J Neurosurg* 76:53–61, 1992.

140. Laitinen LV, Bergenheim AT, Hariz MI. Ventroposterolateral pallidotomy can abolish all parkinsonian symptoms. *Stereotact Funct Neurosurg* 58:14–21, 1992.

141. Larsson B, Leksell L, Rexed B. The high energy proton beam as a neurosurgical tool. *Nature* 182:1222–1223, 1958.

142. Laws ER, Jr., Vance ML. Radiosurgery for pituitary tumors and craniopharyngiomas. *Neurosurg Clin N Am* 10:327–336, 1999.

143. Lederman G, Lowry J, Wertheim S, et al. Acoustic neuroma: Potential benefits of fractionated stereotactic radiosurgery. *Stereotact Funct Neurosurg* 69:175–182, 1997.

144. Leksell L. A stereotaxic apparatus for intracerebral surgery. *Acta Chir Scand* 99:229–233, 1949.

145. Leksell L. The stereotaxic method and radiosurgery of the brain. *Acta Chir Scand* 102:316–319, 1951.

146. Leksell L. Cerebral radiosurgery. I. Gammathalamotomy in two cases of intractable pain. *Acta Chir Scand* 134:585–595, 1968.

147. Levy RM, Bredesen DE, Rosenblum ML. Neurological manifestations of the acquired immunodeficiency syndrome (AIDS): Experience at UCSF and review of the literature. *J Neurosurg* 62:475–495, 1985.

148. Lindquist C, Kihlstrom L, Hellstrand E. Functional neurosurgery—a future for the gamma knife? *Stereotact Funct Neurosurg* 57:72–81, 1991.

149. Lunsford LD. A dedicated CT system for the stereotactic operating room. *Appl Neurophysiol* 45:374–378, 1982.

150. Lunsford LD, Alexander E III, Loeffler JS. General introduction: History of radiosurgery, in, Alexander E III, Loeffler JS, Lunsford LD (ed): *Stereotactic Radiosurgery.* New York: McGraw-Hill, 1993, pp 1–4.

151. Lunsford LD, Maitz A, Lindner G. First United States 201 source cobalt-60 gamma unit for radiosurgery. *Appl Neurophysiol* 50:253–256, 1987.

152. Lunsford LD, Martinez AJ, Latchaw RE. Stereotaxic surgery with a magnetic resonance and computerized tomography-compatible system. *J Neurosurg* 64:872–878, 1986.

153. Madrazo I, Drucker-Colin R, Diaz V. Open microsurgical autograft of adrenal medulla to the right caudate nucleus in two patients with intractable Parkinson's disease. *N Engl J Med* 316:831–834, 1987.

154. Mark VH, Sweet WH. The role of limbic brain dysfunction in aggression. *Res Publ Assoc Res Nerv Ment Dis* 52:186–200, 1974.

155. Mark VH, Gildenberg PL, Franklin PO. Proceedings of the Colloquium on the Use of Embryonic Cell Transplantation for Correction of CNS Disorders. *Appl Neurophysiol* 47:1–76, 1984.

156. Melzack R, Wall PD. Pain mechanisms: A new theory. *Science* 150:971–979, 1965.

157. Meyers R. The modification of alternating tremors, rigidity and festination by surgery of the basal ganglia.
Res Publ Assoc Res Nerv Ment Dis 21:602–665, 1942.

158. Meyers R. Surgical experiments in the therapy of certain 'extrapyramidal diseases.' *Acta Psychiat Neurol*
26:1–42, 1951.

159. Meyers R. Historical background and personal experiences in the surgical relief of hyperkinesia and hyperto-
nus, in Fields W (ed): *Pathogenesis and Treatment of
Parkinsonism.* Springfield, Illinois, Chas C Thomas,
1958, pp 229–270.

160. Meyers R, Fry WJ, Fry FJ, et al. Early experiences
with ultrasonic irradiation of the pallidofugal and nigral complexes in hyperkinetic and hypertonic disorders. *J Neurosurg* 16:32–54, 1959.

161. Mindus, Jenike MA. Neurosurgical treatment of malignant obsessive compulsive disorder. *Psychiatr Clin
North Am* 15:921–938, 1992.

162. Mullan S, Lichtor T. Percutaneous microcompression
of the trigeminal ganglion for trigeminal neuralgia. *J
Neurosurg* 59:1007–1012, 1983.

163. Munari C, Hoffman D, Francione S, et al. Stereo-elec-
troencephalography methodology: Advantages and
limits. *Acta Neurol Scand Suppl* 152:56–67, 1968.

164. Mundinger F, Riechert T. Die stereotaktischen Hirnoperationen zur Behandlung extrapyramidaler Bewegun-
gsstörungen (Parkinsonismus und Hyperkinesen) und
ihre Resultate. Postoperative und Langzeitergebnisse
der stereotaktischen Hirnoperationen bei extrapyrami-
dalmotorischen Bewedunasströrungen. *Teil B Fortsch
Neurol Psychiat* 31:69–120, 1963.

165. Murtagh F, Wycis HT, Robbins R, et al. Visualization
and treatment of cystic brain tumors by stereoencephalotomy. *Acta Radiol* 46:407–414, 1956.

166. Musella R, Short MJ, Wilson WP, et al. Some observations on the physiological mechanisms of "thalamic"
pain. *Electroenceph Clin Neurophysiol* 23:291–292,
1967.

167. Narabayashi H. Stereotaxic instrument for operation
on the human basal ganglia. *Psychiat Neurol Jap* 54:
669–671, 1952.

168. Narabayashi H, Okuma T. Procaine oil blocking of the
globus pallidus for the treatment of rigidity and tremor
of parkinsonism. *Proc Japan Acad* 29:310–318, 1953.

169. Nashold BSJ, Wilson WP. Central pain: Observations
in man with chronic implanted electrodes in the midbrain tegmentum. *Confin Neurol* 27:30–44, 1966.

170. National Commission for the Protection of Human
Subjects of Biomedical and Behavioral Research: Report and Recommendations, Psychosurgery. Washington, DC, DHEW Publications No (05) 77–0001, 1977.

171. Niizuma H, Otsuki T, Johkura H, et al. CT-guided stereotactic aspiration of intracerebral hematoma—Result of a hematoma-lysis method using urokinase. *Appl
Neurophysiol* 48:427–430, 1985.

172. Ohye C, Narabayashi H. Physiological understanding
of the thalamic ventralis intermedius nucleus. *Appl
Neurophysiol* 42:312–312, 1979.

173. Olds J, Milner B. Positive reinforcement produced by
electrical stimulation of the septal area and other regions of the rat brain. *J Comp Physiol Psychol* 47:419,
1954.

174. Pendl G, Eder HG, Schroettner O, et al: Corpus callo-

sotomy with radiosurgery. *Neurosurgery* 45:303–307,
1999.

175. Penn RD, Goetz CG, Tanner CM, et al. The adrenal
medullary transplant operation for Parkinson's disease:
Clinical observations in five patients. *Neurosurgery*
22:999–1004, 1988.

176. Penn RD, Kroin JS. Long-term intrathecal baclofen
infusion for treatment of spasticity. *J Neurosurg* 66:
181–185, 1987.

177. Richardson DE, Akil H. Pain reduction by electrical
brain stimulation in man. II. Chronic self-administra-
tion in the periventricular grey matter. *J Neurosurg* 47:
184–194, 1977.

178. Riechert T, Mundinger F. Indications, technique and
results of the stereotactic operations upon the hypophysis using radio-isotopes. *J Nerv Ment Dis* 13:1–9,
1960.

179. Riechert T, Wolff M. Über ein neues Zielgeraet zur
intrakraniellen elektrischen Abteilung und Ausschaltung. Arch Psychiat Z Neurol 186:225–230, 1951.

180. Riederer P, Rausch WD, Birkmayer W, et al. Dopa-
mine-sensitive adenylate cyclase activity in the caudate
nucleus and adrenal medulla in Parkinson's disease and
in liver cirrhosis. *J Neural Transm Suppl* 14:153–161,
1978.

181. Roberts DW, Strohbehn JW, Hatch JF, et al. A
frameless stereotaxic integration of computerized tomographic imaging and the operating microscope. *J Neurosurg* 65:545–549, 1986.

182. Roeder F, Muller D, Orthner H. Further experiences
in the stereotactic treatment of sexual perversions. J
Neurovisc Relat 10:317–324, 1971.

183. Roessler K, Ungersboeck K, Aichholzer M, et al.
Image-guided neurosurgery comparing a pointer device system with a navigating microscope: A retrospective analysis of 208 cases. *Minim Invasive Neurosurg*
41:53–57, 1998.

184. Sachdev P, Hay P, Cumming S. Psychosurgical treatment of obsessive-compulsive disorder. *Arch Gen Psychiatry* 49:582–584, 1992.

185. Sano K, Sekino H, Mayanagi Y. Results of stimulation
and destruction of the posterior hypothalamus in cases
with violent, aggressive, or restless behaviors, in,
Hitchcock E, Laitinen L, Vaernet K (ed): *Psychosurgery.* Springfield, Ill: Chas C Thomas, 1972.

186. Sano K, Yoshioka M, Ogashiwa M, et al. Thalamolaminotomy: A new operation for relief of intractable pain.
Confin Neurol 27:63–66, 1966.

187. Schwartz HG, O'Leary JL. Section of the spinothalamic tract in the medulla with observations on the
pathways for pain. *Surgery* 9:183–193.

188. Shealy CN, Mortimer JT, Reswick JB. Electrical inhibition of pain by stimulation of the dorsal columns:
Preliminary clinical report. *Anesth Analg (Cleve)* 46:
489–491, 1967.

189. Siegfried J. Is the neurosurgical treatment of Parkinson's disease still indicated? *J Neural Transm Suppl*
195–198, 1980.

190. Siegfried J. Effect of stimulation of the sensory nucleus
of the thalamus on dyskinesia and spasticity. *Rev Neurol (Paris)* 142:380–383, 1986.

191. Siegfried J: Chronic electrical stimulation of the VL-
VPL complex and of the pallidum in the treatment of
extrapyramidal and cerebellar disorders: Personal

experience since 1985. *Stereotact Funct Neurosurg* 62: 71–75, 1994.

192. Sipos EP, Tebo SA, Zinreich SJ, et al. In vivo accuracy testing and clinical experience with the ISG Viewing Wand. *Neurosurgery* 39:194–202, 1996.

193. Smith KR, Frank KJ, Bucholz RD. The NeuroStation—a highly accurate, minimally invasive solution to frameless stereotactic neurosurgery. *Comput Med Imag Graphics* 18:247–256, 1994.

194. Spiegel EA. *Guided Brain Operations.* Basel: Karger, 1982.

195. Spiegel EA, Wycis HT. *Stereoencephalotomy, Part I.* New York: Grune & Stratton, 1952.

196. Spiegel EA, Wycis HT. Thalamotomy and pallidotomy for treatment of choreic movements. *Acta Neurochir* 2:417–422, 1952.

197. Spiegel EA, Wycis HT. Mesencephalotomy in the treatment of ''intractable'' facial pain. Arch Neurol 69: 1–13, 1953.

198. Spiegel EA, Wycis HT. Ansotomy in paralysis agitans. *Arch Neurol Psychiatry* 71:598–614, 1954.

199. Spiegel EA, Wycis HT. First International Symposium on Stereoencephalotomy. *Confin Neurol* 22:165–396, 1962.

200. Spiegel EA, Wycis HT, Baird HW. Effect of thalamic and pallidal lesions upon involuntary movements in choreoathetosis. *Trans Am Neurol Assoc* 75:234, 1950.

201. Spiegel EA, Wycis HT, Baird HW, III. Long range effects of electropallido-ansotomy in extrapyramidal and convulsive disorders. *Neurology* 8:734–740, 1958.

202. Spiegel EA, Wycis HT, Marks M, Lee AStJ. Stereotaxic apparatus for operations on the human brain. *Science* 106:349–350, 1947.

203. Spiegel EA, Wycis HT, Orchinik C. Thalamotomy and hypothalamotomy for the treatment of psychoses. *Res Publ Assoc Res Nerv Ment Dis* 31:379–391, 1953.

204. Spiegel EA, Wycis HT, Szekely EG, et al. Campotomy in various extrapyramidal disorders. *J Neurosurg* 20: 871–881, 1963.

205. Spiegel EA, Wycis HT, Szekely EG, et al. Combined dorsomedial, intralaminar and basal thalamotomy for relief of so-called intractable pain. *J Int Coll Surg* 42: 160–168, 1964.

206. Spiegel EA, Wycis HT, Szekely EG, et al. Role of the caudate nucleus in Parkinsonian bradykinesia. *Confin Neurol* 26:336–341, 1965.

207. Steiner L, Leksell L, Greitz J, et al. Stereotaxic radiosurgery for cerebral arteriovenous malformations. *Acta Chir Scand* 138:459–464, 1972.

208. Steiner L, Pradas D, Lindquist C, et al. Clinical aspects of Gamma Knife stereotactic radiosurgery, in,

Gildenberg PL, Tasker RR (ed): *Textbook of Stereotactic and Functional Neurosurgery.* New York: McGraw-Hill, 1998, pp 757–762.

209. Svennilson E, Torvik A, Lowe R, et al. Treatment of parkinsonism by stereotactic thermolesions in the pallidal region: A clinical evaluation of 81 cases. *Acta Psychiatr Neurol Scand* 35:358–377, 1960.

210. Sweet WH, Wepsic JG. Treatment of chronic pain by stimulation of fibers of primary afferent neuron. *Trans Am Neurol Assoc* 93:103–107, 1968.

211. Uchimura Y, Narabayashi H. Stereoencephalotom. *Psychiat Neurol Jap* (Jap edit) 52:265–265, 1951.

212. Walker AE. Relief of pain by mesencephalic tractotomy. *Arch Neurol Psychiatry* 48:865–883, 1942.

213. Walker AE. Cerebral pedunculotomy for the relief of involuntary movements. I. Hemiballismus. *Acta Psychiatr Neurol Scand* 24:712–729, 1949.

214. Walker AE. Cerebral pedunculotomy for the relief of involuntary movements. II. Parkinsonian tremor. *J Nerv Ment Dis* 116:766–775, 1952.

215. Wall PD, Sweet WH. Temporary abolition of pain in man. *Science* 155:108–109, 1967.

216. Wang JK, Nauss LA, Thomas JE. Pain relief by intrathecally applied morphine in man. *Anesthesiology* 50: 149–151, 1979.

217. Whang CJ, Kwon Y. Long-term follow-up of stereotactic Gamma Knife radiosurgery in epilepsy. *Stereotact Funct Neurosurg* 66(Suppl)1:349–356, 1996.

218. Wilson SAK. An experimental research into the anatomy and physiology of the corpus striatum. *Brain* 36: 427–492, 1914.

219. Winston KR, Lutz W. Linear accelerator as a neurosurgical tool for stereotactic radiosurgery. *Neurosurgery* 22:454–464, 1988.

220. Wycis HT, Spiegel EA. Campotomy in myoclonia. *J Neurosurg* 30:708–713, 1969.

221. Wyss OAM. Hochfrequenz Koagulationsgerät zur reizlosen Ausschaltung. *Helv Physiol Pharmacol Acta* 3: 437–443, 1945.

222. Yeh HS, Taha JM, Tobler WD. Implantation of intracerebral depth electrodes for monitoring seizures using the Pelorus stereotactic system guided by magnetic resonance imaging. Technical note. *J Neurosurg* 78: 138–141, 1993.

223. Young RF, Shumway-Cook A, Vermeulen SS, et al. Gamma knife radiosurgery as a lesioning technique in movement disorder surgery. *J Neurosurg* 89:183–193, 1998.

224. Zamorano L, Dujovny M, Chavantes C, et al. Image-guided stereotactic centered craniotomy and laser resection of solid intracranial lesions. *Stereotact Funct Neurosurg* 54/55:398–403, 1990.

Index